MILD TRAUMATIC BRAIN INJURY REHABILITATION TOOLKIT

For sale by the Superintendent of Documents, U.S. Government Publishing Office
Internet: bookstore.gpo.gov   Phone: toll free (866) 512-1800;   DC area (202) 512-1800
Fax: (202) 512-2104 Mail: Stop IDCC, Washington, DC 20402-0001

ISBN 978-0-16-092676-1

MILD TRAUMATIC BRAIN INJURY REHABILITATION TOOLKIT

Margaret Weightman, PhD, PT

Mary Vining Radomski, PhD, OTR/L

Pauline A. Mashima, PhD, CCC-SLP

Carole R. Roth, PhD, CCC-SLP

Borden Institute

Fort Sam Houston, Texas

Borden Institute
Daniel E. Banks, MD, MS, MACP
LTC MC USA
Director & Editor-in-Chief

Editorial Staff: Ronda Lindsay
Volume Editor

This volume was prepared for military medical educational use. The focus of the information is to foster discussion that may form the basis of doctrine and policy. The opinions or assertions contained herein are the private views of the authors and are not to be construed as official or as reflecting the views of the Department of the Army or the Department of Defense.

Dosage Selection:

The authors and publisher have made every effort to ensure the accuracy of dosages cited herein. However, it is the responsibility of every practitioner to consult appropriate information sources to ascertain correct dosages for each clinical situation, especially for new or unfamiliar drugs and procedures. The authors, editors, publisher, and the Department of Defense cannot be held responsible for any errors found in this book.

Use of Trade or Brand Names:

Use of trade or brand names in this publication is for illustrative purposes only and does not imply endorsement by the Department of Defense.

Neutral Language:

Unless this publication states otherwise, masculine nouns and pronouns do not refer exclusively to men.

Published by the Office of The Surgeon General
Borden Institute
Ft Sam Houston, TX 78234

Library of Congress Cataloging-in-Publication Data

Mild traumatic brain injury rehabilitation toolkit / [edited by] Margaret Weightman, Mary Vining Radomski, Pauline A. Mashima, Carole R. Roth.
    p. ; cm.
  Includes bibliographical references and index.
  I. Weightman, Margaret M., editor. II. Radomski, Mary Vining, editor. III. Mashima, Pauline A., editor. IV. Roth, Carole R., editor.
  [DNLM: 1. Brain Injuries--diagnosis. 2. Brain Injuries--rehabilitation. WL 354]
  RC387.5
  617.4'81044--dc23
                          2014042804
PRINTED IN THE UNITED STATES OF AMERICA

21, 20, 19, 18, 17, 16, 15, 14   5 4 3 2 1

Contents

Contributors

MATTIE ANHELUK, MOT, OTR/L
Occupational Therapist, Instructor Scientist, Comprehensive Outpatient Rehabilitation, Courage Kenny Rehabilitation Institute, United Hospital–Occupational Therapy Department, 33 North Smith Avenue, Saint Paul, Minnesota 55102

CHRISTINE ARULANANTHAM, BOT, OTR/L
Occupational Therapist, Instructor Scientist, Rehabilitation Services, Courage Kenny Rehabilitation Institute / Mercy Hospital, 4050 Coon Rapids Boulevard, Coon Rapids, Minnesota 55433

LESLIE DAVIDSON, PhD, OTR/L
Director, Occupational Therapy, Shenandoah University, 1460 University Drive, Winchester, Virginia 22601

MARSEY WALLER DEVOTO, OTD
Occupational Therapist, Military Share Brain Injury Program, Shepherd Center, 2020 Peachtree Road Northwest, Atlanta, Georgia 30309

SHARI Y.S. GOO-YOSHINO, MS, CCC-SLP
Speech-Language Pathologist, Otolaryngology Service, Department of Surgery, Tripler Army Medical Center, 1 Jarrett White Road, Tripler Army Medical Center, Honolulu, Hawaii 96859

CAROL SMITH HAMMOND, PhD, CCC-SLP
Research Speech Pathologist, Audiology / Speech Pathology, Durham VA Medical Center, #126, 508 Fulton Street, Durham, North Carolina 27705

EMI ISAKI, PhD, CCC-SLP
Associate Professor, Communication Sciences & Disorders, Northern Arizona University, Department of Communication Sciences & Disorders, Building 66, Post Office Box 15045, Flagstaff, Arizona 86011

JANICE P. KEHLER, BPT, MS, MA
Physical Therapist, Physical Medicine and Rehabilitation, VA Medical Center, One Veterans Drive, Room 3R141, Minneapolis, Minnesota 55417

LYNNETTE LEUTY, PT, MA
Supervisor / Staff Therapist, Comprehensive Outpatient Rehabilitation Department, Courage Kenny Rehabilitation Institute, 800 East 28th Street, Mail Stop 12209, Minneapolis, Minnesota 55407

DON MacLENNAN, MA, CCC-SLP
Chief, Speech Pathology Section, Minneapolis VA Health Care System, One Veterans' Drive 127A, Minneapolis, Minnesota 55417

R. KEVIN MANNING, PhD, CCC-SLP
Speech Pathologist, Traumatic Brain Injury Service, San Antonio Military Medical Center–North, 3551 Roger Brooke Drive, Joint-Base Fort Sam Houston, Texas 78234

PAULINE MASHIMA, PhD, CCC-SLP
Chief, Speech Pathology Section, Otolaryngology Service, Department of Surgery, Tripler Army Medical Center, 1 Jarrett White Road, Tripler Army Medical Center, Honolulu, Hawaii 96859

KAREN McCULLOCH, PhD, PT
Professor, Division of Physical Therapy, Department of Allied Health Sciences, School of Medicine, University of North Carolina at Chapel Hill, 321 South Columbia Street, CB 7135 Bondurant Hall, Suite 3024, Chapel Hill, North Carolina 27599

LESLIE NITTA, MS, CCC-SLP
Speech-Language Pathologist, Greater Los Angeles Veterans Affairs Healthcare System, Sepulveda Ambulatory Care Center, 16111 Plumber Street, Building 200, Room 2409 / Gold Team, Sepulveda, California 91343

JENNY OWENS, OTD
Occupational Therapist, Warrior Resiliency and Recovery Center, Blanchfield Army Community Hospital, Building 2543, Room 118, 650 Joel Drive, Fort Campbell, Kentucky 42223

LINDA M. PICON, MCD, CCC-SLP
Speech-Language Pathologist, Veterans' Health Administration, James A. Haley Veterans' Hospital, Audiology and Speech Pathology (ASP 126), 13000 Bruce B. Downs Boulevard, Tampa, Florida 33612; and 4202 East Fowler Avenue, PCD1017, Tampa, Florida 33620

MARY VINING RADOMSKI, PhD, OTR/L
Clinical Scientist, Courage Kenny Research Center, 800 East 28th Street, Mail Stop 12212, Minneapolis, Minnesota 55407

CAROLE R. ROTH, PhD, CCC-SLP, BC-ANCDS
Division Head, Speech Pathology, Naval Medical Center San Diego, 34800 Bob Wilson Drive, Building 2/2, 2K-11R5, San Diego, California 92134

MITCHELL SCHEIMAN, OD
Professor, Associate Dean of Clinical Research, Pennsylvania College of Optometry at Salus University, 8360 Old York Road, Elkins Park, Pennsylvania 19027

MAILE T. SINGSON, MS, CCC-SLP
Speech-Language Pathologist, Traumatic Brain Injury Program, Veterans Affairs Pacific Island Health Care System, Traumatic Brain Injury Clinic, Specialty Clinic Module 8, 459 Patterson Road, Honolulu, Hawaii 96819

SHARON GOWDY WAGENER, OTR/L, BA, MAOT
Occupational Therapist, Instructor Scientist, Rehabilitation Services, Courage Kenny Rehabilitation Institute / Abbott Northwestern Hospital, 800 East 28th Street, Mail Stop 12213, Minneapolis, Minnesota 55407

MARGARET M. WEIGHTMAN, PT, PhD
Clinical Scientist / Physical Therapist, Courage Kenny Research Center, 800 East 28th Street, Mail Stop 12212, Minneapolis, Minnesota 55407

ALINE WIMBERLY, OTR/L, CBIS
Formerly, Occupational Therapist, Warrior Resiliency and Recovery Center, Traumatic Brain Injury Clinic, Fort Campbell, Kentucky

JOETTE ZOLA, BS, OTR/L
Occupational Therapist, Brain Injury Clinic, Courage Kenny Rehabilitation Institute, Allina Health, 800 East 28th Street, Mail Stop 12210, Minneapolis, Minnesota 55407

Foreword

I am pleased to present this volume, entitled *Mild Traumatic Brain Injury Toolkit*, published by the Army Medical Department's Borden Institute. The Borden Institute is the primary outlet for scholarly and peer-reviewed publications by the healthcare providers who take care of our nation's Service Members and Veterans. The Institute's publications to not necessarily represent Army doctrine or the opinion of the Department of Defense (DoD) or the Army; nevertheless, they represent the best work of our providers as they seek to inform future policy and decision-making.

More than a decade of war has underscored the incidence of a common injury that can occur both on and off the battlefield—mild traumatic brain injury (mTBI), also known as concussion. Concussions can occur due to blast events, motor vehicle crashes, training accidents, falls, sports, and general mishaps. Through research, policy, widespread education, and provider training, the Army is working diligently to ensure that those diagnosed with concussion are promptly identified and treated to maximize their recovery.

Rehabilitation professionals provide significant contributions to the recovery, rehabilitation, and reintegration of Service Members who are symptomatic after sustaining an mTBI. In September 2007, the Proponency Office for Rehabilitation and Reintegration (now the Rehabilitation and Reintegration Division) and the Army TBI program lead within the Office of The Surgeon General charged a team of occupational therapists (OTs) and physical therapists (PTs) to develop clinical guidance for state-of-the-art rehabilitative care for post-concussive Service Members.

Civilian and military OTs and PTs collaborated with speech language pathologists to perform a critical review of research and clinical rehabilitation practices in the assessment, treatment, and management of concussions from point of injury to extended rehabilitative care. Rehabilitaion subject matter experts from DoD, the Department of Veterans Affairs, and the civilian sector fully support the resultant Clinical Management Guidance and Toolkit for Rehabilitation Professionals.

In parallel, the rehabilitation community has developed and begun testing a new tool, the Combat Readiness Check (CRC). This tool provides additional objective and reliable data about Service Members' safety and readiness to return to duty after a concussion. The CRC is a compilation of existing instruments and a dual-task test that has undergone clinical applicability testing.

Research is still needed in every area of practice—presenting opportunities to advance outcomes—for Service Members and civilians alike. We invite your comments so future initiatives can meet the greatest need for the largest number of Service Members.

Army Medicine heartily thanks all those involved in this project for their outstanding and tireless commitment to excellence and is proud to add this publication to the scientific body of knowledge. And we are, as ever, Serving to Heal . . . Honored to Serve!

Patricia D. Horoho
Lieutenant General, US Army
The Surgeon General and
Commanding General,
US Army Medical Command

Washington, DC
December 2014

Preface

The wars in Iraq and Afghanistan—Operation Iraqi Freedom (OIF) and Operation Enduring Freedom (OEF)—have mobilized the military and civilian medical and rehabilitation communities to identify best practices in the care of service members with mild traumatic brain injury (mTBI)/concussion. In September 2007, leaders in the Rehabilitation and Reintegration Division at the Army Office of the Surgeon General charged a team of two occupational therapists and three physical therapists (two military and three civilians) to develop occupational therapy (OT) and physical therapy (PT) clinical practice guidance for mTBI in order to help establish, "…state-of-the-art rehabilitative care for Soldiers with mild traumatic brain injuries…[by] completing a critical review of current research and clinical rehabilitative care practices in the assessment, treatment and management of mild TBI at all levels of care (from acute theater to long term life care)." An mTBI guidance document for speech language pathologists (SLPs) was subsequently developed by a team of Department of Defense (DoD), Veterans Affairs (VA), and civilian clinicians. These foundational guidance documents and the contributions of many DoD, VA, and civilian PTs, OTs, and SLPs resulted in this *Mild Traumatic Brain Injury Rehabilitation Toolkit*. As authors and editors who contributed to the guidance documents and Toolkit, we envision that this will be a "work in progress," given the extraordinary advancement in the research and rehabilitation arenas since our work began. The explosion of new research will continue to enhance our recognition and understanding of the effects of single or multiple concussions on service members and civilians alike, and the important contribution of rehabilitation clinicians in treating and measuring progress as service members recover from mTBI.

Margaret Weightman

Acknowledgments

Many people provided critical assistance and guidance for the development of the Rehabilitation Toolkit. LTC(Ret) Lynne Lowe, COL(Ret) Barbara Springer, COL(Ret) Mary Erickson, LTC Sarah Goldman, COL Nikki Butler of the Rehabilitation and Reintegration (R2D) Division (Office of The Surgeon General) identified the need for the Toolkit, consulted on its contents, and offered essential feedback throughout the development process. Ms Diane Flynn crafted the content of the initial version 1 of the OT/PT Toolkit into a format that is readable and consistent and we appreciate this contribution to the project.

Additionally, we gratefully recognize the experts who provided either in-process feedback or who reviewed the final draft of Toolkit sections, including the following individuals: Eleanor Avery, MD (Brooke Army Medical Center, San Antonio, TX); Micaela Cornis-Pop, PhD, CCC-SLP (VA Medical Center, Richmond, VA); Kim Gottshall PhD, PT, ATC (Naval Medical Center, San Diego, CA); Mary RT Kennedy, PhD, CCC-SLP (University of Minnesota, Twin Cities, MN); Lisa Leininger, PT (Courage Kenny Rehabilitation Institute—Abbott Northwestern Hospital, Minneapolis, MN); Imelda Llanos, OTR/L (James A Haley VAMC, Tampa, FL); Nan Musson, MA, CCC-SLP (VA Medical Center, Gainesville, FL); Michelle D Peterson PT, DPT, NCS (VA Medical Center, Minneapolis, MN); MAJ Matthew Scherer, PhD, PT, NCS (Andrew Rader US Army Health Clinic, Ft Myer, VA); McKay Moore Sohlberg, PhD, CCC-SLP (University of Oregon, Eugene, OR); Lyn Turkstra, PhD, CCC-SLP (University of Wisconsin-Madison); Megan Vaught, PT, ScD OCS (Sister Kenny Sports and Physical Therapy Center, Minneapolis, MN); Deborah Voydetich OTR/L (VA Medical Center, Minneapolis, MN); and Orli Weisser-Pike, OTR/L, CLVT, SCLV (Hamilton Eye Institute, Memphis, TN).

We also gratefully acknowledge the individuals who contributed to the development and review of the Clinical Management Guidance: Occupational Therapy and Physical Therapy for Mild Traumatic Brain Injury (Appendix A) and the SLP Clinical Management Guidance for Cognitive-Communication Rehabilitation for Service Members and Veterans with Concussion/Mild Traumatic Brain Injury (Appendix B).

We greatly appreciate the critical assistance of our partners at the Courage Kenny Research Center, especially Roberta Jordan; Jenica Domanico, MAOT; and Michelle Pose, MAOT. We also recognize the important contributions of the team at the Borden Institute to this effort, especially Ronda Lindsay.

Members of the SLP Working Group are grateful to the following individuals who provided invaluable support during the process of developing the SLP CMG and Toolkit: Lei Colon-Yoshimoto (Tripler Army Medical Center, HI); Melissa R. Kolodziej, MS, CCC-SLP (San Antonio Military Medical Center, TX); Gwen Niiya (Tripler Army Medical Center, HI); COL Joseph Sniezek, USA (Tripler Army Medical Center, HI); Amanda Lewis Stephens, MS, CCC-SLP (VA Long Beach Healthcare System); and SGT Samuel Teague, USA (Ft Hood, TX). We appreciate the medical review of the Toolkit provided by Eleanor Avery, MD.

We are grateful for the opportunity to help advance physical and occupational therapy and speech-language pathology practices and outcomes for Service members with c/mTBI.

Margaret Weightman
Mary Vining Radomski
Pauline Mashima
Carole Roth

Chapter 1

INTRODUCTION

MARGARET M. WEIGHTMAN, PhD, PT* and MARY RADOMSKI, PhD, OTR/L†

PURPOSE

CONTENT AND STRUCTURE

RECOMMENDED ASSESSMENTS AND INTERVENTIONS
Assessments
Guidelines for Administering and Interpreting Assessments
Intervention

REHABILITATION AFTER CONCUSSION/MILD TRAUMATIC BRAIN INJURY
General Schema for Physical Therapy
General Schema for Occupational Therapy
General Schema for Speech-Language Pathology

RESEARCH

REFERENCES

*Clinical Scientist/Physical Therapist, Courage Kenny Research Center, 800 East 28th Street, MS 12212, Minneapolis, Minnesota 55407
†Clinical Scientist, Courage Kenny Research Center, 800 East 28th Street, MS 12212, Minneapolis, Minnesota 55407

PURPOSE

This toolkit was designed to help military and civilian physical and occupational therapists and speech-language pathologists gain knowledge of valid and reliable screening tools, patient-oriented outcome instruments, and evidence-informed intervention techniques that are useful in evaluating and treating service members (SMs) with concussion/mild traumatic brain injury (c/mTBI). It also includes general assessment schema for physical and occupational therapists and speech-language pathologists who are new to the population of patients with c/mTBI.

This toolkit is intended to be a companion document to the *Occupational and Physical Therapy Mild Traumatic Brain Injury Clinical Practice Guidance*[1] and *Speech-Language Pathology Clinical Management Guidance for Cognitive-Communication Rehabilitation for Concussion/Mild Traumatic Brain Injury.*[2] These two guidance documents contain full background information on the rationale and document development process as well as a literature review of the evidence for the recommended assessment and intervention processes.

CONTENT AND STRUCTURE

Toolkit content (assessment tools, outcome measures, interventions) was informed by extensive literature review and consultation with subject matter and clinical experts. In recommending specific assessments and interventions, the authors acknowledge that the typical SM at baseline is young, healthy, and physically fit and, even while injured, often performs well on standard assessment tools that may not fully characterize subtle deficits.

Consistent with the guidance documents, the toolkit is organized by problem area. The initial sections focus on impairments of body structure and function and activity limitations (activity intolerance, vestibular deficits, vision deficits, headache, and temporomandibular joint disorders) that are most often addressed before focusing on further functional or cognitive issues. Remediation of pain, dizziness, nausea and vomiting, and vision impairments is often essential to the SM's participation in other therapeutic interventions (Figure 1-1). The later sections of the toolkit deal with cognition; attention and dual-task performance deficits; performance of self-management, work, school, and social roles; participation in fitness activities; and a brief discussion of the participation measurement and health-related quality of life.

In general, the toolkit sections are self-contained so clinicians may select resources from some sections and not others based on individual patient needs. The degree of specificity of clinical instructions varies by topic. Some sections of the toolkit provide pictures and step-by-step directions for carrying out the intervention techniques while other sections provide clinicians with suggestions and guiding principles for designing appropriate treatment interventions based on an individual SM's specific needs. References are located at the end of each section of the toolkit.

RECOMMENDED ASSESSMENTS AND INTERVENTIONS

The toolkit contains ten sections organized around specific problem areas typical of c/mTBI. Appendix Table 1-1 summarizes all assessment and intervention recommendations and indicates the strength of the recommendation and the described International Classification of Functioning, Disability, and Health (ICF) level. It is intended to be used after clinicians have reviewed the specific introductory information for each toolkit section.

Assessments

As an introduction to an assessment, screening tool, or outcome measure, the reader will find a "face sheet" that is designed to help clinicians select, administer, and interpret the most appropriate assessments for specific patients. The face sheet describes the original purpose or description of the tool, followed by a brief narrative on the recommendations or cautions for an instrument's use and a description of the time, equipment, and type of test used. Finally, all the assessments include information on the types of healthy or patient groups that have been tested with the measurement tool. These face sheets do not provide exhaustive reviews but are intended to provide relevant data. The psychometric information provided in the toolkit depends on the type of assessment tool being described.

The following is a summary of key measurement issues that relate to the included instruments, intended as a brief reminder of the definitions and clinical utility of psychometric information in

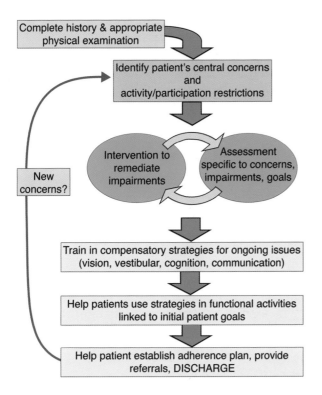

Complete history & appropriate physical examination

Identify patient's central concerns and activity/participation restrictions

New concerns?

Intervention to remediate impairments

Assessment specific to concerns, impairments, goals

Train in compensatory strategies for ongoing issues (vision, vestibular, cognition, communication)

Help patients use strategies in functional activities linked to initial patient goals

Help patient establish adherence plan, provide referrals, DISCHARGE

Figure 1-1. The general process for delivering occupational and physical therapy and speech-language pathology services specific to concussion/mild traumatic brain injury. The therapy schemas are provided for general practice clinicians new to this patient population. Although occupational and physical therapy and speech-language pathology schemas are presented separately for purposes of clarity, it is essential that clinicians collaborate to minimize redundancy and optimize outcomes.

regard to tests and measures and their application to an individual SM. Readers are strongly encouraged to review clinical or rehabilitation research texts, such as Domholdt's *Rehabilitation Research Principles and Applications*[3] and *Foundations of Clinical Research: Applications to Practice*[4] by Portney and Watkins, to refresh their knowledge of pertinent test psychometrics, specifically issues of tests and measure reliability and validity.

Reliability is defined as the extent to which the instrument yields the same results on repeated measures. There are a number of types of reliability important in the use of tests and measures (eg, rater and test-retest reliability). In a practical sense, a test does not provide useable information if it does not result in consistent or stable responses when there have been no changes in the subject, or if two raters scoring the same test responses do not obtain consistent test scores. Depending on the level of measurement, intraclass correlation coefficients

are typically used to evaluate rater reliability, with the values closer to 1.00 representing stronger reliability. For clinical measures, reliability coefficients greater than .90 are considered excellent and supportive of reasonable validity.[4]

An unreliable assessment tool would result in the inability to determine if a change in patient scores reflected a true change or merely resulted from unstable or inconsistent test scoring. According to Domholdt, "An unreliable measure is also an invalid measurement, because measurements with a great deal of error have little meaning or utility."[3(p259)]

In a practical and clinical sense, the evaluating clinician must be consistently aware of the **minimal detectable change (MDC)** for a measurement tool. There is variability and error in all measurement. Clinical test interpretation must recognize that for a true change to occur, the change demonstrated by a SM must be greater than the error variability of a measurement. Haley and Fragala-Pinkham write that the "MDC is considered the minimal amount of change that is not likely to be due to chance variation in measurement."[5] Other measures are used to detect change that is clinically important for the patient, such as minimal clinically important differences (MDICs); however, for this toolkit, we have chosen to report MDC where available.

Measurement of test validity indicates the meaningfulness of test scores as they are used for a specific purpose; that is, it gives usefulness to the inferences made from test scores. Information on face, content, criterion, and construct validity all indicate the extent to which a measurement tool fully measures the construct it is intended to measure. According to Portney and Watkins, validity is not "inherent in an instrument, but must be evaluated within the context of the test's intended use and a specific population."[6(p81)]

Specific to the screening tools used to diagnose a specific condition (eg, benign paroxysmal positional vertigo, unilateral vestibular hypofunction [UVH], or unilateral vision loss [UVL] described in the vestibular section of this toolkit), information is provided on the **sensitivity** (test is positive when the condition is present) and **specificity** (test is negative when the condition is absent) of the test. As Portney and Watkins write, the validity of a diagnostic tool is "evaluated in terms of its ability to accurately assess the presence and absence of the target condition."[6(p93)]

Another critical issue in measurement tools is the **responsiveness to change** of a measurement. Clinicians hope their interventions result in positive and useful change in their patients, and a measurement tool must be able to provide a useful metric that can show change when the client has made a significant clinical improvement.

Guidelines for Administering and Interpreting Assessments

Ideally, assessments and outcome measures would be tested for reliability and validity in the settings and with the raters and specific populations for which they are to be used. This has not yet happened with many of the tests and assessments recommended in this toolkit. Many of the tools have been tested on patients with the problems reported by SMs with c/mTBI (eg, balance complaints or posttraumatic headache). However, most of the instruments have not yet been fully characterized in the young, fit, and healthy population typical of enlisted SMs; specifically those who have some of the pervasive comorbidities found in this population, such as posttraumatic stress disorder or acute stress reaction. This lack of information specific to SMs does not render the test unusable; rather it should caution the evaluating clinician to carefully interpret the data. Again, because of the lack of specific reliability and validity for measurement tools used for SMs with combat-related c/mTBI, the evaluating clinician must consider all factors when interpreting the obtained data.

In addition, measurement tools are not valid and reliable in and of themselves. These qualities depend on the raters (the ability to reliably administer and score a test may require prior training), the patients, the setting, and comorbid conditions (such as posttraumatic stress and acute stress reaction). To optimize the accuracy and interpretability of the assessments, tests and measures must be administered and scored true to the instructions. Attempts to change or invent categories of responses, adapt scoring rubrics, or give "bonus points" or second chances will all reduce the reliability and validity of a tool.

Intervention

Similarly, intervention descriptions begin with a face sheet that is designed to inform clinical reasoning and decision making. The face sheet gives background on the intervention and specifies the strength of recommendation.

Given the scarcity of specific literature to guide recommendations in many of the reported symptom areas, specifically for young and previously healthy SMs, we chose to borrow from Cicerone and colleagues[7] and characterize recommendations as either a **practice standard** or **practice option**.

- Practice standards: recommended practices that are supported by existing c/mTBI guidelines or published, evidence-based reviews concerning the problem area.
- Practice options: potentially beneficial practices that do not have such support but are consistent with current theory, literature, or expert opinion.[7]

REHABILITATION AFTER CONCUSSION/MILD TRAUMATIC BRAIN INJURY

The toolkit specifies clinical practices that are supported by the guidance documents. As such, readers are advised to carefully review the contents of the guidance documents. The guidance documents specify several assumptions about SMs and the clinicians involved in their care and provide several guiding principles for c/mTBI-related rehabilitation across all levels within the military and civilian systems of care. The guidance documents and the toolkit were developed specifically for general practice clinicians whose clinical judgment is fundamental to providing the highest level of care for injured SMs. The guidance documents and toolkit should supplement sound clinical judgment and are premised on the following key assumptions:

- Clinicians use a patient-centered approach in which they communicate an optimistic expectation for an SM's full recovery.

- Clinicians incorporate an SM's goals and priorities into the evaluation process along with evaluating c/mTBI-related symptoms and impairments.
- The scope of practice for the occupational therapist, physical therapist, and speech-language pathologist may vary depending on the level of care, the location of the facility, and access to other healthcare providers (rehabilitation teams and specialists), and military practice may be different from that of civilian practice.
- Whenever feasible, the ICF is used, with problem areas described in terms of body structure/body function, activity, or participation limitations. Clinicians are encouraged to consider all levels of the ICF model when assessing and intervening with SMs or civilians with c/mTBI.

Both personal and environmental factors can impact limitations at each level of the model.

Figure 1-1 outlines a general process for delivery of occupational and physical therapy and speech-language pathology services specific to c/mTBI. The following therapy schemas are provided for general practice clinicians new to this patient population. Although occupational and physical therapy and speech-language pathology schemas are presented separately for purposes of clarity, it is essential that clinicians collaborate to minimize redundancy and optimize outcomes.

General Schema for Physical Therapy

A general plan for physical therapy assessment of an SM with c/mTBI complaints contains both subjective and objective components. It is assumed that physical therapists are aware of relevant background information when taking history (eg, family support, medications, work-related requirements, etc). Initial intake involves taking a thorough history that includes detailed information of the traumatic or causative event (ie, mechanism of injury, occurrence and duration of altered awareness, and duration of posttraumatic amnesia). The patient should be asked for presenting complaints and complete a checklist of current symptoms (eg, Neurobehavioral Symptom Inventory), and should also be asked about prior resolved symptom complaints. A number of patient questionnaires may be appropriate at this time depending on the SM's presenting complaints, such as the:

- Dizziness Handicap Inventory,[8]
- Jaw Functional Limitation Scale,[9,10]
- Patient-specific Functional Scale,[11]
- Headache Disability Inventory,[12]
- Activities-specific Balance Confidence Scale,[13] and
- Numeric Pain Rating Scale.[14]

Additionally, patients should be asked to describe their current activity level, including the type, duration, and intensity of participation in fitness activities; SMs should also be asked to describe their goals for the current physical therapy episode of care. A physical assessment for someone with a history of concussion and ongoing complaints follows the interview segment of the evaluation. It should include the following assessments:

- strength: manual muscle testing; functional strength test using the High Level Mobility Assessment Tool (HiMAT[15,16]) or the Five Times Sit-to-Stand Test[17];
- range of motion;
- range-of-motion screening in major joints, including the neck, and oculomotor mobility;
- sensation;
- gross sensory test for somatosensation, proprioception;
- balance;
- balance screening using a simple balance test, and more extensive balance testing as appropriate (see Chapter 3, Balance Assessment and Intervention);
- coordination (HiMAT may test some gross coordination issues);
- gait velocity;
- comfortable and fast walking speed (consider Functional Gait Assessment); and
- dual-task assessment.

Further physical and functional assessment will depend on the presenting complaints found during the intake interview regarding vestibular and balance complaints, posttraumatic headache, and temporomandibular disorders. Additionally, fitness level may be evaluated using military standards as appropriate at some point during the episode of care. As always, clinician judgment is key to deciding when additional assessment is needed.

Based on history and assessment findings, provide appropriate intervention, education, and discharge planning, including home programming, appropriate referrals and follow-up, exercise recommendations, and planning for resumption of military and social roles.

General Schema for Occupational Therapy

Therapists should acquaint themselves with the patient's diagnosis, comorbidities, and past medical, social, educational, and service history by careful review of the patient's chart. This information is critical to selecting assessment tools and interpreting assessment results. Assessment follows this general sequence.

- Interview the patient (and family members, if available) to discover background information that may be not be included in the medical record. Therapists may also use the interview to better understand the patient's most pressing concerns, problem areas, and priorities specific to interventions. The Canadian Occupational Performance Measure[18] is recommended for initial interview and periodic progress reassessment.

- Screen for vision problems. Administer the College of Optometrists in Vision Development (COVD) Quality of Life Assessment[19] (a symptom questionnaire). If the patient has vision complaints, conduct a full vision assessment, including visual acuity, visual fields, oculomotor control, and binocular vision. Refer patients with vision impairments to an ophthalmologist or optometrist who specializes in TBI for more in-depth evaluation.

- Implement vision remediation intervention as directed by a neuro-ophthalmologist or optometrist and help the patient identify and implement vision compensations to optimize functioning.

- Collaborate with other team members to address potential problems with sleep and structure-recommended changes in sleep hygiene.

- Identify potential cognitive inefficiencies. Observe the patient's functional performance under circumstances that require varying degrees of memory, attention, and executive functioning and consider a standardized functional assessment, such as the Mortera-Cognitive Screening Measure[20,21] or the Dynamic Observation of Function Checklist (see Chapter 7, Cognitive Assessment and Intervention). If a full neuropsychological battery has been recently performed, review the results to obtain information about the patient's cognitive status. If not, administer cognitive assessments based on problem areas evident during functional task performance. Options include the following:
  - Behavioural Assessment of Dysexecutive Syndrome,[22]
  - Cognistat,[23]
  - Repeatable Battery for the Assessment of Neuropsychological Status,[24]
  - Behavior Rating Inventory of Executive Function–Adult (BRIEF–A),[25]
  - Contextual Memory Test,[26]
  - Rivermead Behavioral Memory Test,[27] and
  - Test of Everyday Attention.[28]

- Instruct the patient in compensatory cognitive strategies (attention, memory, and executive function) based on the nature of patient complaints and assessment results. Collaborate with patients to identify the compensatory strategies they are most likely to adopt and benefit from.

- Structure clinical and nonclinical opportunities for the patient to rehearse the new skill or strategy, and help the patient implement the new skill or strategy within the context of personally relevant self-management tasks, such as medication management or bill paying and budgeting.

- Continue to develop additional compensatory strategies as indicated. As patients adopt and employ an array of successful compensatory strategies, help them use those skills to resume social, work, and school roles; schedule a regimen of declining contact with patients so they remain supported while increasingly and successfully resuming these roles.

- Set up a discharge plan that includes problem solving with the patient regarding long-term adherence to therapy recommendations and resources if new problems arise.

General Schema for Speech-Language Pathology

Begin the SLP focus by reviewing the patient's chart. As with the OT approach, clinicians should acquaint themselves with the patient's diagnosis, comorbidities, and past medical, social, educational, and vocational and military service history. This information is critical for selecting assessment tools and interpreting assessment results. Also as with OT, interview the patient (and family members, if available) to obtain additional background information that may not be included in the medical record and to better understand the patient's most pressing concerns, problem areas, self-help strategies, priorities, goals, and expectations specific to rehabilitation.

Refer the patient to an audiologist for evaluation to determine if auditory symptoms are associated with c/mTBI. Collaborate with other team members to address comorbidities such as pain, sensory impairments, fatigue, stress, sleep deprivation, drug effects, and psychosocial concerns that can contribute to cognitive and communication inefficiencies, and identify potential cognitive-communication inefficiencies. If a full neuropsychological battery has been recently performed, review the results to obtain information about the patient's cognitive status, strengths and weaknesses, and measures of effort.

If not, consider referral to a neuropsychologist to obtain the necessary information. Assess problem areas using standardized instruments (eg, broad assessment of cognitive-communication abilities, domain-specific assessments, and functional performance assessments) and self-report measures.

Observe the patient's functional performance under circumstances that require varying degrees of attention, speed of information processing, memory, self-regulation, social communication, and executive function. Instruct the patient in compensatory cognitive-communication strategies (attention, memory, speed of information processing, executive functions, social communication, and conversational disfluencies) based on the nature of patient complaints and assessment results. Collaborate with the patient to identify the compensatory strategies most likely to be beneficial in real-life contexts; structure functional and meaningful tasks within clinical sessions for the patient to practice and habituate the new skill or strategy.

Perform ongoing assessment to determine the effectiveness of intervention and modify compensatory strategies as appropriate to optimize function. As the patient adopts and employs an array of successful compensatory strategies, facilitate generalization of the new skill or strategy to personally relevant contexts—including new settings, people, and situations—to enable the patient to resume social, work, and school roles.

Schedule a regimen of declining contact so the patient remains supported while increasingly and successfully resuming personal, social, work, and school roles. Discharge the patient from therapy and formulate a plan for follow-up that includes problem solving with the patient regarding long-term adherence to therapy recommendations and resources if new problems arise.

RESEARCH

Published research and guidelines are constantly being updated. The guidance documents and toolkit are based on currently available evidence. Where appropriate, the guidelines, tools, and interventions recommended incorporate clinical expertise and may be biased by the consulted expert panel. With this in mind, the authors welcome feedback and recommendations for omissions, updates, and future inclusions in this toolkit.

REFERENCES

1. Radomski MV, Weightman MM, Davidson L, Rodgers M, Bolgla R. *Clinical Practice Guidance: Occupational Therapy and Physical Therapy for Mild Traumatic Brain Injury*. US Army Office of the Surgeon General: Falls Church, VA; 2010.

2. Cornis-Pop M, Mashima PA, Roth CR, et al. Guest editorial: cognitive-communication rehabilitation for combat-related mild traumatic brain injury. *J Rehabil Res Dev*. 2012;49(7):xi–xxxii.

3. Domholdt E. *Rehabilitation Research Principles and Applications*. 3rd ed. St. Louis, MO: Elsevier Saunders; 2005.

4. Portney LG, Watkins MP. *Foundations of Clinical Research: Applications to Practice*. 3rd ed. Upper Saddle River, NJ: Pearson/Prentice Hall; 2008.

5. Haley SM, Fragala-Pinkham MA. Interpreting change scores of tests and measures used in physical therapy. *Phys Ther*. 2006;86(5):735–743.

6. Portney LG, Watkins MP. *Foundations of Clinical Research: Applications to Practice*. 2nd ed. Upper Saddle River, NJ: Prentice Hall; 2000.

7. Cicerone KD, Dahlberg C, Kalmer K, et al. Evidence-based cognitive rehabilitation: recommendations for clinical practice. *Arch Phys Med Rehabil*. 2000;81:1596–1615.

8. Whitney SL, Marchetti GF, Morris LO. Usefulness of the dizziness handicap inventory in the screening for benign paroxysmal positional vertigo. *Otol Neurotol*. 2005;26(5):1027–1033.

9. Ohrbach R, Granger C, List T, Dworkin S. Preliminary development and validation of the Jaw Functional Limitation Scale. *Community Dent Oral Epidemiol*. 2008;36:228–236.

10. Ohrbach R, Larsson P, List T. The Jaw Functional Limitation Scale: development, reliability, and validity of 8-item and 20-item versions. *J Orofac Pain*. 2008;22:219–230.

11. Stratford P, Gill C, Westaway M, Binkley J. Assessing disability and change on individual patients: a report of a patient specific measure. *Physio Canada*. 1995;47(4):258–263.

12. Jacobson GP, Ramadan NM, Aggarwal SK, Newman CW. The Henry Ford Hospital Headache Disability Inventory (HDI). *Neurology*. 1994;44(5):837–842.

13. Powell LE, Myers AM. The Activities-specific Balance Confidence (ABC) Scale. *J Gerontol Med Sci*. 1995;50(1):M2834.

14. Jenson MP Karoly P Braver S. The measurement of clinical pain intensity: a comparison of six methods. Pain 1986; 27:117–26.

15. Williams G, Robertson V, Greenwood K, Goldie P, Morris ME. The high-level mobility assessment tool (HiMAT) for traumatic brain injury. Part 1: item generation. *Brain Inj*. 2005;19(11):925–932.

16. Williams G, Robertson V, Greenwood K, Goldie P, Morris ME. The high-level mobility assessment tool (HiMAT) for traumatic brain injury. Part 2: content validity and discriminability. *Brain Inj*. 2005;19(10):833–843.

17. Csuka M, McCarty DJ. Simple method for measurement of lower extremity muscle strength. *Am J Med*. 1985;78:77–81.

18. Law M, Baptiste S, McColl MA, Carswell A, Polatajko H, Pollock N. *Canadian Occupational Performance Measure*. 2nd ed. Toronto, Ontario: Canadian National Organisation of Occupational Therapists–ACE Publications; 1994.

19. Maples WC. Test-retest reliability of the College of Optometrists in Vision Development Quality of Life Outcomes Assessment short form. *J Optom Vis Dev*. 2002;33:126–134.

20. Mortera MH. Instrument development in brain injury rehabilitation: Part I. *Physical Disabilities Special Interest Section Quarterly*. 2006a;29(3):1–4.

21. Mortera MH. Instrument development in brain injury rehabilitation: Part II. *Physical Disabilities Special Interest Section Quarterly*. 2006b;29(4):1–2.

22. Wilson BA, Evans JJ, Alderman N, Burgess P. The development of an ecologically valid test for assessing patients with a dysexecutive syndrome. *Neuropsychol Rehabil*. 1998;8:213–228.

23. Kiernan RJ, Mueller J, Langston JW, Van Dyke C. The Neurobehavioral Cognitive Status Examination: a brief but quantitative approach to cognitive assessment. *Ann Intern Med*. 1987;107(4):481–485.

24. Randolph C. *Repeatable Battery for the Assessment of Neuropsychological Status: Manual*. San Antonio, TX: Psychological Corporation; 1998.

25. Roth R, Isquith P, Gioia G. *Behavior Rating Inventory of Executive Function-Adult version (BRIEF-A)*. Lutz, FL: Psychological Assessment Resources, Inc; 2005.

26. Toglia JP. *The Contextual Memory Test*. San Antonio, TX: Harcourt Assessments; 1993.

27. Wilson BA, Cockburn J, Baddeley AD, Hiorns R. The development and validation of a test battery for detecting and monitoring everyday memory problems. *J Clin Exp Neuropsychol*. 1989;11(6):855–870.

28. Robertson IH, Ward T, Ridgeway V, Nimmo-Smith I. The structure of normal human attention: The Test of Everyday Attention. *J Int Neuropsychol Soc*. 1996;2(6):525–534.

Chapter 2

VESTIBULAR ASSESSMENT AND INTERVENTION

MARGARET M. WEIGHTMAN, PhD, PT[*] AND LYNNETTE LEUTY, PT, DPT, NCS[†]

[*]Clinical Scientist/Physical Therapist, Courage Kenny Research Center, 800 East 28th Street, Mail Stop 12212, Minneapolis, Minnesota 55407
[†]Supervisor/Staff Therapist, Comprehensive Outpatient Rehabilitation Department, Courage Kenny Rehabilitation Institute, 800 East 28th Street, Mail Stop 12209, Minneapolis, Minnesota 55407

INTRODUCTION

Vestibular deficits that arise in conjunction with concussion/mild traumatic brain injury (c/mTBI) can have complex etiologies; thus, treatment is individualized and specific to the cause. Initial assessment to characterize history, postural control, and basic vestibular functions will help determine possible etiology and direct intervention. Physical and occupational therapists who have not previously seen vestibular patients may need education in the techniques and assessments beyond what is described here and in Appendix A of the toolkit[1]; however, certain basic assessment and intervention principles are appropriate for initial consideration.

Several references are provided to guide problem solving to determine possible causes of vestibular dysfunction. Figure 2-1 and Table 2-1[2] provide an initial point of reference for considering an injury sustained in a combat or military context, where c/mTBI consideration is also an important focus of assessment. For those with clear vestibular complaints, clinicians should refer to Figure 16-1 in Herdman's *Vestibular Rehabilitation, Third Edition*,[3(p230)] to determine possible causes of the complaint. Of the possible causes Herdman outlines, benign paroxysmal positional vertigo (BPPV) and unilateral vestibular hypofunction or loss (UVH/L) may occur in the military c/mTBI population and are appropriate for the generalist clinician to evaluate and treat.[2,4]

If the complaint is consistent with episodes of vertigo (a sense of spinning), an algorithm for assessing BPPV may help determine the injury location and best treatment options. An additional important resource for information on treating BPPV is the Clinical Practice Guideline: Benign Paroxysmal Positional Vertigo.[4]

Although not represented in Herdman's[3(p230)] flow diagram, reports of other vestibular complaints have been described in military populations, including exercise-induced and blast-induced dizziness (unsteadiness) with or without vertigo.[5,6]

For assessing and treating complex etiologies such as perilymphatic fistula, bilateral vestibular hypofunction or loss, Ménière disease, or other dizziness complaints, service members should be referred to an ear, nose, and throat specialist; otolaryngologist; or neurologist for further evaluation and for treatment by therapists with specialized vestibular training.

This assessment section is intended to help a generalist therapist determine the possible cause of a vestibular complaint. The full components of a vestibular clinical examination, including the history and specialized vestibular tests, are beyond the scope of this toolkit. The reader is referred to Herdman[3] for full information and is encouraged to seek consultation from therapists with specialized vestibular training.

The intervention section of this toolkit provides information on canalith repositioning maneuvers (CRMs) for BPPV of the posterior canal and of the horizontal (lateral) canal.[4] Vestibular rehabilitation program elements included in the toolkit focus on adapting vestibular ocular reflex (VOR) mechanisms and improving gaze stability, improving postural control, and performing exercises that encourage habituation of symptoms associated with vestibular impairment. These principles may be applied to individuals with residual complaints after treatment for BPPV, UVH/L, as well as to individuals with migraine-associated dizziness (MAD).

This section of the toolkit provides assessments and interventions that are considered **practice standards** for BPPV and UVH/L based on the level of evidence available at this time. The vestibular rehabilitation protocols as described for UVH/L and MAD are considered **practice options**. Evidence for these practice recommendations is derived primarily from studies of the civilian population.

VESTIBULAR ASSESSMENT

Taking a history is the initial step in assessing a patient who complains of dizziness; the next step is a systems evaluation. Common mechanisms of vestibular injury in the warfighter often differ from those that cause civilian vestibular injury. Following a combat situation where a blast event occurs, initial assessment focuses on evaluation for alteration in consciousness consistent with a brain injury, and ensuring no red flags are present that indicate the need for emergent care to manage a life-threatening condition. If signs and symptoms are more consistent with blast-induced dizziness, refer to the recommended physical therapy clinical evaluation found in Scherer and Schubert (see Figure 2-1).[2]

A number of clinical and laboratory tests are beneficial to further define possible vestibular pathology (see Table 2-1).[2] Although laboratory tests

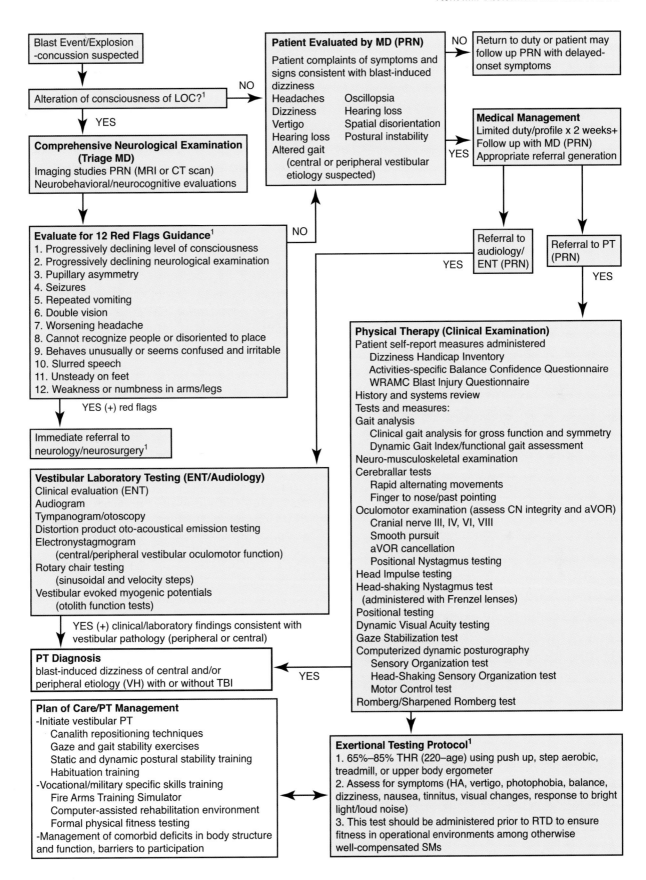

Figure 2-1. Traumatic brain injury and vestibular pathology after blast exposure.

Figure 2-1 caption *continues*

aVOR: angular vestibulo-ocular reflex
CT: computed tomography
HA: headache
MD: medical doctor
PRN: as needed/indicated by provider
RTD: return to duty
TBI: traumatic brain injury
VH: vestibular hypofunction

CN: cranial nerve
ENT: ear, nose, and throat (otolaryngology MD)
LOC: loss of consciousness
MRI: magnetic resonance imaging
PT: physical therapy
SM: service member
THR: target heart rate
WRAMC: Walter Reed Army Medical Center

1. Wrisley D, Marchetti G, Kuharsky D, Whitney S. Reliability, internal consistency, and validity of data obtained with the Functional Gait Assessment. *Phys Ther*. 2004;84:906–918.

Reproduced with permission from: Scherer MR, Schubert MC. Traumatic brain injury and vestibular pathology as a comorbidity after blast exposure. *Phys Ther*. 2009;89:988. Copyright 2009, American Physical Therapy Association. Any further reproduction or distribution requires written permission from APTA.

TABLE 2-1

CLINICAL AND LABORATORY TESTS FOR VESTIBULAR PATHOLOGY IN SUBJECTS EXPOSED TO BLASTS

Tests	Structures, Pathways, or Process Assessed	Applications	Abnormal Findings	Interpretation
Head impulse test[1] (clinical)	Horizontal semicircular canals, superior branch of vestibular nerve	High-acceleration, moderate-velocity, low-amplitude head rotation with subject maintaining gaze on fixed target	Corrective saccade to target after head rotation	Abnormal angular vestibulo-ocular reflex (aVOR) attributable to peripheral vestibular hypofunction
Electronystagmography[2] (laboratory)	Extraocular muscles, horizontal semicircular canals, superior branch of vestibular nerve, vestibular and oculomotor pathways within central nervous system	Exposure to aural and visual stimulation (eg, calorics, moving targets)	Abnormal nystagmus, abnormal eye movements	Abnormal 8th cranial nerve, abnormal smooth pursuit or saccades attributable to pathology within peripheral or central vestibular pathways, oculomotor pathways, or both
Rotary chair test[2] (laboratory)	Horizontal semicircular canals, superior branch of vestibular nerve	Sinusoidal rotation at frequencies of 0.01–0.64 Hz; clockwise and counterclockwise rotation at 60°/s and 240°/s	Abnormal nystagmus, abnormal eye movements	Abnormal aVOR gain or phase attributable to pathology within peripheral or central vestibular or oculomotor pathways
Positional test[2,3] (clinical or laboratory)	Semicircular canals involved canal	Movement into gravity-dependent position	Patient-reported complaints of vertigo and pathologic nystagmus	Abnormal presence of otoconia in semicircular canal (ie, benign paroxysmal positional vertigo)

Table 2-1 *continues*

(Table 2-1 *continued)*

Tests	Structures, Pathways, or Process Assessed	Applications	Abnormal Findings	Interpretation
Dynamic visual acuity Test[2,4] (clinical)	Horizontal semicircular canals, vestibular nerve	Active or passive head movement while visualizing optotype direction	Inability to identify target during head movement	Abnormal aVOR attributable to peripheral vestibular hypofunction; uncompensated aVOR
Computerized dynamic posturography,[5] sensory organization test (SOT), motor control test (MCT) (clinical or laboratory)	Integration of multi-sensory input for balance	Challenge of balance with equipment and software under different conditions	SOT: inappropriate responses to inaccurate sensory inputs; MCT: delayed motor responses to unpredictable perturbations	SOT: age- and height-referenced responses to sway in sagittal plane; MCT: balance dysfunction and impaired reactive latencies
Balance Manager Dynamic inVision System*,[6] gaze stability, perception time, target acquisition, target tracking (clinical)	Horizontal semicircular canals, vestibular nerve, vestibular and oculomotor pathways	Head movement while visualizing letters; tracking of moving targets	Abnormal oculometric features compared with those of subjects who were healthy and matched for age	Behavioral measure suggesting cerebellar dysfunction; damage to central oculomotor pathways, vestibular pathways, or both

aVOR: angular vestibulo-ocular reflex
SOT: sensory organization test
MCT: motor control test
*The Balance Manager Dynamic inVision System (NeuroCom International Inc, Clackamas, OR) provides oculomotor and vestibular testing not available in other NeuroCom systems. Novel assessments include perception time, target acquisition, and target tracking. Gaze stability testing is provided in commercially available models such as the SMART Equi-Test System (NeuroCom International Inc). Visual testing typically is performed in a darkened room with a viewing distance of 390 cm (13 ft). Perception time is measured by calculating the time (in milliseconds) that a randomly presented target must be on the screen before accurate recognition by a subject. Target acquisition is the time (in milliseconds) required to make a saccade from the center of the screen to the new optotype position. Target tracking is the speed (in degrees per second) at which a subject can accurately track a symbol. Gaze stabilization is the speed (in degrees per second) at which a subject can move his or her head and accurately hold a target in view.[6]

1. Halmagyi GM, Curthoys IS. A clinical sign of canal paresis. *Arch Neurol.* 1988;45:737–739. 2. Fife T, Tusa R, Furman J, et al. Assessment: vestibular testing techniques in adults and children—report of the Therapeutics and Technology Assessment Subcommittee of the American Academy of Neurology. *Neurology.* 2000;55:1431–1441. 3. Roberts R, Gans R. Background, technique, interpretation, and usefulness of positional/position testing. In: Jacobsen J, Shepherd N, eds. *Balance Function Assessment and Management.* San Diego, CA: Plural Publishing; 2008: 171–196. 4. Herdman SJ, Tusa RJ, Blatt PJ, et al. Computerized dynamic visual acuity test in the assessment of vestibular deficits. *Am J Otol.* 1998;19:790–796. 5. Shepard N, Janky K. Interpretation and usefulness of computerized dynamic posturography. In: Jacobsen J, Shepherd N, eds. *Balance Function Assessment and Management.* San Diego, CA: Plural Publishing; 2008: 359–378. 6. Gottshall, K. Vestibular-visual-cognitive interaction tests in patients with blast trauma. In: *Association for Research in Otolaryngology Midwinter Meeting;* February 14–19, 2009; Baltimore, MD. Abstract 180.

(eg, electronystagmography, rotary chair, computerized dynamic posturography, Balance Manager InVision system [NeuroCom, Clackamas, OR]) would not be initiated or interpreted by a generalist therapist, awareness of these tests is beneficial.

Other clinical tests are described in this section that are appropriate for a generalist to administer. According to Herdman,[3] specific information is obtained on the temporal quality (onset and duration) and nature of the person's complaints to clarify whether the complaint is vertigo (an illusion of movement, typically a sense of spinning) or disequilibrium (sense of being off balance; see Herdman, Figure 16-1).[3(p230)] Some individuals with vestibular dysfunction experience symptoms only during particular head movements.

Individuals in combat situations may sustain c/mTBI with vestibular deficits as a result of blunt injury or blast exposure. Positional vertigo is associated with trauma in the civilian population, but has also been described following blast injury in a military population.[5] Hoffer et al[6] have described MAD in association with blunt trauma, with symptoms including migraine headache, episodic vertigo, and balance disorder (although the headache and vertigo need not be simultaneous). Injury sustained in a blast incident has been associated with various patterns of symptoms, including positional vertigo, exercise-induced dizziness, and blast-induced dizziness with or without episodes of vertigo.[5,7,8]

Basic clinical examinations are similar for all vestibular complaints. A thorough history is the initial

TABLE 2-2

TRAUMATIC BRAIN INJURY AND VESTIBULAR PATHOLOGY AFTER BLAST EXPOSURE*

Position	Nystagmus Elicited	Does Nystagmus Last < 60 Seconds?	Possible Diagnosis	Recommendation
Left Dix-Hallpike Test	Upbeating, leftward torsional	Yes	Left posterior canalithiasis	Left posterior canal CRT
		No	Left posterior cupulothiasis	Referral to vestibular specialist
	Downbeating, rightward/ leftward torsional	Yes	Right/left anterior canalithiasis	Anterior canal CRT initiate maneuver toward torsional direction/nystagmus
		No	Right/left anterior cupulothiasis	Referral to vestibular specialist
Right Dix-Hallpike Test	Upbeating, rightward torsional	Yes	Right posterior canalithiasis	Right posterior canal CRT
		No	Right posterior canal cupulothiasis	Referral to vestibular specialist
	Downbeating, rightward/ leftward torsional	Yes	Right/left anterior canalithiasis	Anterior canal CRT initiate maneuver toward torsional direction
		No	Right/left anterior cupulothiasis	Referral to vestibular specialist
Right/Left Roll Test	Geotrophic[+]	Yes	Horizontal canalithiasis	Horizontal canal CRT initiate maneuver toward side with most intense nystagmus
	Ageotrophic[‡]	No	Horizontal cupulothiasis	Referral to vestibular specialist

CRT: canalith repositioning therapy

*This is a guide for testing clients who have a history of episodic vertigo that is of short duration (< 1 min) indicating benign paroxysmal positional vertigo as a diagnosis. These recommendations are for general practice therapists with basic knowledge of vestibular interventions.

[+]"Geotropic" means nystagmus that beats toward the ground. Typically the affected ear is tested down toward the mat. This is nystagmus with the slow phase beating toward the ground (toward the mat table if affected ear is down) and fast correction away from the ground.

[‡]"Ageotrophic" nystagmus beats away from the ground or "towards the sky."

component of any vestibular examination. A history of episodic vertigo of short duration suggests the need for positional testing for BPPV (Table 2-2). Tests of the VOR (eg, dynamic visual acuity, head impulse testing, and head-shaking nystagmus [HSN]) and postural control (See Chapter 3: Balance and Functional Abilities Assessment and Intervention) clarify the extent of impairment and possible targets for intervention. Testing for body and position changes that may provoke symptoms (Motion Sensitivity Quotient [MSQ] Test, exertional testing; see Chapter 10: Fitness Assessment and Intervention) may be necessary to determine baseline symp-

tom intensity. Assessing self-perception of disability (Dizziness Handicap Inventory [DHI] or Vestibular Activities of Daily Activity Scale) from vestibular complaints allows for understanding of the impact of these deficits on quality-of-life issues. Videos of a number of the vestibular tests can be found in the Geriatric Examination Toolkit from the University of Missouri (web.missouri.edu/~proste/tool/vest/index.htm) and on the webpage of the Vestibular Special Interest Group of the Neurology Section of the American Physical Therapy Association (www.neuropt.org/special-interest-groups/vestibular-rehabilitation/resources).

DIX-HALLPIKE MANEUVER

Purpose/Description

The Dix-Hallpike maneuver is a diagnostic, clinical provocation test that attempts to reproduce positional vertigo with associated nystagmus. A positive test is indicative of posterior canal BPPV.[3,4] The maneuver is used as part of a vestibular examination for imbalance, dizziness, and vertigo. It is indicated in clients who have a history of repeated episodes of vertigo with changes in head position relative to gravity.[9] Typically the side with the suspected involved canal is tested first and, if found positive, the patient may be directly treated with CRM. This combination of assessment and treatment is often done to avoid repeated provocation of patients who have significant symptoms.

Administration Protocol/Equipment/Time

Administration time is less than 5 minutes. Interpretation is enhanced by Frenzel lenses or infrared goggles.

Factors that may affect diagnostic accuracy of the Dix-Hallpike maneuver include the speed of movements during the test, time of day, and the angle of the plane of the occiput during the maneuver.[10] Because fixation on a visual target can suppress nystagmus, patients undergoing Dix-Hallpike testing may benefit from having their vision blocked.

Groups Tested With This Measure

Groups tested with this measure include those that present with characteristics of BPPV, such as brief, episodic, positional vertigo that is acquired spontaneously or may follow head trauma, labyrinthitis, or ischemia of the anterior vestibular artery.[11]

Interpretability

The Dix-Hallpike maneuver is considered the gold standard in diagnosing posterior canal BPPV.[4] Posterior canal BPPV is diagnosed when the client has a history of positional vertigo and, upon completion of the Dix-Hallpike maneuver, develops a provoked vertigo with a mixed torsional and vertical nystagmus. The vertigo and nystagmus begin within 5 to 20 seconds of the completion of the Dix-Hallpike maneuver and last less than 60 seconds.[4]

Sensitivity

- 50%–88% in a review article on the diagnostic evaluation of dizziness[12]
- 82% in patients with posterior canal BPPV primarily tested by specialty clinicians[13]
- 79% in a critically appraised topic review (95% confidence interval: 65%–94%)[14]

Specificity

- 71% in patients with posterior canal BPPV primarily tested by specialty clinicians[13]
- 75% in a critically appraised review[14]

Procedure

Use the following steps to test for suspected posterior canal BPPV (Figure 2-2):

- Help the patient into an initial position of long sitting on a mat so when the patient is moved into a supine position, only the trunk and shoulders are supported by the mat and the patient's head is supported by the examiner's hands over the edge of the mat.

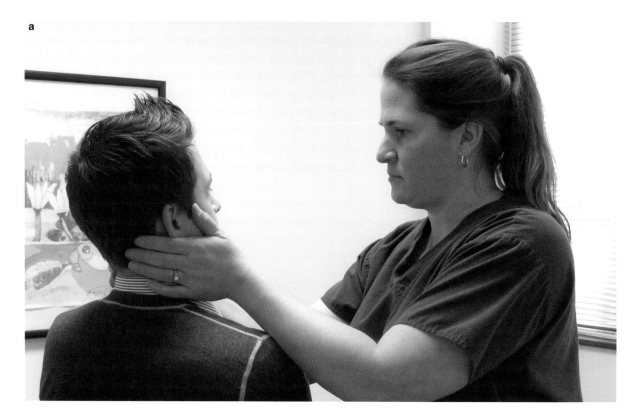

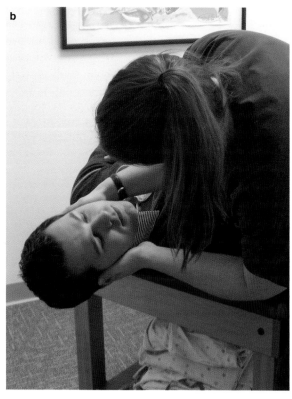

Figure 2-2. Administration of the Dix-Hallpike maneuver. **(a)** For the right Dix-Hallpike, move the client's head to 45 degrees or rotation to the right side. **(b)** Quickly move the client into a supine position, maintaining 45 degrees of rotation, to where the patient's head is hanging in 20 degrees of extension and is supported by the examiner.

- Quickly move the client into a supine position, maintaining 45 degrees of rotation, to where the patient's head is hanging in 20 degrees of extension and is supported by the examiner.
- Hold this position for 1 minute. Observe the patient's eyes for a mixed torsional and vertical jerk nystagmus; the vertigo and nystagmus will begin within 5 to 20 seconds of movement into the test position and will last less than 60 seconds.
- Return the patient to the original long sit position.
- For the left Dix-Hallpike maneuver, the client's head is placed into 45 degrees of rotation to the left. Then follow the sequence above.

- For the right Dix-Hallpike, move the client's head to 45 degrees of rotation to the right side.

The direction of the nystagmus indicates the posterior versus anterior canal (see Table 2-2 and refer to the Herdman text).[2(p252)]

RECORD OF FINDINGS FOR DIX-HALLPIKE MANEUVER

Dix-Hallpike (circle): Right: positive/negative   Left: positive/negative
Description of observed nystagmus:
Onset (sec): _____
Duration (sec): _____
Description of observed nystagmus: _____

Selected References

Dix R, Hallpike CS. The pathology, symptomatology and diagnosis of certain common disorders of the vestibular system. *Ann Otol Rhinol Laryngol.* 1952;6:987–1016.

Bhattacharyya N, Baugh RF, Orvidas L, et al. Clinical practice guideline: benign paroxysmal positional vertigo. *Otolaryngol Head Neck Surg.* 2008;139:S47–S81.

ROLL TEST

Purpose/Description

The roll test is a diagnostic, clinical provocation test that attempts to reproduce positional vertigo associated with nystagmus. A positive test is indicative of horizontal (lateral) canal BPPV.[4,15,16] The roll test is used as part of a vestibular examination for imbalance, dizziness, and vertigo. It is indicated if the patient has a history compatible with BPPV and the Dix-Hallpike maneuver gives negative results. Typically, the side with the suspected involved canal is tested first and, if found positive, the patient may be directly treated with the roll maneuver (also called the Lempert maneuver or barbecue roll maneuver). This combination of assessment and treatment is often done to avoid repeated provocation of patients who have significant symptoms.

Administration Protocol/Equipment/Time

Administration time is less than 5 minutes, and interpretation is enhanced by Frenzel lenses or infrared goggles. Patients undergoing the roll test may benefit from having their vision blocked with lenses or goggles because fixation on a visual target can suppress nystagmus.

Groups Tested With This Measure

Those that present with characteristics of BPPV, including brief, episodic, positional vertigo that is acquired spontaneously or may follow head trauma, labyrinthitis, or ischemia of the anterior vestibular artery should be tested using this method.[3,4,11,16]

Interpretability

Horizontal (lateral) canal BPPV is diagnosed when the client has a history of positional vertigo and, upon completion of the roll test, develops a provoked vertigo that is geotropic (canalithiasis).[3] The vertigo and nystagmus tend to begin within 5 to 20 seconds after completion of the roll test and last less than 60 seconds.[4,16] The side involved is considered the side with the most intense nystagmus. A positive supine roll test is the most frequently used test for diagnosing horizontal (lateral) canal BPPV.[4] If nystagmus persists for greater than 60 seconds, this may be indicative of a more severe form of BPPV (cupulolithiasis or central origin) and the client should be referred to a vestibular specialist (see Table 2-2).

Sensitivity

Not determined

Specificity

Not determined

Procedure

To perform the roll test for suspected horizontal (lateral) canal BPPV (Figure 2-3):

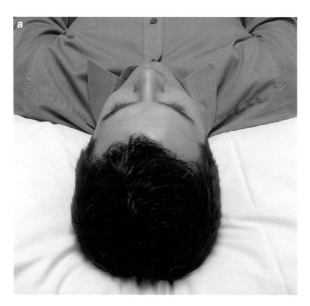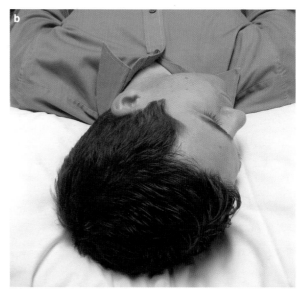

Figure 2-3. Administration of roll test. **(a)** Position the client supine with his or her head at 20 degrees flexion, supported by a pillow or by the therapist. **(b)** Quickly rotate the patient's head toward the right side 90 degrees and hold for 1 minute, or if the patient's orthopaedic limitations warrant, the entire trunk and head can be rolled (it is the head position in space that is important for this maneuver).

- Position the client supine with his or her head at 20 degrees flexion, supported by a pillow or by the therapist.
- Quickly rotate the patient's head toward the right side 90 degrees and hold for 1 minute, or if the patient's orthopaedic limitations warrant, the entire trunk and head can be rolled (it is the head position in space that is important for this maneuver).
- Observe the patient's eyes for geotropic (beats toward downward ear) or ageotropic (beats toward upper ear) nystagmus.

The vertigo and nystagmus will begin within 5 to 20 seconds of movement into the test position and last less than 60 seconds.
- When nystagmus subsides (or if no nystagmus is elicited), return the patient's head to a neutral rotation or "face-up" position.
- For the left roll test, the client's head is rapidly rotated 90 degrees to the left. The above sequence is then followed (see Table 2-2 and the Herdman text).[3(p252)]

RECORD OF FINDINGS FOR ROLL TEST

Roll Test (circle):   **Right:** positive/negative   **Left**: positive/negative

Description of observed nystagmus:_____

Onset (seconds):_____

Duration (seconds): _____

Direction of nystagmus (circle):   geotropic (bottom ear)

ageotropic (upper ear)

Selected References

Bhattacharyya N, Baugh RF, Orvidas L, et al. Clinical practice guideline: benign paroxysmal positional vertigo. *Otolaryngol Head Neck Surg.* 2008;139:S47–S81.

Fife TD. Recognition and management of horizontal canal benign positional vertigo. *Am J Otol.* 1998;19:345–351.

DYNAMIC VISUAL ACUITY TEST (CLINICAL)

Purpose/Description

The clinical Dynamic Visual Acuity Test is a procedural test that measures eye gaze stabilization with active head movement. It is a performance measure of the VOR[17,18] that can be used in patients with suspected vestibular hypofunction as part of a vestibular examination for imbalance, dizziness, vertigo, and oscillopsia (blurred vision with head movement).[16,19]

Administration Protocol/Equipment/Time

Administration takes less than 5 minutes and requires a Snellen eye chart or clinical equivalent, such as the Early Treatment Diabetic Retinopathy Study chart.

Groups Tested With This Measure

Those suspected of having UVH/L should be tested with this measure, including patients with vestibular neuronitis, Ménière disease, vestibular schwannoma, vascular lesions affecting the vestibular nerve, or TBI.[19,20]

Interpretability

A two-line difference is considered normal; greater than two-line difference is a positive sign for oscillopsia.[18,21]

Sensitivity

- < 50% of 115 clients with dizziness (for UVH, bilateral vestibular hypofunction, and dizziness)[22]

Specificity

- 100% in clients with dizziness[22]

Procedure

Perform the Dynamic Visual Acuity test (Figure 2-4) following these steps:

- The patient may be seated or standing. If the patient uses prescription glasses, the glasses should be worn during testing.
- Test static visual acuity by having the patient read the lowest line on a standard

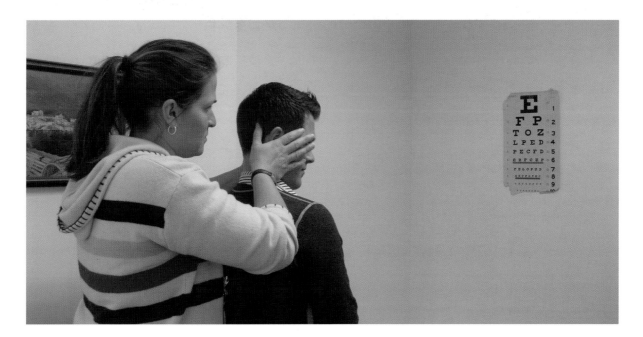

Figure 2-4. Administration of the Dynamic Visual Acuity Test.

Snellen (or clinical equivalent) eye chart, keeping his or her head still. The lowest line readable is the line in which three or fewer errors are made. Record this line and identify the number of errors.

- Test dynamic visual acuity by having the patient read the lowest line possible on a standard Snellen (or clinical equivalent) eye chart while tilting the patient's head 30

degrees forward (to orient the horizontal canals with the horizontal plane) and passively oscillating the head horizontally at 2 Hz. The lowest line readable is the line in which three or fewer errors are made. Record this line and identify the number of errors.

- Note the difference between the lines read in the static and dynamic tests.

RECORD OF FINDINGS FOR DYNAMIC VISUAL ACUITY TEST (CLINICAL)

Lowest readable line (static): _____   Errors: _____

Lowest readable line (2 Hz passive movement): _____   Errors: _____

Line change between static and dynamic condition: _____

Selected References

Barber HO. Vestibular neurophysiology. *Otolaryngol Head Neck Surg.* Feb 1984;92(1):55–58.

Burgio DL, Blakley RW, Myers SF. The high-frequency oscillopsia test. *J Vestib Res.* 1992;2:221–226.

Schubert MC, Minor LB. Vestibulo-ocular physiology underlying vestibular hypofunction. *Phys Ther.* Apr 2004;84(4):373–385.

HEAD IMPULSE TEST (HEAD THRUST TEST)

Purpose/Description

The head impulse test is a clinical test that assesses the integrity of the VOR.[23] It may be used in a patient with suspected vestibular hypofunction as part of a vestibular examination for imbalance, dizziness, vertigo, and oscillopsia.[16,24]

Administration Protocol/Equipment/Time

Administration takes less than 1 minute and no special equipment is required. The sensitivity of the head impulse test appears to be improved when the patient's head is pitched 30 degrees downward and the thrust is done with an unpredictable timing and direction.[24]

Groups Tested With This Measure

Those suspected of having UVH/L, including patients with vestibular neuronitis, Ménière disease, vestibular schwannoma, vascular lesions affecting the vestibular nerve, or TBI may benefit from this test.[20,24]

Interpretability

The head impulse test is considered positive when, after a small, high-speed movement of the head, a refixation saccade is noted.[23,25] A client with vestibular hypofunction may use a refixation saccade after the head is moved toward the side of the hypofunction. With bilateral hypofunction, a refixation saccade may be seen with both the right and left tests. Individuals with normal vestibular function do not use corrective saccades after the head impulse test; their eyes stay fixed on the target (eg, examiner's nose). The head impulse test is only positive in vestibular loss or hypofunction, not in cerebellar stroke or migraine, so it may be useful in a differential diagnosis.

Sensitivity (35%–71%; enhanced when following specific protocol)

- 45% in 265 patients evaluated for symptoms of vertigo[26]
- 35% in 105 patients who presented for evaluation of dizziness[27]

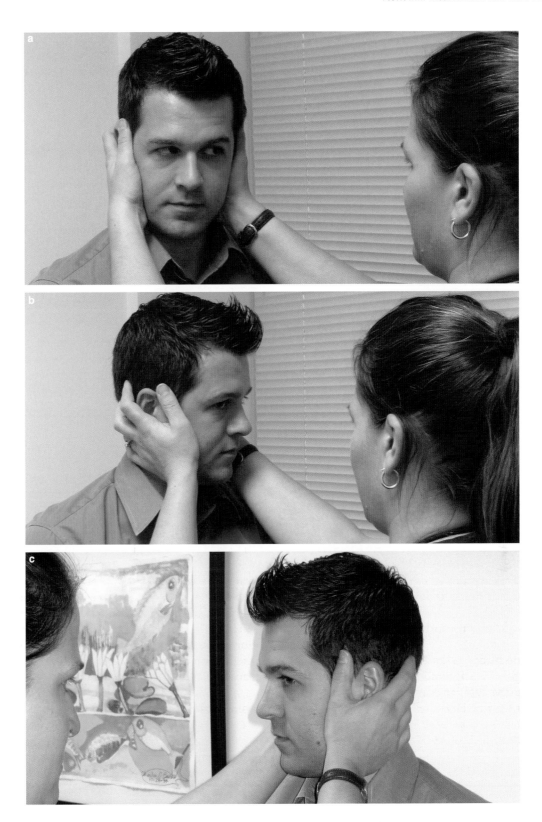

Figure 2-5. Administration of the head impulse test. **(a)** With the patient in a sitting position, passively tilt the patient's head forward 30 degrees to orient the horizontal semicircular canals parallel to the horizontal plane. Instruct the patient to look at a target (eg, the examiner's nose). **(b)** Passively and slowly move the patient's head in right and left rotation (approximately 20-degree to 30-degree arc of motion) to assess that the patient is relaxed. **(c)** Quickly (3,000 degrees to 4,000 degrees/sec/sec) move the patient's head from neutral rotation to 5 degrees–10 degrees of rotation in one direction and stop.

- 71% for identifying vestibular hypofunction in persons with UVH (176 persons with and without vestibular dysfunction)[24]

Specificity (82%–95%)

- 91% in 265 patients evaluated for symptoms of vertigo[26]
- 95% in 105 patients who presented for evaluation of dizziness[28]
- 82% for UVH or BVH, 176 persons with and without vestibular dysfunction[29]

Procedure

Perform the head impulse test following these steps (Figure 2-5):

- With the patient in a sitting position, passively tilt the patient's head forward 30 degrees to orient the horizontal semicircular canals parallel to the horizontal plane.

- Instruct the patient to look at a target (eg, the examiner's nose). Passively and slowly move the patient's head in right and left rotation (approximately 20-degree to 30-degree arc of motion) to assess that the patient is relaxed.
- Quickly (3,000 degrees to 4,000 degrees/sec/sec) move the patient's head from neutral rotation to 5 degrees–10 degrees of rotation in one direction and stop.
- Observe the patient's eyes for a corrective saccade. The corrective saccade is a rapid eye motion that returns the eyes toward the target (eg, examiner's nose) and indicates a decreased gain of the VOR.
- Complete this test three times in each direction (if corrective saccade is noted in at least two of three thrusts, result is positive).

Note that ensuring the head is pitched 30 degrees down and the thrust is performed with an unpredictable timing and direction appears to improve the sensitivity of the head impulse test.[30]

HEAD IMPULSE TEST RECORD OF FINDINGS

Circle findings:

Right impulse: Trial 1: _____ Trial 2: _____ Trial 3: _____ positive/negative

Left impulse: Trial 1: _____ Trial 2: _____ Trial 3: _____ positive/negative

---

HEAD-SHAKING NYSTAGMUS TEST

Purpose/Description

The HSN test is a clinical test that assesses for dynamic asymmetry in the vestibular system.[3] It is used in patients with suspected vestibular hypofunction and is a simple screening evaluation for peripheral vestibular system disease. It is used as part of a vestibular examination for imbalance, dizziness, vertigo, and oscillopsia.[16,19,31]

Administration Protocol/Equipment/Time

Administration takes less than 1 minute. Interpretation is enhanced by use of Frenzel lenses or infrared goggles. Therapists must screen for spontaneous nystagmus prior to testing for HSN. Patients undergoing HSN testing must have their vision blocked with lenses or goggles because fixation on a visual target can suppress nystagmus.

Groups Tested With This Measure

HSN is used to test those suspected of having UVH/L. These may be individuals with vestibular neuronitis, Ménière disease, vestibular schwannoma, vascular lesions affecting the vestibular nerve, or TBI.[19,20]

Interpretability

When head movements stop, nystagmus that beats toward the more active (intact) side or away from the side of a unilateral peripheral vestibular lesion indicates a positive response. Three consecutive beats of nystagmus is considered a positive response. This test indicates an imbalance between the right and left sides; it does not define the source of imbalance. Those with symmetric peripheral vestibular input will *not* have HSN.

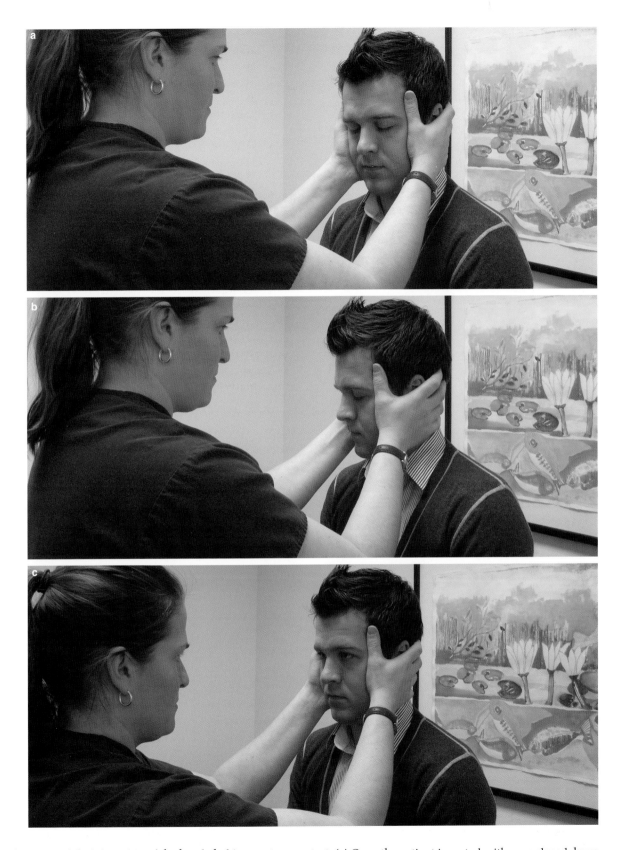

Figure 2-6. Administration of the head-shaking nystagmus test. **(a)** Once the patient is seated with eyes closed, have the patient tilt his or her head forward 30 degrees. **(b)** Rotate or shake the patient's head back and forth 20 times in 10 seconds (2 Hz) in approximately 45 degrees of rotation to either side. **(c)** Stop the movement and ask the patient to open his or her eyes and look straight ahead.

Sensitivity (Range 27%–66%)

- 66% for detecting greater than 20% canal paresis in 132 patients referred for full otologic and neuro-otologic examination with complaints of dizziness and balance problems[32]
- 38% in 196 patients with peripheral vestibular dysfunction[33]
- 27% in 116 consecutive dizzy patients seen for balance function testing[34]
- 31% in 53 patients with unilateral peripheral hypofunction[35]
- 35% in 105 outpatients who presented for evaluation of dizziness (ages 13–87 years)[27]

Specificity (Range 77%–96%)

- 77% for detecting greater than 20% canal paresis, 132 patients referred for full otologic and neuro-otologic examination with complaints of dizziness and balance problems[32]
- 79% in 196 patients with peripheral vestibular dysfunction[33]
- 85% in 116 consecutive dizzy patients seen for balance function testing[36]
- 92% in 105 outpatients who presented for evaluation of dizziness (ages 13–87 years)[27]

- 96% in 53 patients with unilateral peripheral hypofunction[35]

Procedure

Perform the test as follows (Figure 2-6):

- Once the patient is seated with eyes closed, have the patient tilt his or her head forward 30 degrees.
- Rotate or shake the patient's head back and forth 20 times in 10 seconds (2 Hz) in approximately 45 degrees of rotation to either side.
- Stop the movement and ask the patient to open his or her eyes and look straight ahead. Observe for nystagmus.
- When the head movements stop, nystagmus that beats toward the more active side or away from the side of a unilateral peripheral vestibular lesion indicates a positive response. Three consecutive beats of nystagmus is considered a positive response.

This test can also be completed with infrared goggles or Frenzel lenses. Signs of central etiology include prolonged nystagmus, vertical nystagmus, and dysconjugate nystagmus.[37]

HORIZONTAL HEAD-SHAKING INDUCED NYSTAGMUS RECORD OF FINDINGS

Circle findings:

Positive / Negative

Horizontal nystagmus: right-beating / left-beating

Selected References

Angeli SI, Velandia S, Snapp H. Head-shaking nystagmus predicts greater disability in unilateral peripheral vestibulopathy. *Am J Otolaryngol.* Nov 2011;32(6):522–527.

Jacobson GP, Newman CW, Safadi I. Sensitivity and specificity of the head-shaking test for detecting vestibular system abnormalities. *Ann Otol Rhinol Laryngol.* Jul 1990;99(7 Pt 1):539–542.

Goebel JA, Garcia P. Prevalence of post-headshake nystagmus in patients with caloric deficits and vertigo. *Otolaryngol Head Neck Surg.* 1992;106:121–127.

Schubert MC, Minor LB. Vestibulo-ocular physiology underlying vestibular hypofunction. *Phys Ther.* Apr 2004;84(4):373–385.

DIZZINESS HANDICAP INVENTORY

Purpose/Description

The DHI is a 25-item questionnaire—with a total possible score of 100—designed to measure self-perception of disability from vestibular system dysfunction (Exhibit 2-1).[36,38,39] The emotional scale (9 items) is 36 points, the functional scale (9 items) is 36 points, and the physical scale (7 items) is 28 points. Each question provides a choice of three responses: yes (4 points), sometimes (2 points), or no (0 points).

The DHI is the standard disease-specific tool used to assess health status and quality of life in individuals with vestibular disorders.[40] It is recommended for use at the initial evaluation and at follow-up after an episode of care for service members with vestibular complaints.

Administration Protocol/Equipment/Time

The DHI may be administered via a paper-and-pencil self-test or computerized answer self-test; each takes about 5 minutes to administer and 5 minutes to score.

Groups Tested With This Measure

The DHI is used to assess the effects of vestibular rehabilitation for dizziness of various origins.[40-42] Military populations tested with this measure included those with dizziness after brain injury[43] and exercise-induced dizziness.[8,44]

Interpretability

- Norms: a score of "0" indicated no handicap. The higher the point total (either total score or a subscale) a patient scores, the greater the perceived disability due to dizziness.
- Minimal detectable change (MDC): +/- 9.32 (standard error of the mean for 95% confidence interval) for persons in a vestibular rehabilitation program.[40] The standard error would be 6.23 between pre- and posttreatment scores, indicating the scores would have to differ by at least 18 points (95% confidence interval) for a true change.[36] If the patient's score is less than the MDC value, it was considered indistinguishable from measurement error.

The DHI was found to be more responsive to change than the SF-36 questionnaire in patients with vestibular disorders. Guyatt's responsiveness statistic (mean change divided by the standard deviation of change in subjects who remained unchanged) was 1.66 for total DHI, 1.89 for functional subscale, 0.75 for physical subscale, and 1.14 for emotional subscale.[40]

Reliability Estimates

- Internal consistency: high internal consistency reliability (Chronbach's alpha = 0.78–0.89)[36]
- Interrater: not applicable
- Intrarater: not applicable
- Test-Retest: 14 subjects (age range 26–71 years) were administered DHI face to face within a few days of each other. The total scores were as follows: r = .97, degrees of freedom = 12, P < .001, functional subscale (r = .94), emotional (r = .97), and physical (r = .92). These scores reflect excellent

---

EXHIBIT 2-1

DIZZINESS HANDICAP INVENTORY RESOURCES

This instrument can be obtained from the original publication:

Jacobson GP, Newman CW. The development of the dizziness handicap inventory. *Arch Otolaryngol Head Neck Surg.* 1990;116:424–427.

It can also be found in the Geriatric Examination Toolkit from the University of Missouri at: web.missouri.edu/~proste/tool/vest/index.htm, or from the Southampton Hospitals website, at: www.southamptonhospital.org/Resources/10355/FileRepository/Forms/Dizziness%20Hanicap%20Inventory%20-%20English.pdf.

test-retest reliability, with internal consistency (Chronbach's alpha) for DHI at .89 for total score (.85 functional subscale, .72 emotional subscale, .78 physical subscale).[36] Twenty subjects (age range 36–78 years) with vestibular disorders who took DHI twice, 24 to 48 hours apart, showed excellent retest reliability with intraclass correlation coefficient (ICC) (2,1) = .94.[40]

Validity

- Content/Face: established with an initial 37 questions developed empirically from case history reports of patients with dizziness and was reduced to 25 items by removing items that showed low-corrected item-total correlations or because of similarity in content to included items.[36]
- Criterion: in a group of 367 adults seen consecutively for balance function evaluations (mean age 48.8 years; standard deviation 14.5 years) the DHI correlated with a patient's ability to remain upright as quantified by platform posturography (r = 0.40–0.58).[45]

- Construct: 106 consecutive patients categorized as occasionally, frequently, or continuously experiencing dizziness had significantly different total DHI scores. The patient's age had no significant effect on self-perceived handicap as indicated by the total DHI score.[36] High correlations coefficients were found between total DHI score and the eight dimensions of the SF-36 questionnaire in ENT outpatients.[46] The construct validity of the sections of the DHI have not been fully studied.[47]

In a group of 15 patients with symptoms of exercise-induced motion intolerance (nausea, disequilibrium, and "dizziness") brought on by exercise involving head motion, such as sit-ups, push-ups, running, or swimming, an individualized exercise program was administered to provoke and allow habituation to symptoms of motion intolerance. Mean time of return to duty was 4.6 weeks. Statistically significant improvement in DHI scores were noted, with a decrease of 17.3 points after treatment, coincident with significant improvements in the Activities-specific Balance Confidence Scale, Dynamic Gait Index, and computerized dynamic posturography.[8]

Selected References

Enloe LJ, Shields RK. Evaluation of health-related quality of life in individuals with vestibular disease using disease-specific and general outcome measures. *Phys Ther.* Sep 1997;77(9):890–903.

Gottshall KR, Moore RJ, Hoffer ME, et al. Exercise induced motion intolerance: role in operational environments. Paper presented at: Spatial Disorientation in Military Vehicles: Causes, Consequences and Cures; April 15–17, 2002; La Coruña, Spain.

Gottshall KR, Drake A, Gray N, McDonald E, Hoffer ME. Objective vestibular tests as outcome measures in head injury patients. *Laryngoscope.* 2003;113(10):1746–1750.

Jacobson GP, Newman CW, Hunter L, Balzer GK. Balance function test correlates of the Dizziness Handicap Inventory. *J Am Acad Audiol.* Oct 1991;2(4):253–260.

MOTION SENSITIVITY QUOTIENT TEST

Purpose/Description

The MSQ Test is a clinical technique to measure motion-provoked dizziness using a series of 16 quick changes to head or body position (Exhibit 2-2).[48] The severity and duration of the dizziness are recorded in each position and a cumulative score is calculated. The test was developed by Shepard and Telian[49] to establish individualized exercise programs for patients with chronic UVH. The 16 head and body movements in the MSQ protocol

described by Smith-Wheelock and colleagues[49] include:

1. sitting to supine,
2. supine to left side,
3. supine to right side,
4. supine to sitting,
5. left Dix-Hallpike (sitting to supine, head hanging to the left),
6. head up from left Dix-Hallpike,
7. right Dix-Hallpike (sitting to supine, head

EXHIBIT 2-2

MOTION SENSITIVITY QUOTIENT TEST RESOURCES

This instrument can be obtained from the original publication:

Smith-Wheelock M, Shepard NT, Telian SA. Physical therapy program for vestibular rehabilitation. *Am J Otol.* 1991;12(3):218–225. Figure 1.

It can also be found in the Geriatric Examination Toolkit from the University of Missouri at: web.missouri.edu/~proste/tool/vest/index.htm.

---

hanging to the right),
8. head up from right Dix-Hallpike,
9. sitting with head tipped to left knee,
10. head up from left knee,
11. sitting with head tipped to right knee,
12. head up from right knee,
13. head turns while sitting,
14. sitting head tilts,
15. 180 degrees turn to right while standing, and
16. 180 degrees turn to left while standing.

Scoring is based on symptom intensity via patient verbal report (0–5 scale) and symptom duration on a 0 to 3 scale (0–4 sec = 0; 5–10 sec = 1 point; 11–30 sec = 2 points; > 30 sec = 3 points). Symptom improvement on the MSQ Test is indicated by decreased number of provoking positions, increased number of repetitions before symptom onset, decreased intensity of symptoms, and shorter duration of symptoms.

Administration Protocol/Equipment/Time

The MSQ requires a mat table and chair. Administration time is less than 10 to 15 minutes, depending on the patient's tolerance and need for rest.

Groups Tested With This Measure

The MSQ was used in one study for those with motion-provoked dizziness (ages 43–86) and normal controls (ages 37–79)[48] to predict older driver safety in an on-road driving assessment,[50] and for those undergoing vestibular rehabilitation.[49]

Interpretability

- Norms:
  - 0%: normal
  - 0–10%: mild motion sensitivity

- 11%–30%: moderate motion sensitivity
  - 31%–100%: severe motion sensitivity[32]
- Sensitivity: 100%[46]
- Specificity: 80% for patients with motion sensitivity[46]
- MDC: 8.5% (test-retest ICC = .98, SD 25.9).[46] If the patient's score is less than the MDC value, it is considered to be indistinguishable from measurement error.
- Responsiveness estimates: not available
- Reliability estimates:
  - Internal consistency: not available
  - Interrater: 15 subjects with motion provoked dizziness (ages 43–86 years), two examiners, ICC = 0.99[46]
  - Intrarater: not available
  - Test-Retest: 15 subjects with motion provoked dizziness (ages 43–86 years) and 10 control subjects (ages 37–79 years) were tested at baseline and 24 hours later (8 subjects were also tested 90 minutes after baseline). ICC at 90 minutes = 0.98, ICC at 24 hours = 0.96[46]
- Validity estimates:
  - Content/Face: not available
  - Criterion: not available
  - Construct: 100% of community-dwelling individuals from regional senior citizen centers who complained of motion-provoked dizziness during routine movements associated with daily living reported symptoms on the MSQ Test. Only 2 of 10 (test specificity of 80%) of community-dwelling individuals from regional senior citizen centers without complaints of motion-provoked dizziness during routine movements associated with daily living reported dizziness in either right or left up from Dix-Hallpike.[46]

Selected References

Smith-Wheelock M, Shepard NT, Telian SA. Physical therapy program for vestibular rehabilitation. *Am J Otol.* May 1991;12(3):218–225.

Akin FW, Davenport MJ. Validity and reliability of the Motion Sensitivity Test. *J Rehab Res Dev.* Sep–Oct 2003;40(5):415–421.

VESTIBULAR DISORDERS ACTIVITIES OF DAILY LIVING SCALE

Purpose/Description

The Vestibular Disorders Activities of Daily Living (VADL) Scale is a 28-item questionnaire developed to assess self-perceived disablement and quality of life in patients with vestibular impairment.[51] The functional, or basic, self-maintenance subscale includes 12 items; the ambulatory, or mobility, skills subscale has 9 items; and the instrumental subscale (more socially complex tasks outside the home) includes 7 items (Exhibit 2-3). This self-administered checklist uses a 10-point qualitative scale, but also includes a "not applicable" option if a subject wants to refrain from answering a question or if a question does not apply.[50(p883)] Scale ratings range from 1 (independent) to 10 (not participating in the activity). The VADL Scale, which includes tasks like driving a car and using an elevator, may be more responsive to higher levels of impairment and therefore more useful for higher functioning individuals. It has been suggested that the VADL Scale is also more responsive to lesser levels of independence, given the 10-point scale in comparison to the 3-point scale on the DHI.[51]

Administration Protocol/Equipment/Time

The test consists of a paper-and-pencil self-test or a computerized answer self-test, each of which takes about 5 to 10 minutes to administer and 5 minutes to score.

Groups Tested With This Measure

The VADL is used to assess the effects of rehabilitation on chronic vestibular impairment for dizziness of peripheral origin.[52,53] This questionnaire has been used to assess service members with acute (within 72 hours), subacute (4–30 days), and chronic (> 30 days) vestibular complaints following blast exposure.[5,51]

Interpretability

- Norms: healthy subjects were independent (scale rating of "1") on the items on the VADL.[48]

Scale ratings range from 1 (independent) to 10 (too difficult to perform, not participating in the activity).

- MDC: not available. If the patient's score is less than the MDC value, it is considered indistinguishable from measurement error.
- Responsiveness estimates: not available
- Reliability estimates:
  - Internal consistency: alpha = 0.97 (total score), r = 0.92–0.97 (dimensions).[48]
  - Interrater: not available
  - Test-Retest: tested over a 2-hour time period; rc = 1 (concordance coefficient), rc = 0.87–0.97 (dimensions).[48]
- Validity estimates:
  - Content/Face: face validity established by a group of experts from a list of items taken from existing scales of self-perceived disablement in patients with vestibular impairment.[48]
- Criterion: moderately correlates with the Dizziness Handicap Inventory, Spearman's rho = 0.66.[48]
- Construct: differentiates healthy adults from patients with BPPV or chronic vestibulopathy.[48]

Selected References

Cohen HS, Kimball KT. Development of the vestibular disorders activities of daily living scale. *Arch Otolaryngol Head Neck Surg.* Jul 2000;126(7):881–887.

Cohen HS, Kimball KT. Increased independence and decreased vertigo after vestibular rehabilitation. *Otolaryngol Head Neck Surg.* Jan 2003;128(1):60–70.

> **EXHIBIT 2-3**
>
> **RESOURCES FOR THE VESTIBULAR DISORDERS ACTIVITIES OF DAILY LIVING SCALE**
>
> This instrument can be obtained from the original publication:
>
> Cohen HS, Kimball KT. Development of the Vestibular Disorders of Daily Living Scale. *Arch Otolaryngol Head Neck Surg.* 2000;126:881–887.
>
> It can also be found on a number of external websites through internet search engines.

VESTIBULAR INTERVENTION

Intervention strategies must be tailored to the symptom profile of the patient with vestibular dysfunction. Interventions designed to address positional vertigo are very specific, with particular maneuvers based on the semicircular canal that is involved. The use of repositioning maneuvers is often effective for positional vertigo symptoms. The CRM is used to treat BPPV of the posterior semicircular canal (posterior canal canalithiasis) with an 83% to 93% rate of remission of reported BPPV.[4,54,55] The roll maneuver (barbecue roll) is used to move canaliths from the horizontal (lateral) canal into the vestibule to treat horizontal (lateral) canal BPPV. The effectiveness of this maneuver is approximately 75%, according to summary information provided in the *Clinical Practice Guideline on BPPV.*[4]

Home instructions for precautions following the CRM and instruction in Brandt-Daroff habituation exercises for milder residual complaints of dizziness or vertigo have been suggested.[3] Herdman also suggests instructing patients in the appropriate CRM so they may repeat the maneuver on their own, as long as they are experiencing vertigo during treatment.[3] It has been suggested that posttraumatic BPPV is different from the idiopathic form. Gordon et al reported that 67% of patients with traumatic BPPV required repeated treatment before complete symptom resolution, compared to 14% of patients with idiopathic BPPV. This group also reported that posttraumatic patients had significantly more frequent recurrences.[56]

Intervention for UVH includes exercises designed to facilitate central nervous system compensation or adaptation rather than alter underlying vestibular disease. Service members can learn to compensate for UVH with appropriate vestibular rehabilitation and gaze stability exercises.[57] Exercise-based interventions can be applied to patients with a range of vestibular issues and are categorized in three main areas: 1) gaze stabilization exercises that address VOR functions and gaze stability as a means to facilitate adaptation and improvement of vestibular function; 2) motion-sensitivity exercises for individuals who have increased complaints associated with conditions of visual conflict or increased optic flow, or associated with exercise-induced dizziness to structure practice for habituation to provoking stimuli; and 3) postural stability exercises to improve balance and postural control (see also Chapter 3: Balance and Functional Abilities Assessment and Intervention).

The characteristics of vestibular dysfunction as a result of combat exposure have been described by Gottshall and Hoffer.[5,7] In addition to possible positional vertigo, symptoms could include exertional (or exercise-induced) dizziness, blast-induced disequilibrium, and blast-induced disequilibrium with vertigo. Components of a comprehensive exercise program for service members in this context include the following:

- exercises that target vestibulo-ocular and cervico-ocular reflexes;
- activities that challenge somatosensory and depth perception by manipulating head motion, visual, and surface conditions;
- integrating challenges to dynamic gait; and
- graded aerobic exercise (see Chapter 10: Fitness Assessment and Intervention).

MAD has been described in a military population and is characterized by episodic vertigo with periods of unsteadiness, headaches, and abnormalities in VOR testing.[6] The use of medication and control of dietary triggers is helpful in controlling MAD.[58] Vestibular rehabilitation has also been effective for MAD,[58,59] especially when combined with an antimigraine medication and physical therapy intervention.[60,61] Rehabilitation strategies are similar to those for UVH/L and include habituation exercises, balance retraining, and daily aerobic exercises.

CANALITH REPOSITIONING MANEUVERS

Background

Individuals with BPPV frequently report positional dizziness, disrupted vision, nausea, imbalance and general motion intolerance, and falls. Typically, positional vertigo occurs with activities of daily living (rolling in bed, looking up, tying shoes), with the dizziness impacting the person's postural stability and interrupting daily activities.[62,63] The characteristics that distinguish vertigo of BPPV are a history of episodic vertigo of short duration (< 60 seconds) that has a brief delay (seconds) in onset when a person moves into a provoking position and is fatigable.[3]

Strength of Recommendation: Practice Standard

Posterior semicircular canal CRM (also called Epley maneuver) is the gold standard for treatment of posterior semicircular canal BPPV.[3,4,64] Standard treatment for horizontal (lateral) semicircular canal BPPV is the horizontal CRM (barbecue roll).[3]

Intervention

- See specific instruction sheets for CRM for the posterior or for the horizontal (lateral) canal.
- A firm surface, such as a treatment table or mat table, is needed, and Frenzel lenses or infrared goggles are helpful.
- The treatment takes about 5 to 10 minutes to administer.
- Following appropriate CRM, residual postural control impairments and fitness limitations are addressed as indicated for the individual patient.

Once the CRM procedures are completed, patients should:

- try to remain upright for the rest of the day (patients can be taught to complete the CRM at home),
- be reassessed in 1 month or less after the initial treatment to confirm symptom resolution, and
- be referred to a vestibular specialist for further assessment if initial treatment is unsuccessful.

CANALITH REPOSITIONING MANEUVER FOR POSTERIOR CANAL BENIGN PAROXYSMAL POSITIONAL VERTIGO (EPLEY MANEUVER)

Treatment for posterior canal BPPV canalithiasis (ie, otoconia is free-floating) is via the CRM.[3,4] The affected ear is identified as the side that causes dizziness with rolling and turning and results in a positive Dix-Hallpike test. Perform the following steps for right-sided posterior semicircular canal BPPV (Figure 2-7):

- Place the patient in a long sitting position with his or her head turned 45 degrees toward the affected (eg, right) ear (see Figure 2-7a).
- Quickly move the patient to the supine supported position, with the patient's head in 45 degrees right rotation and 20 degrees extension over the edge of the bed or table. Maintain this position until the dizziness stops, plus an additional 20 seconds (see Figure 2-7b).
- Continue to support the patient's head and turn it 45 degrees in the opposite (eg, left) rotation, maintaining 20 degrees of extension over the edge of the mat or table. Hold this position until the dizziness stops, plus an additional 20 seconds (see Figure 2-7c).

- Continue to support the patient's head and turn it so the 45 degrees rotation (eg, left) is maintained and the client is rolled onto the same-side shoulder (eg, left). The head should be turned 45 degrees down toward the floor. Hold this position until the dizziness stops, plus an additional 20 seconds (see Figure 2-7d).
- Slowly bring the patient to the upright sitting position, head still rotated 45 degrees to the opposite side (eg, left; see Figure 2-7e).

Patients should be informed that:

- they should keep their eyes open during the treatment;
- they may experience vertigo during the treatment;
- they must remain in the treatment positions until the vertigo has stopped;
- if they absolutely cannot remain in the treatment position, the therapist will help them slowly return to a sitting position; and
- the therapist will not let them fall.

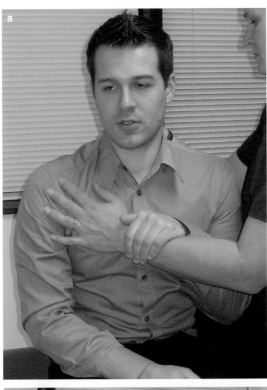

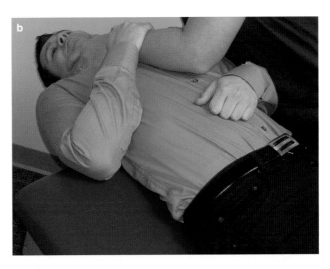

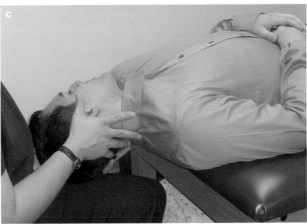

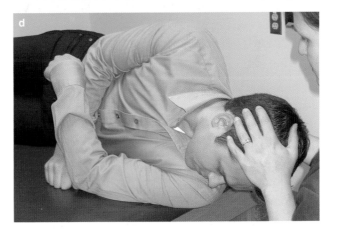

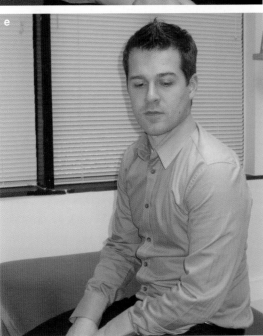

Figure 2-7. Administration of the canalith repositioning maneuver for posterior canal benign paroxysmal positional vertigo. **(a)** Place the patient in a long sitting position with his or her head turned 45 degrees toward the affected (eg, right) ear. **(b)** Quickly move the patient to the supine supported position, with the patient's head in 45 degrees right rotation and 20 degrees extension over the edge of the bed or table. Maintain this position until the dizziness stops, plus an additional 20 seconds. **(c)** Continue to support the patient's head and turn it 45 degrees in the opposite (eg, left) rotation, maintaining 20 degrees of extension over the edge of the mat or table. Hold this position until the dizziness stops, plus an additional 20 seconds. **(d)** Continue to support the patient's head and turn it so the 45 degrees rotation (eg, left) is maintained and the client is rolled onto the same-side shoulder (eg, left). The head should be turned 45 degrees down toward the floor. Hold this position until the dizziness stops, plus an additional 20 seconds. **(e)** Slowly bring the patient to the upright sitting position, head still rotated 45 degrees to the opposite side (eg, left).

Selected References

Bhattacharyya N, Baugh RF, Orvidas L, et al. Clinical practice guideline: benign paroxysmal positional vertigo. *Otolaryngol Head Neck Surg.* 2008;139:S47–S81.

Hilton MP, Pinder DK. The Epley (canalith repositioning) manoeuvre for benign paroxysmal positional vertigo. *Cochrane Database Syst Rev.* 2004;2:CD003162.

CANALITH REPOSITIONING MANEUVER FOR HORIZONTAL (LATERAL) CANAL BENIGN PAROXYSMAL POSITIONAL VERTIGO (BARBECUE ROLL MANEUVER)

The barbecue roll maneuver is the most commonly used maneuver for horizontal (lateral) canalithiasis (ie, otoconia is free-floating).[3,4] The affected ear is identified as the side that causes more nystagmus and vertigo during the roll test (Figure 2-8). Perform the following steps:

- Lie supine on the examination table or bed with the affected ear down (see Figure 2-8a).
- Slowly roll your head away from the affected ear to the face-up position; maintain this position until dizziness stops plus an additional 20 seconds (see Figure 2-8b).
- Continue to roll the head in the same direction until the affected ear is pointed up; maintain this position until dizziness stops plus an additional 20 seconds (see Figure 2-8c).
- Roll your head and body in the same direction until your face is down and remain in this position until dizziness stops plus an additional 20 seconds. You may support your forehead with your hands. If the treatment has been effective, your vertigo should be resolved (see Figure 2-8d).
- Continue to roll in the same direction (completing a 360 degrees roll) until returning to the supine position with your head turned to the initial position (see Figure 2-8e).

Selected References

Bhattacharyya N, Baugh RF, Orvidas L, et al. Clinical practice guideline: benign paroxysmal positional vertigo. *Otolaryngol Head Neck Surg.* 2008;139:S47–S81.

Hilton MP, Pinder DK. The Epley (canalith repositioning) manoeuvre for benign paroxysmal positional vertigo. *Cochrane Database Syst Rev.* 2004;2:CD003162.

REHABILITATION FOR UNILATERAL VESTIBULAR HYPOFUNCTION OR LOSS

Background

Unilateral peripheral vestibular dysfunction can occur postoperatively or as a result of disease or trauma. Clients with UVH/L frequently report problems with visual acuity (blurring) during head movement (oscillopsia) and reduced postural stability[65] that affects ambulation[66] and the ability to participate in activities of daily living. Visual acuity complaints can be particularly devastating for a service member in a deployed setting. Interventions follow a problem-based approach and are driven by the specific impairments identified during the physical therapy examination as well as by the client's goals. Intervention for this disorder includes exercises designed to facilitate central nervous system compensation by adaptation, substitution, or habituation.[3,67]

Strength of Recommendation: Practice Standard

In a Cochrane review, Hillier and Holohan[57] found moderate to strong evidence that vestibular rehabilitation is a safe, effective management for unilateral peripheral vestibular dysfunction.

Intervention

Acute: Individuals with acute UVH/L typically have prolonged continuous vertigo even at rest, severe nausea and vomiting, and spontaneous nystagmus (beating away from the affected [lesioned] side) seen in room light during the first several days to a week following the onset or causative incident.[21] A person may have bilateral vestibular hypofunction with one side more involved than the other and will exhibit similar symptoms. Treatment considerations:

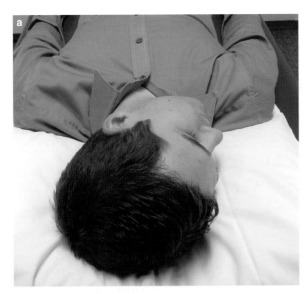

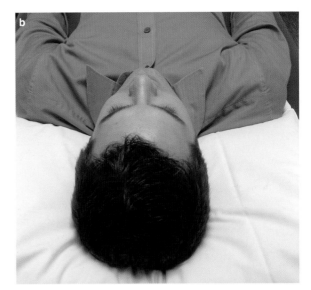

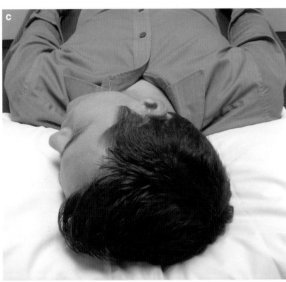

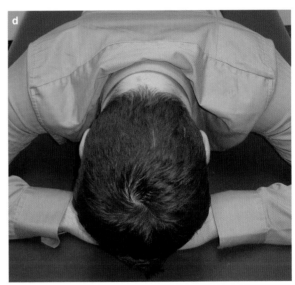

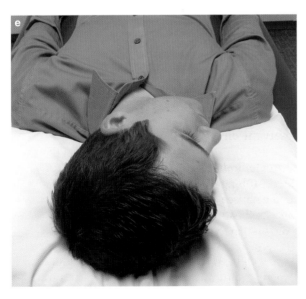

Figure 2-8. Administration of the canalith repositioning maneuver for horizontal canal benign paroxysmal positional vertigo. **(a)** Lie supine on the examination table or bed with the affected ear down. **(b)** Slowly roll your head away from the affected ear to the face-up position; maintain this position until dizziness stops plus an additional 20 seconds. **(c)** Continue to roll the head in the same direction until the affected ear is pointed up; maintain this position until dizziness stops plus an additional 20 seconds. **(d)** Roll your head and body in the same direction until your face is down and remain in this position until dizziness stops plus an additional 20 seconds. You may support your forehead with your hands. If the treatment has been effective, your vertigo should be resolved. **(e)** Continue to roll in the same direction (completing a 360 degrees roll) until returning to the supine position with your head turned to the initial position.

EXHIBIT 2-4

GAZE STABILITY: X1 VIEWING EXERCISES

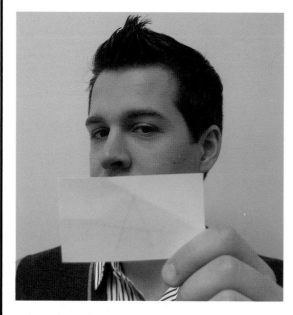 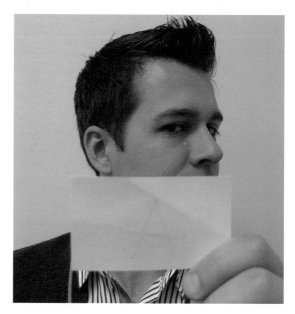

- Start out looking straight ahead at a stationary target (eg, a letter, number, or word written on an index card) held in your hand or placed on a wall 12 to 18 inches from your face.
- Move your head back and forth (45° in either direction) while trying to keep the target in focus.
- Slowly increase the speed of your head turns as you are able, always keeping the target in focus. Your symptoms will likely return with this exercise.
- Practice for up to 60 seconds, then rest.
- Complete these X-1 exercises in a horizontal direction, 4 to 5 times per day in each direction.
- Advance to the following background: _____.

- Antiemetics and vestibular suppressants may be useful acutely but should be withdrawn as soon as possible (preferably after the first several days).
- Prolonged use of vestibular suppressants may impede the process of central vestibular compensation.[68]
- Early resumption of normal activity should be encouraged to promote compensation.
- Patient education regarding diagnosis, prognosis, and the process and rationale for vestibular rehabilitation is important throughout treatment.
- There is some evidence that a supervised vestibular rehabilitation program in combination with vestibular suppressants may be more beneficial than vestibular suppressants alone in addressing vestibular ataxia.[69,70]

Chronic: For individuals with chronic UVH/L, interventions address chronic dizziness and disequilibrium, the dynamic aspects of gaze stability, and postural control.[3,21] Goals of treatment include:

- improvement in the ability to see clearly during head movements,
- improvement in balance and ambulation during functional tasks,
- decreased sensitivity to head movements,
- improvement in general conditioning and fitness, and
- a return to normal occupational and social roles and participation.[3,21,71]

Treatment Considerations:

- continued rapid tapering and discontinuation of vestibular suppressant medication[72,73];

EXHIBIT 2-5

GAZE STABILITY: X1 VIEWING EXERCISES PERFORMED IN A VERTICAL ORIENTATION

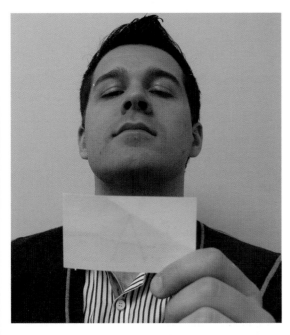 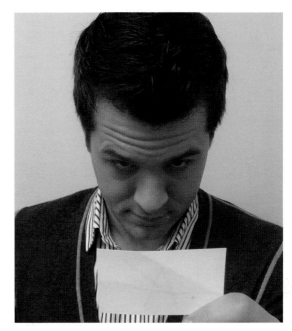

- Start out looking straight ahead at stationary target (eg, a letter, number, or word written on an index card) held in your hand or placed on a wall 12 to 18 inches from your face.
- Move your head up and down (45 degrees in either direction) while trying to keep the target in focus.
- Slowly increase the speed of your head movement upward and downward as you are able, keeping the target in focus. Your symptoms will likely return with this exercise.
- Practice for up to 60 seconds, then rest.
- Complete the exercise in a vertical direction, 4 to 5 times per day in each direction.
- Advance to the following background: _____.

- continued patient education regarding diagnosis, prognosis, and the process and rationale for vestibular rehabilitation throughout the treatment episode; and
- initiation of vestibular exercises.[3,57,74,75]

Oscillopsia is addressed through visual-vestibular exercises such as the VOR X1, VOR X2, imaginary targets, and gaze shifting, eye-head movement exercises (see Exhibits 2-4–2-8).[18,71,74,75]

These exercises are performed with a visual target (beginning large, with progression to smaller targets), with the head moving either horizontally or vertically. Exercises need to include near and far targets, with particular focus on near targets.[76] The three main goals of gaze exercises are to "1) improve visual acuity during head movements, 2) improve visual-vestibular interactions during head movements, and 3) decrease the individual's sensitivity to head movements."[77(p501)]

Viewing exercises should advance through more difficult postures; for example, progressing from sitting, to standing, to standing on foam or other compliant surfaces, to standing on a trampoline, to bouncing on trampoline, and so on. Gait tasks can be advanced using level surfaces, inclines, varying speeds, jogging and treadmill activities.

Viewing exercises should also advance through progressively busier environments. Patients should exercise in a quiet area initially, then progress to busier and louder environments. Distracting backgrounds, including horizontal lines and checkerboard patterns,[78] can be used to change visual target complexity.

Viewing exercises should advance in number of repetitions, time, frequency, and speed. Work

EXHIBIT 2-6

GAZE STABILITY EXERCISES: X2 VIEWING EXERCISES

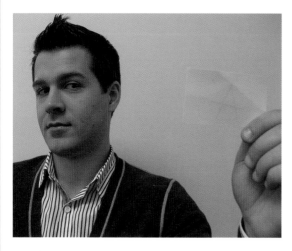 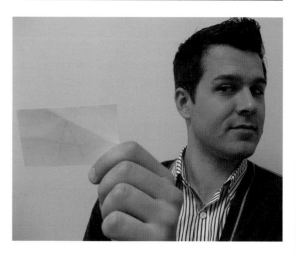

In this activity you will view a target that moves in the opposite direction from your head. This is a difficult activity to coordinate and will require practice.

- Start out by turning your head 45 degrees to the right and positioning the target 45 degrees from midline to the left.
- View the target. The target could be a letter, number, or word on an index card and should be held in your hand about 12 to 18 inches from your face.
- Then move your head to the left and the card to the right, while trying to keep the target in focus.
- Once your head is 45 degrees to the left and the target is 45 degrees to the right, reverse the directions and return to the original position.
- Repeat, slowly increasing the speed of your head turns with the goal of keeping the target in focus. It is expected that you will get a return of your symptoms with this exercise.
- Practice for 60 seconds, then rest.
- Complete in horizontal and vertical directions.
- Try to do these X2 exercises 4 to 5 times per day in each direction.
- Advance to the following background:_____

EXHIBIT 2-7

GAZE STABILITY: HEAD-EYE MOVEMENT BETWEEN TWO TARGETS*

- Place two targets in front of you about an arm's length away and slightly wider than shoulder width apart. The first target should be positioned so that when you look at one target, you can see the other target in your peripheral vision without difficulty.
- Begin with your head and eyes turned to directly face the target on the right.
- Shift your eye gaze to the target on the left and immediately follow your gaze with a head turn toward the target on the left. Repeat going toward the right (eye gaze followed by a head turn), and continue back and forth between the targets.
- Vary the speed of your head movement, making sure to keep the target in focus. Attempt to perform this gaze exercise as quickly as possible.
- Practice for 60 seconds and increase the time, as tolerated, up to 5 minutes.
- This exercise can also be performed with targets placed vertically (one target above the other).

*These exercises are most often used for individuals with bilateral vestibular hypofunction. They may be used at the therapist's discretion for those with unilateral vestibular hypofunction or loss.

EXHIBIT 2-8

GAZE STABILITY: HEAD-EYE MOVEMENT BETWEEN TWO TARGETS (GAZE SHIFTING)[*]

- Place two targets in front of you about an arm's length away and slightly wider than shoulder width apart. The first target should be positioned so that when you look at one target, you can see the other target in your peripheral vision without difficulty.
- Begin with your head and eyes turned to directly face the target on the right.
- Shift your eye gaze to the target on the left and immediately follow your gaze with a head turn toward the target on the left. Repeat going toward the right (eye gaze followed by a head turn), and continue back and forth between the targets.
- Vary the speed of your head movement, making sure to keep the target in focus. Attempt to perform this gaze exercise as quickly as possible.
- Practice for 60 seconds and increase the time, as tolerated, up to 5 minutes.
- This exercise can also be performed with targets placed vertically (one target above the other).

---

*These exercises are most often used for individuals with bilateral vestibular hypofunction. They may be used at the therapist's discretion for those with unilateral vestibular hypofunction or loss.

---

toward completing an exercise up to 1 minute at a time, 4 to 5 times daily.[3,74] Initially, a metronome may be used to promote increased head speed. As soon as tolerated, unpredictable head movements should be introduced.[79] Demonstrable improvement may take up to 6 weeks[74,80]; recovery optimization may take up to 1 year.[71]

Points to Remember

- It is important that patients do the exercises and movements quickly enough and through sufficient range of motion to elicit at least mild symptoms.[81] Vestibular rehabilitation should simulate rotational head perturbations during functional activities such as ambulation (0.5–5.0 Hz).[82]
- The patient should begin with a lower frequency and duration of exercise and progress as tolerated, particularly if he or she has increased motion sensitivity.
- It may take at least 4 weeks before symptoms begin to decrease; a conditioning program should be introduced as soon as tolerated to counteract physical deconditioning from inactivity (see also Chapter 10: Fitness Assessment and Intervention).
- Practitioners should also consider referring patients to occupational therapy for a driving assessment. Patients should not drive if they cannot see clearly during head movements or if head movements result in significant dizziness or disorientation.
- A home-based physical therapy program is typically followed by periodic clinical follow-up (eg, weekly to monthly).
- Referral to a therapist specializing in vestibular rehabilitation may be indicated if the patient does not progress.

TREATMENT OF MOTION SENSITIVITY AND EXERCISE-INDUCED DIZZINESS

Sensitivity to motion (dizziness and nausea), especially head motion, is a common finding in those with vestibular disorders as well as those with dizziness complaints following TBI. Patients may also have visual motion sensitivity with increasing symptoms in busy and crowded environments.[77]

The provoking positions found on the MSQ Test (see Motion Sensitivity Quotient Test Purpose/Description above) may be used to design a treatment program based on the concept of habituation by repeated exposure to the symptom-provoking posi-

tions and movements. Three or four test movements are selected from the Motion Sensitivity Test, typically ones that caused a mild to moderate increase in symptoms (not a severe increase). The patient should then perform those motions 2 to 3 times, twice daily. After each performance of the exercise, the patient should wait for the symptoms to resolve or return to baseline. This program is advanced by increasing movement speed or altering the movement activity. Improvements may take 6 to 8 weeks. If no progress is made within 2 months, patients may need to alter their lifestyle or vocation.[3] The

TABLE 2-3

POSTURAL CONTROL ACTIVITIES: GENERAL SUGGESTIONS

Static Activities	Wide base of support standing Narrowed base of support standing Modified tandem stance Tandem stance Single-leg stance	Advance to compliant surfaces Advance by adding perturbations and distractions

Dynamic Activities	Weight shifts in:
	  - wide base of support standing
	  - narrowed base of support standing
	  - modified tandem stance
	  - tandem stance
	  - single-leg stance
		Advance to compliant surfaces, unstable surfaces
		Advance by adding head movements
		Advance by adding upper extremity activities
		  - reaching
		  - throwing/catching a ball, throw outside of midline
		Advance by adding lower extremity activities
		  - marching
		  - kicking ball

Gait Activities	Braiding Sidestepping Tandem ambulation Heel walking Toe walking Lunging Running Skipping	Advance by changing surfaces, inclines Advance by adding head movement Advance by adding dual task activity (motor or cognitive)*

*See Chapter 8: Dual Task Assessment and Intervention.

program should be updated periodically based on patient response.

Another example of a generalized program to address motion sensitivity problems is found in Shepard et al.[77(p504)] In addition to activities similar to those based on findings from the MSQ Test, the therapist can choose from functional activities that are symptom provoking for an individual patient.

Exertional, or exercise-induced, dizziness results in nausea, disequilibrium, and feeling "dizzy" or unsteady during or immediately following exercise. These symptoms appear to be a form of motion intolerance, as they are associated with exercise that involves head motion (sit-ups, push-ups, running, swimming), but not with exercise that is more stable (eg, riding a stationary bike). Exercise-induced dizziness has been described in a military population as having a disabling effect because physical training and active duty often require individuals to be very physically active.[8] These symptoms may be missed if more basic motion sensitivity testing is conducted that does not require repetitive and rapid head movement or physical exertion.

Interventions may include exercises using vestibular rehabilitation principles that include an exertional component to provoke vestibular symptoms by requiring maximal tolerable effort. Some have advocated for exercise that includes diagonal and spiral movement patterns, use of gravity, acceleration, resistance, and an unstable base of support to simulate operational conditions. One particular program included progressive conditioning that began with a timed walk that progressed to a 3-mile run.[8] Improvements in clinical measures of balance and self-report of dizziness handicap were noted for all patients, with an average of 4.6 weeks to return to active duty.[7] See Chapter 10, Fitness Assessment and Intervention, for further evidence supporting a progressive fitness program in cases where complaints linger beyond 2 or 3 weeks after c/mTBI.

Postural Stability Exercise Progression

A postural stability exercise program should also be initiated and advanced.[21,83] A typical and generalized postural stability exercise program can be found in *Brain Injury Medicine Principles and Practice*, by Zasler, Katz, Zafonte[84] (see Table 28-3 in that text); exercises are assigned at the therapist's discretion (Table 2-3). If cervical range-of-motion limitations are identified, range of motion, stretching, or manual therapy may be indicated. Fitness and conditioning programs should be introduced as soon as tolerated, including a walking program, or stationary cycling program as strategies to combat fatigue secondary to deconditioning.

Postural control is addressed throughout the vestibular rehabilitation program by advancing the patient through a paradigm such as the following:

- Advance viewing exercises (X1, X2, imaginary targets, etc.) through more difficult postures.
  - Progress from sitting to standing, to standing on foam or other compliant surfaces, standing on trampoline, bouncing on trampoline, etc.
  - Progress gait tasks on level surfaces; use varying speeds, inclines, treadmill, jogging.
- Advance viewing exercises through progressively busier environments.
  - Exercise in a quiet area initially; progress to busier and louder environments.
  - Use distracting backgrounds, including horizontal lines or checkerboard patterns.[78]
- Advance the number of repetitions, time, frequency, and speed of viewing exercises.

The patient can still have postural stability impairments after improvement with gaze stability. Refer to the section of this toolkit on higher-level balance and functional abilities (Chapter 3: Balance and Functional Abilities Assessment and Intervention) for additional interventions.

FITNESS AND CONDITIONING PROGRAM FOR BALANCE RETRAINING FOLLOWING VESTIBULAR DYSFUNCTION

A fitness and conditioning program should be introduced as soon as tolerated. This program should include balance retraining and a walking or stationary cycling program to combat fatigue secondary to deconditioning. All healthy adults aged 18 to 65 years need moderate-intensity aerobic physical activity for a minimum of 30 minutes 5 days a week and activities to increase muscular strength and endurance for a minimum of 2 days each week.[85] Exercise may improve mood and aspects of health status in individuals with TBI.[86] The following are some key points to remember when designing an exercise program:

- Start slowly and increase the duration and intensity of exercises over time.
- Monitor heart rate or rate of perceived exertion.
- Vary the exercise program to keep from becoming bored.
- Use a calendar or notebook to keep track of exercise days and times.
- When cleared by the referring physician, progress from walking or stationary cycling to other aerobic exercises, such as running and swimming.[86]
- Include avocational activities that are fun and challenge balance and vision simultaneously, such as golf, bowling, tennis, racquetball, ping-pong, cycling, cross-country skiing, and hiking.
- Alternative balance activities can include yoga, tai chi, and other non-contact martial arts.
- Incorporate service-specific physical fitness requirements for running, push-ups, and sit-ups (see Chapter 10: Fitness Assessment and Intervention, for service-specific websites).

REFERENCES

1. Radomski MV, Weightman MM, Davidson L, Rodgers M, Bolgla R. *Clinical Practice Guidance: Occupational Therapy and Physical Therapy for Mild Traumatic Brain injury.* Falls Church, VA: Army Office of the Surgeon General; 2010.

2. Scherer MR, Schubert MC. Traumatic brain injury and vestibular pathology as a comorbidity after blast exposure. *Phys Ther.* Sep 2009;89(9):980–992.

3. Herdman SJ. *Vestibular Rehabilitation.* Vol 3. Philadelphia, PA: FA Davis Company; 2007.

4. Bhattacharyya N, Baugh RF, Orvidas L, et al. Clinical practice guideline: benign paroxysmal positional vertigo. *Otolaryngol Head Neck Surg.* 2008;139:S47–S81.

5. Hoffer ME, Balaban C, Gottshall KR, Balough BJ, Maddox MR, Penta JR. Blast exposure: vestibular consequences and associated characteristics. *Otol Neurotol.* Feb 2010;31(2):232–236.

6. Hoffer ME, Gottshall KR, Moore R, Balough BJ, Wester D. Characterizing and treating dizziness after mild head trauma. *Otol Neurotol.* 2004;25(2):135–138.

7. Gottshall KR, Hoffer ME. Tracking recovery of vestibular function in individuals with blast-induced head trauma using vestibular-visual-cognitive interaction tests. *J Neurol Phys Ther.* Jun 2010;34(2):94–97.

8. Gottshall KR, Moore RJ, Hoffer ME, et al. Exercise induced motion intolerance: role in operational environments. Paper presented at: Spatial Disorientation in Military Vehicles: Causes, Consequences and Cures; April 15–17, 2002; La Coruña, Spain.

9. Dix R, Hallpike CS. The pathology, symptomatology and diagnosis of certain common disorders of the vestibular system. *Ann Otol Rhinol Laryngol.* 1952;6:987–1016.

10. Nunez RA, Cass SP, Furman JM. Short- and long-term outcomes of canalith repositioning for benign paroxysmal positional vertigo. *Otolaryngol Head Neck Surg.* May 2000;122(5):647–652.

11. Baloh RW, Honrubia V, Jacobson K. Benign positional vertigo: clinical and oculographic features in 240 cases. *Neurology.* Mar 1987;37(3):371–378.

12. Hoffman RM, Einstadter D, Kroenke K. Evaluating dizziness. *Am J Med.* Nov 1999;107(5):468–478.

13. Lopez-Escamez JA, Lopez-Nevot A, Gamiz MJ, et al. [Diagnosis of common causes of vertigo using a structured clinical history]. *Acta Otorrinolaringol Esp.* Jan-Feb 2000;51(1):25–30.

14. Halker RB, Barrs DM, Wellik KE, Wingerchuk DM, Demaerschalk BM. Establishing a diagnosis of benign paroxysmal positional vertigo through the Dix-Hallpike and side-lying maneuvers: a critically appraised topic. *Neurologist.* May 2008;14(3):201–204.

15. Fife TD. Recognition and management of horizontal canal benign positional vertigo. *Am J Otol.* May 1998;19(3):345–351.

16. Fife TD, Tusa RJ, Furman JM, et al. Assessment: vestibular testing techniques in adults and children: report of the Therapeutics and Technology Assessment Subcommittee of the American Academy of Neurology. *Neurology.* Nov 28, 2000;55(10):1431–1441.

17. Barber HO. Vestibular neurophysiology. *Otolaryngol Head Neck Surg.* Feb 1984;92(1):55–58.

18. Herdman SJ, Hall CD, Schubert MC, Das VE, Tusa RJ. Recovery of dynamic visual acuity in bilateral vestibular hypofunction. *Arch Otolaryngol Head Neck Surg.* Apr 2007;133(4):383–389.

19. Schubert MC, Minor LB. Vestibulo-ocular physiology underlying vestibular hypofunction. *Phys Ther.* Apr 2004;84(4):373–385.

20. Basford JR, Chou LS, Kaufman KR, et al. An assessment of gait and balance deficits after traumatic brain injury. *Arch Phys Med Rehabil.* Mar 2003;84(3):343–349.

21. Shepard NT, Telian SA. *Practical Management of the Balance Disorder Patient.* New York, NY: Thomson Delmar Learning; 1996.

22. Burgio DL, Blakley RW, Myers SF. The high-frequency oscillopsia test. *J Vestib Res.* 1992;2:221–226.

23. Halmagyi GM, Curthoys IS. A clinical sign of canal paresis. *Arch Neurol.* Jul 1988;45(7):737–739.

24. Schubert MC, Tusa RJ, Grine LE, Herdman SJ. Optimizing the sensitivity of the head thrust test for identifying vestibular hypofunction. *Phys Ther.* Feb 2004;84(2):151–158.

25. Beynon GJ, Jani P, Baguley DM. A clinical evaluation of head impulse testing. *Clin Otolaryngol Allied Sci.* Apr 1998;23(2):117–122.

26. Perez N, Rama-Lopez J. Head-impulse and caloric tests in patients with dizziness. *Otol Neurotol.* Nov 2003;24(6):913–917.

27. Harvey SA, Wood DJ, Feroah TR. Relationship of the head impulse test and head-shake nystagmus in reference to caloric testing. *Am J Otol.* Mar 1997;18(2):207–213.

28. Bryant RA, Harvey AG. Acute stress disorder: a critical review of diagnostic issue. *Clinical Psychol Rev.* 1997;17:757–773.

29. Hall CD, Schubert MC, Herdman SJ. Prediction of fall risk reduction as measured by dynamic gait index in individuals with unilateral vestibular hypofunction. *Otol Neurotol.* Sep 2004;25(5):746–751.

30. Schubert MC, Das V, Tusa RJ, Herdman SJ. Cervico-ocular reflex in normal subjects and patients with unilateral vestibular hypofunction. *Otol Neurotol.* Jan 2004;25(1):65–71.

31. Goebel JA, Garcia P. Prevalence of post-headshake nystagmus in patients with caloric deficits and vertigo. *Otolaryngol Head Neck Surg.* Feb 1992;106(2):121–127.

32. Iwasaki S, Ito K, Abbey K, Murofushi T. Prediction of canal paresis using head-shaking nystagmus test. *Acta Otolaryngol.* Sep 2004;124(7):803–806.

33. Asawavichianginda S, Fujimoto M, Mai M, Rutka J. Prevalence of head-shaking nystagmus in patients according to their diagnostic classification in a dizziness unit. *J Otolaryngol.* Feb 1997;26(1):20–25.

34. Jacobson GP, Newman CW, Safadi I. Sensitivity and specificity of the head-shaking test for detecting vestibular system abnormalities. *Ann Otol Rhinol Laryngol.* Jul 1990;99(7 Pt 1):539–542.

35. Angeli SI, Velandia S, Snapp H. Head-shaking nystagmus predicts greater disability in unilateral peripheral vestibulopathy. *Am J Otolaryngol.* Nov 2011;32(6):522–527.

36. Jacobson GP, Newman CW. The development of the Dizziness Handicap Inventory. *Arch Otolaryngol Head Neck Surg.* Apr 1990;116(4):424–427.

37. Goebel JA. The ten-minute examination of the dizzy patient. *Semin Neurol.* Dec 2001;21(4):391–398.

38. University of Missouri School of Health Professions, Department of Physical Therapy. Geriatric Examination Toolkit. http://web.missouri.edu/~proste/tool/vest/Dizziness-Handicap-Inventory.pdf. Accessed April 8, 2013.

39. Southampton Hospital. Dizziness Handicap Inventory. http://www.southamptonhospital.org/Resources/10355/FileRepository/Forms/Dizziness%20Hanicap%20Inventory%20-%20English.pdf. Accessed April 8, 2013.

40. Enloe LJ, Shields RK. Evaluation of health-related quality of life in individuals with vestibular disease using disease-specific and general outcome measures. *Phys Ther.* Sep 1997;77(9):890–903.

41. Cowand JL, Wrisley DM, Walker M, Strasnick B, Jacobson JT. Efficacy of vestibular rehabilitation. *Otolaryngol Head Neck Surg.* Jan 1998;118(1):49–54.

42. Gill-Body KM, Beninato M, Krebs DE. Relationship among balance impairments, functional performance, and disability in people with peripheral vestibular hypofunction. *Phys Ther.* Aug 2000;80(8):748–758.

43. Gottshall KR, Drake A, Gray N, McDonald E, Hoffer ME. Objective vestibular tests as outcome measures in head injury patients. *Laryngoscope.* 2003;113(10):1746–1750.

44. Gottshall KR, Gray NL, Drake AI, Tejidor R, Hoffer ME, McDonald EC. To investigate the influence of acute vestibular impairment following mild traumatic brain injury on subsequent ability to remain on activity duty 12 months later. *Mil Med.* Aug 2007;172(8):852–857.

45. Jacobson GP, Newman CW, Hunter L, Balzer GK. Balance function test correlates of the Dizziness Handicap Inventory. *J Am Acad Audiol.* Oct 1991;2(4):253–260.

46. Fielder H, Denholm SW, Lyons RA, Fielder CP. Measurement of health status in patients with vertigo. *Clin Otolaryngol Allied Sci.* Apr 1996;21(2):124–126.

47. Duracinsky M, Mosnier I, Bouccara D, Sterkers O, Chassany O. Literature review of questionnaires assessing vertigo and dizziness, and their impact on patients' quality of life. *Value Health.* Jul–Aug 2007;10(4):273–284.

48. Akin FW, Davenport MJ. Validity and reliability of the Motion Sensitivity Test. *J Rehab Res Dev.* Sep–Oct 2003;40(5):415–421.

49. Smith-Wheelock M, Shepard NT, Telian SA. Physical therapy program for vestibular rehabilitation. *Am J Otol.* May 1991;12(3):218–225.

50. Wood JM, Anstey KJ, Kerr GK, Lacherez PF, Lord S. A multidomain approach for predicting older driver safety under in-traffic road conditions. *J Am Geriatr Soc.* Jun 2008;56(6):986–993.

51. Cohen HS, Kimball KT. Development of the vestibular disorders activities of daily living scale. *Arch Otolaryngol Head Neck Surg.* Jul 2000;126(7):881–887.

52. Cohen HS, Kimball KT. Increased independence and decreased vertigo after vestibular rehabilitation. *Otolaryngol Head Neck Surg.* Jan 2003;128(1):60–70.

53. Shah PS, Kale JS. A study of the effects of a vestibular rehabilitation program on patients with peripheral vestibular dysfunctions. *Indian J Occup Ther.* 2004;36(1):11–16.

54. Herdman SJ, Tusa RJ, Zee DS, Proctor LR, Mattox DE. Single treatment approaches to benign paroxysmal positional vertigo. *Arch Otolaryngol Head Neck Surg.* 1993;119(4):450–454.

55. Wolf JS, Boyev KP, Manokey BJ, Mattox DE. Success of the modified Epley maneuver in treating benign paroxysmal positional vertigo. *Laryngoscope.* Jun 1999;109(6):900–903.

56. Gordon CR, Levite R, Joffe V, Gadoth N. Is posttraumatic benign paroxysmal positional vertigo different from the idiopathic form? *Arch Neurol.* 2004;61(10):1590–1593.

57. Hiller SL, Holohan V. Vestibular rehabilitation for unilateral peripheral vestibular dysfunction. *Cochrane Database Syst Rev.* 2007(4):CD005397.

58. Cass SP, Furman JM, Ankerstjerne K, Balaban C, Yetiser S, Aydogan B. Migraine-related vestibulopathy. *Ann Otol Rhinol Laryngol.* 1997;106(3):182–189.

59. Johnson GD. Medical management of migraine-related dizziness and vertigo. *Laryngoscope.* 1998;108(Supplement 85):1–28.

60. Gottshall KR, Moore RJ, Hoffer ME. Vestibular rehabilitation for migraine-associated dizziness. *Intl Tinnitus J.* 2005;11(1):81–84.

61. Whitney SL, Wrisley DM, Brown KE, Furman JM. Physical therapy for migraine-related vestibulopathy and vestibular dysfunction with history of migraine. *Laryngoscope.* 2000;110(9):1528–1534.

62. Li JC, Li CJ, Epley J, Weinberg L. Cost-effective management of benign positional vertigo using canalith repositioning. *Otolaryngol Head Neck Surg.* Mar 2000;122(3):334–339.

63. Von Brevern M, Radtke A, Lezius F. Epidemiology of benign paroxysmal positional vertigo: a population-based study in Olmsted County, Minnesota. *Mayo Clin Proc.* 1991;66:596–601.

64. Hilton MP, Pinder DK. The Epley (canalith repositioning) manoeuvre for benign paroxysmal positional vertigo. *Cochrane Database Syst Rev.* 2004;2:CD003162.

65. Horak FB. Postural compensation for vestibular loss. *Ann N Y Acad Sci.* May 2009;1164:76–81.

66. Whitney SL, Marchetti GF, Pritcher M, Furman JM. Gaze stabilization and gait performance in vestibular dysfunction. *Gait Posture.* Feb 2009;29(2):194–198.

67. Kasai T, Zee DS. Eye-head coordination in labyrinthine-defective human beings. *Brain Res.* 1978;144(1):123–141.

68. Zuccaro TA. Pharmacological management of vertigo. *J Neurol Phys Ther.* 2003;27(3):118–121.

69. Fujino A, Tokumasu K, Okamoto M, et al. Vestibular training for acute unilateral vestibular disturbances: its efficacy in comparison with antivertigo drug. *Acta Otolaryngol Suppl.* 1996;524:21–26.

70. Teggi R, Caldirola D, Fabiano B, Recanati P, Bussi M. Rehabilitation after acute vestibular disorders. *J Laryngol Otol.* Apr 2009;123(4):397–402.

71. Clendaniel RA, Tucci DL. Vestibular rehabilitation strategies in Meniere's disease. *Otolaryngol Clin North Am.* Dec 1997;30(6):1145–1158.

72. Robertson D, Ireland D. Evaluation and treatment of uncompensated unilateral vestibular disease. *Otolaryngol Clin North Am.* Oct 1997;30(5):745–757.

73. Shepard NT, Telian SA, Smith-Wheelock M. Habituation and balance training therapy: a retrospective review. *Neurol Clin.* 1990;8:469–475.

74. Herdman SJ, Schubert MC, Das VE, Tusa RJ. Recovery of dynamic visual acuity in unilateral vestibular hypofunction. *Arch Otolaryngol Head Neck Surg.* 2003;129(8):819–824.

75. Szturm T, Ireland DJ, Lessing-Turner M. Comparison of different exercise programs in the rehabilitation of patients with chronic peripheral vestibular dysfunction. *J Vestib Res.* Nov–Dec 1994;4(6):461–479.

76. Peters BT, Bloomberg JJ. Dynamic visual acuity using "far" and "near" targets. *Acta Otolaryngol.* Apr 2005;125(4):353–357.

77. Shepard NT, Clendaniel RA, Ruckenstein M. Balance and Dizziness. In: Zasler ND, Katz DI, Zafonte R, eds. *Brain Injury Medicine Principles and Practice.* New York, NY: Demos; 2007: 491–510.

78. Horning E, Gorman S. Vestibular rehabilitation decreases fall risk and improves gaze stability for an older individual with unilateral vestibular hypofunction. *J Geriatr Phys Ther.* 2007;30(3):121–127.

79. Herdman SJ, Schubert MC, Tusa RJ. Role of central preprogramming in dynamic visual acuity with vestibular loss. *Arch Otolaryngol Head Neck Surg.* Oct 2001;127(10):1205–1210.

80. Whitney SL, Rossi MM. Efficacy of vestibular rehabilitation. *Otolaryngol Clin North Am.* Jun 2000;33(3):659–672.

81. Borello-France DF, Gallagher JD, Redfern M, Furman JM, Carvell GE. Voluntary movement strategies of individuals with unilateral peripheral vestibular hypofunction. *J Vestib Res.* 1999;9(4):265–275.

82. Grossman GE, Leigh RJ. Instability of gaze during locomotion in patients with deficient vestibular function. *Ann Neurol.* May 1990;27(5):528–532.

83. Horak FB, Jones-Rycewicz C, Black FO, Shumway-Cook A. Effects of vestibular rehabilitation on dizziness and imbalance. *Otolaryngol Head Neck Surg.* Feb 1992;106(2):175–180.

84. Zasler ND, Katz DI, Zafonte RD. *Brain Injury Medicine Principles and Practice.* Vol 1. New York, NY: Demos Medical Publishing; 2007.

85. Haskell WL, Lee IM, Pate RR, et al. Physical activity and public health: updated recommendations for adults from the American College of Sports Medicine and the American Heart Association. *Med Sci Sports Exer.* 2007;39(8):1423–1434.

86. Gordon WA, Sliwinski M, Echo J, McLoughlin M, Sheerer MS, Meili TE. The benefits of exercise in individuals with traumatic brain injury: a retrospective study. *J Head Trauma Rehabil.* 1998;13(4):58–67.

Chapter 3

BALANCE AND FUNCTIONAL ABILITIES ASSESSMENT AND INTERVENTION

MARGARET M. WEIGHTMAN, PhD, PT*

*Clinical Scientist/Physical Therapist, Courage Kenny Research Center, 800 East 28th Street, Mail Stop 12212, Minneapolis, Minnesota 55407

INTRODUCTION

Balance deficits that arise in conjunction with concussion/mild traumatic brain injury (c/mTBI) typically occur as a result of vestibular dysfunction.[1,2] Residual balance deficits often follow treatment for a vestibular disorder, and treatment is individualized and specific to the cause. Several assessments[1,3–5] attempt to identify systems that may contribute to residual balance deficits.

The assessment section of this chapter includes evaluation of body structure/function, activity, and participation level of functioning. Therapists are encouraged to use a battery of assessments to clarify the causes and impacts of balance deficits on an individual service member, with the understanding that no currently available tool focuses on the impact of balance on military-related skills. The intervention section of this chapter provides a tip sheet of options and considerations for balance intervention.

Although assessing balance and functional abilities is considered a **practice standard**, the choice of which specific assessment tools to use is up to the individual therapist (**practice option**). Therapists are encouraged to measure both static and dynamic balance to fully characterize deficits in the complex military population. Measuring comfortable and fast gait speed, which has been considered by some to be a vital sign and correlates to levels of function in many areas, is the one method considered a practice standard.[6] Support for balance deficit treatment is based on evidence for specific populations, such as the elderly, but remains lacking specific to individuals in the age range and with the comorbidities of the typical military population. Support for vestibular rehabilitation programs to address residual balance deficits, especially following blast exposure, is expanding.[1] The intervention suggestions described here are considered practice options.

SECTION 1: BALANCE ASSESSMENT

INTRODUCTION

Because balance issues that result from c/mTBI are often related to vestibular deficits, a vestibular deficit screen is recommended, with more thorough testing recommended if findings suggest vestibular impairment.[1,2] Tests commonly used to assess balance in the elderly or in those with other medical disorders are often not sensitive to the high-level functional abilities of service members with c/mTBI and demonstrate a "ceiling effect" (ie, subjects score at the upper limit of an instrument's range, therefore actual variation in data is not reflected in scores).[7–10] Tests such as the High-Level Mobility Assessment Tool (HiMAT), the Functional Gait Assessment (FGA), and the Illinois Agility Test (IAT), in addition to the use of dynamic posturography where available, may provide the appropriate level of challenge for this population.[7–10] For those service members with complex deficits, the more time-intensive Balance Evaluation Systems Test (BESTest) may be considered to clarify the underlying systems contributing to the service member's deficits.[4] A mini-BESTest has been developed to measure the

single dimension of "dynamic balance."[11] Although both BESTest versions have been used primarily in older adults, they may be useful in a service member population. Therapists should consider military-relevant obstacle courses and activities, possibly using completion time as a measurement. However, there are no standardized balance assessments for that level of challenge at this time.

Therapists should be aware that many of the assessment tools included in this section have limited or no psychometric information on individuals of typical military age and with the customary fitness level required for military readiness. Data is provided for the younger population if available, although most information is found for middle-aged and older adults or those with specific neurological disorders. The choice of tools used to assess balance and functional deficits is up to the individual therapist. A range of psychometric information is provided to allow therapists to make informed decisions related to the needs of the individual service member.

ACTIVITIES-SPECIFIC BALANCE CONFIDENCE SCALE

Purpose/Description

The Activities-Specific Balance Confidence (ABC) Scale was developed as an evaluative measure to assess balance confidence in ambulatory community-dwelling older adults (Exhibit 3-1). Each activity requires position changes or walking in progressively more difficult situations. The ABC

EXHIBIT 3-1

ADDITIONAL RESOURCES FOR THE ACTIVITIES-SPECIFIC BALANCE CONFIDENCE SCALE

This instrument can be obtained from the original publication:

- Powell LE, Myers AM. The Activities-specific Balance Confidence (ABC) Scale. *J Gerontol Med Sci.* 1995;50 (1):M2834.

It can also be found at the following:

- Rehabilitation Institute of Chicago, Center for Rehabilitation Outcomes Research, Northwestern University Feinberg School of Medicine Department of Medical Social Sciences Informatics Group. Rehabilitation Measures Database. www.rehabmeasures.org/Lists/RehabMeasures/DispForm.aspx?ID=949&Source=http%3A%2F%2Fwww%2Erehabmeasures%2Eorg%2Frehabweb%2Fallmeasures%2Easpx%3FPageView%3DShared. Accessed July 8, 2013.
- University of Missouri, School of Health Professions, Department of Physical Therapy. Geriatric Examination Toolkit. web.missouri.edu/~proste/tool/vest/index.htm. Accessed July 8, 2013.
- Southampton Hospital website. www.southamptonhospital.org/Resources/10355/FileRepository/Forms/Dizziness%20Hanicap%20Inventory%20-%20English.pdf. Accessed July 8, 2013.

Scale uses an 11-point scale, ranging from 0 (no confidence) to 11 (complete confidence).[12]

Recommended Instrument Use

The ABC Scale is a participation-level measure of balance. Situations are more related to home and community environment and may not be relevant to military activities; however, this self-test is typically used to assess the impact of balance deficits on daily functioning.

Administration Protocol/Equipment/Time

This is a paper-and-pencil self-test that takes about 5 minutes to administer and 5 minutes to score.

Groups Tested With This Measure

The ABC Scale has been used in community-dwelling elderly adults,[12] retirement home residents, and those undergoing hip and knee replacements[13]; in persons with vestibular disorders, including migraine-related vestibulopathy[14-16]; and in persons with stroke.[17]

Interpretability

- Norms: 100% corresponds to complete balance confidence. According to the developers, individuals who score above the mid-80s tend to be highly functioning and physically active.[13]
- Minimal detectable change (MDC): Information is not available on persons with concussion/mTBI. MDC based on a 95% confidence interval ($MDC_{95\%}$) = 21.7 in 60 community-dwelling seniors.[12] $MDC_{95\%}$ = 17.5 in 50 lower-extremity amputees in an outpatient setting.[18] If the patient's score is less than the MDC value, it is considered indistinguishable from measurement error.

Responsiveness Estimates

- Patients with vestibular diagnoses with migraine had a mean change of 12%, and those with vestibular diagnoses without history of migraine had a mean change of 25%.[19]
- A mean change of 10% was found in patients with moderate to severe loss of vestibular function following physical therapy intervention.[20]

- The ABC Scale was found not responsive to change (mean change – 1.1) in 213 noninstitutionalized women aged 70 and over, undergoing a 12-week, home-based, fall prevention program of exercise, education, and individualized risk-reduction counseling; however, the finding may have been related to a ceiling effect in high-functioning women.[21]

Reliability Estimates

- Internal consistency: Chronbach's alpha = 0.95[21]
- Interrater: not applicable, questionnaire
- Intrarater: not applicable, questionnaire
- Test-Retest: total ABC Scale scores r = 0.92 in community-dwelling elderly[12]; intraclass correlation (ICC) (3,1) = 0.91 in 50 outpatients with lower extremity amputation[18]

Validity Estimates

- Content/Face: Items for the ABC Scale were generated by 15 clinicians and 12 elderly outpatients using the Falls Efficacy Scale, with the addition of more situation-specific measures of balance confidence.[12]
- Criterion: correlation between ABC Scale and the Survey of Activities and Fear of Falling in older women: r = – 0.65[21]; correlation with Dizziness Handicap Inventory (DHI) in patients in a balance and vestibular clinic (ages 26–88), r = – 0.64.[15] In 167 patients with mild balance impairment, the odds ratio for frequent falling (adjusted for age and gender) was not significant (OR = 0.71).[22] The average ABC Scale score for persons who fall was 38% and for nonfallers was 81%.[12] In 287 persons (270 females, 17 males) in senior living facilities, persons with ABC Scale scores less than 50% were 2.6 times more likely to be depressed, 3.8 times more likely to walk slower than 0.9 m/s, 4.4 times more likely to use an assistive device for walking, and 5.4 times more likely to have impaired gait and balance than persons with ABC Scale scores over 50%.[23]
- Construct: ABC Scale correlated with tandem stance time (r = 0.59), with single-leg stance time (r = 0.59), with tandem walking (r = – 0.52), with the 6-minute walk test (r = 0.63), and with Tinetti's Performance Oriented Mobility Assessment (r = 0.64) in 1,767 mildly balance-impaired older adults involved in a balance-training and fall-reduction program (Form 3-1).[22]

Administration

The ABC Scale can be self-administered or conducted via personal or telephone interview. Larger font size should be used for self-administration testing, while an enlarged version of the rating scale on an index card will facilitate interviews. Each respondent should be queried concerning their understanding of the instructions, and probed regarding difficulty answering any specific items.

Instructions to Respondents

Instruct respondents as follows: "For each of the following, please indicate your level of confidence in doing the activity without losing your balance or becoming unsteady by choosing one of the percentage points on the scale from 0% to 100%. If you do not currently do the activity in question, try to imagine how confident you would be if you had to do the activity. If you normally use a walking aid to do the activity or hold onto someone, rate your confidence as if you were using these supports. If you have any questions about answering any of the items, please ask the administrator."

Instructions for Scoring

Total the ratings (possible range 0–1,600) and divide by 16 (or the number of items completed) to get each person's ABC Scale score. If a person qualifies his or her response to items 2, 9, 11, 14, or 15 (different ratings for up versus down or onto versus off), solicit separate ratings and use the lowest confidence rating of the two, which will limit the entire activity (eg, likelihood of using stairs). Total scores can be computed if at least 12 of the items are answered. Note that internal confidence (alpha) does not decrease appreciably with the deletion of item 16 (icy sidewalks) for administration in warmer climates.[13]

Development and Psychometric Properties

The ABC Scale was developed inductively with older adults and therapists, with evidence for test-retest reliability, hierarchical ordering, ability to discriminate between fallers and nonfallers, and high- versus low-mobility groups, and

FORM 3-1

THE ACTIVITIES-SPECIFIC BALANCE CONFIDENCE (ABC) SCALE

For <u>each</u> of the following activities, please indicate your level of self-confidence by choosing a corresponding number from the following rating scale:

0%	10	20	30	40	50	60	70	80	90	100%

No Confidence   **Completely Confident**

How confident are you that you can maintain your balance and remain steady when you . . .

1. walk around the house? _____ %

2. walk up or down stairs? _____ %

3. bend over and pick up a slipper from the front of a closet floor? _____ %

4. reach for a small can off a shelf at eye level? _____ %

5. stand on your tip toes and reach for something above your head? _____ %

6. stand on a chair and reach for something? _____ %

7. sweep the floor? _____ %

8. walk outside the house to a car parked in the driveway? _____ %

9. get into or out of a car? _____ %

10. walk across a parking lot to the mall? _____ %

11. walk up or down a ramp? _____ %

12. walk in a crowded mall where people rapidly walk past you? _____ %

13. are bumped into by people as you walk through the mall? _____ %

14. step onto or off of an escalator while holding onto a railing? _____ %

15. step onto or off an escalator while holding onto parcels such that you cannot hold onto the railing? _____ %

16. walk outside on icy sidewalks? _____ %

association with balance performance measures.[12] ABC Scale scores above 50 and less than 80 are indicative of a moderate level of functioning characteristic of persons with chronic conditions. Scores above 80 indicate higher functioning, usually in active older adults, and are achievable through exercise and rehabilitative therapy.[12] The ABC Scale (and its cultural adaptations) continues to be widely used for various populations (eg, stroke).

Selected Reference

Powell LE, Myers AM. The Activities-specific Balance Confidence (ABC) Scale. *J Gerontol Med Sci*. 1995;50(1):M2834.

SINGLE-LIMB STANCE TEST

Purpose/Description

The Single-Limb Stance (SLS) Test, also called the Unipedal Stance Test, is a simple physical performance test of static balance ability.

Recommended Instrument Use

This simple test of static equilibrium is typically used as part of a battery of balance assessments.

Administration Protocol/Equipment/Time

The SLS Test requires a stopwatch and a flat surface. It takes less than 5 minutes, depending on the number of trials and limbs tested (Exhibit 3-2).

Groups Tested With This Measure

This test has been used to predict falls; to assess patients with chronic pain, peripheral neuropathy, Parkinson's disease, multiple sclerosis, and vestibular disorders; in community-dwelling elderly; as a measure of frailty; following ankle fracture, brain injury, stroke, and concussion; and for testing health-related fitness.[24]

Interpretability

Norms: Table 3-1 is a subset of the data most relevant to the ages of typical military personnel taken from Table 1 in Springer et al.[24] Testing was done for a maximum of 45 seconds. Subjects crossed their arms and were asked to look at a spot on the wall. Table 3-2 provides additional norms for 30-second maximum test times from Bohannon et al (1984; Tables 3-1 and 3-2).

MDC: eyes open = 5.3 seconds; eyes closed = 16.8 seconds (patients with acute unilateral vestibular loss). These minimal detectable change estimates were calculated from data from Kammerlind et al using patients with unilateral vestibular loss.[25]

MDC was not available for normal subjects or those with concussion. If the patient's score is less than the MDC value, it is considered indistinguishable from measurement error.

Responsiveness Estimates

An effect size of 0.57 and a response mean of 0.79 for change over 8 weeks were found in patients with non-peripheral vertigo and unsteadiness.[25]

Reliability Estimates

- Internal consistency: not available
- Interrater: ICC = 0.99 for eyes open and eyes closed in 50 healthy subjects between 19 and over 80 years old for the best of three trials; ICC = 0.95 for the mean of three trials for eyes closed; ICC = 0.83 for eyes closed mean of 3 trials[24]
  - ICC = 0.98 in 30 patients with acute unilateral vestibular loss with eyes open.
  - ICC = 1.0 in 30 patients with acute unilateral vestibular loss with eyes closed.
  - ICC = 1.0 in 20 patients with central neurological dysfunction with eyes open.
  - ICC = 0.99 in 20 patients with central neurological dysfunction with eyes closed.[25]
- Intrarater: r = 0.93 on retest within 1 week[26]
- Test-Retest
  - ICC = 0.92 in 30 patients with acute unilateral vestibular loss with eyes open.
  - ICC = 0.56 in 30 patients with acute unilateral vestibular loss with eyes closed.
  - ICC = 0.96 in 20 patients with central neurological dysfunction with eyes open.

EXHIBIT 3-2

RECORD OF FINDINGS FOR SINGLE-LIMB STANCE TEST

- Subject should stand on a flat surface without shoes, or with firm-bottomed shoes with no or low heels.
- Arms should be at the subject's sides, at hips.
- Timing begins on lifting of the nonstance limb.
- Timing ends:
  - with floor contact of the raised limb, or
  - touching of the raised limb to the stance leg, or
  - touching of wall or other support to prevent a fall.
- Timing stops at 45 seconds.
- Use the best of three trials.

Note: Patient can be tested with eyes open and again with eyes closed. One or both limbs may be assessed.

EYES OPEN:

Trial 1 _____   Trial 1 _____

Trial 2 _____   Trial 2 _____

Trial 3 _____   Trial 3 _____

Right (seconds to 0.1) _____ Left (seconds to 0.1) _____

EYES CLOSED:

Trial 1 _____   Trial 1 _____

Trial 2 _____   Trial 2 _____

Trial 3 _____   Trial 3 _____

Right (seconds to 0.1) _____ Left (seconds to 0.1) _____

TABLE 3-1

UNIPEDAL STANCE TIME NORMATIVE VALUES

Age	Gender	Eyes Open, Best of 3 Trials (sec) Mean (SE)	Eyes Open, Mean of 3 Trials (sec) Mean (SE)	Eyes Closed, Best of 3 Trials (sec) Mean (SE)	Eyes Closed, Mean of 3 Trials (sec) Mean (SE)
18–39	Female (n = 44)	45.1 (0.1)	43.5 (3.8)	13.1 (12.3)	8.5 (9.1)
	Male (n = 54)	44.4 (4.1)	43.2 (6.0)	16.9 (13.9)	10.2 (9.6)
40–49	Female (n = 47)	41.6 (0.1)	40.4 (10.1)	13.5 (12.4)	7.4 (6.7)
	Male (n = 51)	41.9 (9.9)	40.1 (11.5)	12.0 (13.5)	7.3 (7.4)

SE: standard error
Reproduced with permission from: Springer BA, Marin R, Cyhan T, Roberts H, Gill NW. Normative values for the unipedal stance test with eyes open and closed. *J Geriatr Phys Ther*. 2007;30(1):8–15.

TABLE 3-2

SUMMARY STATISTICS FROM ONE-LEGGED TIMED BALANCE TESTS OF SUBJECTS*

Decade	Eyes	$\overline{X} \pm s$	Minimum	First Quartile	Median	Third Quartile	Maximum	< 30 sec (%)
20–29	Opened	30.0±	•••	•••	•••	•••	•••	0
	Closed	28.8±2.3	22.5	28.6	•••	•••	•••	25
30–39	Opened	30.0±	•••	•••	•••	•••	•••	0
	Closed	27.8±5.0	8.4	29.9	•••	•••	•••	23
40–49	Opened	29.7±1.3	23.0	•••	•••	•••	•••	6
	Closed	24.2±8.4	3.5	18.9	•••	•••	•••	24
50–59	Opened	29.4±2.9	14.3	•••	•••	•••	•••	6
	Closed	21.0±9.5	5.1	11.9	24.8	•••	•••	57
60–69	Opened	22.5±8.6	4.8	17.0	24.6	•••	•••	57
	Closed	10.2±8.6	2.1	4.5	7.1	12.5	•••	90
70–79	Opened	14.2±9.3	1.2	4.9	12.2	21.6	•••	90
	Closed	4.3±3.0	0.7	2.3	3.4	5.4	12.7	100

*Time in seconds. Best of five trials used with counting stopping at 30 seconds. 30–32 subjects in each decade.
Reproduced with permission from: Bohannon RW, Larkin PA, Cook AC, Gear J, Singer J. Decrease in timed balance test scores with aging. *Phys Ther.* Jul 1984;64(7):1067–1070. The American Physical Therapy Association. This material is copyrighted and any further reproduction or distribution requires written permission from APTA.

○ ICC = 0.72 in 20 patients with central neurological dysfunction with eyes closed.[25]

Validity Estimates

- Content/Face: SLS is a component of a number of other balance scales.[27]
- Criterion: SLS time correlates significantly with ABC Scale (r = 0.41), tandem stance (r = 0.55), and Timed Up and Go (r = –0.38), in 167 independent-living residents.[28]
- Construct: SLS time distinguishes between age groups[24,29]; distinguishes patients with known pathologies (ie, peripheral neuropathy) that would be expected to negatively affect balance.[30] SLS time identifies fallers.[30] SLS time correlates significantly with the Timed Up and Go without (r = 0.40) and with concurrent cognitive tasks (r = 0.27) in community-dwelling women over 70 years old.[31]

Selected Reference

Springer BA, Marin R, Cyhan T, Roberts H, Gill NW. Normative values for the unipedal stance test with eyes open and closed. *J Geriatr Phys Ther.* 2007;30(1):8–15.

ROMBERG AND SHARPENED ROMBERG

Purpose/Description

The Romberg and Sharpened Romberg tests are physical performance Tests used to assess a person's ability to maintain an upright posture with a stable and then a narrowed base of support (Exhibit 3-3).

Recommended Instrument Use

Neurologists are familiar with this test. The original Romberg has been used clinically for balance testing since the 1850s.[32]

Groups Tested With This Measure

This test has been used on healthy men and women,[33,34] for predicting falls,[35,36] on persons with dizziness and unsteadiness,[37] on persons with Parkinsonism,[38] and on those with vestibular disorders after traumatic brain injury.[39]

Administration Protocol/Equipment/Time

Subjects may cross their arms or hold their arms by their sides; timing begins after the subject

EXHIBIT 3-3

PROTOCOL RECORD OF FINDINGS FOR ROMBERG/SHARPENED ROMBERG TEST

Testing Protocol:

- Subject should stand without shoes on.
- Subjects may cross their arms or hold their arms by their sides.
- Timing begins after the subject assumes the proper position.
- Timing is stopped:
    - if subjects move their feet from the original (proper) position,
    - if they open their eyes on the eyes-closed trials, or
    - if they reach the maximum balance time of 60 seconds (record to the 0.1 second).
- Four conditions are measured. The four test positions include:

Romberg	TRIAL 1	TRIAL 2	Average
1. Feet together, eyes open, 60 seconds (R-EO)	_____	_____	_____
2. Feet together, eyes closed, 60 seconds (R-EC)	_____	_____	_____

Sharpened Romberg	TRIAL 1	TRIAL 2	Average
3. Feet heel to toe, eyes open, 60 seconds (SR-EO) (dominant foot behind nondominant foot)	_____	_____	_____
4. Feet heel to toe, eyes closed, 60 seconds (SR-EC) (dominant foot behind nondominant foot)	_____	_____	_____

Patient Instructions (Eyes Open, Romberg)

Stand with both anklebones touching each other, with your hands crossed and touching the opposite shoulders. Stand without shoes on, if possible, and look straight ahead at a target about 3 feet in front of you. Try to stay in this position for 60 seconds.

Instructions for the Patient (Eyes Closed, Romberg)

Stand with both anklebones touching each other, with your hands crossed and touching the opposite shoulders. Stand without shoes on, if possible, and look straight ahead with your eyes closed. Try to stay in this position for 60 seconds.
Note: These tests can also be done with a 30-second maximum limit.

R-EC: Romberg, eyes closed
R-EO: Romberg, eyes open
SR-EC: Sharpened Romberg, eyes closed
SR-EO: Sharpened Romberg, eyes open

assumes the proper position. Four conditions are measured. Timing is stopped if subjects move their feet from the original (proper) position, if they open their eyes on the eyes-closed trials, or if they reach the maximum balance time of 60 seconds (note that some scenarios use a maximum balance time of 30 seconds).[40] Two trials can be given and the longest balance time recorded. The test positions are as follows: for Romberg, 1) feet together, eyes open, 60 seconds (Romberg, eyes open); 2) feet together, eyes closed, 60 seconds (Romberg, eyes closed); and for sharpened Romberg, 1) feet heel to toe, eyes open, 60 seconds (Sharpened Romberg, eyes open; dominant foot behind nondominant foot); 2) feet heel to toe, eyes closed, 60 seconds (Sharpened Romberg, eyes closed; dominant foot behind nondominant foot).

TABLE 3-3

TANDEM ROMBERG (EYES CLOSED)

Decade	Mean	Standard Deviation	Median	Percent 30 Sec	Percent 10 Sec
3 (n = 58)	29.94	.43	30.00	98	100
4 (n = 42)	30.00	.00	30.00	100	100
5 (n = 32)	28.82	4.66	30.00	94	97
6 (n = 28)	28.03	4.87	30.00	82	100

Data source: Vereeck L, Wuyts F, Truijen S, Van de Heyning P. Clinical assessment of balance: normative data, and gender and age effects. *Int J Audiol.* Feb 2008;47(2):67–75.

Interpretability

Norms: Table 3-3 provides a subset of the normative values on tandem Romberg tested with eyes closed.[37] Additional normative values for older adults (50 years of age and older) can be found in Steffen and Mollinger (Table 3-4).[41] No younger groups were tested.

$MDC_{95\%}$: 9 to 10 seconds in sharpened Romberg with eyes open and 3 to 9 seconds with eyes closed in subjects with central and peripheral vestibular dysfunction.[25] If the patient's score is less than the MDC value, it is considered indistinguishable from measurement error.

Responsiveness Estimates

Twenty nonexercising community dwellers (ages 58–68) showed a 4.9-second improvement in Sharpened Romberg following a 3-month program of 1 hour, twice weekly Caribbean dance exercise, compared to 20 community dwellers with no physical activity.[42]

Reliability Estimates

- Internal consistency: not applicable

- Interrater: eyes open r = 0.75, eyes closed r = 0.97[34]; 30 patients with acute vestibular loss[25]; Sharpened Romberg, eyes open, ICC = 1.00; Sharpened Romberg, eyes closed, ICC = 0.99
- Intrarater: 45 women with eyes open and eyes closed ICC (2,1) = 0.99[34]
- Test-Retest: 30 subjects with unilateral vestibular loss doing Sharpened Romberg, eyes closed ICC = 0.63; Sharpened Romberg, eyes open ICC = 0.76[25]; 19 subjects between 24 and 39 years old (examining aviation simulator sickness): ICC (2,1) = 0.72 with eyes closed and ICC (2,1) = 0.90 with eyes open[43]

Validity Estimates

- Content/Face: The sharpened Romberg came to be used in the 1940s as a posture requiring a higher-level skill than the Romberg.[44]
- Criterion: Elderly females with a history of falls had significantly lower scores on sharpened Romberg with eyes open than did elderly female nonfallers.[36]
- Construct: not available

TABLE 3-4

TANDEM ROMBERG: OLDER ADULTS

Age/Gender	Sharpened Rhomberg, Eyes Open			Sharpened Rhomberg, Eyes Closed		
50–59	Mean	SD	CI (95%)	Mean	SD	CI (95%)
Male (n = 9)	60	0	60-60	51	18	37-60
Female (n = 15)	56	15	48-64	37	22	24-49

CI: confidence interval
SD: standard deviation
Data source: Steffen TM, Mollinger LA. Age- and gender-related test performance in community-dwelling adults. *J Neurol Phys Ther.* Dec 2005;29(4):181–188.

Selected References

Romberg MH. Manual of Nervous System Diseases of Man. London, England: Sydenham Society. 1853:395–401.

Black FO, Wall C, Rockette HE, Kitch R. Normal subject postural sway during the Romberg test. *Am J Otolaryngol.* 1982;3(5):309–315.

BALANCE ERROR SCORING SYSTEM

Purpose/Description

The Balance Error Scoring System (BESS) is a physical performance test that uses modified Romberg stances on different surfaces to assess postural stability (Exhibit 3-4). It was developed as a practical and cost-effective method of assessing balance at the sidelines in athletes, primarily to assist in return-to-play decisions following concussion.[45]

Recommended Instrument Use

The BESS can be used for a quick evaluation of postural control in service members as a component of a battery of tests to determine return-to-duty status.[46] A practice effect has been reported on repeat administrations of the BESS, particularly with the single-leg stance on foam.[47] The environment for baseline testing may affect the BESS score. Baseline testing for postural control using the BESS should be conducted "in the setting or environment in which post injury testing will most likely take place," as it has been shown that normal subjects' performance was worse when tested at the sideline versus in a clinical environment.[48]

Administration Protocol/Equipment/Time

The test consists of three stance conditions (double leg, single leg, and tandem) and two surfaces (firm and foam) assessed for 20 seconds each; each stance condition is completed with eyes closed. A stopwatch and a medium-density foam square (50 cm × 41 cm × 6 cm thick) are the only equipment needed. Scoring is done by counting the number of errors during each trial. Each error counts as one point and the total score is the sum of all the errors. Depending on a subject's ability and the number of errors, testing takes 5 to 10 minutes. No formal training is required to administer the BESS. A higher score indicates a poorer performance, with the very best performance resulting in a score of 0.[45]

Groups Tested With This Measure

Those tested with the BESS include high school and college athletes,[47–49] young athletes between the ages of 9 and 14,[50] and community-dwelling adults between the ages of 29 and 65.[51]

Interpretability

- Norms: Iverson et al have recently presented normative data for community-dwelling adults from age 20 to 69.[52] Data most relevant to service members are presented in Table 3-5.
- MDC: Reliable change indices are as follows[50]:
  - 90% CI = − 9.4 or + 5.3 points
  - 80% CI = − 7.9 or + 3.8 points
  - 70% CI = − 6.8 or + 2.6 points
  - 7.3 points (videotaped athletes–intrarater reliability data)[53]

If the patient's score is less than the MDC value, it is considered indistinguishable from measurement error.

Responsiveness Estimates

In collegiate football players following concussion, BESS scores changed from baseline, on average 5.7 points (95% CI) when measured immediately following the game or practice in which the injury occurred.[49]

Reliability Estimates

- Internal consistency: not available
- Interrater: ICC = 0.78–0.93 in control subjects for BESS subscores[54]; ICC = 0.57 for total BESS score (errors) using videotape of 30 athletes.[53] A lack of errors in some conditions (eg, double-leg stance on firm surface) did not allow calculation of rater reliability for that condition.
- Intrarater: ICC = 0.74 for total BESS score (errors) using videotape of 30 athletes.[53] ICC = 0.87–0.98 for total BESS and BESS subscores with a single tester viewing 20 videotaped subjects on two different days.[50]

EXHIBIT 3-4

BALANCE ERROR SCORING SYSTEM INSTRUCTIONS

Developed by researchers and clinicians at the University of North Carolina's Sports Medicine Research Laboratory, Chapel Hill, NC 27599-8700. The following is reproduced with permission from K Guskiewicz, April 26, 2010.[45]

The Balance Error Scoring System provides a portable, cost-effective, and objective method of assessing static postural stability. In the absence of expensive, sophisticated postural stability assessment tools, the BESS can be used to assess the effects of mild head injury on static postural stability. Information obtained from this clinical balance tool can be used to assist clinicians in making return-to-play decisions following mild head injury.

The BESS can be performed in nearly any environment and takes approximately 10 minutes to conduct.

Materials

1. Testing surfaces
   Two testing surfaces are needed: floor/ground and foam pad.
   1a. Floor/ground: any level surface is appropriate.
   1b. Foam pad: Power Systems Airex Balance Pad 81000 (Power Systems, Inc, Knoxville, TN); dimensions: length: 10 inches; width: 10 inches; height: 2.5 inches

The purpose of the foam pad is to create an unstable surface and a more challenging balance task, which varies by body weight. It has been hypothesized that as body weight increases the foam will deform to a greater degree around the foot. The heavier the person, the more the foam will deform. As the foam deforms around the foot, there is an increase in support on the lateral surfaces of the foot. The increased contact area between the foot and foam has also been theorized to increase the tactile sense of the foot, also helping to increase postural stability. The increase in tactile sense will cause additional sensory information to be sent to the CNS [central nervous system]. As the brain processes this information it can make better decisions when responding to the unstable foam surface.

2. Stopwatch
   Necessary for timing the subjects during the six 20-second trials

3. An assistant to act as a spotter
   The spotter is necessary to assist the subject should they become unstable and begin to fall. The spotter's attention is especially important during the foam surface.

4. BESS Testing Protocol
   These instructions should be read to the subject during administration of the BESS.

5. BESS Score Card

BESS Test Administration

1. Before administering the BESS, the following materials should be present:
   - foam pad
   - stopwatch
   - spotter
   - BESS Testing Protocol
   - BESS Score Card
2. Before testing, instruct the individual to remove shoes and any ankle taping if necessary. Socks may be worn if desired.
3. Read the instructions to the subject as they are written in the BESS Testing Protocol.
4. Record errors on the BESS Score Card as they are described below.

(**Exhibit 3-4** *continues*)

Exhibit 3-4 *continued*

BALANCE ERROR SCORING SYSTEM (SCORE CARD)

Types of Errors

1. Hands lifted off iliac crest
2. Opening eyes
3. Step, stumble, or fall
4. Moving hip into greater than 30 degrees abduction
5. Lifting forefoot or heel
6. Remaining out of test position greater than 5 seconds

SCORE CARD		
Error	Firm Surface	Foam Surface
Double leg stance (feet together)		
Single leg stance (nondominant foot)		
Tandem stance (nondominant foot in back)		
Total score		
BESS TOTAL		

The BESS is calculated by adding one error point for each error during the 6-20 second test.

Scoring the BESS

Each of the 20-second trials is scored by counting the errors, or deviations from the proper stance, accumulated by the subject. The examiner will begin counting errors only after the individual has assumed the proper testing position.

Errors: An error is credited to the subject when any of the following occur:

- moving the hands off of the iliac crests
- opening the eyes
- step stumble or fall
- abduction or flexion of the hip beyond 30°
- lifting the forefoot or heel off of the testing surface
- remaining out of the proper testing position for greater than 5 seconds

The maximum total number of errors for any single condition is 10.

Normal Scores for Each Possible Testing Surface (Table)

Maximum Number of Errors Possible for Each Testing Surface (Table)

If a subject commits multiple errors simultaneously, only one error is recorded. For example, if an individual steps or stumbles, opens their eyes, and removes their hands from their hips simultaneously, then they are credited with only one error.

(**Exhibit 3-4** *continues*)

Exhibit 3-4 *continued*

Subjects that are unable to maintain the testing procedure for a minimum of 5 seconds are assigned the highest possible score, 10, for that testing condition.

Double-leg stance: standing on a firm surface with feet side by side (touching), hands on the hips and eyes closed (Figures 1 and 2).

Single-leg stance: standing on a firm surface on the nondominant foot (defined below), the hip is flexed to approximately 30° and knee flexed to approximately 45°. Hands are on the hips and eyes closed (Figures 3 and 4).

*Nondominant foot: the nondominant foot is defined as the opposite leg of the preferred kicking leg.

Tandem stance: standing heel to toe on a firm surface with the nondominant foot (defined above) in the back. Heel of the dominant foot should be touching the toe of the nondominant foot. Hands are on the hips and their eyes are closed (Figures 5 and 6).

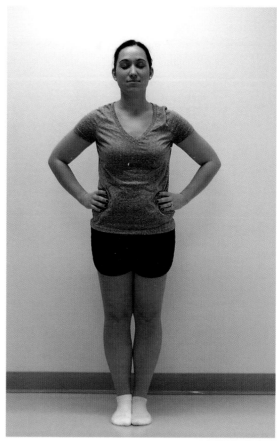

Figure 1. Balance Error Scoring System, double-leg stance, flat surface.

Script for the BESS Testing Protocol

<u>**Direction to the subject**</u>: *I am now going to test your balance.*

Please take your shoes off, roll up your pant legs above ankle (if applicable), and remove any ankle taping (if applicable).

This test will consist of six 20-second tests with three different stances on two different surfaces. I will describe the stances as we go along.

Double-Leg Stance

<u>**Direction to the subject**</u>: *The first stance is standing with your feet together like this.* [Administrator demonstrates two-legged stance.]

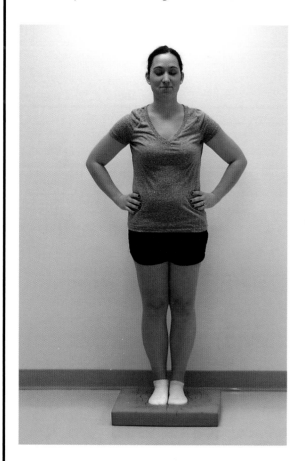

Figure 2. Balance Error Scoring System, double-leg stance, foam surface.

(Exhibit 3-4 *continues*)

Exhibit 3-4 *continued*

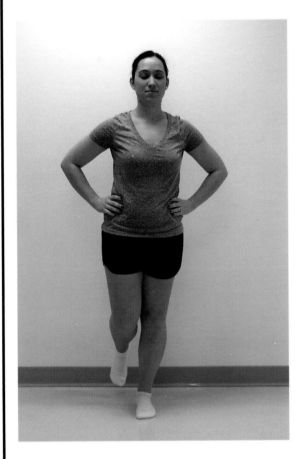

Figure 3. Balance Error Scoring System, single-leg stance, flat surface.

Single-Leg Stance

Direction to subject: *If you were to kick a ball, which foot would you use?* [This will be the dominant foot.]

Now stand on your nondominant foot.

[Before continuing the test, assess the position of the dominant leg as such: the dominant leg should be held in approximately 30° of hip flexion and 45° of knee flexion.]

Again, you should try to maintain stability for 20 seconds with your eyes closed. I will be counting the number of times you move out of this position.

Place your hands on your hips. When you close your eyes the testing time will begin.
[Start timer when subject closes their eyes.]

Direction to the spotter: *You are to assist the subject*

You will be standing with your hands on your hips with your eyes closed. You should try to maintain stability in that position for entire 20 seconds. I will be counting the number of times you move out of this position. For example: if you take your hands off your hips, open your eyes, take a step, lift your toes or your heels. If you do move out of the testing stance, simply open your eyes, regain your balance, get back into the testing position as quickly as possible, and close your eyes again.

There will be a person positioned by you to help you get into the testing stance and to help if you lose your balance.

Direction to the spotter: *You are to assist the subject if they fall during the test and to help them get back into the position.*

Direction to the subject: *Put your feet together, put your hands on your hips and when you close your eyes the testing time will begin.* [Start timer when subject closes their eyes.]

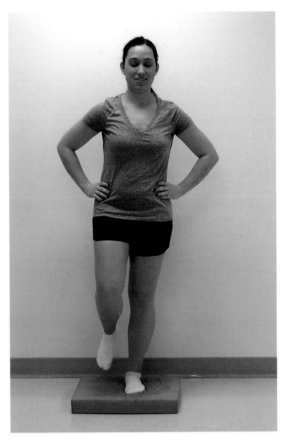

Figure 4. Balance Error Scoring System, single-leg stance, foam surface.

(Exhibit 3-4 *continues*)

Exhibit 3-4 *continued*

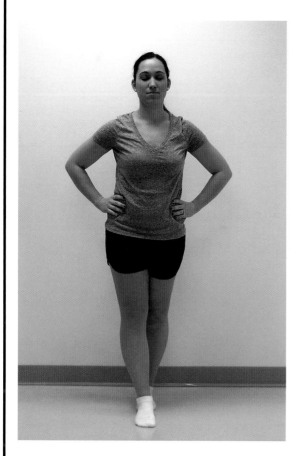

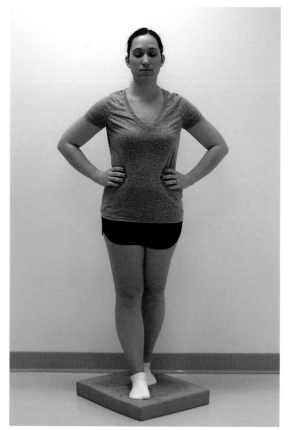

Figure 5. Balance Error Scoring System, tandem stance, flat surface.

Figure 6. Balance Error Scoring System, tandem stance, foam surface.

if they fall during the test and to help them get back into the position.

Tandem Stance

    <u>**Directions to the subject**</u>: *Now stand heel to toe with your nondominant foot in back. Your weight should be evenly distributed across both feet.*

    Again, you should try to maintain stability for 20 seconds with your eyes closed. I will be counting the number of times you move out of this position.

    Place your hands on your hips. When you close your eyes the testing time will begin.
[Start timer when subject closes their eyes.]

    <u>**Direction to the spotter**</u>: *You are to assist the subject if they fall during the test and to help them get back into the position.*

    *** Repeat each set of instructions for the foam pad
Note which foot was tested: . . . Left . . . Right (ie, which is the **nondominant** foot)

TABLE 3-5

NORMATIVE DATA FOR BALANCE ERROR SCORING SYSTEM (ERRORS)[*]

Age	Mean	Median	Standard Deviation	Superior (> 90th Percentile)	Broadly Normal (25–75 Percentile)	Poor (2nd–9th Percentile)
20–29 (n = 65)	11.3	11.0	4.8	0–5	8–14	18–23
30–39 (n = 173)	11.5	11.0	5.5	0–4	8–15	19–26
40–49 (n = 352)	12.5	11.5	6.2	0–5	9–16	21–28

[*]Iverson and Koehle recently presented normative data for community-dwelling adults from ages 20 to 69. Data most relevant to service members is presented here.
Data source: Iverson GL, Koehle MS. Normative data for the balance error scoring system in adults. *Rehabil Res Practice*. 2013;2013:846418.

- Test-Retest: In fifty 9- to 14-year-old athletes, BESS (errors) ICC (2,1) = 0.70, (SEM = 3.17).[50]

Validity Estimates

- Content/Face: not available
- Criterion: There are significant correlations between the BESS and force platform sway measures using normal subjects.[45]
- Construct: There is a small to medium correlation between age and BESS (r = 0.36).[51]

Selected References

Guskiewicz KM. Postural stability assessment following concussion: one piece of the puzzle. *Clin J Sport Med*. 2001;11:182–189.

Bell, DR, Guskiewicz KM, Clark MA, Padua DA. Systematic review of the Balance Error Scoring System. *Sports Health: A Multidisciplinary Approach*. 2011;3(3)287–295.

MODIFIED CLINICAL TEST OF SENSORY INTERACTION ON BALANCE

Purpose/Description

The Modified Clinical Test of Sensory Interaction on Balance (mCTSIB) is a physical performance test that attempts to differentiate the relative contribution of the somatosensory, visual, and vestibular systems to maintaining standing balance.[5] The original test was modified from six conditions to four.

Recommended Instrument Use

The mCTSIB is a useful screening tool for identifying persons with abnormal postural control and abnormal use of sensory inputs for balance control in standing.

Administration Protocol/Equipment/Time

The mCTSIB requires a stopwatch and dense foam pad (typically a 16-inch square, 3 to 4 inches high, medium-density foam that does not bottom out). Testing is done under four conditions, with a maximum of three trials per condition, each up to 30 seconds. Scoring involves recording the time (in seconds) to complete each trial. The times are then summed for a total mCTSIB score (maximum score 120 seconds for all four conditions). Higher scores indicate better performance of sensory interaction and balance. Depending on the subject's ability and how many trials are needed, testing takes 5 to 15 minutes. No formal training is required to administer the mCTSIB.

Groups Tested With This Measure

The mCTSIB has been used to evaluate individuals undergoing vestibular physical therapy,[55] physical therapy students and faculty, community-dwelling elderly, and those with vestibular disorders.[56] It has also been used to determine fall risk in older adults[57] and to assess those with peripheral neuropathy.[58]

Interpretability

- Norms: Subjects between the ages of 20 and 24, 25 and 44, and 45 and 64 years of age were able to maintain balance for 30 seconds in all four conditions.[56] Subjects in the 65-to-84-year-old range were able to stand on a firm surface with eyes open and closed for 30 seconds. These older subjects had significantly lower time when on foam with eyes open and eyes closed.
  Thirty subjects between 23 and 81 years old (mean 58.1 +/− 17.1) with both peripheral and central vestibular disorders, with a mean DHI score of 43.0 (+/− 19.6) showed the following time (in seconds) during the mCTSIB with feet shoulder-width apart[55]:
  - Firm surface with eyes open: 30.0 +/−0.0
  - Firm surface with eyes closed: 29.0 +/−3.9
  - Foam with eyes open: 29.0 +/− 4.1
  - Foam with eyes closed: 25.2 +/− 9.3
    Using the Sensory Organization Test (SOT) total scores as criterion, the mCTSIB had a sensitivity of 88% in both open (feet shoulder-width apart) and closed (feet together) stance, with a specificity of 50% when performed in a closed stance and a specificity of 44% when performed in an open stance.[59]
- MDC: not available. If the patient's score is less than the MDC value, it is considered indistinguishable from measurement error.

Responsiveness Estimates

This test is a screening tool that assesses a person's ability to use sensory inputs for balance control in standing. The mCTSIB, in combination with single-leg stance, and tandem Romberg in eyes open and closed conditions, has been used to monitor change over time in a group of vestibular patients[60]; however, studies that use the mCTSIB alone for responsiveness to change were not found.

Reliability Estimates

- Internal consistency: not available
- Interrater: r =0.99 with testing done on five physical therapy students (ages 20–24 years)[56]; r = 0.75 in older, community-dwelling adults[57]
- Intrarater: not available
- Test-Retest: r = 0.99 with testing done on five physical therapy students (ages 20–24 years)[56]

Validity Estimates

- Content/Face: not available
- Criterion: In a group of 50 patients with vestibular complaints, foam posturography demonstrated a significant correlation (P < 0.005) with moving platform posturography as the gold standard (90% agreement). A sensitivity of 95% and specificity of 90% were found between the foam posturography and the gold standard of the SOT on the moving platform.[61] In a group of patients undergoing vestibular rehabilitation, correlations between CTSIB and SOT range from 0.41 to 0.89 tested over the duration of the treatment.[60] The mCTSIB performed with feet together was slightly more sensitive than the mCTSIB performed with feet apart and correlated better with the SOT in persons with vestibular disorders.[59]
- Construct: The mCTSIB has been used to determine fall risk in older adults.[57] When subjects were age matched, no differences were found on condition 4 (eyes open on foam) between asymptomatic subjects and vestibular-impaired subjects.[56]

Performing the Test

This test provides a preliminary assessment of how well a person can integrate vestibular, visual, and somatosensory input for maintaining postural balance and how well the person can compensate when one or more of these senses is compromised.

Condition 1: three sensory systems available for balance (vision, vestibular, somatosensory)

Condition 2: vestibular and somatosensory available, vision absent

Condition 3: vestibular and vision available, somatosensory compromised

Condition 4: vestibular available, vision absent, somatosensory compromised

Equipment

Necessary equipment includes a stopwatch and dense foam pad, typically a 16-inch square, 3 to 4 inches high, medium-density foam that does not bottom out.

Starting Position

The subject stands on foam with his or her feet shoulder-width apart and arms crossed over the chest.

Protocol

Use the stopwatch to time a 30-second trial. Time is stopped and recorded if the subject:

- deviates from initial crossed-arm position,
- opens eyes during an "eyes closed" trial condition, or
- moves feet (takes a step) or requires manual assistance to prevent loss of balance.

A successful trial is recorded if the subject independently maintains the starting position for 30 seconds. Perform a maximum of three trials, or until the subject either maintains the starting position for 30 seconds or completes three 30-second attempts.

Scoring

Record the time (in seconds) that the subject was able to maintain the starting position up to the maximum of 30 seconds. The total score is the time recorded for each condition (maximum 120 seconds for all four conditions), or if more than one trial was performed for each condition, add the average times of each condition (maximum 120 seconds for all four conditions, Exhibit 3-5).

EXHIBIT 3-5

MODIFIED CLINICAL TEST OF SENSORY INTERACTION ON BALANCE

 # A -EYES OPEN, FIRM SURFACE

Trial 1:_____sec

Trial 2:_____sec   Average score (Total 3 trials / 3): _____ sec

Trial 3:_____sec

 # B -EYES CLOSED, FIRM SURFACE

Trial 1:_____sec

Trial 2:_____sec   Average score (Total 3 trials / 3): _____ sec

Trial 3:_____sec

 # C -EYES OPEN, FOAM SURFACE

Trial 1:_____sec

Trial 2:_____sec   Average score (Total 3 trials / 3):_____sec

Trial 3:_____sec

 # D -EYES CLOSED, FOAM SURFACE

Trial 1:_____sec

Trial 2:_____sec   Average score (Total 3 trials / 3):_____sec

Trial 3:_____sec

Total score: _____ / 120 sec

(Use the average score for each condition if more than one trial was required).

Data source: Shumway-Cook A, Horak FB, Assessing the influence of sensory interaction on balance. *Phys Ther*. 1986;66:1548–1550.

Selected Reference

Shumway-Cook A, Horak FB. Assessing the influence of sensory interaction on balance. *Phys Ther*. 1986;66:1548–1550.

BALANCE EVALUATION SYSTEMS TEST

Purpose/Description

The BESTest is a physical performance test developed to differentiate balance deficits by identifying the underlying postural control systems responsible for poor functional balance. The premise is that by identifying the underlying systems contributing to different types of balance deficits, an appropriate and specific rehabilitation approach can be developed.[4] The areas of assessment include biomechanical constraints, stability limits/verticality, anticipatory postural movements, postural responses, sensory orientation, and stability in gait. The test is available at the developer's website (www.bestest.us) free of charge; a training disk is available for a fee and is highly recommended.

Recommended Instrument Use

The BESTest was developed to assess and treat patients (primarily the elderly) with different types of balance problems. Its purpose is to identify deficits in the six targeted balance control systems and develop intervention strategies based on the findings. The therapist may consider using the BESTest for service members with complex balance complaints.

Administration Protocol/Equipment/Time

The BESTest consists of 36 items grouped into 6 systems. These are measured using a stopwatch, tape measure, 10-degree incline ramp, foam block, performance, or observation. Measures obtained on each item are scored on a scale from 0 (worst performance) to 3 (best performance). Scores for each section and the total test are provided as a percentage of total points. Testing takes 30 minutes by an experienced therapist. Training for inexperienced raters (those with no physical therapy experience) is recommended. Learning to score the BESTest requires prior review and 45 minutes of instruction with demonstration.[4] Training can be obtained via DVD or by attending a training course (see www.ohsu.edu/xd/research/centers-institutes/neurology/parkinson-center/research/horak-lab-balance/bestest.cfm; or www.ohsu.edu/tech-transfer/portal/technology.php?technology_id=217191).

Groups Tested With This Measure

The BESTest has been used on 22 subjects with and without balance disorders, ranging in age from 50 to 88 years,[4] and on subjects with Parkinson's disease.[62]

Interpretability

- Norms: not available. Some portions of the BESTest are drawn from existing clinical tests and there may be normative data available on individual parts, but none is available on the BESTest in its entirety.
- MDC: not available. If the patient's score is less than the MDC value, it is considered indistinguishable from measurement error.

Responsiveness Estimates: not available

Reliability Estimates

- Internal consistency: not available
- Interrater: ICC = 0.91 on total score, with the ICC for six sections ranging from r = 0.79 to 0.96[4]
- Intrarater: not available
- Test-Retest: not available

Validity Estimates

- Content/Face: Many subcomponents are taken from existing balance assessments and placed in the theoretical framework. Thousands of therapists responded to early versions of the BESTest through a large number of continuing education courses.[4]
- Criterion: r = 0.636, correlation between the BESTest and the ABC scale in subjects (age 50 to 88 years old) with and without balance disorders.[4]
- Construct: not available

Selected References

Horak FB, Wrisley DM, James F. The Balance Evaluation Systems Test (BESTest) to differentiate balance deficits. *Phys Ther*. 2009;89(5):484–498.

Horak F. BESTest-Balance Evaluation-Systems Test. http://www.ohsu.edu/xd/research/centers-institutes/neurology/parkinson-center/research/horak-lab-balance/bestest.cfm. Accessed July 16, 2013.

MINI-BALANCE EVALUATION SYSTEMS TEST OF DYNAMIC BALANCE

The Mini-BESTest is a 14-item scale used to measure dynamic balance. It was developed following factor and Rasch analysis to eliminate redundant or insensitive items on the original BESTest[11] and to improve scoring and make the test shorter to administer. The 14 items in the mini-BESTest include tests in four of the six original targeted balance control systems: (1) anticipatory transitions, (2) postural responses, (3) sensory orientation, and (4) dynamic gait. The Rasch analysis and refinement was done to focus on "dynamic balance" and to separate psychometric analyses of parts I, "biomechanical constraints," and II, "stability limits" of the original BESTest.[11]

Recommended Instrument Use

The Mini-BESTest has been used primarily in older adults with different types of balance problems,[11] especially those with Parkinson's disease.[63,64] A therapist may consider using the Mini-BESTest for service members with subtle balance deficits, as it has shown promise in discerning subtle balance deficits in patients with early Parkinson's disease[65] without the same ceiling effects as the Berg Balance Test in this population.

Administration Protocol/Equipment/Time

The Mini-BESTest consists of 14 items grouped into four systems. It takes 10 to 15 minutes to administer and requires a stopwatch, tape measure, 10-degree incline ramp, shoe box, chair, and foam block (medium-density memory foam, 4 inches thick). It requires patient performance be observed by the therapist. Measures obtained on each item are scored on a scale of 0 (poor balance) to 2 (normal, no impairment of balance), with a maximum score of 28. Two of the test items score both the right and left sides by recording the worse side.[65]

Groups Tested With This Measure

The Mini-BESTest has been tested on a convenience sample of 115 subjects (mean age 62.7 years; 53 men, 62 women) with balance disorders of various etiologies (primarily hemiparesis, Parkinson's disease, other neuromuscular diseases, hereditary ataxia, and multiple sclerosis, etc).[11] The Mini-BESTest was more accurate in predicting falls than the Berg Balance Scale or the FGA during 6-month and 12-month prospective analyses in a group of 80 participants with idiopathic Parkinson's disease,[63] and identified those with mild Parkinson's disease better than the Berg Balance Scale.[65] Data on subjects with c/mTBI have not yet been published. The Mini-BESTest can be downloaded from the Internet (www.bestest.us/files/7413/6380/7277/MiniBEST_revised_final_3_8_13.pdf).

Interpretability

- Norms: not available; however, some portions of the Mini-BESTest are drawn from existing clinical tests and there may be normative data available on individual parts, but none is available on the Mini-BESTest in its entirety.
- MDC: not available. If the patient's score is less than the MDC value, it is considered indistinguishable from measurement error.

Responsiveness Estimates: not available

Reliability Estimates

- Internal consistency: not available
- Interrater: ICC r ≥ 0.91 on total score (n = 15 between three raters) in persons with Parkinson's disease[64]
- Intrarater: not available
- Test-Retest: ICC r ≥ 0.92 (n = 24) in persons with Parkinson's disease[64]

Validity Estimates

- Content/Face: Many subcomponents of the original BESTest are taken from existing balance assessments and placed in the theoretical framework. Thousands of therapists responded to early versions of the BESTest through a large number of continuing education courses.[4]
- Criterion: Tested on 97 persons with Parkinson's disease, the Mini-BESTest correlated significantly with the Berg Balance Scale (r = 0.79, P < 0.001).[65]
- Construct: The Mini-BESTest was able to distinguish between fallers and nonfallers in persons with Parkinson's disease.[63]
- Sensitivity/Specificity: A cut-off point for the Mini-BESTest to differentiate "those with and without postural response deficits ≥ 21, yielding (sensitivity, specificity) = (89%, 81%)."[65]

Selected Reference

Franchignoni F, Horak F, Godi M, Nardone A, Giordano A. Using psychometric techniques to improve the balance evaluations systems test: the Mini-BESTest. *J Rehab Med*. 2010;42:323–331.

COMPUTERIZED DYNAMIC POSTUROGRAPHY

Computerized dynamic posturography (CDP) involves the use of a sophisticated force platform system to study the contributions of the visual, vestibular, and somatosensory systems to maintaining postural stability. The protocols described in this toolkit are proprietary to NeuroCom (Clackamas, OR; www.resourcesonbalance.com/program/role/cdp/index.aspx), but there are other balance platform systems available (eg, Micromedical Balance Quest, Chatham, IL; www.micromedical.com/balancequest.html).

Using the NeuroCom platform, CDP includes the SOT, Motor Control Test (MCT), and Adaptation Test. The assessments described here for use in service members with c/mTBI are the SOT and the MCT.

Sensory Organization Test

The SOT portion of CDP systematically removes one or more sensory components of balance (vision, somatosensory, vestibular) to evaluate which component the client is reliant upon for balance. Certain patterns of dysfunction are associated with specific deficits and indicate a person's ability to suppress inappropriate visual and proprioceptive information. Patterns of response may also indicate a person's inability to weight appropriate sensory input to the specific test condition. The six evaluation conditions are as follows:

1) Condition 1: stable platform with eyes open in a stable visual environment (patient has full use of all information: visual, vestibular, and somatosensory).
2) Condition 2: stable platform with eyes closed (patient must rely on vestibular and somatosensory information).
3) Condition 3: stable platform with moving visual surround (patient must suppress a false sense of visually induced movement and rely on vestibular and somatosensory inputs).
4) Condition 4: unstable platform with eyes open in a stable visual environment (patient must rely on vestibular and visual inputs).
5) Condition 5: unstable platform with eyes closed (patient must rely on vestibular input only because visual and somatosensory feedback have been eliminated).
6) Condition 6: unstable platform and unstable visual environment (patient must rely on vestibular input alone and suppress a false sense of visually induced movement).[66]

The SOT report provides a composite equilibrium score, sensory analysis ratios, strategy analysis, and center of gravity alignment. The composite equilibrium score characterizes the subject's overall level of balance performance. The sensory analysis ratios help identify impairments of or reliance on individual sensory systems, including the somatosensory, visual, and vestibular systems. The strategy analysis evaluates the subject's appropriate use of hip or ankle strategies in response to support surface changes. Finally, the center-of-gravity position data provides information on the location of the subject's center of gravity relative to the base of support (see NeuroCom user's manual[67]).

Motor Control Test

The MCT measures a person's ability to reflexively recover from unexpected external surface provocations. The MCT report provides information on weight symmetry and the latency and amplitude of a patient's response to a perturbation. Weight symmetry evaluates the relative distribution of weight during perturbations, while latency and amplitude quantify the onset time and amplitude of response to small, medium, and large perturbations in forward and backward directions (see NeuroCom user's manual[67]).

Recommended Instrument Use

CDP should not be used in isolation, but in conjunction with clinical measures of balance to obtain a comprehensive view of a service member's balance deficits. Although there remain issues with fully characterizing the reliability, validity, and responsiveness of CDP for service members with c/mTBI, CDP, where available, can assist in a full description of and the progress or course of balance complaints can help practitioners describe and assess the progress of balance complaints. The American Academy of Otolaryngology—Head and Neck Surgery recognizes dynamic platform posturography as medically indicated and appropriate in evaluating those with suspected balance or dizziness disorders.

CDP protocols are often used to evaluate patients for aphysiologic responses, malingering, or exaggerated patterns of responses to testing. A number of criteria have been developed[68–70] to address the issue of sway patterns and postural responses that are out of proportion to the clinical assessments and laboratory findings of postural and gait control, given the presenting mechanism and severity of injury or diagnosis. These criteria include such findings as high intertrial variability, performance on "easier" SOT conditions (1 and 2) being worse than performance on more difficult conditions (5 and 6), and exaggerated motor responses to small translations that do not appropriately increase with the larger forward-and-backward translations and include the therapist's clinical judgment.[70]

Administration Protocol/Equipment/Time

The information provided here for the SOT and the MCT is only available through use of the NeuroCom Balance Master System. Testing takes 10 to 20 minutes.

Other companies that provide dynamic posturography that can allow testing of the modified clinical test of sensory organization on balance include Micromedical's Balance Quest (http://www.micromedical.com/balancequest.html)/

Groups Tested With This Measure

In addition to testing individuals with vestibular and other causes of balance disorders,[71,72] CDP has been used to quantify abnormalities in sensory weighting and postural sway in persons with mild to severe traumatic brain injury.[10,73,74] The SOT portion of CDP was used to assess balance deficits in 10 subjects with mild to severe TBI and in 10 control subjects without TBI.[75]

Interpretability

Norms: The documentation and software from NeuroCom provides comparison to normative data for subjects in the age ranges of 20 to 59, 60 to 69, and 70 to 79. Wrisley et al studied the learning effects of the equilibrium scores on SOT conditions in 13 healthy subjects (6 men, 7 women) between the ages of 21 and 36 years (mean age 24 +/− 4 years) to determine clinically meaningful change scores for the SOT. Subjects were tested five times over a 2-week period, with a retention test 1 month later. The first three conditions did not demonstrate a learning effect, while the increase in scores for conditions 4, 5, and 6 plateaued after the third session. Therefore, data for the fourth trial is an example of normative values in the young, healthy population (composite score: 89.2 ± 2.1):

1. eyes open, firm surface (%): 95.8 ± 0.8
2. eyes closed, firm surface (%): 93.0 ± 1.9
3. sway reference vision, firm surface (%): 93.6 ± 2.0
4. eyes open, sway reference surface (%): 92.8 ± 1.9
5. eyes closed, sway reference surface (%): 83.6 ± 3.1
6. sway reference vision and surface (%): 82.8 ± 5.6[76]

MDC: A learning effect has been demonstrated in healthy young adults. An improvement of greater than 8 points on the composite score "would be considered a change greater than the learning of the task."[76] In a study to assess sensitivity and specificity of the CDP and SOT variables, Broglio et al, using the reliable change index, developed cut scores for each SOT variable using a range of confidence intervals from 70% to 95%.[77(p150)] This work involved NeuroCom SOT assessments completed

TABLE 3-6

RELIABLE CHANGE AND CUT SCORES FOR SOT VARIABLES IN HEALTHY AND CONCUSSED YOUNG ADULTS

Change Scores	RCI Value	Composite Balance	Somatosensory Ratio	Visual Ratio	Vestibular Ratio
95% CI	1.96	9.75	10.08	11.93	25.69
90% CI	1.65	8.48	8.46	9.99	22.41

CI: confidence interval
RCI: reliable change index
SOT: Sensory Organization Test
Data source: Broglio SP, Ferrara MS, Sopiarz K, Kelly MS. Reliable change of the sensory organization test. *Clin J Sport Med*. Mar 2008;18(2):148–154.

twice on 66 healthy (age 20.1 +/– 1.96 years) and 63 concussed (age 20.3 +/– 1.35 years) young adults. Findings for the 90% and 95% confidence interval cut scores are found in Table 3-6.

Responsiveness Estimates: Data could not be located for persons with c/mTBI.

Sensitivity and Specificity

Broglio et al found the highest sensitivity (57%) and specificity (80%) at the 75% confidence interval using estimates of reliable change on the Neuro-Com SOT to distinguish between healthy (n = 66) and concussed (n = 63) young adults.[77] DiFabio completed a metaanalysis of the sensitivity and specificity of platform posturography and found an overall sensitivity and specificity of about 50%.[78] Individual diagnostic categories were found to influence the predictive value of abnormal results (73% for benign paroxysmal positional vertigo and Ménèiere disease, and 41% for peripheral vestibular disease).[78]

In a review of the literature by DiFabio,[79] dynamic posturography (SOT and MCT) were found to be highly specific for detecting vestibular dysfunction (specificity over 90%). The sensitivity of either static or dynamic posturography was low, but improved to 61% to 89% in detecting vestibular deficits if combined with tests of horizontal vestibulo-ocular reflex function.[79]

Reliability Estimates

- Test-Retest:
  - SOT: In 13 healthy adults (ages 21 to 36), composite SOT score was 0.67 (ICC [2,3]) when tested an average of 1.7 days apart. According to Wrisley et

al, individual equilibrium scores for all conditions except condition 3 (stable surface, sway referenced vision) were also fair to good, with scores ranging from 0.43 to 0.79 from session 1 to session 2. Condition 3 showed poor test-retest reliability with an ICC (2,3) of 0.35.[76]

Test-retest reliability in 66 healthy participants (39 men, 27 women, ages 20.1+/–1.96 years) tested an average of 49.1 days apart resulted in a composite balance of r = 0.56, somatosensory ratio of r = 0.10, visual ratio of r = 0.27, and vestibular ratio of r = 0.51.[77]
  - MCT: not available in healthy young adults or those with c/mTBI. In a study of 98 middle-aged and elderly adults, latency and response strength measures of the MCT showed good test-retest reliability (ICCs 0.66–0.98).[80] Procedures for manually marked latencies must be consistently established within clinics.[81]

Validity Estimates

- Content/Face: SOT and MCT test the sensory systems that contribute to balance and postural reactions to external perturbations that allow balance recovery.
- Criterion: CDP discriminated between patients with dizziness (n = 37) and normal controls (n = 22) with dizzy patients classified by audiometry, bithermal calorics, electronystagmography, tympanography, and rotational chair testing.
- Construct: NeuroCom has documented validity in multiple populations, such as vestibular injury, Parkinson's disease,

and multiple sclerosis. SOT scores of college athletes suffering mild head injuries showed significant deficits lasting 3 to 7 days when all other tests were normal and when compared to their preinjury baselines.[82] The concussion group had reductions in SOT scores over the first week, while neuropsychological tests were normal.

Postural stability deficits outlasted most neuropsychological and self-report symptoms in 24 subjects with sport-related concussion versus normal control subjects.[83] A systematic review of the published literature on the evidence of validity, reliability, and responsiveness of CDP measurements systems used in rehabilitation found that most of the studies were of poor design, making clinically meaningful decisions based on CDP findings difficult.[84]

Selected Reference

Balance Manager Systems, Clinical Interpretation Guide. NeuroCom International, Inc: Clackamas, OR: 2008.

HIGH-LEVEL MOBILITY ASSESSMENT TOOL

Purpose/Description

The HiMAT is a physical performance test used to assess high-level mobility deficits following TBI and to quantify therapy outcomes following intervention (Figure 3-1).[85,86]

Recommended Instrument Use

This test, which includes activities such as running and jumping, may be considered to assess higher-level mobility prior to using the service-specific fitness tests or obstacle courses. Note that it has not yet been specifically tested on persons with c/mTBI only, and there may be a ceiling effect given the normative value findings for males.[87]

Administration Protocol/Equipment/Time

The HiMAT consists of 13 items that are measured using either a stopwatch or tape measure. Measures obtained on each item are scored on a 0-to-5 scale based on time or distance and summed for a total HiMAT score (maximum score 54). Higher scores indicate better mobility performance. Depending on the client's ability and how many items he or she can perform, testing takes 5 to 15 minutes. No formal training is required to administer the HiMAT.

Groups Tested With This Measure

In one study, 103 ambulatory persons with TBI, recruited from inpatients, outpatients, and annual review clinics, were evaluated using HiMAT.[85,86] In another, 103 young, healthy adults ages 18 to 25 years old were tested, as were 28 people with chronic acquired brain injury undergoing a 3-month, high-level mobility program of strengthening exercises, prerunning and running drills,

and agility exercises supplemented with a gym or home exercise program.[87] The HiMAT is available on the Internet (www.tbims.org/combi/list.html).

Interpretability

- Norms: 103 young, healthy adults ages 18 to 25.[87] The median HiMAT score in males was 54/54 (interquartile range 53–54), and the 5th percentile was 50. A ceiling effect was evident for males, as 52.1% achieved the maximum score. The median HiMAT score in females was 51/54 (interquartile range 48–53), and the 5th percentile was 44.
- MDC: MDC_{95} +/– 2.66 points. If the patient's score is less than the MDC value, it is considered indistinguishable from measurement error. Given test and retest mean difference (1 point) to be 95% confident that clinically important change has occurred, persons have to improve by 4 points or deteriorate by at least 2 points.[88]

Responsiveness Estimates

Fourteen persons with TBI were initially tested less than 12 months after injury and were tested again 3 months later. These subjects were still considered to be in the acute recovery phase and were expected to improve over the 3-month interval. The individuals improved an average of 12.1 points (range 3–25 points) on the HiMAT.[89]

Reliability Estimates

- Internal consistency: Chronbach's alpha of 0.99 indicating that the extent to which the items measure the same domain was very high.

HiMAT: HIGH-LEVEL MOBILITY ASSESSMENT TOOL

DATE......................

DATE OF ACCIDENT....................

DIAGNOSIS....................

AFFECTED SIDE   LEFT/RIGHT

PATIENT ID LABEL

		SCORE					
ITEM	PERFORMANCE	0	1	2	3	4	5
WALK	sec	X	> 6.6	5.4–6.6	4.3–5.3	< 4.3	X
WALK BACKWARD	sec		> 13.3	8.1–13.3	5.8-8.0	< 5.8	X
WALK ON TOES	sec		> 8.9	7.0–8.9	5.4–6.9	< 5.4	X
WALK OVER OBSTACLE	sec		> 7.1	5.4–7.1	4.5–5.3	< 4.5	X
RUN	sec		> 2.7	2.0–2.7	1.7–1.9	< 1.7	X
SKIP	sec		> 4.0	3.5–4.0	3.0–3.4	< 3.0	X
HOP FORWARD (AFFECTED)	sec		> 7.0	5.3–7.0	4.1–5.2	< 4.1	X
BOUND (AFFECTED)	1) cm 2) cm 3) cm		< 80	80–103	104–132	> 132	X
BOUND (LESS AFFECTED)	1) cm 2) cm 3) cm		< 82	82–105	106–129	> 129	X
UP STAIRS	sec		> 22.8	14.6–22.8	12.3–14.5	< 12.3	X

Figure 3-1. High-Level Mobility Assessment Tool (continued on next page)

DEPENDENT (Rail **OR** not reciprocal; if not, score 5 and rate below)							
UP STAIRS INDEPENDENT (No rail **AND** reciprocal; if not, score 0 and rate above)	sec		> 9.1	7.6–9.1	6.8–7.5	< 6.8	X
DOWN STAIRS DEPENDENT (Rail **OR** not reciprocal; if not, score 5 and rate below)	sec		> 24.3	17.6–24.3	12.8–17.5	< 12.8	X
DOWN STAIRS INDEPENDENT (No rail **AND** reciprocal; if not, score 0 and rate above)	sec		> 8.4	6.6–8.4	5.8–6.5	< 5.8	X
	SUBTOTAL						

TOTAL HiMAT SCORE   **/54**

Figure 3-1. (continued on next page)

HiMAT: High-Level Mobility Assessment Tool

Subject suitability: The HiMAT is appropriate for assessing people with high-level balance and mobility problems. The minimal mobility requirement for testing is independent walking over 20 m without gait aids. Orthoses are permitted.

Item testing: Testing takes 5–10 minutes. Patients are allowed 1 practice trial for each item.

Instructions: Patients are instructed to perform at their maximum safe speed except for the bounding and stair items.

Walking: The middle 10 m of 20-m trial is timed.

Walk backward: As for walking.

Walk on toes: As for walking. Any heel contact during the middle 10 m is recorded as a fail.

Walk over obstacle: As for walking. A house brick is placed across the walkway at the midpoint. Patients must step over the brick without contacting it. A fail is recorded if patients step around the brick or make contact with the brick.

Run: The middle 10 m of a 20-m trial is timed. A fail is recorded if patients fail to have a consistent flight phase during the trial.

Skipping: The middle 10 m of a 20-m trial is timed. A fail is recorded if patients fail to have a consistent flight phase during the trial.

Hop forward: Patients stand on their more affected leg and hop forward. The time to hop 10 m is recorded.

Bound (affected): A bound is a jump from one leg to the other with a flight phase. Patients stand behind a line on their less affected leg, hands on hips, and jump forward **landing on their more affected leg**. Each bound is measured from the line to the heel of the landing leg. The average of three trials is recorded.

Bound (less affected): Patients stand behind a line on their more affected leg, hands on hips, and jump forward **landing on their less affected leg**. The average of three trials is recorded.

Up stairs: Patients are asked to walk up a flight of 14 stairs as they normally would and at their normal

Figure 3-1. (continued on next page)

speed. The trial is recorded from when the patient starts until both feet are at the top. Patients who use a rail or nonreciprocal pattern are scored on **Up Stairs Dependent**. Patients who ascend the stairs reciprocally without a rail are scored on **Up Stairs Independent** and get an additional 5 points in the last column of Up Stairs Dependent.

Down stairs: As for Up stairs.

Scoring: All times and distances are recorded in the "performance" column. The corresponding score for each item is then circled and each column is then subtotaled. Subtotals are then added to calculate the HiMAT score.

Figure 3-1. High-Level Mobility Assessment Tool (HiMAT) and instructions.
Reproduced with permission from Gavin Williams. Please notify Gavin Williams at gavin.williams@epworth.org.au or gavin@neuro-solutions.net so the use of the HiMAT can be tracked.

- Interrater: Three experienced physical therapists (two of whom had no prior knowledge of the HiMAT) concurrently and independently scored performances of 17 persons with TBI.[86]
  - ICC (2,1) = 0.99 for individual items.
  - ICC (2,1) = 0.99 for total scores.
- Intrarater: Twenty people with TBI occurring at least 18 months prior to testing were retested 2 days after their initial test. The retest ICC (2,1) was 0.99.[88]
- Test-Retest: The mean difference between test and retest 2 days later was 1 point. Standard error of measurement (SEM) was calculated to determine the 95% confidence interval for determining MDC. MDC was calculated to be +/− 2.66 points, indicating 95% confidence that clinically important change has occurred if individuals have improved by 4 points or deteriorated by at least 2 points.[88]

Validity Estimates

- Content/Face: Content was initially generated from a review of existing mobility scales and by surveys of experts.[85]

- Criterion: 103 persons with TBI were concurrently scored on the HiMAT, motor Functional Independence Measure (FIM), and gross function Rivermead Motor Assessment (RMA). Correlations (using Pearson r) were calculated between the HiMAT, the motor FIM, and the gross function component of the RMA to investigate concurrent validity. The correlation between the HiMAT and the motor FIM was only moderately strong (r = 0.53, P < 0.01) due to a substantial ceiling effect the motor FIM suffers when compared to the HiMAT. More specifically, the motor FIM was unable to discriminate motor performance for 90 (87.4%) of the 103 patients, yet these patients had a mean score on the HiMAT of only 32.6/54 (SD 13.8, range 5–54).[89] The HiMAT and gross function RMA had a much stronger correlation (r = 0.87, P < 0.01), but the gross function RMA also had a substantial ceiling effect when compared to the HiMAT. Of the 103 subjects, 53 (51.5%) scored the maximum score of 13/13 on the gross function RMA, yet had a mean score of only 41.7/54 on the HiMAT (SD 8.8, range 24–54).[89]
- Construct: not available

Selected References

Williams G, Robertson V, Greenwood K, Goldie P, Morris ME. The High-level Mobility Assessment Tool (HiMAT) for traumatic brain injury. Part 1: Item generation. *Brain Inj*. 2005;19(11):925–932.

Williams G, Robertson V, Greenwood K, Goldie P, Morris ME. The High-level Mobility Assessment Tool (HiMAT) for traumatic brain injury. Part 2: Content validity and discriminability. *Brain Inj*. 2005;19(10):833–843.

REVISED HIGH-LEVEL MOBILITY ASSESSMENT TOOL

The revised HiMAT is a modification of the original HiMAT (Figure 3-2). Rausch analysis was used to delete items and develop a unidimensional measure of "high-level mobility limitations" in persons with TBI.[90] This revised test no longer requires stairs.

Recommended Instrument Use

With test items such as running and jumping, this test may be considered for use to assess higher-level mobility prior to using the service-specific fitness tests or obstacle courses. It has not yet been specifically tested on persons with c/mTBI only, and there may be a ceiling effect given the normative value findings for males.[91] It may be considered for use in clinics or deployed settings where no stairs are available.

Administration Protocol/Equipment/Time

The revised HiMAT consists of eight items measured using either a stopwatch (to 1/10th second) or tape measure (in centimeters); a house brick is required as an obstacle. Measures obtained on each item are scored on a 0-to-4 scale based on time or distance and summed for a total HiMAT score (maximum score is 32). Higher scores indicate better mobility performance. Depending on the client's ability and how many items he or she can perform, testing takes 5 to 10 minutes; 1 practice trial is given for each item. No formal training is required to administer the HiMAT.

Groups Tested With This Measure

Data was reanalyzed for the original 103 ambulatory persons with primarily moderate and severe TBI recruited from inpatients, outpatients, and annual review clinics.[85,86,90]

Interpretability

- Norms: The original HiMAT tested 103 young, healthy adults ages 18 to 25.[91] Given that males demonstrated a ceiling effect and the interquartile range of 53 to 54, the norms for healthy, 18- to 25-year-old males would be expected to be 32 (see information for the full HiMAT[91]). Females were not retested for the revised HiMAT; see information on normative values for the full HiMAT.[91]
- MDC: MDC_{95} +/− 2 points. If the patient's score is less than the MDC value, it is considered indistinguishable from measurement error.

Responsiveness Estimates: not specifically retested for the revised HiMAT; see information on the full HiMAT.

Reliability Estimates

- Internal consistency: Revised HiMAT showed excellent internal consistency for high-level mobility (Pearson separation index = 0.96).[87] The information on rater reliability and retest reliability are from the original HiMAT, as the original dataset was reanalyzed.
- Interrater: Three experienced physical therapists (two of whom had no prior knowledge of the HiMAT) concurrently and independently scored performances of 17 persons with TBI.[88]
  - ICC (2,1) = 0.99 for individual items
  - ICC (2,1) = 0.99 for total scores
- Intrarater: Twenty people with TBI occurring at least 18 months prior to testing were retested 2 days after the initial test. The retest ICC (2,1) was 0.99.[88]
- Test-Retest: The mean difference between test and retest 2 days later was 1 point. SEM was calculated to determine the 95% confidence interval for determining MDC. MDC was calculated to be +/− 2.66 points, indicating 95% confidence that clinically important change has occurred if individuals have improved by 4 points or deteriorated by at least 2 points.[88]

Validity Estimates

- Content/Face: Content was initially generated from a review of existing mobility scales and by surveys of experts.[85]
- Criterion: See information under the original HiMAT; testing has not been redone using the revised HiMAT.
- Construct: not available

REVISED HiMAT (NO STAIR ITEMS)

DATE......................

DATE OF ACCIDENT.....................

DIAGNOSIS....................

AFFECTED SIDE   LEFT/RIGHT

PATIENT ID LABEL

ITEM	PERFORMANCE		0	1	2	3	4
WALK		sec	X	> 6.6	5.4–6.6	4.3–5.3	< 4.3
WALK BACKWARD		sec		> 13.3	8.1–13.3	5.8-8.0	< 5.8
WALK ON TOES		sec		> 8.9	7.0–8.9	5.4–6.9	< 5.4
WALK OVER OBSTACLE		sec		> 7.1	5.4–7.1	4.5–5.3	< 4.5
RUN		sec		> 2.7	2.0–2.7	1.7–1.9	< 1.7
SKIP		sec		> 4.0	3.5–4.0	3.0–3.4	< 3.0
HOP FORWARD (AFFECTED)		sec		> 7.0	5.3–7.0	4.1–5.2	< 4.1
BOUND (LESS AFFECTED)	1) cm 2) cm 3) cm			< 82	82–105	106–129	> 129
	SUBTOTAL						

*Note: When using the Revised HiMAT, the MDC score is +/− 2 points. This means that a 2-point score change is required to be 95% confident that true change has occurred.

TOTAL HiMAT SCORE   **/32**

Figure 3-2. Revised High-Level Mobility Assessment Tool (continued on next page)

HiMAT: High-Level Mobility Assessment Tool

Subject suitability:	The HiMAT is appropriate for assessing people with high-level balance and mobility problems. The minimal mobility requirement for testing is independent walking over 20 m without gait aids. Orthoses are permitted.
Item testing:	Testing takes 5–10 minutes. Patients are allowed 1 practice trial for each item.
Instructions:	Patients are instructed to perform at their maximum safe speed except for the bounding and stair items.
Walking:	The middle 10 m of 20-m trial is timed.
Walk backward:	As for walking.
Walk on toes:	As for walking. Any heel contact during the middle 10 m is recorded as a fail.
Walk over obstacle:	As for walking. A house brick is placed across the walkway at the midpoint. Patients must step over the brick without contacting it. A fail is recorded if patients step around the brick or make contact with the brick.
Run:	The middle 10 m of a 20-m trial is timed. A fail is recorded if patients fail to have a consistent flight phase during the trial.
Skipping:	The middle 10 m of a 20-m trial is timed. A fail is recorded if patients fail to have a consistent flight phase during the trial.
Hop forward:	Patients stand on their more affected leg and hop forward. The time to hop 10 m is recorded.
Bound (less affected):	A bound is a jump from one leg to the other with a flight phase. Patients stand behind a line on their more affected leg, hands on hips, and jump forward **landing on their less affected leg**. The average of three trials is recorded.
Scoring:	All times and distances are recorded in the "performance" column. The corresponding score for each item is then circled and each column is then subtotaled. Subtotals are then added to calculate the HiMAT score.

Figure 3-2. Revised High-Level Mobility Assessment Tool (HiMAT; no stairs) and instructions.

Selected Reference

Williams G, Pallant J, Greenwood K. Further development of the High-level Mobility Assessment Tool (HiMAT). *Brain Inj.* 2010;24(7–8):1027–1031.

GAIT SPEED

Purpose/Description

Gait speed is a physical performance test derived directly from measuring the parameters of distance and time. It has been used as a gold standard to validate outcome measures in various patient populations.

Recommended Instrument Use

Gait speed is a standard measure that should be used for all ambulatory patients. It has been proposed as a sixth vital sign.[6]

Administration Protocol/Equipment/Time

Testing takes less than 5 minutes, depending on the number of trials and speeds tested. Equipment includes a stopwatch that can record to tenths of a second, a tape measure, and a level surface of at least 9.1 meters (30 ft). Shoes are recommended and the use of a subject's habitual assistive device is permitted and indicated.

Groups Tested With This Measure

Gait speed testing has been used to assess the following individuals:

- those who have sustained stroke,[92]
- those with multiple sclerosis,[93]
- healthy adults,[94]
- amputees,
- those with rheumatoid arthritis,
- children with traumatic brain injury,[95-97]
- individuals with osteoarthritis,
- the elderly,
- those who have sustained spinal cord injury,
- individuals with Parkinson's disease,[38] and
- individuals with cerebral palsy.[98]

Interpretability

Norms: Tables 3-7–3-9[99]

MDC: In 37 community-dwelling adults with Parkinsonism, MCD (95%)was 0.18 m/s for comfortable gait speed, and 0.25 m/s for fast gait speed.[38] Steffen and Seney[38] summarize the literature on test-retest reliability in stroke and TBI and report MDC (95%) values of 0.11 to 0.24 m/s for comfortable gait speed and 0.24 m/s for fast gait speed. MDC values could not be found for persons with c/mTBI. If the patient's score is less than the MDC value, it is considered indistinguishable from measurement error (Table 3-10).

TABLE 3-7

GAIT SPEED (MEN)*

Age	N	Comfortable Pace cm/s	m/s	ft/s	Fast Pace cm/s	m/s	ft/s
20	15	139.3	1.393	4.57	253.3	2.533	8.31
30	13	145.8	1.458	4.78	245.6	2.456	8.06
40	22	146.2	1.462	4.80	246.2	2.462	8.08
50	22	139.3	1.393	4.57	206.9	2.069	6.79
60	18	135.9	1.359	4.46	193.3	1.933	6.34
70	22	133.0	1.330	4.36	207.9	2.079	6.82

*See data source for height normalized gait speed factor for each age group.
Data source: Bohannon RW. Comfortable and maximum walking speed of adults aged 20–79 years: reference values and determinants. *Age and Ageing* 1997;26:15–19. Table 4.

TABLE 3-8

GAIT SPEED (WOMEN)*

Age	N	Comfortable Pace cm/s	m/s	ft/s	Fast Pace cm/s	m/s	ft/s
20	22	140.7	1.407	4.61	246.7	2.467	8.09
30	23	141.5	1.415	4.64	234.2	2.342	7.68
40	21	139.1	1.391	4.56	212.3	2.123	6.96
50	21	139.5	1.395	4.58	201.0	2.010	6.59
60	18	129.6	1.296	4.25	177.4	1.774	5.82
70	20	127.2	1.272	4.17	174.9	1.749	5.74

*See data source for height normalized gait speed factor for each age group.
Data source: Bohannon RW. Comfortable and maximum walking speed of adults aged 20–79 years: reference values and determinants. *Age and Ageing* 1997;26:15–19. Table 4.

TABLE 3-9

GAIT SPEED IN SINGLE TASK AND DUAL TASK CONDITIONS IN YOUNG ADULTS

Group (N = 14 in all groups)	Day 2 (m/s) Single Task	Day 2 (m/s) Dual Task
Concussed Athletes	1.227 ± 0.150	1.101 ± 0.174
Concussed Nonathlete	1.270 ± 1.127	1.321 ± 0.114
Normal Athlete	1.217 ± 0.134	1.196 ± 0.152
Normal Nonathlete	1.381 ± 0.107	1.391 ± 0.142

Data source: Parker TM, Osternig LR, van Donkelaar P, Chou LS. Balance control during gait in athletes and non-athletes following concussion. *Med Eng Phys.* Oct 2008;30(8):959–967.

TABLE 3-10

MINIMAL DETECTABLE CHANGE IN GAIT SPEED FOR MEN AND WOMEN IN THEIR 20S DURING COMFORTABLE AND FAST WALKING

MDC 90%	Comfortable m/s	Comfortable ft/s	Fast m/s	Fast ft/s
Men	0.11	0.36	0.20	0.67
Women	0.13	0.41	0.18	0.60

Data source: Bohannon RW. Comfortable and maximum walking speed of adults aged 20–79 years: reference values and determinants. *Age Ageing.* 1997;26(1):15–19.

Responsiveness Estimates

- Functional walking categories[92]
  - physiologic walker: 0.1 m/s
  - limited household walker: 0.23 m/s
  - unlimited household walker: 0.27 m/s
  - most limited household walker: 0.4 m/s
  - least limited household walker: 0.58 m/s
  - community walker: 0.8 m/s

Reliability Estimates

- Internal consistency: not applicable
- Interrater: In a group of 12 ambulatory subjects an average of 15.8 months after TBI (initial mean Glasgow Come Scale score of 5.8), interrater reliability (IRR) of five trials of comfortably paced walking speed was 0.99, and IRR of fast-paced walking speed was 0.99. In persons with stroke, r = 1.0.[100]
- Intrarater: not available
- Test-Retest: comfortable walking speed ICC (3,1) = 0.903. Fast walking speed ICC (3,1) = 0.910 (adults)[101]

Validity Estimates

- Content/Face: not applicable

- Criterion: In a group of 12 ambulatory subjects, an average of 15.8 months after TBI (initial mean Glasgow Come Scale score of 5.8), correlation of a stopwatch measure over a known distance to measurement with infrared timing gates indicated a perfect concurrent validity.[96]
- Construct: Age, height, and hip, knee, and ankle muscle strength correlated significantly (P < 0.05) with both comfortable and maximum gait speed. Gender correlated significantly with maximum gait speed. Leisure activity and work activity were not significantly correlated with either comfortable or maximum gait speed.[101]
- Within the first 48 hours following concussion, gait velocity was found to be significantly slower in concussed subjects than in normal subjects in both single- and dual-task conditions.[102]
- Following TBI, 10 subjects (4 with mild TBI, with GCS scores greater than 12, 9 subjects evaluated within 2 years after their injury) walked with a significantly slower gait speed (1.15 +/− .17 m/s) than 10 age-, gender-, height-, and weight-matched controls (1.31 +/− 1.1).[103]

Selected References

van Loo MA, Moseley AM, Bossman JM, de Bie RA, Hassett L. Inter-rater reliability and concurrent validity of walking speed measurement after traumatic brain injury. *Clinical Rehab.* 2003;17:775–779.

van Loo MA, Moseley AM, Bossman JM, de Bie RA, Hassett L. Test-retest reliability of walking speed, step length and step width measurement after traumatic brain injury: a pilot study. *Brain Inj.* 2004;18(10):1041–1048.

GAIT SPEED

General Instructions

- Mark off a 20-ft (6.1-m) unobstructed walkway on the floor with colored tape.
- Mark an additional 5 ft (0.91 m) from the start and end of the walkway (total 30 ft) for acceleration and deceleration and place a cone, pylon, or other marker at the finish line (before the 5-ft deceleration zone).
- Start the subject at the beginning of the acceleration zone. Begin timing when the subject's first foot crosses the start line marker. Stop timing when the subject's first foot crosses the finish line marker.
- Record the time to the tenths of a second. Record the faster of two trials.
- Gait speed is measured in distance walked in a given time (gait speed = distance / time; eg, 20 ft / 4.1 seconds = 4.88 ft / sec = 1.49 m / sec), typically measured in meters per second or feet per second.
- The time in distance (meters or feet) is divided by the number of seconds recorded (Exhibit 3-6).
- Therapist should walk next to the subject and use a gait belt if there are any safety concerns.

Standardized Instructions to Give at the Start Line

- *Walk at a comfortable walking speed to the cone at the end of the walkway.*
- *Walk as fast as you can safely walk to the cone at the end of the walkway.*

Note: If space considerations warrant, any standard distance can be used with markers at the start and finish line and 3 to 5 feet before and after the lines for acceleration and deceleration. Gait speed is usually reported in meters per second but can be reported in feet per second as long as the comparisons are consistent.

EXHIBIT 3-6

GAIT SPEED RECORDING

Comfortable Speed:
  Trial 1 _____ seconds   Trial 2 _____ seconds

Fast Speed:
  Trial 1 _____ seconds   Trial 2 _____ seconds

FUNCTIONAL GAIT ASSESSMENT

The FGA is a ten-item gait assessment based on the Dynamic Gait Index (DGI) developed to avoid the ceiling effect of the DGI in persons with vestibular disorders. Items added to the DGI were gait with narrow base of support, ambulating backwards, and gait with eyes closed.[8] The maximum FGA total score is 30, with each item measured on a 0-to-3 scale (Exhibit 3-7).

Recommended Instrument Use

A standardized measure of gait ability is recommended. Options include the FGA in addition to a measure of gait speed.

Administration Protocol/Equipment/Time

The FGA takes approximately 20 minutes and requires a marked, 20-ft (6-m) walkway with a marked 12-inch (30.48-cm) width.

Groups Tested With This Measure

Groups tested with this measure include 6 patients with vestibular disorders[8]; 200 adults, ages 40 to 89 years, living independently[104]; 35 subjects with balance deficits (mean age 66.6 with SD 13.9) and 39 control subjects (mean age of 32.2 with SD 15.1)[105]; and 35 older adults aged 60 to 90 years.[106]

Interpretability

- Norms: See Table 3-11. In a comparison of the FGA and the SOT for 39 control subjects (nonfallers) with mean age of 32.2 (SD 15.1), the mean FGA score was 24.8 (SD 4.6), with a 95% confidence interval of 23.6 to 26.1[105]
- MDC: not available. If the patient's score is less than the MDC value, it is considered indistinguishable from measurement error.

EXHIBIT 3-7

ADDITIONAL RESOURCES FOR FUNCTIONAL GAIT ASSESSMENT

This instrument can be obtained from the original publication:

Wrisley DM, Marchetti GF, Kuharsky DK, Whitney SL. Reliability, internal consistency and validity of data obtained with the Functional Gait Assessment. *Phys Ther*. 2004;84:906–918.

It can be found through links at the following websites:

- Rehabilitation Measures Database www.rehabmeasures.org/rehabweb/allmeasures. aspx?PageView=Shared
- Geriatric Examination Toolkit (University of Missouri) web.missouri.edu/~proste/tool/vest/index. htm

---

Responsiveness Estimates: not available

Reliability Estimates (tested with experienced and student therapists)

- Internal consistency: Chronbach's alpha = 0.79 across two trials. Item-to-corrected-item correlations ranged from 0.12 to 0.80.[8]
- Interrater
  - Total score: ICC = 0.84
  - Percent agreement:0 58%
  - Individual items: 40%–90%
  - Kappa: 0.50
  - Individual items 0.16–0.83[8] This study involved raters who were not trained on the FGA.
  - ICC (model 2) = 0.93 for 200 adults, ages 40–89 years old, living independently.[104] This study involved raters who were trained on the FGA.
- Intrarater
  - Total score: ICC = 0.83
  - Percent agreement: 67%
  - Individual items: 60%–90%
  - Kappa: 0.50
  - Individual items: 0.37–0.78 (raters were not trained on the FGA)[8]
- Test-Retest: not available

Validity Estimates

- Content/Face: FGA is based on the DGI, which was developed to assess postural stability during gait tasks in older adults

at risk of falling. Because of the ceiling effect of the DGI in younger patients with vestibular disorders who still report gait difficulties, the FGA was constructed as a modified version of the DGI with one item removed and three items added.[8]

- Criterion: FGA scores were correlated with the ABC Scale scores (r = 0.64), DHI scores (r = –0.64), perception of dizziness symptoms on a Visual Analog Scale (r = – 0.70), number of falls (r = – 0.66), Timed Up and Go scores (r = 0.50), and DGI scores (r = 0.80).[104]

  FGA scores demonstrated high correlation with the SOT (r = 0.713), high negative correlation between the FGA and age (r = – 0.786), and moderate negative correlation between the FGA and fall history (r = – 0.573) in 35 subjects with balance deficits (mean age 66.6 with SD 13.9) and 39 control subjects (mean age of 32.2 with SD 15.1).[105]

  In 35 older adults aged 60 to 90 years, the FGA correlated with the ABC Scale (r = 0.053), Berg Balance Scale (r = 0.84), and Timed Up and Go Test (r = – 0.84).[106]

- Construct: Mean total scores for the FGA show a systematic decrease with increased age, especially in subjects aged 70 years and older.[104] According to Wrisley and Kumar, the "FGA (scores 22/30) provided 100% sensitivity, 72% specificity, positive likelihood ratio of 3.6, and negative likelihood ratio of 0 to predict prospective falls."[106]

TABLE 3-11

FUNCTIONAL GAIT ASSESSMENT TOTAL SCORES BY DECADE

Age (y)	N	Minimum Score	Maximum Score	Mean	Standard Deviation	95% Confidence Interval
40–49	27	24	30	28.9	1.5	28.3–29.5
50–59	33	25	30	28.4	1.6	27.9–29.0
60–69	63	20	30	27.1	2.3	26.5–27.7
70–79	44	16	30	24.9	3.6	23.9–26.0
80–89	33	10	28	20.8	4.7	19.2–22.6
Total	**200**	**10**	**30**	**26.2**	**4.0**	**25.5–26.6**

Reproduced with permission from: Walker ML, Austin AG, Banke GM, et al. Reference group data for the Functional Gait Assessment. *Phys Ther*. 2007;87(11):1468–1477. Used with permission of the American Physical Therapy Association. This material is copyrighted, and any further reproduction or distribution is prohibited.

ILLINOIS AGILITY TEST

Purpose/Description

The IAT requires a person to run short distances while navigating obstacles; it involves speeded cutting and direction changes.[9]

Recommended Instrument Use

A standardized measure of agility that was developed for physical fitness testing in healthy populations, this test is relevant for service members because it tests high-level mobility on a course that requires maneuvering with fast directional changes.

Administration Protocol/Equipment/Time

The IAT takes approximately 5 minutes to administer. It requires a flat, nonslip surface, stopwatch, eight cones, and a measuring tape to set up the course. The course is 10 m in length by 5 m in width. Four cones mark the corners of the perimeter of the course: the start line is marked by two cones on one end, and the turning line is marked by two cones on the opposite side of the 10-m length. The additional four cones are positioned equidistant (3.3 m apart) along the center of the 10-m length at the 2.5-m mark.

A "jog-through" of the course and the pattern that is traversed is necessary prior to timed testing. Use Figure 3-3 to set up the course and to instruct service members in the expected pattern. Initial testing protocol requires the service member to start positioned at the left of the starting line in a push-up position, with the vertex of the head in line with the starting line (position A). When given the "go" signal, the service member stands and runs to touch the base of the cone on the far left of the course (position B), then returns to the center cone that is closest to the starting line, proceeding in a serpentine pattern around each of the four cones in the center of the course. At the fourth cone, the service member continues the serpentine pattern back to the first cone near the start line. After rounding that cone for the second time, the service member runs quickly to the cone on the far right of the course (position C), touches the base of it, and returns to the starting line as quickly as possible (position D). Starting position may be modified to standing; however, norms would no longer apply. If the required-size space is not available in a clinical environment, a smaller course could be created; however, norms would not be translatable to a different course.

The test is administered twice and the fastest of the two times is recorded.

Groups Tested With This Measure

Details of data gathered to establish norms are unpublished, but are presumed to include healthy, active college students from a textbook by Getchell.[9] These values are reproduced in numerous other sources.[107,108] Additional studies have focused on elite soccer athletes,[109] law enforcement officers,[110] and US Army Soldiers who were active and healthy.[111] This group also studied service members with transtibial and transfemoral amputation.[112]

Interpretability

- Norms: Mean IAT time for a group of active duty service members (97 male soldiers, mean age 26.2 years, mean number of physical training days per week 5.0) was 18.17 seconds (SD 1.14 s).[111] Law enforcement officer standards[110] suggest a police academy entrance standard of 22.3 seconds, requiring scores of 18.6 on average for men and 20.2 seconds for women to meet performance standards following training. FitForce Guidelines[113] suggest median scores for federal and municipal agencies at 18.1 to 18.2 seconds (Table 3-12).
- MDC: no data available

Responsiveness Estimates: no data available

Reliability Estimates

- Internal consistency: not available
- Interrater: ICC values for a battery of balance and fitness tests including the IAT ranged from 0.924 to 0.995 for healthy service members, and 0.97 to 0.99 for service members with amputation.[114]
- Intrarater: no data available
- Test-Retest: ICC values were higher for service members with amputation than for a healthy comparison group.[114] Serial tests for elite soccer athletes over the course of a season showed average scores varied slightly, but remained on average in the range of 14.63 to 14.97 seconds (SD 0.38 s).[109]

Validity Estimates

- Content/Face: The IAT is commonly used in athletic populations to assess speed and agility while running with direction changes and obstacle avoidance. The prone starting position has face validity: the ability to rapidly move from prone to running is similar to rapid transitions necessary in combat situations.
- Criterion: IAT performance times were highly correlated with times for two tests of agility, the T-test and the modified Edgren side-step test in a sample of 97 active duty, male, US Army soldiers (mean age 26.2 years, SD 5.5 years; mean number of

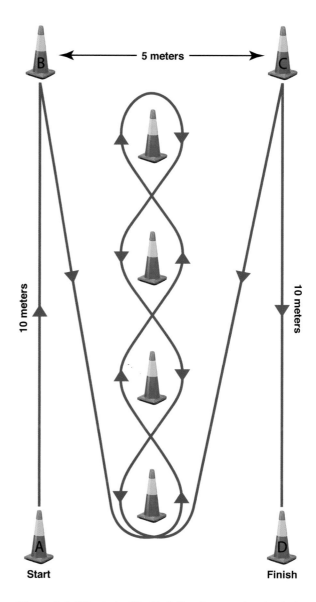

Figure 3-3. Illinois Agility Test. Service member to starts positioned at the left of the starting line in a push-up position, vertex of the head in line with the starting line (position A). When given the "go" signal, the service member stands and runs to touch the base of the cone on the far left of the course (position B), then returns to the center cone closest to the starting line, proceeding in a serpentine pattern around each of the four cones in the center of the course. At the fourth cone, the service member continues the serpentine pattern back to the first cone near the start line. After rounding that cone for the second time, the service member runs quickly to the cone on the far right of the course (position C), touches the base of it, and returns to the starting line as quickly as possible (position D). The test is administered twice and the fastest of the two times is recorded.

physical training days per week 5.0, SD .8 days; mean height 70.0 in., SD 2.5 in.; mean weight 181.4 lb, SD 23.2 lb).[111]

- Construct: Known groups comparison: a study of 97 active duty soldiers and 62 service members with amputation (42 with unilateral transtibial amputation, 20 with unilateral transfemoral amputation) performed three speed and agility tests. Analysis of variance showed significant group differences for active duty and amputee service members on the tests. Individuals with transtibial amputation performed better than those with transfemoral amputation, although 51% of the unilateral transtibial amputees performed within the range of values seen in the active duty control group. None of the transfemoral amputees completed tests in the active duty range.[112]

TABLE 3-12

TYPICAL ILLINOIS AGILITY TEST TIMES AND RATINGS*

Rating	Male	Female
Excellent	< 15.2	< 17.0
Good	16.1–15.2	17.9–17.0
Average	18.1–16.2	21.7–18.0
Fair	18.3–18.2	23.0–21.8
Poor	> 18.3	> 23.0

*This chart is available from multiple sources[1–3] but original data were not published, so specifics of test population age, size, and testing methods are not available. Clinicians using this test on a regular basis suggest the values for higher-level skill are rarely observed in practice, even with uninjured individuals. Therefore the accuracy of the ratings is debatable. Test results may be better interpreted as an evaluative measure for an individual gauging his or her improvement over time.
Data sources: 1) Getchell B. *Physical Fitness: A Way of Life*. 4th ed. 4th ed. New York, NY: Macmillan Publishing Company; 1992. 2) Roozen M. Illinois Agility Test. *National Strength and Conditioning Association's Performance Training Journal*. 2004;3(5):5–6. 3) Reiman MP, Manske RC. *Functional Testing in Human Performance*. Champaign, Il: Human Kinetics; 2009.

Selected References

Caldwell BP, Peters DM. Seasonal variation in physiological fitness of a semiprofessional soccer team. *J Strength Conditioning Res*. 2009;23(5):1370–1377.

Gaunaurd Ignacio A. The Comprehensive High-level Activity Mobility Predictor (CHAMP): a performance-based assessment instrument to quantify high-level mobility in service members with traumatic lower limb loss. *Open Access Dissertations*. 2012: Paper 712.

Getchell B. *Physical Fitness: A Way of Life*. 4th ed. New York, NY: Macmillan Publishing Company; 1992: 69–72.

Hoffman & Associates. Physical readiness standards validation of the Nevada P.O.S.T. Category I Peace Officers in Total Fitness for Public Safety: Executive Summary. 2009. http://apps.post.nv.gov/Administration/Cat2%20Physical%20Readiness%20Standards%20Validation%20Report.pdf. Accessed March 7, 2014.

Integrated Fitness Systems/FitForce. Fitness Tests, Standards and Norms. What is Valid? What is Legal? Salem, MA: FitForce; 2007: 8. http://fitforce.org/documents/Microsoft_Word_-_Whitepaper_-_CIAR.0307.pdf. Accessed July 17, 2013.

Raya MA, Jayne D, Linberg A, Manrique P, Gagne E, Muller D, Tucker C. Criterion validity of the modified Edgren side-step and the Illinois agility test in a healthy athletic population. *JOSPT*. 2009;39(1):A116.

Reiman MP, Manske RC. *Functional Testing in Human Performance*. Champaign, IL: Human Kinetics; 2009: 199, 208.

Roozen M. Illinois Agility Test. *NCSA's Performance Training Journal*. 2004;3(5):3–5.

FIVE TIMES SIT-TO-STAND TEST

Purpose/Description

The Five Times Sit-To-Stand Test (FTSST) is a physical performance test initially developed to measure lower-extremity muscle strength.[3] It has also been used to examine functional status, balance, and vestibular dysfunction, and to distinguish between fallers and nonfallers.[115–119] Other versions include the Timed Stands Test and the Ten Chair Stands Test.

Recommended Instrument Use

The FTSST is a functional strength test option. Therapists should consider using it in addition to other strength screening tests.

Administration Protocol/Equipment/Time

Stopwatch and armless chair (height 43 cm, depth 47.5 cm) are required for the FTSST. The test takes less than 1 minute to administer. A practice trial can be given.

Groups Tested With This Measure

The FTSST has been used to test healthy males and females,[3] older adults,[119] and persons with balance deficits,[119] vestibular loss,[118] arthritis, renal disease,[120] and stroke.[115] The FTSST and other versions (Timed Stands, the Ten Times Sit-to-Stand Test) have been used as outcome measures after intervention.[119]

Interpretability

- Norms: 16 men and 16 women healthy normal subjects (age range 23-57 years) had a mean of 8.2 seconds (SD 0.3s), a range of 4.9 to 12.7 seconds, and a 95% CI of 7.5 to 8.8 seconds.[119]
  Using a time cutoff of 13 seconds, the FTSST identified subjects with balance dysfunction with a sensitivity (66%) and specificity (67%) in subjects 23 to 90 years old (both normal controls and subjects with balance dysfunction). For just those subjects less than 60 years old, the sensitivity (87%) and specificity (84%) was optimal at a cutoff point of 10 seconds.[119]
- MDC (95% CI): estimates vary depending on variability of test population. In 12 normal controls (adults ages 18–55 years old), using a 90% confidence interval Blake and O'Meara (2004) found a MDC of 0.4 seconds.[120] In 30 older adults after hip fracture, using a 90% confidence interval Sherrington and Lord (2005) found a MDC of 6.7 seconds.[121] If the patient's score is less than the MDC value, it is considered indistinguishable from measurement error.

Responsiveness Estimates

One hundred and seventeen patients (45 men, 72 women), mean age 62.7 years, with peripheral, central, or mixed vestibular dysfunction underwent vestibular rehabilitation. Logistic regression showed that an improvement in the FTSST of greater than 2.3 seconds resulted in an odds ratio of 4.67 for demonstrating clinical improvement in DHI, compared to a change less than 2.3 seconds.[118] Subjects with central vestibular dysfunction (n = 12) showed an improvement of 6.8 seconds (+/− 6.3) in the FTSST from before to after rehabilitation.[122]

Reliability Estimates

- Internal consistency: not available
- Interrater: in individuals ages 60 and older ICC = 0.71 (n = 392)[123]
- Intrarater: in individuals ages 60 and older ICC = 0.64 (n = 392).[123] In 12 renal patients (ages 18–55 years old) and 12 age-matched controls, ICC = 0.98.[120]
- Test-Retest: ICC (3,1) = 0.92 (95% CI 0.84–0.97) for 27 inpatients and outpatients who had suffered a hip fracture.[121]

Validity Estimates

- Content/Face: The sit-to-stand task is a functional skill that requires lower-extremity strength.
- Criterion: For 72 subjects with balance or vestibular disorders and 81 control subjects (age range 23–90 years), the Spearman rho between the FTSST and DGI was –0.68 (P < 0.001), and between the FTSST and the ABC Scale was –0.58 (P < 0.001).[119]
- Construct: In 89 control- and balance-impaired subjects younger than 60 years old, the FTSST correctly identified subjects with balance disorders 81% of the time.[119]

Selected Reference

Csuka M, McCarty DJ. Simple method for measurement of lower extremity muscle strength. *Am J Med*. 1985;78:77–81.

FIVE TIMES SIT-TO-STAND TEST ADMINISTRATION

Purpose/Description

This test provides an assessment of lower-extremity muscle strength.[3] It may also be used to examine functional status, balance, and vestibular dysfunction.

Equipment

Stopwatch and armless chair (43 cm high, 47.5 cm deep). Use consistent chair when monitoring change over time so that the chair seat height remains constant. Testing takes less than 1 minute. A practice trial may be given.

Administration

- Subjects sit in the armless chair with their trunk against the back.
- Subjects cross their arms over their chest.

- Subjects are allowed to place their feet comfortably under them during testing.
- Timing begins when examiner says "go" and stops when the subject's buttocks touch the chair on the fifth repetition.

Instructions From Examiner

- *I want you to stand up and sit down five times as quickly as you can when I say "go."*
- *Stand up fully between repetitions and to not touch the back of the chair during each repetition of sitting down.*

Test Results: Time _____ seconds (to 0.1 second)

Developers: Csuka M, McCarty DJ. Simple method for measurement of lower extremity muscle strength. *Am J Med*. 1985;78:77–81.

SECTION 2: BALANCE INTERVENTION

Intervention

Balance issues that result from c/mTBI are often related to vestibular deficits. Balance retraining programs improved symptoms in military personnel with dizziness associated with TBI.[124,125] Task and environmental conditions may influence balance when impairments are present. Therapists should consider modifying the complexity of balance tasks (simplify to allow success) and analyze the effects of reducing environmental complexity on balance as a part of the examination and intervention process. Typically, a program begins with simple balance tasks done in a quiet environment and slowly progresses the task demands and task environment so as to avoiding overwhelming a service member with a balance disorder, especially if it occurs in connection with vestibular deficits. Balance retraining programs include progressively more challenging tasks and environments,[126] including sports and martial arts activities to make them relevant for service members. Additionally, posturography platforms may be considered in treatment situations to provide practice adjusting to altered platform stability and sensory conditions.[124] The expectation for carryover from posturography platform training to improvement in functional abilities should be examined in c/mTBI. While the use of posturography in persons with stroke has resulted in improved static standing balance, improvement did not carry over to functional activities in the stroke population.[127]

For a progressive balance intervention program related to residual vestibular deficits, see Chapter 2: Vestibular Assessment and Intervention. For those complex patients who have been assessed using the BESTest, the identified subsystems can be used as the basis for designing an individualized treatment program. For example, deficits in biomechanical constraints may indicate a need for specific strengthening or stretching, or for further assessment in footwear.

Background

Given that balance deficits that arise in conjunction with c/mTBI typically occur as a result of vestibular dysfunction, a vestibular rehabilitation program (see Chapter 2: Vestibular Assessment and Intervention) often resolves the balance deficits. Significant improvements in balance after vestibular rehabilitation are reported and are believed to be "related to habituation or adaptation of the central nervous system, sensory substitution, or reweighting of the sensory systems."[128] Information on recovery of balance issues following c/mTBI is primarily available as it relates to return to sports.[129] High-level balance dysfunction may be more evident after the service member has been stressed by exercise or intense work. Therapists should be aware of the need to increase task challenges progressively and monitor perception of exertion accordingly. Note that factors such as specific diagnosis, emotional state, age, and symptom duration may all affect the outcome of intervention for balance deficits.[128]

Strength of Recommendation: Practice Option

Descriptive studies have shown that balance retraining programs improve symptoms in military personnel with dizziness associated with TBI.[124] Evidence for precise balance retraining interventions has not been found specific to individuals with c/mTBI. Suggestions presented here are taken from the literature regarding vestibular rehabilitation, motor learning, stroke, and the elderly.[128] Balance retraining as part of a vestibular rehabilitation program is considered a **practice standard**. The use of CDP platforms has been suggested for balance retraining, though evidence for carryover for improvements in abilities on CDP have not yet been shown in persons with c/mTBI as it relates to clinical measures of balance.

Intervention Methods

- Provide education and training on a graded exercise program with a slow, symptom-free return to full activity. Encourage the symptom-free implementation of a progressive fitness program as tolerated, incorporating activities and sports that challenge balance while recognizing the need for safety and the avoidance of a second injury (see Chapter 2: Vestibular Assessment and Intervention).
- Educate the service member regarding adaptability of the nervous system and the need to challenge the nervous system to facilitate recovery. The service member should understand that avoiding activity because of symptom provocation may delay recovery.
- A "Points to Remember" sheet is included for therapists designing balance and strengthening intervention programs.
- When appropriate, the specific subsystems identified on the BESTest[4] or Mini-BESTest[11] as contributing to balance or strength deficits can be used as the basis for designing an individualized treatment program.

HIGHER-LEVEL BALANCE AND FUNCTIONAL ABILITIES: THERAPIST POINTS TO REMEMBER

- The ability to avoid reinjury (impaired visual-spatial skills and postural control) is often diminished for weeks to a few months following c/mTBI, even when clinic-based assessments are normal. Design of an individualized balance retraining program **must** take into account safety and avoidance of a second injury.
- Dual tasks that combine cognitive and physical abilities may more closely simulate the complexities of service member duties. For a service member, individual task components may test as normal, but a problem emerges when multiple tasks are combined.
- Studies on specific balance retraining programs following c/mTBI are limited because function typically returns to baseline within a few weeks to 3 months following c/mTBI. Many of the suggestions for balance interventions come from studies on moderate to severe TBI, stroke, and other patient populations.[130,131] Chapter 10: Fitness Assessment and Intervention, in this toolkit, and new Return to Activity Clinical guidelines published by the Defense and Veterans Brain Injury Center (2013) should be reviewed prior to initiating intensive balance retraining programs where heart rate and blood pressure significantly increase.[132]
- Given that balance deficits following c/mTBI (specifically blast-related c/mTBI) are often related to vestibular deficits, initial balance retraining activities should be graded and interventions designed to avoid sensory overload. Tasks that require

head turning or gaze stability while moving may be especially challenging if there are vestibular deficits. The service member who becomes overly symptomatic during balance exercises will likely not comply with a retraining program.

- As with all learning tasks, important variables to consider when retraining postural control are the quantity, duration, and intensity of training sessions.[133] Evidence on the optimum frequency and duration of practice for balance activities specifically following c/mTBI is not yet available.
- Learning and retraining are enhanced by training specificity, motivating activities important to the individual (leisure or work related), and varied feedback schedules. Eventual progression of activities that include military occupation-related tasks, such as climbing into and over vehicles and walls, completing obstacle courses, negotiating uneven terrain, crawling, altering speeds, and adapting to environmental complexity are encouraged, as long as safety and avoidance of a second injury are considered.
- When designing and analyzing tasks for

progression of balance programs, the therapist may want to consider Gentile's taxonomy[134] and evaluate the environment (stationary or in motion), the body (body is stable or in transport), and whether or not there is manipulation (hand use). Advancing all three contexts or components of tasks simultaneously may overwhelm some service members.

- Virtual-reality–based games and activities may provide the intensity and motivation important to retraining balance in this population.[133]
- Preliminary evidence indicates that exercise programs such as Tai Chi Chuan (commonly known as tai chi) provide at least short-term benefits in health status, mood, and self-esteem in persons with TBI,[131] as well as improved balance and reduced risk of falls in older persons.[135,136]
- Consider a water-based, balance retraining program as an adjunct to land-based therapies; there may be reduced fear of falling and injury while in an aquatic environment during challenging balance tasks[137] (ensure the environment does not exacerbate vestibular complaints).

Selected References

Gordon WA, Sliwinski M, Echo J, McLoughlin M, Sheerer MS, Meili TE. The benefits of exercise in individuals with traumatic brain injury: a retrospective study. *J Head Trauma Rehabil*. 1998;13(4):58–67.

Haskell WL, Lee IM, Pate RR, et al. Physical activity and public health: updated recommendations for adults from the American College of Sports Medicine and the American Heart Association. *Med Sci Sports Exerc*. 2007;39(8):1423–1434.

FITNESS AND CONDITIONING PROGRAM FOR BALANCE RETRAINING FOLLOWING VESTIBULAR DYSFUNCTION

A fitness and conditioning program should be introduced as soon as tolerated. This program should include balance retraining or a walking or stationary cycling program to combat fatigue secondary to deconditioning. All healthy adults aged 18 to 65 years need moderate-intensity aerobic physical activity for a minimum of 30 minutes on 5 days each week, and activities to increase muscular strength and endurance for a minimum of 2 days each week.[138] Exercise may improve mood and aspects of health status in individuals with TBI.[139]

The following specific suggestions may be made to the service member:

- Start slowly and increase the duration and intensity of your exercises over time.
- Monitor your heart rate or rate of perceived exertion.
- Vary your exercise program to keep from becoming bored.
- Use a calendar, notebook, or smartphone to keep track of your exercise days and times.

Activity suggestions include:

- Walking or stationary cycling to combat fatigue secondary to deconditioning. When cleared by the referring physician, progress to other aerobic exercises, such as running and swimming.[140]

- Avocational activities that are fun and that challenge balance and vision simultaneously, such as:
  - golf,
  - bowling,
  - tennis,
  - racquetball,
  - ping-pong,
  - dancing,
  - cycling,
  - cross-country skiing, or
  - hiking.
- Alternative balance activities, such as tai chi or other noncontact martial arts or yoga.
- Incorporate service-specific physical fitness requirements for running, pushups, and sit-ups (see Chapter 10, Fitness Assessment and Intervention, for service-specific websites).

Selected References

Gordon WA, Sliwinski M, Echo J, McLoughlin M, Sheerer MS, Meili TE. The benefits of exercise in individuals with traumatic brain injury: a retrospective study. *J Head Trauma Rehabil.* 1998;13(4):58–67.

Haskell WL, Lee IM, Pate RR, et al. Physical activity and public health: updated recommendations for adults from the American College of Sports Medicine and the American Heart Association. *Med Sci Sports Exer.* 2007;39(8):1423–1434.

REFERENCES

1. Gottshall KR. Vestibular rehabilitation after mild traumatic brain injury with vestibular pathology. *NeuroRehabilitation.* 2011;29:167–171.

2. Scherer MR, Schubert MC. Traumatic brain injury and vestibular pathology as a comorbidity after blast exposure. *Phys Ther.* Sep 2009;89(9):980–992.

3. Csuka M, McCarty DJ. Simple method for measurement of lower extremity muscle strength. *Am J Med.* Jan 1985;78(1):77–81.

4. Horak FB, Wrisley DM, Frank J. The Balance Evaluation Systems Test (BESTest) to differentiate balance deficits. *Phys Ther.* May 2009;89(5):484–498.

5. Shumway-Cook A, Horak FB. Assessing the influence of sensory interaction of balance. Suggestion from the field. *Phys Ther.* Oct 1986;66(10):1548–1550.

6. Cleland JA, Fritz JM, Whitman JM, Palmer JA. The reliability and construct validity of the Neck Disability Index and patient specific functional scale in patients with cervical radiculopathy. *Spine.* 2006;31(5):598–602.

7. Podsiadlo D, Richardson S. The time "Up & Go": a test of basic functional mobility for frail elderly persons. *J Am Geriatr Soc.* Feb 1991;39(2):142–148.

8. Wrisley DM, Marchetti GF, Kuharsky DK, Whitney SL. Reliability, internal consistency, and validity of data obtained with the functional gait assessment. *Phys Ther.* 2004;84(10):906–918.

9. Getchell B. *Physical Fitness: A Way of Life, 4th ed.* 4th ed. New York, NY: Macmillan Publishing Company; 1992.

10. Pickett TC, Radfar-Baublitz LS, McDonald SD, Walker WC, Cifu DX. Objectively assessing balance deficits after TBI: role of computerized posturography. *J Rehabil Res Dev.* 2007;44(7):983–990.

11. Franchignoni F, Horak F, Godi M, Nardone A, Giordano A. Using psychometric techniques to improve the Balance Evaluation Systems Test: the mini-BESTest. *J Rehabil Med.* Apr 2010;42(4):323–331.

12. Powell LE, Myers AM. The activities-specific Balance Confidence (ABC) scale. *J Gerontol A Biol Sci Med Sci.* Jan 1995;50A(1):M28.

13. Myers AM, Fletcher PC, Myers AH, Sherk W. Discriminative and evaluative properties of the activities-specific balance confidence (ABC) scale. *J Gerontol A Biol Sci Med Sci.* Jul 1998;53(4):M287–294.

14. Gottshall KR, Moore RJ, Hoffer ME. Vestibular rehabilitation for migraine-associated dizziness. *Int Tinnitus J.* 2005;11(1):81–84.

15. Whitney SL, Hudak MT, Marchetti GF. The activities-specific balance confidence scale and the dizziness handicap inventory: a comparison. *J Vestib Res.* 1999;9(4):253–259.

16. Whitney SL, Wrisley DM, Brown KE, Furman JM. Physical therapy for migraine-related vestibulopathy and vestibular dysfunction with history of migraine. *Laryngoscope.* 2000;110(9):1528–1534.

17. Botner EM, Miller WC, Eng JJ. Measurement properties of the Activities-specific Balance Confidence Scale among individuals with stroke. *Disabil Rehabil.* Feb 18 2005;27(4):156–163.

18. Miller WC, Deathe AB, Speechley M. Psychometric properties of the Activities-specific Balance Confidence Scale among individuals with a lower-limb amputation. *Arch Phys Med Rehabil.* May 2003;84(5):656–661.

19. Wrisley DM, Whitney SL, Furman JM. Vestibular rehabilitation outcomes in patients with a history of migraine. *Otol Neurotol.* 2002;23(4):483–487.

20. Brown KE, Whitney SL, Wrisley DM, Furman JM. Physical therapy outcomes for persons with bilateral vestibular loss. *Laryngoscope.* Oct 2001;111(10):1812–1817.

21. Talley KM, Wyman JF, Gross CR. Psychometric properties of the activities-specific balance confidence scale and the survey of activities and fear of falling in older women. *J Am Geriatr Soc.* Feb 2008;56(2):328–333.

22. Cho BL, Scarpace D, Alexander NB. Tests of stepping as indicators of mobility, balance, and fall risk in balance-impaired older adults. *J Am Geriatr Soc.* Jul 2004;52(7):1168–1173.

23. Kressig RW, Wolf SL, Sattin RW, et al. Associations of demographic, functional, and behavioral characteristics with activity-related fear of falling among older adults transitioning to frailty. *J Am Geriatr Soc.* Nov 2001;49(11):1456–1462.

24. Springer BA, Marin R, Cyhan T, Roberts H, Gill NW. Normative values for the unipedal stance test with eyes open and closed. *J Geriatr Phys Ther.* 2007;30(1):8–15.

25. Kammerlind AS, Larsson PB, Ledin T, Skargren E. Reliability of clinical balance tests and subjective ratings in dizziness and disequilibrium. *Adv Physiother.* 2005;7(3):96–107.

26. Balogun JA, Ajayi LO, Alawale F. Determinants of single limb stance balance performance. *Afr J Med Med Sci.* Sep-Dec 1997;26(3–4):153–157.

27. Berg KO, Wood-Dauphinee SL, Williams JI, Maki B. Measuring balance in the elderly: validation of an instrument. *Can J Public Health.* Jul-Aug 1992;83(suppl 2):S7–11.

28. Cyarto EV, Brown WJ, Marshall AL, Trost SG. Comparative effects of home- and group-based exercise on balance confidence and balance ability in older adults: cluster randomized trial. *Gerontology.* 2008;54(5):272–280.

29. Bohannon RW, Larkin PA, Cook AC, Gear J, Singer J. Decrease in timed balance test scores with aging. *Phys Ther.* Jul 1984;64(7):1067–1070.

30. Hurvitz EA, Richardson JK, Werner RA, Ruhl AM, Dixon MR. Unipedal stance testing as an indicator of fall risk among older outpatients. *Arch Phys Med Rehabil.* May 2000;81(5):587–591.

31. Vaillant J, Vuillerme N, Martigne P, et al. Balance, aging, and osteoporosis: effects of cognitive exercises combined with physiotherapy. *Joint Bone Spine.* Jul 2006;73(4):414–418.

32. Romberg MH. *Manual of Nervous System Diseases of Man.* London, England: Sydenham Society; 1853.

33. Black FO, Wall C 3rd, Rockette HE Jr, Kitch R. Normal subject postural sway during the Romberg test. *Am J Otolaryngol.* Sep–Oct 1982;3(5):309–318.

34. Franchignoni F, Tesio L, Martino MT, Ricupero C. Reliability of four simple, quantitative tests of balance and mobility in healthy elderly females. *Aging (Milano).* Feb 1998;10(1):26–31.

35. Bloem BR, Grimbergen YA, Cramer M, Willemsen M, Zwinderman AH. Prospective assessment of falls in Parkinson's disease. *J Neurol.* Nov 2001;248(11):950–958.

36. Heitmann DK, Gossman MR, Shaddeau SA, Jackson JR. Balance performance and step width in noninstitutionalized, elderly, female fallers and nonfallers. *Phys Ther.* Nov 1989;69(11):923–931.

37. Vereeck L, Wuyts F, Truijen S, Van de Heyning P. Clinical assessment of balance: normative data, and gender and age effects. *Int J Audiol.* Feb 2008;47(2):67–75.

38. Steffen TM, Seney M. Test-retest reliability and minimal detectable change on balance and ambulation tests, the 36-item short-form health survey, and the unified Parkinson disease rating scale in people with parkinsonism. *Phys Ther.* Jun 2008;88(6):733–746.

39. Roland PS, Otto E. Vestibular dysfunction after traumatic brain injury: evaluation and management. In: Ashly MJ, Krych DK, eds. *Traumatic Brain Injury Rehabilitation.* Boca Raton, FL: CRC Press. 1995; 131–170. Chap 6.

40. Horak FB. Clinical measurement of postural control in adults. *Phys Ther.* Dec 1987;67(12):1881–1885.

41. Steffen TM, Mollinger LA. Age- and gender-related test performance in community-dwelling adults. *J Neurol Phys Ther.* Dec 2005;29(4):181–188.

42. Federici A, Bellagamba S, Rocchi MB. Does dance-based training improve balance in adult and young old subjects? A pilot randomized controlled trial. *Aging Clin Exp Res.* Oct 2005;17(5):385–389.

43. Hamilton KM, Kantor L, Magee LE. Limitations of postural equilibrium tests for examining simulator sickness. *Aviat Space Environ Med.* Mar 1989;60(3):246–251.

44. Briggs RC, Gossman MR, Birch R, Drews JE, Shaddeau SA. Balance performance among noninstitutionalized elderly women. *Phys Ther.* Sep 1989;69(9):748–756.

45. Guskiewicz KM. Postural stability assessment following concussion: one piece of the puzzle. *Clin J Sport Med.* Jul 2001;11(3):182–189.

46. Defense and Veterans Brain Injury Center. *DVBIC Working Group on the Acute Management of Mild Traumatic Brain Injury in Military Operational Settings: Clinical Practice Guideline and Recommendations.* DVBIC: Silver Spring, MD: 2006.

47. Valovich TC, Perrin DH, Gansneder BM. Repeat administration elicits a practice effect with the balance error scoring system but not with the standardized assessment of concussion in high school athletes. *J Athl Train.* 2003;38(1):38, 51–56.

48. Onate JA, Beck BC, Van Lunen BL. On-field testing environment and balance error scoring system performance during preseason screening of healthy collegiate baseball players. *J Athl Train.* Oct–Dec 2007;42(4):446–451.

49. McCrea MA, Guskiewicz KM, Marshall SW, et al. Acute effects and recovery time following concussion in collegiate football players: the NCAA Concussion Study. *JAMA.* Nov 19 2003;290(19):2556–2563.

50. Valovich McLeod TC, Barr WB, McCrea M, Guskiewicz KM. Psychometric and measurement properties of concussion assessment tools in youth sports. *J Athl Train.* Oct–Dec 2006;41(4):399–408.

51. Iverson GL, Kaarto ML, Koehle MS. Normative data for the balance error scoring system: implications for brain injury evaluations. *Brain Inj.* Feb 2008;22(2):147–152.

52. Iverson GL, Koehle MS. Normative data for the balance error scoring system in adults. *Rehabil Res Pract.* 2013;2013:846418.

53. Finnoff JT, Peterson VJ, Hollman JH, Smith J. Intrarater and interrater reliability of the Balance Error Scoring System (BESS). *PM R.* Jan 2009;1(1):50–54.

54. Riemann B, Guskiewicz K, Shields E. Relationship between clinical and force plate measures of postural stability. *J Sport Rehab.* 1999;8:71–78.

55. Whitney SL, Wrisley DM. The influence of footwear on timed balance scores of the modified clinical test of sensory interaction and balance. *Arch Phys Med Rehabil.* Mar 2004;85(3):439–443.

56. Cohen HS, Blatchly CA, Gombash LL. A study of the clinical test of sensory interaction and balance. *Physical Ther.* Jun 1993;73(6):346–351; discussion 351–344.

57. Anacker SL, Di Fabio RP. Influence of sensory inputs on standing balance in community-dwelling elders with a recent history of falling. *Phys Ther.* Aug 1992;72(8):575–581; discussion 581–574.

58. Dickstein R, Shupert CL, Horak FB. Fingertip touch improves postural stability in patients with peripheral neuropathy. *Gait Posture.* Dec 2001;14(3):238–247.

59. Wrisley DM, Whitney SL. The effect of foot position on the modified clinical test of sensory interaction and balance. *Arch Phys Med Rehabil.* Feb 2004;85(2):335–338.

60. El-Kashlan HK, Shepard NT, Asher AM, Smith-Wheelock M, Telian SA. Evaluation of clinical measures of equilibrium. *Laryngoscope.* Mar 1998;108(3):311–319.

61. Weber PC, Cass SP. Clinical assessment of postural stability. *Am J Otol.* Nov 1993;14(6):566–569.

62. Leddy AL, Crowner BE, Earhart GM. Functional gait assessment and balance evaluation system test: reliability, validity, sensitivity, and specificity for identifying individuals with Parkinson disease who fall. *PhysTher.* Jan 2011;91(1):102–113.

63. Duncan RP, Leddy AL, Cavanaugh JT, et al. Accuracy of fall prediction in Parkinson disease: six-month and 12-month prospective analyses. *Parkinsons Dis.* 2012;2012:237673.

64. Leddy AL, Crowner BE, Earhart GM. Utility of the Mini-BESTest, BESTest, and BESTest sections for balance assessments in individuals with Parkinson disease. *J Neurol Phys Ther.* Jun 2011;35(2):90–97.

65. King LA, Priest KC, Salarian A, Pierce D, Horak FB. Comparing the Mini-BESTest with the Berg Balance Scale to evaluate balance disorders in Parkinson's disease. *Parkinsons Dis.* 2012;2012:375419.

66. Peltier J. Evaluation of Vestibular Function, Grand Rounds Presentation, UTMB, Dept. of Otolaryngology. In: Quinn FB Jr, ed. *Dr. Quinn's Online Textbook of Otolaryngology: Grand Rounds Archive.* Galveston, TX: The University of Texas Medical Branch; 2005: http://www.utmb.edu/otoref/grnds/GrndsIndex.html. Accessed July 17, 2013.

67. Balance Manager Systems. *Clinical Interpretation Guide, Computerized Dynamic Posturography.* Clackamas, OR: NeuroCom International, Inc.

68. Cevette MJ, Puetz B, Marion MS, Wertz ML, Muenter MD. Aphysiologic performance on dynamic posturography. *Otolaryngol Head Neck Surg.* Jun 1995;112(6):676–688.

69. Longridge NS, Mallinson AI. "Across the board" posturography abnormalities in vestibular injury. *Otol Neurotol.* Jul 2005;26(4):695–698.

70. Mallinson AI, Longridge NS. A new set of criteria for evaluating malingering in work-related vestibular injury. *Otol Neurotol.* Jul 2005;26(4):686–690.

71. Goebel JA, Paige GD. Dynamic posturography and caloric test results in patients with and without vertigo. *Otolaryngol Head Neck Surg.* Jun 1989;100(6):553–558.

72. Hamid MA, Hughes GB, Kinney SE. Specificity and sensitivity of dynamic posturography. A retrospective analysis. *Acta Otolaryngol Suppl.* 1991;481:596–600.

73. Geurts AC, Ribbers GM, Knoop JA, van Limbeek J. Identification of static and dynamic postural instability following traumatic brain injury. *Arch Phys Med Rehabil.* Jul 1996;77(7):639–644.

74. Guskiewicz KM. Assessment of postural stability following sport-related concussion. *Curr Sports Med Rep.* Feb 2003;2(1):24–30.

75. Basford JR, Chou LS, Kaufman KR, et al. An assessment of gait and balance deficits after traumatic brain injury. *Arch Phys Med Rehabil.* Mar 2003;84(3):343–349.

76. Wrisley DM, Stephens MJ, Mosley S, Wojnowski A, Duffy J, Burkard R. Learning effects of repetitive administrations of the sensory organization test in healthy young adults. *Arch Phys Med Rehabil.* Aug 2007;88(8):1049–1054.

77. Broglio SP, Ferrara MS, Sopiarz K, Kelly MS. Reliable change of the sensory organization test. *Clin J Sport Med.* Mar 2008;18(2):148–154.

78. Di Fabio RP. Meta-analysis of the sensitivity and specificity of platform posturography. *Arch Otolaryngol Head Neck Surg.* Feb 1996;122(2):150–156.

79. Di Fabio RP. Sensitivity and specificity of platform posturography for identifying patients with vestibular dysfunction. *Phys Ther.* Apr 1995;75(4):290–305.

80. Ikai T, Kamikubo T, Nishi M, Miyano M. Dynamic postural control in middle-aged and elderly people. *Japanese J Rehabil Med.* 2002;39:311–316.

81. *Balance Manager Systems, Clinical Interpretation Guide.* Clackamas, OR: NeuroCom International, Inc; 2008.

82. Guskiewicz KM, Riemann BL, Perrin DH, Nashner LM. Alternative approaches to the assessment of mild head injury in athletes. *Med Sci Sports Exerc.* Jul 1997;29(7 suppl):S213–221.

83. Peterson CL, Ferrara MS, Mrazik M, Piland S, Elliott R. Evaluation of neuropsychological domain scores and postural stability following cerebral concussion in sports. *Clin J Sport Med.* Jul 2003;13(4):230–237.

84. Harstall C. Computerized dynamic posturography in rehabilitation: has its reliability and validity been established? *Physiother Can.* 2000;52(1):56–63.

85. Williams GP, Robertson V, Greenwood KM, Goldie P, Morris ME. The high-level mobility assessment tool (HiMAT) for traumatic brain injury. Part 1: item generation. *Brain Inj.* Oct 2005;19(11):925–932.

86. Williams GP, Robertson V, Greenwood KM, Goldie PA, Morris ME. The high-level mobility assessment tool (HiMAT) for traumatic brain injury. Part 2: content validity and discriminability. *Brain Inj.* Sep 2005;19(10):833–843.

87. Williams GP, Morris ME. High-level mobility outcomes following acquired brain injury: a preliminary evaluation. *Brain Inj.* Apr 2009;23(4):307–312.

88. Williams GP, Greenwood KM, Robertson VJ, Goldie PA, Morris ME. High-Level Mobility Assessment Tool (HiMAT): Interrater reliability, retest reliability, and internal consistency. *Phys Ther.* 2006a;86(3):395–400.

89. Williams GP, Robertson V, Greenwood KM, Goldie P, Morris ME. The concurrent validity and responsiveness of the high-level mobility assessment tool for measuring the mobility limitations of people with traumatic brain injury. *Arch Phys Med Rehabil.* 2006b;87(3):437–442.

90. Williams GP, Pallant J, Greenwood KM. Further development of the High-level Mobility Assessment Tool (HiMAT). *Brain Inj.* 2010;24(7–8):1027–1031.

91. Williams GP, Rosie J, Densienko S, Taylor D. Normative values for the high-level mobility assessment tool (HiMAT). *Int J Ther Rehabil.* 2009;16(7):370–374.

92. Fritz S, Lusardi M. White paper: "Walking speed: the sixth vital sign." *J Geriatr Phys Ther.* 2009;32(2):2–5.

93. Perry J, Garrett M, Gronley JK, Mulroy SJ. Classification of walking handicap in the stroke population. *Stroke.* Jun 1995;26(6):982–989.

94. Paltamaa J, Sarasoja T, Leskinen E, Wikstrom J, Malkia E. Measuring deterioration in international classification of functioning domains of people with multiple sclerosis who are ambulatory. *Phys Ther.* Feb 2008;88(2):176–190.

95. Oberg T, Karsznia A, Oberg K. Basic gait parameters: reference data for normal subjects, 10–79 years of age. *J Rehabil Res Dev.* 1993;30(2):210–223.

96. Moseley AM, Lanzarone S, Bosman JM, et al. Ecological validity of walking speed assessment after traumatic brain injury: a pilot study. *J Head Trauma Rehabil.* Jul–Aug 2004;19(4):341–348.

97. van Loo MA, Moseley AM, Bosman JM, de Bie RA, Hassett L. Inter-rater reliability and concurrent validity of walking speed measurement after traumatic brain injury. *Clin Rehabil.* 2003;17(7):775–779.

98. van Loo MA, Moseley AM, Bosman JM, de Bie RA, Hassett L. Test-re-test reliability of walking speed, step length and step width measurement after traumatic brain injury: a pilot study. *Brain Inj.* Oct 2004;18(10):1041–1048.

99. Finch E, Brooks D, Stratford PW, Mayo N. *Physical Rehabilitation Outcome Measures Second Edition, A Guide to Enhanced Clinical Decision Making.* 2nd ed. Hamilton, Ontario: BC Decker, Inc; 2002.

100. Parker TM, Osternig LR, van Donkelaar P, Chou LS. Balance control during gait in athletes and non-athletes following concussion. *Med Eng Phys.* Oct 2008;30(8):959–967.

101. Holden MK, Gill KM, Magliozzi MR, Nathan J, Piehl-Baker L. Clinical gait assessment in the neurologically impaired. Reliability and meaningfulness. *Phys Ther.* Jan 1984;64(1):35–40.

102. Bohannon RW. Comfortable and maximum walking speed of adults aged 20–79 years: reference values and determinants. *Age Ageing.* Jan 1997;26(1):15–19.

103. Parker TM, Osternig LR, VAN Donkelaar P, Chou LS. Gait stability following concussion. *Med Sci Sports Exerc.* Jun 2006;38(6):1032–1040.

104. Chou LS, Kaufman KR, Walker-Rabatin AE, Brey RH, Basford JR. Dynamic instability during obstacle crossing following traumatic brain injury. *Gait Posture.* Dec 2004;20(3):245–254.

105. Walker ML, Austin AG, Banke GM, et al. Reference group data for the functional gait assessment. *Phys Ther.* Nov 2007;87(11):1468–1477.

106. Anson E, Cronan N. The Functional Gait Assessment and Sensory Organization Test: a Comparison. Poster presented at: PT 2009: The Annual Conference and Exposition of the APTA, Baltimore, 2009. http://apps.apta.org/Custom/abstracts/pt2009/abstractsPt.cfm?m_id=19661

107. Wrisley DM, Kumar NA. Functional gait assessment: concurrent, discriminative, and predictive validity in community-dwelling older adults. *Phys Ther.* May 2010;90(5):761–773.

108. Roozen M. Illinois Agility Test. *NSCA's Performance Training Journal.* 2004;3(5):5–6.

109. Reiman MP, Manske RC. *Functional Testing in Human Performance.* Champaign, Il: Human Kinetics; 2009.

110. Caldwell BP, Peters DM. Seasonal variation in physiological fitness of a semiprofessional soccer team. *J Strength Cond Res.* Aug 2009;23(5):1370–1377.

111. Hoffman and Associates. *Physical Readiness Standards Validation of the Nevada P.O.S.T. Category I Peace Officers in Total Fitness for Public Safety: Executive Summary.* 2009. http://apps.post.nv.gov/Administration/Cat1%20 Physical%20Readiness%20Standards%20Validation%20Report.pdf

112. Raya MA, Jayne D, Linberg A, et al. Criterion validity of the modified Edgren side-step and the Illinois agility test in a healthy athletic population. *J Orthop Sports Phys Ther.* 39;2009:A116.

113. Gaunaurd K, Gailey RS, Raya MS, Campbell SM, Roach KR. Speed and agility testing of military service members with traumatic limb loss. Paper presented at: 13th International Society for Prosthetics and Orthotics World Congress; May 12, 2010; Leipzig, Germany.

114. Integrated Fitness Systems/FitForce. Fitness Tests, Standards and Norms. What is Valid? What is Legal? Salem, MA: FitForce; 2007: 8. http://fitforce.org/documents/Microsoft_Word_-_Whitepaper_-_CIAR.0307.pdf. Accessed July 17, 2013.

115. Gaunaurd IA. The Comprehensive High-level Activity Mobility Predictor (CHAMP): a performance-based assessment instrument to quantify high-level mobility in service members with traumatic lower limb loss. *Open Access Dissertations.* 2012; Paper 712.

116. Belgen B, Beninato M, Sullivan PE, Narielwalla K. The association of balance capacity and falls self-efficacy with history of falling in community-dwelling people with chronic stroke. *Arch Phys Med Rehabil.* Apr 2006;87(4):554–561.

117. Chandler JM, Duncan PW, Kochersberger G, Studenski S. Is lower extremity strength gain associated with improvement in physical performance and disability in frail, community-dwelling elders? *Arch Phys Med Rehabil.* Jan 1998;79(1):24–30.

118. Lord SR, Murray SM, Chapman K, Munro B, Tiedemann A. Sit-to-stand performance depends on sensation, speed, balance, and psychological status in addition to strength in older people. *J Gerontol A Biol Sci Med Sci.* Aug 2002;57(8):M539–543.

119. Meretta BM, Whitney SL, Marchetti GF, Sparto PJ, Muirhead RJ. The five times sit to stand test: responsiveness to change and concurrent validity in adults undergoing vestibular rehabilitation. *J Vestib Res.* 2006;16(4–5):233–243.

120. Whitney SL, Wrisley DM, Marchetti GF, Gee MA, Redfern MS, Furman JM. Clinical measurement of sit-to-stand performance in people with balance disorders: validity of data for the Five-Times-Sit-to-Stand Test. *Physical Ther.* Oct 2005;85(10):1034–1045.

121. Blake C, O'Meara YM. Subjective and objective physical limitations in high-functioning renal dialysis patients. *Nephrol Dial Transplant.* Dec 2004;19(12):3124–3129.

122. Sherrington C, Lord SR. Reliability of simple portable tests of physical performance in older people after hip fracture. *Clin Rehabil.* Aug 2005;19(5):496–504.

123. Brown KE, Whitney SL, Marchetti GF, Wrisley DM, Furman JM. Physical therapy for central vestibular dysfunction. *Arch Phys Med Rehabil.* 2006;87(1):76–81.

124. Ostchega Y, Harris TB, Hirsch R, Parsons VL, Kington R, Katzoff M. Reliability and prevalence of physical performance examination assessing mobility and balance in older persons in the US: data from the Third National Health and Nutrition Examination Survey. *J Am Geriatr Soc.* Sep 2000;48(9):1136–1141.

125. Hoffer ME, Balough BJ, Gottshall KR. Posttraumatic balance disorders. *Int Tinnitus J.* 2007;13(1):69–72.

126. Hoffer ME, Gottshall KR, Moore R, Balough BJ, Wester D. Characterizing and treating dizziness after mild head trauma. *Otol Neurotol.* 2004;25(2):135–138.

127. Zasler ND, Katz DI, Zafonte RD. *Brain Injury Medicine Principles and Practice.* Vol 1. New York, NY: Demos Medical Publishing; 2007.

128. Barclay-Goddard R, Stevenson T, Poluha W, Moffatt ME, Taback SP. Force platform feedback for standing balance training after stroke. *Cochrane Database Syst Rev.* 2004;(4):CD004129.

129. Wrisley DM, Pavlou M. Physical therapy for balance disorders. *Neurol Clin.* Aug 2005;23(3):855–874, vii–viii.

130. McCrory P, Johnston K, Meeuwisse W, et al. Summary and agreement statement of the 2nd International Conference on Concussion in sport. *Br J Sports Med.* 2005;39:196–204.

131. Gemmell C, Leathem JM. A study investigating the effects of Tai Chi Chuan: individuals with traumatic brain injury compared to controls. *Brain Inj.* Feb 2006;20(2):151–156.

132. Pollock A, Baer G, Pomeroy V, Langhorne P. Physiotherapy treatment approaches for the recovery of postural control and lower limb function following stroke. *Cochrane Database Syst Rev.* 2007;(1):CD001920.

133. Defense and Veterans Brain Injury Center. New Clinical Recommendations Released for Traumatic Brain Injuries. http://dvbic.dcoe.mil/press/2014/new-clinical-recommendations-released-traumatic-brain-injuries. Accessed August 28, 2014.

134. Adamovich SV, Fluet GG, Tunik E, Merians AS. Sensorimotor training in virtual reality: a review. *NeuroRehabilitation.* 2009;25(1):29–44.

135. Gentile A. Skill acquisition: action, movement, and neuromotor processes. In: Carr J, Shepherd R, Gordon J, eds. *Movement Science: Foundations for Physical Therapy in Rehabilitation.* Rockville, MD: Aspen Systems; 1987: 115.

136. Wolf SL, Barnhart HX, Ellison GL, Coogler CE. The effect of Tai Chi Quan and computerized balance training on postural stability in older subjects. Atlanta FICSIT Group. Frailty and Injuries: Cooperative Studies on Intervention Techniques. *Phys Ther.* Apr 1997;77(4):371–381; discussion 382–374.

137. Wolf SL, Barnhart HX, Kutner NG, McNeely E, Coogler C, Xu T. Reducing frailty and falls in older persons: an investigation of Tai Chi and computerized balance training. Atlanta FICSIT Group. Frailty and Injuries: Cooperative Studies of Intervention Techniques. *J Am Geriatr Soc.* May 1996;44(5):489–497.

138. Degano AC, Geigle PR. Use of aquatic physical therapy in the treatment of balance and gait impairments following traumatic brain injury: a case report. *J Aquatic Phys Ther.* Spring 2009;17(1):16–21.

139. Haskell WL, Lee IM, Pate RR, et al. Physical activity and public health: updated recommendations for adults from the American College of Sports Medicine and the American Heart Association. *Med Sci Sports Exer.* 2007;39(8):1423–1434.

140. Gordon WA, Sliwinski M, Echo J, McLoughlin M, Sheerer MS, Meili TE. The benefits of exercise in individuals with traumatic brain injury: a retrospective study. *J Head Trauma Rehabil.* 1998;13(4):58–67.

Chapter 4

VISION ASSESSMENT AND INTERVENTION

SHARON GOWDY WAGENER, OTR/L, BA, MAOT*; MATTIE ANHELUK, MOT, OTR/L[†]; CHRISTINE ARULANANTHAM, BOT, OTR/L[‡]; AND MITCHELL SCHEIMAN, OD[§]

*Occupational Therapist, Instructor Scientist, Rehabilitation Services, Courage Kenny Rehabilitation Institute/Abbott Northwestern Hospital, 800 East 28th Street, Mail Stop 12213, Minneapolis, Minnesota 55407
[†] Occupational Therapist, Instructor Scientist, Comprehensive Outpatient Rehabilitation, Courage Kenny Rehabilitation Institute, United Hospital–Occupational Therapy Department, 33 North Smith Avenue, Saint Paul, Minnesota 55102
[‡] Occupational Therapist, Instructor Scientist, Rehabilitation Services, Courage Kenny Rehabilitation Institute/Mercy Hospital, 4050 Coon Rapids Boulevard, Coon Rapids, Minnesota 55433
[§] Professor, Associate Dean of Clinical Research, Pennsylvania College of Optometry at Salus University, 8360 Old York Road, Elkins Park, Pennsylvania 19027

SECTION 1: VISION ASSESSMENT

INTRODUCTION

Vision is the most far-reaching of our sensory systems. Changes to this system can affect patients' ability to participate in therapy as well as to function in everyday life.[1] Combat troops with blast-related concussion/mild traumatic brain injury (c/mTBI) are at risk for visual dysfunction.[2] Occupational therapists are often the first-line clinicians who can identify visual impairment. The occupational therapist's roles include the following[3]:

- evaluating vision function through vision screening and functional observations.
- determining if and how visual impairment may be affecting the patient's functional performance.

If visual impairment is suspected, the occupational therapist:

- refers the patient to the staff optometrist with expertise in vision and traumatic brain injury (TBI) or neuro-ophthalmologist for further evaluation and intervention management,
- educates the patient and the rehabilitation team about how the impairment is affecting the patient functionally, and
- provides both compensatory and remedial (in collaboration with an optometrist) treatment, as appropriate.

Occupational therapists provide a basic vision screening that includes the following elements:

- symptom questionnaire,
- visual acuity,
- visual fields,
- ocular motor (pursuits, saccades, convergence),
- binocular vision, and
- glare/photophobia.

The specific screening tool or method used will be dictated by available resources and therapist's expertise and preferences; assessments included in the toolkit are considered options.

General Instructions for Vision Assessment

- Set up in a well-lit, glare- and clutter-free room. Minimal distractions (physical, visual, or auditory) are optimal.

- Make sure the patient is seated comfortably with his or her head vertically erect.
- If the patient is wearing glasses, ensure they fit properly and that the patient uses the appropriate section of the glasses for the task (Figure 4-1).
  ◦ Upper portion of the lens is for distance.
  ◦ Trifocal for mid-distance (18–24 inches), such as a computer monitor.
  ◦ Lower portion for near distance (~16 inches), for example, reading distance.
  ◦ Some people wear progressive lenses that do not have obvious segments, but placement should be similar.
- Another factor to consider is that many people are now using monovision contacts: one eye is used for distance and the other for near vision. Be sure to ask about this and adapt your assessment accordingly.

Assessment Sequence and Methods

- Begin the assessment with a questionnaire of symptoms to help determine if and how the patient is experiencing visual stress or impairment.
- It is also possible to piece together the areas of assessment with a variety of tests. The order of assessment should follow that of the above list as it moves from basic visual components to more complex tasks (ie, start with acuity to determine if the patient is able to see functionally to participate).

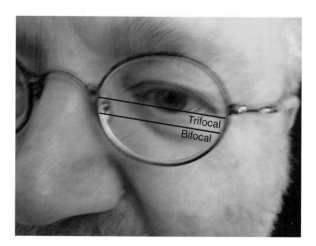

Figure 4-1. Segments in progressive lenses.

TABLE 4-1

RECOMMENDED COMPONENTS OF VISION SCREEN

Components of Vision Screen*	Corrective Lenses Use During Testing
Functional performance/behavioral vision checklist concurrent with or complementary to tests	SM wears corrective lenses (if appropriate)
Symptom self-report: COVD-QOL Outcomes Assessment + photosensitivity interview question	
Far/near acuity: CPAC	
Accommodation: Accommodative Amplitude Test	
Convergence: near point of convergence	
Eye alignment & binocular: eye alignment test	
Saccades: A-DEM	
Pursuits: NSUCO	SM is tested without his/her corrective lenses
Confrontation: finger counting	

* In order of administration
A-DEM: Adult Developmental Eye Movement Test
COVD-QOL: College of Optometrists in Vision Development Quality of Life Assessment
CPAC: Chronister Pocket Acuity Chart
NSUCO: Northeastern State College of Optometry Eye Movement Test
SM: service member

- The occupational therapist observes how the patient is using his or her eyes and the functional implications. The therapist should look for the following:
  ○ facial expressions, head turning or slanting, squinting;
  ○ fatigue, frustration, complaints of headaches, etc;
  ○ complaints of losing one's place when reading;
  ○ quality of eye movements;
  ○ smooth versus jerky movements;
  ○ eyes missing or losing the targets; and
  ○ over- and undershooting.

These symptoms, along with the patient's ability to perform the tasks or tests, will help the occupational therapist determine whether the patient is experiencing visual impairment.

General Equipment to Have on Hand

- Occluders or eye patches
- Penlight
- Ruler
- Pen and paper
- Dowels with small balls or objects attached to the ends

Preferred Methods

Because the visual system is central to participation in therapy and functioning in everyday life, occupational therapists perform a vision screen on service members with TBI to identify suspected deficits, refer to vision specialists, and better understand patients' functional performance problems. The utility of this process, however, is impeded by the fact that there is no gold standard for a vision screen on adults with TBI. This issue will be resolved if and when psychometric data are collected and published on this population.

To address the need to specify preferred practices until such time, a consensus panel comprised of occupational therapy and optometry vision experts was convened in July 2011 by the US Army Office of the Surgeon General—Rehabilitation and Reintegration Division. The panel was charged with examining existing options and using a modified Delphi process to achieve consensus as to the composition of a brief occupational therapy vision screen for SMs with c/mTBI (Table 4-1); the tools and methods considered are further described in this chapter. Note that, like most assessments in this section, methods endorsed by the panel are considered **practice options** because they have not been fully evaluated on adults with c/mTBI; however, given their selection from many alternatives, those methods recommended by the panel might be considered "better" practice options. Do not under-estimate the importance of your own observation skills and look for functional implications.

Additional Resources for Occupational Therapy and Vision

Gillen G. *Cognitive and Perceptual Rehabilitation: Optimizing Function.* St Louis, MO: Mosby; 2009.

Scheiman M. *Understanding and Managing Vision Deficits: A Guide for Occupational Therapists.* 3rd ed. Thorofare, NJ: SLACK Incorporated; 2011.

Zoltan B. *Vision, Perception, and Cognition: A Manual for the Evaluation and Treatment of the Adult With Acquired Brain Injury.* 4th ed. Thorofare, NJ: SLACK Incorporated; 2007.

SYMPTOMS SELF-REPORT: COLLEGE OF OPTOMETRISTS IN VISION DEVELOPMENT QUALITY OF LIFE ASSESSMENT

Purpose/Description

The College of Optometrists in Vision Development Quality of Life Outcomes (COVD-QOL) Assessment was developed in 1995 to describe and measure changes resulting from optometric intervention, including vision therapy. This 30-item, self-report survey addresses four areas: (1) physical/occupational function, (2) psychological well-being, (3) social interaction, and (4) somatic sensation. The short form, the S-COVD-QOL, includes 19 items and test-retest reliability suggests the short form is a satisfactory substitute.[4] This assessment may be used to identify problems, provide treatment, and make referrals. It is **not** intended to replace a comprehensive vision evaluation by an optometrist.

The questionnaire may be a helpful inclusion in an initial occupational therapy evaluation when:

- the patient has not had a comprehensive visual assessment by an optometrist or ophthalmologist to identify visual impairments, and
- the patient has mild-to-moderate brain injury or c/mTBI, and observation of functional performance suggests the possibility of visual dysfunction in a number of domains.

This questionnaire should be used in conjunction with a full vision screen.

Administration Protocol/Equipment/Time

Maples[5] recommended use of this assessment at optometric initial assessment, during therapy, at completion of therapy, and at a predetermined time after intervention. Patients rate each statement on a 0-to-4 scale (with 0 indicating that the symptom is never present and 4 indicating the symptom is always present). The questionnaire is to be completed by the patient or therapist via interview with patient, family members, and caregivers. Administration time is less than 10 minutes. The questionnaire is available at no cost and can be obtained by contacting the College of Optometrists in Vision Development (215 West Garfield Road, Suite 200, Aurora, OH 44202).

Groups Tested With This Measure

The COVD-QOL Assessment has been used in children and adults with various types of vision disorders. Diagnoses including strabismus, amblyopia, TBI, autism spectrum, sports vision, vision skills, vision perception, and reading dysfunction were included in a multisite study, which concluded that patients reported significantly fewer symptoms after vision therapy using the COVD-QOL Assessment.[6] Shin, Park, and Park[7] used the COVD-QOL Assessment with parents and their children ages 9 to 13 years old to explore the prevalence and types of nonstrabismic accommodative or vergence dysfunctions. Farrar, Call, and Maples[8] compared the visual symptoms between attention deficit disorder (ADD)/attention deficit-hyperactivity disorder (ADHD) and non-ADD/ADHD children. There is no literature describing the use of the COVD-QOL Assessment in adults with c/mTBI.

Interpretability

- Norms: not available
- Minimal detectable change 95% (MDC_{95}): 0.193 for the item mean score on the

COVD-QOL. This means a patient's posttreatment score needs to change by at least .193 from the pretreatment score for the 30 items to be 95% confident that true change occurred (rather than measurement error). MDC_{95} was calculated based on Maples.[5]

- Responsiveness estimates: not available

Reliability Estimates

- Internal consistency: not available
- Interrater: not available
- Intrarater: not available
- Test-Retest: Maples[5] determined test-retest by testing 19 optometry students with administrations separated by 2 weeks. Wilcoxon Signed Rank Analysis showed no significant differences. A paired t-test and item analysis were insignificant. Spearman's rho correlation for test-retest of each subject was 0.878. In total, 89% of subjects scored insignificantly different, while 90% of items were found to vary insignificantly.

Validity Estimates

- Content/Face: not available
- Criterion: not available
- Construct: Daugherty, Frantz, Allison, and Gabriel[9] demonstrated quality-of-life changes after vision therapy with subjects diagnosed with binocular vision who ranged from 7 to 45 years of age. White and Major[10] compared subjects with convergence insufficiency and subjects with normal binocular vision using this measure and found two of the 30 items were statistically higher for convergence insufficiency than for normal binocular vision. Farrar, Call, and Maples[8] compared the visual symptoms between ADD/ADHD and non-ADD/ADHD children and noted that 14 of the 33 symptoms were significantly more severe in the ADD/ADHD group.

Selected References

Daugherty KM, Frantz KA, Allison CL, Gabriel HM. Evaluating changes in quality of life after vision therapy using the COVD Quality of Life Outcomes Assessment. *Optom Vis Dev*. 2007;38:75–81.

Maples WC. Test-retest reliability of the College of Optometrists in Vision Development Quality of Life Outcomes Assessment Short Form. *J Optom Vis Dev*. 2002;33:126–134.

Maples WC. Test-retest reliability of the College of Optometrists in Vision Development Quality of Life Outcomes Assessment. *Optometry*. 2000;71(9):579–585.

DYNAMIC FUNCTIONAL TASK OBSERVATION: VISION

Purpose/Description

Functional task observation is a critical component of a comprehensive cognitive and visual assessment. Many standardized tests do not pose the same challenges to patients as trying to function in unstructured tasks or environments; therefore, systematic observation of functional task performance provides unique opportunities to further understand patients' challenges and strengths. By observing patients as they perform functional tasks, occupational therapists assess the extent to which task, environment, and personal characteristics interact to impact performance. Furthermore, therapists modify task and environmental variables to right-fit challenges specific to an individual's goals and to determine under which circumstances the patient's performance is optimized. Occupational therapists design patient-relevant functional tasks and use an observation worksheet, like the Dynamic Functional Task Observation Checklist (Form 4-1), to analyze task and environmental characteristics and to catalog the associated personal characteristics and overall performance.

Recommended Instrument Use: Practice Option

The Dynamic Functional Task Observation Checklist may be used to structure patient performance observations during the assessment phase and throughout the episode of care.

FORM 4-1

SISTER KENNY DYNAMIC VISUAL TASK OBSERVATION CHECKLIST

Task description: _____

Component	Descriptions of characteristics			Notes
Task characteristics	Perceived degree of difficulty		☐ Easy ☐ Moderate ☐ Difficult	
	Perceived degree of familiarity		☐ Familiar ☐ Familiar with new challenges ☐ Unfamiliar	
	Type of instruction provided		☐ Verbal ☐ Written ☐ Demonstrated ☐ Pictorial	
	Physical demands		☐ Sedentary ☐ Active ☐ Gross motor ☐ Fine motor ☐ Other: ☐ Other:	
	Cognitive demands		Attention Memory Executive skills	
	Visual demands	Acuity	Size font	
		Scanning	☐ Scanning	
		Visual attention	Table top Environmental scanning Static Dynamic ☐ Smooth pursuits ☐ Convergence/Divergence Other:	
Environment characteristics	Performance setting		☐ Clinic ☐ Community	
	Stimulus-arousal properties		☐ Little to no distracters ☐ Auditory distracters ☐ Visual distracters	
	Visual/auditory considerations		☐ Lighting needs ☐ Glasses, patches ☐ Hearing device	
	Physical considerations		☐ None ☐ Pain ☐ Decreased endurance ☐ U/E limitations ☐ L/E limitations ☐ Decreased balance	
	Emotional considerations		☐ None ☐ Seems anxious ☐ Seems depressed	
	Self-awareness associated with the task at-hand		☐ Anticipatory ☐ Emergent ☐ Intellectual ☐ Little to none	

(**Form 4-1** *continues*)

Form 4-1 *continued*

Functional observations related to vision	Patient makes accommodations via head position	☐ Tilted to one side ☐ Turned to one side ☐ Other	
	Patient makes accommodations via trunk posture	☐ Leaning in toward activity ☐ Leaning to one side or the other ☐ Other:	
	Patient makes accommodations via eyes	☐ Squinting ☐ Closing one eye ☐ Other:	
	Hand/eye coordination	☐ Reaching accuracy ☐ Ability to write on a line accurately	
Task performance	Task accuracy (use of forms is accurate, writing is legible, organized, found all components without cues)	☐ Totally accurate ☐ Somewhat accurate ☐ Not accurate	
	Activity tolerance	☐ Functional with no breaks ☐ Functional with self-initiated breaks ☐ Impaired, needed breaks and cues to take them ☐ Lethargic/unable ☐ Complaints of eye strain ☐ Complaints of headaches ☐ Other:	
	Self-prediction-reflection of visual challenge and ability to manage	☐ Able to accurately predict performance ☐ Able to reflect on performance ☐ Needed cues to predict performance ☐ Needed cues to reflect on performance	
	Response to feedback	☐ Responsive to feedback; uses feedback ☐ Defensive and reluctant ☐ Refusal to listen/argues	
	Visual strategy use	Strategy: ☐ Independently initiated ☐ Cues required Strategy: ☐ Independently initiated ☐ Cues required Strategy: ☐ Independently initiated ☐ Cues required Strategy: ☐ Independently initiated ☐ Cues required	

Administration Protocol/Equipment/Time

These dimensions vary depending on the task developed by the clinician. See Chapter 9, Performance and Self-Management, Work, Social, and School Roles, for examples of vision-demanding tasks, including the following: job-specific tactical simulation 1 (dynamic visual scanning activity), job-specific tactical simulation 2 (target detection on visual scanning activity), class-A error detection, topographical symbols on a military map, and grid coordinates of a point on a military map.

Groups Tested With This Measure

These methods have not been formally tested on any groups. This description proposes methods by which occupational therapists can standardize observational tasks for their own use.

Interpretability

- Norms: There are no norms for this process, but as individual therapists craft and frequently use a core set of observational tasks, they will readily identify abnormalities, errors, or discrepancies in performance.
- MDC: not applicable
- Responsiveness estimates: not applicable

Reliability and Validity Estimates: not applicable

DISTANCE VISUAL ACUITY TESTING

Purpose/Description

Distance visual acuity testing is used to determine the patient's ability to focus on and distinguish fine detail at a distance of 20 feet.

Recommended Instrument Use: Practice Option

Administration Protocol/Equipment/Time

Equipment required includes Chronister Pocket Acuity Chart (CPAC; Gulden Ophthalmics, Elkins Park, PA), a flip-pocket chart of 22 pages of targets.

Setup

- Provide adequate lighting on the test card.
- Glasses or contacts should be worn during testing if the patient normally wears them. Make sure the patient uses the appropriate glasses and portion of the glasses for the test (ie, if he or she has bifocal, trifocals, or progressive lenses; see Figure 4-1).
- Although visual acuity is traditionally measured with one eye covered, it is recommended that the patient keeps both eyes open during testing, as the goal is to determine if there is a visual acuity problem that could interfere with how the patient functions with both eyes open.

Administration Protocol

- Position the CPAC 20 feet away from the patient. Instruct the patient to verbally identify all the letters on the 20/40 line (note the "40" in lower left corner of the chart).
- To pass the screening, the patient must be able to correctly read three of the four 20/40 letters. Patients who fail the screening should be referred to a vision specialist (email communication, Mitchell Scheiman, OD, Chief, Pediatric/Binocular Vision Service and Professor, Salus University, The Eye Institute of the Pennsylvania College of Optometry, Philadelphia, PA, January 12, 2012). It is unnecessary for the patient to read the larger letters unless the therapist wants to determine exact visual acuity.
- If the patient has problems reading letters, visual acuity may be assessed using the Lea Symbols Test (Good-Lite Co, Elgin, IN).

Groups Tested With This Measure: not available

Interpretability

- Norms: Expect to see at least 20/40 with both eyes together.
- Although 20/20 visual acuity is considered "normal," in a screening format it is only necessary to determine whether a patient has a loss of visual acuity that might interfere with function; thus, for screening purposes, visual acuity worse than 20/40 is used as the criterion for referral.
- MDC: not applicable
- Responsiveness estimates: not applicable

Reliability and Validity Estimates: not available

Selected Reference

Scheiman M. *Understanding and Managing Vision Deficits: A Guide for Occupational Therapists*. 3rd ed. Thorofare, NJ: SLACK Incorporated; 2011.

ACCOMMODATIVE AMPLITUDE TEST

Purpose/Description

Accommodative amplitude is defined as the "closest near focusing response that can be produced with maximal voluntary effort in the fully corrected eye."[11(p128)] An accommodative amplitude screen may be used to identify problems, provide treatment, and make referrals. It is not intended to replace a comprehensive vision evaluation by an optometrist.

Recommended Instrument Use: Practice Standard

This test may be a helpful inclusion in an initial occupational therapy evaluation when:

- the patient has not had a comprehensive visual assessment by an optometrist or ophthalmologist to identify visual impairments, and
- the patient has mild-to-moderate brain injury or c/mTBI and observation of functional performance suggests the possibility of visual dysfunction in a number of domains.

This test can be used in conjunction with a full vision screen to assess for accommodation problems.

Administration Protocol/Equipment/Time

See below for the modified push-up method instructions. Administration time is less than 2 minutes. Equipment needs include a fixation stick such as the Gulden fixation stick, eye patch, and ruler. Positioning is important and the occupational therapist should try to find the best position that permits the patient to attend and concentrate on the task. The patient's head will ideally be vertically erect. If the patient wears corrective lenses, they should be used during this test.

Modified Push-Up Method

Preliminary Steps
- If glasses have been prescribed for both far and near distance, the glasses should be worn for this test; however, if glasses were only prescribed for reading, they should not be used for this test. In addition, if the patient wears a bifocal or progressive lens, the patient's accommodative amplitude must be measured through the top portion of the glasses, not the reading portion of the glass.
- Make sure there is no glare and that illumination is adequate.
- Position the patient to optimize attention.

Testing
- Place patch over the patient's left eye.
- Hold the fixation stick with the 20/30 target about 1 inch in front of the patient's right eye (use the small single letter on top of the stick).
- Slowly move the fixation stick away from the eye until the patient can identify the letter (it does not have to be perfectly clear).
- Measure distance from eye to target when the patient can identify the letter.

Scoring
- Record the distance from the patient's eye to the target when the patient can identify the letter (Exhibit 4-1).
- Divide 40 by this number to determine the patient's amplitude of accommodation (eg, if the patient can see the letter at 8 inches: $40 \div 8 = 5D$).
- Use norms tables to interpret results (see Interpretability).

Groups Tested With This Measure

Green et al[12] used the push-up accommodative amplitude method as a measure of accommodation when testing 12 adult patients with c/mTBI compared to 10 control subjects with no visual impairment. A significant difference between the mean push-up accommodative amplitudes was indicated for subjects with c/mTBI when compared to age-appropriate normative values. Conclusions indicated use of the push-up accommodative amplitude method as a visual screening tool for

---

EXHIBIT 4-1

ACCOMMODATION RESULTS

Distance at which patient can identify letter: _____ inches

40 / (# of inches) = 40 / _____ = _____ D* (amplitude of accommodation)

Possible impairment of accommodation: Yes____ No ____

---
*Compare this result with the expected amplitude of accommodation by age.
Expected mean amplitude: 18.5D – [0.30D × (age in years)] or, for expected mean amplitude, see Scheiman M. *Understanding and Managing Vision Deficits: A Guide for Occupational Therapists*. 3rd ed. Thorofare, NJ: SLACK Incorporated; 2011.

---

hospital technical and therapy staff, including occupational therapists. Chen and O'Leary[13] showed high reliability between the conventional and modified push-up methods testing children and adults. Rouse, Borsting, and Deland[14] evaluated interrater and intrarater reliability of the monocular push-up accommodative amplitude with children and found reliability repeatable in children.

Interpretability

- Norms: Hofstetter created formulas for the expected mean accommodative amplitudes based on normative data of Duane and Donders.[11(p396)]
- Expected mean amplitude: 18.5D – [0.30D × (age in years)]. Also, see Scheiman[15] for expected values of amplitude of accommodation by age.
- If the patient's amplitude of accommodation is more than 2D below the expected finding, it is considered a problem. If a patient's amplitude of accommodation is greater than expected, it suggests the patient has excellent accommodation.
- MDC: not available
- Responsiveness estimates: not available

Reliability Estimates

- Internal consistency: not available
- Interrater: Good interrater reliability with children indicated by intraclass correlation (ICC) ranges 0.81 to 0.85.[14]
- Intrarater: Intrarater within-session reliability was excellent with children with ICC's ≥ 0.88.[14] Rouse and colleagues also determined fair-to-good between-session intrarater reliability with ICC 0.89 and 0.69.[14]
- Test-Retest: Repeatability of the modified push-up method for two occasions was high for both monocular and binocular testing with young adult subjects.[13]

Validity Estimates

- Content/Face: not available
- Criterion: Chen and O'Leary[13] compared the modified push-up to the conventional push-up method with children and adult subjects and found the tests to be interchangeable.
- Construct: Green et al[12] found significant difference between the mean push-up accommodative amplitudes for subjects with c/mTBI when compared to age-appropriate normative values.

Selected References

Chen AH, O'Leary DJ. Validity and repeatability of the modified push-up method for measuring the amplitude of accommodation. *Clin Exp Optom*. 1998;81:63–71.

Green W, Ciuffreda KJ, Thiagarajan P, Szymanowicz D, Ludlam DP, Kapoor N. Accommodation in mild traumatic brain injury. *J Rehabil Res Dev*. 2010;47(3):183–199.

Scheiman M. *Understanding and Managing Vision Deficits: A Guide for Occupational Therapists*. 3rd ed. Thorofare, NJ: SLACK Incorporated; 2011.

NEAR POINT OF CONVERGENCE

Purpose/Description

Convergence is defined as the ability to maintain eye alignment as an object approaches the eyes. This test of near point convergence (NPC) may be used to identify problems, provide treatment, and make referrals. It is not intended to replace a comprehensive vision evaluation by an optometrist.

Recommended Instrument Use: Practice Standard

This test may be a helpful inclusion in an initial occupational therapy evaluation when:

- the patient has not had a comprehensive visual assessment by an optometrist/ophthalmologist to identify visual impairments, and
- the patient has mild-to-moderate brain injury or complicated c/mTBI and observation of functional performance suggests the possibility of visual dysfunction in a number of domains.

This test can be used in conjunction with a full vision screen to assess for convergence.

Administration Protocol/Equipment/Time

Equipment needed includes a penlight or pencil and a ruler. Administration time is less than 2 minutes.

Procedure

- Stand or sit face to face with the patient in a location that optimizes the patient's ability to attend to the task.
- Begin with the pencil tip or penlight approximately 12 inches away from the pa-

tient at eye level. Ask if the patient sees one pencil or penlight. If not, move the pencil or penlight further away until the patient sees one pencil.
- Slowly move the pencil tip or penlight toward the patient at eye level and between the patient's eyes.
- Instruct the patient to keep his/her eyes on the tip of the pencil or penlight for as long as possible.
- Ask the patient to tell you when he/she sees a split image (ie, two pencil tips).
- Once diplopia occurs, move the pencil tip or penlight toward the patient another inch or two and then begin to move it away.
- Ask the patient to try to see "one" again.
- Watch the eyes carefully and observe whether they stop working together as a team. One eye will usually drift out.

Scoring

The therapist should record the distance (in inches) between the patient and pencil point or penlight at which the patient reports double vision and the distance at which the patient reports recovery of single vision (Exhibit 4-2).

Normal performance. When the eyes lose alignment, it is referred to as a "break." When a break occurs, one will eye drift outward, and when the patient recovers fusion, the eyes will move back into alignment.[15] Patients with normal convergence will report double vision and lose alignment when the pencil tip or penlight moves toward them to within 2 to 4 inches of their eyes.[15] Those with normal convergences will recover single vision when the target is 4 to 6 inches as it is moved away from them.[15]

Abnormal performance. Patients with significant problems with binocular vision may or may not actually report double vision because some

---

EXHIBIT 4-2

NEAR POINT OF CONVERGENCE RESULTS

Breaking point*: _____
Recovery of fusion†: _____
Possible impairment of convergence: Yes____   No____

*As identified by patient or observation of break by therapist, clinical cutoff value of 5 cm or ~ 2 inches
†As identified by patient or observation of eye realignment by therapist, clinical cutoff value of 7 cm or ~ 3.5 inches

may be able to suppress the eye that turns out. Therefore, the therapist must watch the patient's eyes to determine when the break and recovery occur.

Groups Tested With This Measure

NPC testing is used in both children and adults in routine eye care examinations and during vision screenings. Scheiman et al[16] investigated normative data for adults and determined clinical cut off values. Reliability of the NPC test has been established with elementary school children.[14] Thiagarajan et al report a significant difference of NPC break and recovery values were found between c/mTBI and normal groups.[17(p460)]

Interpretability

- Norms: In a study involving optometric diagnosing, Scheiman and colleagues[16] suggested the value of 5 cm (~ 2 inches) for the NPC break and 7 cm (~ 3–3.5 inches)

for the convergence recovery in adults using an accommodative target or a penlight with red and green glasses.
- MDC: not available
- Responsiveness estimates: not applicable

Reliability Estimates

- Internal consistency: not available
- Interrater: Rouse and colleagues report excellent interrater reliability with children.[14]
- Intrarater: Rouse and colleagues report excellent within-session intrarater reliability of the NPC, with ICC 0.94 to 0.98 and good between-session reliability, with ICC 0.92 to 0.89.[14] Subjects were children.
- Test-Retest: not available

Validity Estimates

- Content/Face: not available
- Criterion: not available
- Construct: not available

Selected References

Scheiman M. *Understanding and Managing Vision Deficits: A Guide for Occupational Therapists*. 3rd ed. Thorofare, NJ: SLACK Incorporated; 2011.

Scheiman M, Gallaway M, Frantz KA, et al. Nearpoint of convergence: test procedure, target selection, and normative data. *Optom Vis Sci*. Mar 2003;80(3):214–225.

Thiagarajan P, Ciuffreda KJ, Ludlam DP. Vergence dysfunction in mild traumatic brain injury (mTBI): a review. *Ophthalmic Physiol Opt*. 2011;31:456–468.

BINOCULAR VISION: EYE ALIGNMENT TEST

Purpose/Description

Binocular vision is the ability of the visual system to fuse or combine the information from the right and left eyes to form one image.[1] The images that arrive from each eye must be identical, and for this to occur, both eyes must be aligned so they point at the same object at all times. The terms "heterophoria" and "phoria" are used to describe eyes that turn in, out, or up.[15] There are three common types of phoria: (1) exophoria (eyes have a tendency to turn out), (2) esophoria (eyes have tendency to turn in), and (3) hyperphoria (one eye has a tendency to turn up).[1] The Eye Alignment Test employs the methods of the Modified Thorington method and may be used to identify problems, provide treatment, and make referrals. It is not intended to replace a comprehensive vision evaluation by an optometrist.

Recommended Instrument Use: Practice Option

This test may be a helpful inclusion in an initial occupational therapy evaluation when:

- the patient has not had a comprehensive visual assessment by an optometrist/ophthalmologist to identify visual impairments, and
- the patient has mild-to-moderate brain injury or c/mTBI and observation of functional performance suggests the possibility of visual dysfunction in a number of domains.

This test can be used in conjunction with a full vision screen to screen for accommodation problems.

Administration Protocol/Equipment/Time

This test is only performed once with the Maddox rod before the right eye. It is not necessary to repeat the test. Administration time is less than 5 minutes. As stated in several studies, including Goss et al,[18] this test is quick and simple to perform and easy for patients to understand.

Equipment

Adult Screening Kit (Gulden Ophthalmics, Elkins Park, PA), which includes eye alignment near card, Maddox rod, penlight, and the Chronister Pocket Acuity Card.

Setup

If the patient typically wears corrective lenses for reading, they should be used for this test. Position the patient to optimize concentration, preferably sitting comfortably.

Procedure

- Place the penlight into the black plastic holder behind the eye alignment card.
- Examiner should hold the Maddox rod horizontally before the right eye.
- Hold the eye alignment card 16 inches from the patient, perpendicular to the face, with the light at eye level.
- Tell the patient to look at the light and report through which letter or number the red line is passing. If the patient is unable to verbally respond, ask him/her to point to where the red line is passing.
- Orient the Maddox rod vertically before the right eye.
- Tell the patient to look at the light and report through which letter or number the red line is passing. If the patient is unable to verbally respond, ask him/her to point to where the red line is passing.

Scoring

Record the letter or number reported by the patient for both horizontal and vertical alignment (Exhibit 4-3). Compare this to the norms printed on the lower right-hand side of the eye alignment card.

Expected Findings

- Exophoria less than 8
- Esophoria less than 4

Possible Problems

- The patient only sees the red line or the white light, but never both together. This indicates suppression.
- The patient sees the red line moving (it is unstable). This indicates a possible accommodative problem (unstable accommodation).
- The patient reports that the red line is not horizontal or vertical (it is oblique). This indicates the examiner is not holding the Maddox rod horizontally or vertically.

Groups Tested With This Measure

This test has been studied on healthy young adults[18–20] and children.[21] There are no published data on use of this test with adults with c/mTBI.

Interpretability

- Norms: not available for adults
- MDC: not appropriate
- Responsiveness estimates: not available

EXHIBIT 4-3

EYE ALIGNMENT TEST RESULTS

Horizontal alignment[*]: _____
Vertical alignment[†]: _____
Possible impairment of eye alignment: Yes _____ No _____

[*]As identified by patient, clinical cutoff value of less than 8 for exophoria (left of center), and less than 4 for esophoria (right of center)
[†]As identified by patient, clinical cutoff value of less than 2

Reliability Estimates

- Internal consistency: not appropriate
- Interrater: Strong interrater correlation found with the modified Thorington method (r = 0.92).[19]
- Intrarater: Among the subjective tests, the modified Thorington test was the most repeatable.[22] However, no difference between the results of the various tests was "statistically significant" for repeatability.
- Test-Retest: not available

Validity Estimates

- Content/Face: not available
- Criterion: Antona and colleagues compared the modified Thorington test with three others (von Graefe technique, Maddox rod test, and prism cover test) and concluded that due to the low level of agreement observed between these tests, interchangeability is not recommended in clinical practice.[22]
- Construct: not available

Selected References

Antona B, Gonzalez E, Barrio A, Barra F, Sanchez I, Cebrian JL. Strabometry precision: intra-examiner repeatability and agreement in measuring the magnitude of the angle of latent binocular ocular deviations (heterophorias or latent strabismus). *Binocul Vis Strabolog Q Simms Romano.* 2011;26(2):91–104.

Goss DA, Moyer BJ, Teske MC. A Comparison of Dissociated Phoria Test Findings with Von Graefe Phorometry & Modified Thorington Testing. *J Behav Optom.* 2008;19(6):145–149.

Lyon DW, Goss DA, Horner D, Downey JP, Rainey B. Normative data for modified Thorington phorias and prism bar vergences from the Benton-IU study. *Optometry.* Oct 2005;76(10):593–599.

Rainey BB, Schroeder TL, Goss DA, Grosvenor TP. Inter-examiner repeatability of heterophoria tests. *Optom Vis Sci.* Oct 1998;75(10):719–726.

Scheiman M. *Understanding and Managing Vision Deficits.* Thorofare, NJ: SLACK Incorporated; 1997.

Scheiman M. *Understanding and Managing Vision Deficits: A Guide for Occupational Therapists.* 3rd ed. Thorofare, NJ: SLACK Incorporated; 2011.

SACCADES: DEVELOPMENTAL EYE MOVEMENT TEST

Purpose/Description

The Developmental Eye Movement (DEM) test is a number-naming saccadic eye movement test that was originally developed to address saccadic movements in children. There is a need for a similar assessment in adults, as saccadic eye movements are also a concern in adults with acquired brain injuries such as stroke or TBI, and one has been developed. However, it is not available publically and there are questions whether the adult test may be considered a parallel test to the DEM due to the use of double digit numbers which may make a difference in test performance.[23] Due to the lack of support that is truly evidence based, it is recommend to use the DEM using the age 13 norms, even if the test will under-identify impairment in saccadic eye movements.[24]

The purpose of this test is to assess fixational and saccade activity during reading and nonreading tasks. Saccade control is the ability of the eye to move from one point of interest to another after an appropriate period of fixation.[24] These rapid, jumping movements enable the subject's image to be projected onto the fovea of the eye, the sharpest point of visual acuity highly concentrated with receptors and nerve cells. Saccadic and fixational activity is important for word recognition and for processing larger units of printed language.[24]

Recommended Instrument Use: Practice Option

This test may be a helpful inclusion in an initial occupational therapy evaluation when:

- the patient has not had a comprehensive visual assessment by an optometrist/ophthalmologist to identify visual impairments, and
- the patient has mild-to-moderate brain injury or c/mTBI and observation of

functional performance suggests the possibility of visual dysfunction in a number of domains.

The vertical subtest is used to evaluate automaticity of number calling (language function) and evaluate children at risk for reading disability (this skill is significantly correlated with reading achievement).[25] The test can be used in conjunction with a full vision screen to screen for accommodative and binocular vision problems.

Administration Protocol/Equipment/Time

One of the main advantages of the DEM is the ease of administration without the need for sophisticated instrumentation. Therefore, it is a useful instrument for patients with decreased attention and concentration.[24] The oculomotor performance is assessed by verbal naming speed and accuracy. The DEM is composed of two parts, the horizontal and vertical tests. Both tests require rapid, continuous naming.

The DEM consists of timing the patient reading aloud 80 double-digit numbers arranged vertically and the same numbers arranged horizontally. The vertical test uses two test plates with two columns on each page and 20 evenly spaced numbers in each column. The test plate for the horizontal test is comprised of 16 rows with five unevenly spaced numbers in each row. After adjusting for errors, the horizontal time is divided by the vertical time. The resulting ratio score is a comparison of the speed of reading material that compares performance of a number-naming task with a higher saccadic eye movement component (ie, the horizontal test results) to performance of the same number naming task with a lower saccadic eye movement requirement (ie, the vertical test results). This comparison allows for adjustment for number-naming speed and results in a measurement of the efficiency of horizontal saccadic eye movements.

Equipment

- DEM test (consists of three subtests)
- Vertical test A (contains 40 single digits)
- Vertical test B (contains 40 single digits)
- Horizontal test C (contains 80 single digits)
- Stopwatch

Setup and Procedure

- The patient views the test cards at 40 cm (~ 16 inches) away

- Ask the patient to call out the numbers on vertical tests A and B as quickly as possible from top to bottom without using his or her finger.
- Record time and errors (addition, omission, substitution).
- Ask the patient to call out the numbers on the horizontal test C as quickly as possible without using his or her finger. The patient calls out the numbers across the page.
- Record time and errors (addition [A], omission [O], substitution).
- Calculate the score to determine whether or not to refer the patient to a vision specialist.

Scoring

- *V* equals the total completion time for vertical tests A and B (in seconds).
- Determine the horizontal adjusted (*HA*) response time as follows (where horizontal time [*HT*] is in seconds): $HT \times 80 / (80 - O + A)$.
- Determine the ratio score by dividing the *HA* time by the vertical time (ratio = *HA/V*).
- Compare the service member's score to the referral cut point based on the age 13 norm (Exhibit 4-4). Refer accordingly.

Groups Tested With This Measure

The DEM was initially normed and administered to 556 elementary school students ranging in age from 6-13 years.[25] The authors were unaware of any sample selection biases.[25] Tassinari and DeLand addressed its reliability and associated symptomatology.[25] This instrument has not been tested on adults with c/mTBI.

Interpretability

- Norms: determined by using the norms for age 13 by Garcia et al[25] (see Exhibit 4-4). Service members whose ratio scores are one standard deviation above the mean (eg, above the cut point) should be referred to a vision specialist.
- MDC: not available
- Responsiveness estimates: not available

Reliability Estimates

- Internal consistency: Garcia et al found that the correlations between all subtests were

---

EXHIBIT 4-4

DEVELOPMENTAL EYE MOVEMENT TEST RESULTS

Test A Vertical: _____ seconds
Test B Vertical: _____ seconds
  Adjusted Vertical Time (V) = (tests A + B) = _____ seconds
Test C – Horizontal (HT): _____ seconds
  Errors: additions (A) _____   omissions (O) _____   substitutions _____   transposition _____
  Horizontal Adjusted Time $(HA) = HT \times 80/(80 - O + A) =$
Ratio score: $HA / V =$ _____
Compare score to cut point below*: Possible impairment of saccades: Yes_____ No _____

---

*Clinical cutoff value is a ratio score greater than 1.22. Cutoff for screening is determined as 1 standard deviation above the mean norm for age 13 (ratio mean = 1.12, standard deviation = 0.10 [no adult norms available]).
Data source: Richman JE. *DEM Manual: The Developmental Eye Movement Test: Examiner's Manual.* Version 2.0. Mishawaka, IN: Bernell Corporation; 2009.

---

significant $(P < 0.001)$ except vertical time and ratio score $(r = -0.05)$[25]

- Interrater: Testing the interrater reliability found vertical time, r = 0.81, horizontal time, r = 0.91, ratio r = 0.57 $(P < 0.01)$.[25]
- Intrarater: Testing the intrarater reliability found vertical time, r = 0.89, horizontal time, r = 0.86, ratio r = 0.57 $(P < 0.01)$.[25]
- Test-Retest: There are several studies that address this in children with varying results. Vertical time, r = 0.85; horizontal time, r = 1.89; ratio scores (corrected for attenuation), r = 0.66.[25] There are two reliability studies that show poor test-retest

reliability for vertical, horizontal, and ratio.[26]

Validity Estimates

- Content/Face: not available
- Criterion: not available
- Construct: The Wide Range Achievement Test was compared to the DEM. The results indicated moderate to high negative correlations with all DEM subtests that were significant at the P < 0.001 level (vertical time r = -0.79; horizontal time r = -0.78; ratio = -0.55).[25]

Selected References

Garcia RP, Richman JE, Nicholson SB, Gaines CS. A new visual-verbal saccade test: The Developmental Eye Movement test (DEM). *J Behavioral Optom.* 1990;61:124-135.

Powell JM, Birk K, Cummings EH, Col MA. The need for adult norms on the Developmental Eye Movement test. *J Behavioral Optom.* 2005;16(2):38–41.

Tassinari JT, DeLand P. Developmental Eye Movement test: reliability and symptomatology. *Optometry.* Jul 2005;76(7):387–399.

PURSUITS AND SACCADES: NORTHEASTERN STATE UNIVERSITY COLLEGE OF OPTOMETRY OCULOMOTOR TEST

Purpose/Description

The Northeastern State University College of Optometry (NSUCO) Oculomotor Test is a direct observational test for screening saccades and pursuits to determine if a patient demonstrates impairment with these visual skills. Saccades are quick eye movements that occur when the eyes fix on various targets in the visual field,[27] and pursuits are "eye movements that maintain continued fixation on a moving target."[27(p241)]

The purpose of this standardized test is to assess four aspects of pursuits and saccades, including: (1) ability (sustaining power), (2) accuracy, (3) degree of head movement the patient uses to perform the task, and (4) degree of body movement. It may be used to identify problems, provide treatment, and make referrals; it is not intended to replace a comprehensive vision evaluation by an optometrist/ophthalmologist.

Recommended Instrument Use: Practice Option

This test may be a helpful inclusion in an initial occupational therapy evaluation when:

1. the patient has not had a comprehensive visual assessment by an optometrist/ophthalmologist to identify visual impairments, and
2. the patient has mild-to-moderate brain injury or c/mTBI and observation of functional performance suggests the possibility of visual dysfunction in a number of domains.

This test can be used in conjunction with a full vision screen to assess saccades and pursuits and can be used for patients ages 5 to adulthood.

Administration Protocol/Equipment/Time

Required equipment includes two small (approximately a 1/2-inch diameter), colored, reflective spheres (balls) mounted on dowel sticks. Administration time is less than 5 minutes. The limited verbal interaction required by the examiner together with objective observations enables this to be an advantageous direct observational test.

Groups Tested With This Measure

Although the NSUCO Oculomotor Test is widely used with adult patients, it has not been formally tested on adults with or without brain injury. It has been tested extensively on children up to the age of 14, including interrater and intrarater reliability, and test-retest reliability,[28] construct validity,[29,30] and norms.[31]

Interpretability

This test has not been normed on adults. Because oculomotor development is believed to plateau by age 14, clinicians may consider using the norms reported by Maples, Atchley, and Ficklin (Tables 4-2 and 4-3). To do so, the clinician assigns a score of 1 through 5 based on the scoring criteria, then compares each score to the failure criteria. Scores that fall below the minimal levels may indicate impairment. Beyond assigning scores, therapists may use the NSUCO Oculomotor Test as a venue for observing patient performance in areas of ability, accuracy, and head and body movement and use these observations to decide whether to refer the patient to a vision specialist for more in-depth evaluation.

- MDC: not available; however, repeat testing over time with changes in performance would give different scores.
- Responsiveness estimates: not available

Reliability Estimates

- Internal consistency: not available
- Interrater: 21 elementary students tested with 24 student clinicians scoring:
  - Average exact agreement of the four scores of the pursuits test: 73.5%.[28]
  - Average exact agreement of the four scores of the saccades test: 75%.[28]
- Intrarater: 21 elementary students tested with 24 student clinicians scoring:
  - Average exact agreement of the four scores of the pursuits test: 90%.[28]

TABLE 4-2

SACCADES: NORMS FOR INDIVIDUALS 14 YEARS OF AGE AND OLDER*

		SACCADES		
	Ability	**Accuracy**	**Head Movement**	**Body Movement**
Male	Less than 5	Less than 4	Less than 3	Less than 5
Female	Less than 5	Less than 3	Less than 4	Less than 5

*Scores indicate failure.
Adapted with permission from: Maples WC, Atchley J, Ficklin T. Northeastern State University College of Optometry's oculomotor norms. *J Behav Optom.* 1992;3:149.

TABLE 4-3

PURSUITS: NORMS FOR INDIVIDUALS 14 YEARS OF AGE AND OLDER*

	PURSUITS			
	Ability	Accuracy	Head Movement	Body Movement
Male	Less than 5	Less than 5	Less than 4	Less than 5
Female	Less than 5	Less than 4	Less than 4	Less than 5

*Scores indicate failure.
Adapted with permission from: Maples WC, Atchley J, Ficklin T. Northeastern State University College of Optometry's oculomotor norms. *J Behav Optom.* 1992;3:149.

- ○ Average exact agreement of the four scores of the saccades test: 83%.[28]
- Test-Retest: 21 elementary students tested with two paired scores on each scale (8 observations × 21 patients = 168 possible significant differences). 87% reliability with 22 significant differences found at the .05 level.[31]

This test did not show significant improvement on retest except for improvement in saccade head movement.[31]

Validity Estimates

- Content/Face: not available
- Criterion: not available
- Construct: NSUCO Oculomotor Test was used to compare academic performance in normal, learning-disabled, and gifted children. The difference between gifted and learning-disabled children was statistically significant in two tests out of eight; however, three tests approached significance. Gifted and normal children were found to be very similar.[29,31] The NSUCO Oculomotor Test was also used to compare good readers and poor readers in a third grade class as determined by the Gates McGinitie or Science Research Association Achievement Reading Test Achievement Reading Test. Videotapes were made of the oculomotor behavior of both good readers (average 1 year, 9 months above grade placement) and poor readers (average 1 year, 3 months below grade placement). All eight categories for pursuits and saccades tested at a significantly different performance at the 0.5 level or better.[30,31]

Selected References

Maples WC, Atchley J, Ficklin TW. Northeastern State University College of Optometry's oculomotor norms. *J Behav Optom.* 1992;3:143–150.

Maples WC, Ficklin TW. Inter-rater and test-rater reliability of pursuits and saccades. *J Am Optom Assoc.* 1988;59:549-552.

Quintana LA. Assessing Abilities and Capacities: Vision, Visual Perception and Praxis. In: Radomsk MV, Trombly Latham CA, eds. *Occupational Therapy for Physical Dysfunction.* Philadelphia, PA: Lippincott, Williams & Wilkins; 2008:234–259.

Standard Setup

- Posture: position patient standing, with feet shoulder-width apart, directly in front of the examiner.
- Head: no instructions are given to the patient to move or not to move his or her head.
- Target characteristics: small (approximately 1/2-inch diameter), colored, reflective spheres (balls) mounted on dowel sticks. One target is used for pursuits, two for saccades.

Movement of the Target

Directional

- Saccades are performed in the horizontal meridian only.
- Pursuits are performed rotationally, both clockwise and counterclockwise.

Extent

- Saccade extent should be at approximately 4 inches on each side of the patient's midline (8 inches total).
- Pursuit path should be approximately 8 inches in diameter. The upper and lower extent of the circular path should coincide with the patient's midline.
- Test distance from the patient: no more than 15.5 inches and no less than the Harmon distance (the distance from the subject's middle knuckle to his or her elbow).
- Ocular condition: binocular only
- Age of the patient: 5 years to adult[31]

Instructions

- Saccades: "When I say 'red,' look at the red ball. When I say 'green,' look at the green ball. Remember, don't look until I tell you to."
- Pursuits: "Watch the ball as it goes around. Try to see yourself in the ball. Don't ever take your eyes off the ball."[31]

Scoring

- **Ability**: can the patient keep his or her attention under control to complete five round trips for saccades and two clockwise and then two counterclockwise rotations for pursuits?
  - **Saccades**
    1. Completes less than two round trips
    2. Completes two round trips
    3. Completes three round trips
    4. Completes four round trips
    5. Completes five round trips
  - **Pursuits**
    1. Cannot complete 1/2 rotations in either the clockwise or counterclockwise direction

    2. Completes 1/2 rotation in either direction
    3. Completes one rotation in either direction
    4. Completes two rotations in one direction but less than two rotations in the other direction
    5. Completes two rotations in each direction
- **Accuracy (pursuits and saccades are graded alike)**: can the patient accurately and consistently fixate so no noticeable correction is needed in the case of saccades, or track the target so no noticeable refixation is needed when doing pursuits?
  - **Saccades**
    1. Large over- or undershooting is noted one or more times.
    2. Moderate over- or undershooting is noted one or more times.
    3. Constant slight over- or undershooting is noted (greater than 50% of the time).
    4. Intermittent slight over- or undershooting is noted (less than 50% of the time).
    5. No over- or under-shooting is noted.
  - **Pursuits**
    1. No attempt to follow the target, or requires greater than 10 refixations
    2. Refixations 5–10 times
    3. Refixations 3–5 times
    4. Refixations 2 times or less
    5. No refixations
- **Head and body movement:** can the patient accomplish the saccade or pursuit test without moving his or her head or body? Both saccade and pursuit scoring use the same criteria for this aspect of the testing.
    1. Large movement of the head or body at any time
    2. Moderate movement of the head or body at any time
    3. Slight movement of the head or body greater than 50% of the time
    4. Slight movement of the head or body less than 50% of the time
    5. No movement of the head or body

Record results and compare to norms (Exhibit 4-5, see Tables 4-2 and 4-3).[31]

EXHIBIT 4-5

PURSUITS AND SACCADES: NORTHEASTERN STATE COLLEGE OF OPTOMETRY EYE MOVEMENT TEST

	Pursuits	Saccades
Ability		
Accuracy		
Head Movement		
Body Movement		

Data source: Maples WC, Atchley J, Ficklin TW. Northeastern State University College of Optometry's oculomotor norms. *J Behav Optom.* 1992;3:143–150.

CONFRONTATION FIELD TEST

Purpose/Description

Visual field deficit is a visual concern associated with acquired brain injury.[15] Confrontation field testing enables the therapist to screen for gross peripheral visual field loss.

Recommended Instrument Use: Practice Option

There are several confrontation field tests and the choice of tests may affect the likelihood of identifying a visual field defect.[32] The confrontation field test should be used as a screen only because it lacks adequate sensitivity[33]; therefore, if the screening results are negative but the patient's behavior suggests field loss, he or she should still be referred to a vision specialist.[15] This test may be a helpful inclusion in an initial occupational therapy evaluation when:

- the patient has not had a comprehensive visual assessment by an optometrist/ophthalmologist to identify visual impairments, and
- the patient has mild-to-moderate brain injury or complicated c/mTBI and observation of functional performance suggests the possibility of visual dysfunctional in a number of domains.

Administration Protocol/Equipment/Time

Required equipment includes two eye patches/occluders and a target white sphere, 3 mm or less in diameter, mounted on a nonglossy wand. Administration time is less than 5 minutes.

Groups Tested With This Measure

Kerr et al[32] investigated the accuracy of confrontation visual field testing with adult subjects with visual deficit etiologies including: glaucoma, optic neuropathies, optic neuritis, glioma, stroke, and chiasmal tumors. Trobe et al[33] compared various finger and color confrontation tests in identifying chiasmal and optic nerve visual field defects. Subjects included persons with chiasmal hemianopias and neuropathy-related nerve-fiber-bundle defects. Age was not specified. Shahinfar, Johnson, and Madsen[34] reported specificity on various visual field defects, including hemianopias. This test has not been validated on adults with c/mTBI.

Interpretability

Kerr et al[32] investigated the accuracy of confrontation visual field testing and concluded that when performed individually, confrontation visual field tests are insensitive at detecting visual field loss. When confrontation tests were combined, sensitivity improved. Finger counting combined with static finger wiggle achieved 44.6% sensitivity and 97.2% specificity. Use of a kinetic red target resulted in the highest sensitivity and specificity.

- Norms: there are no norms for this test and total score is not calculated.
  - In Part 1, the patient should be able to see the target at approximately the same point at which you can see it. If there appears to be a significant discrepancy,

a visual field deficit may be present and a referral is necessary for a more precise measurement of the patient's visual field.

- ◦ In Part 2, you are testing the patient's ability to see two objects simultaneously. Patients with visual neglect will have problems with the task even if they do well with Part 1.
- MDC: not available
- Responsiveness estimates: not available

Reliability Estimates: not available

Validity Estimates

- Content validity: not available
- Criterion validity: Kerr et al[32] found confrontation testing to be insensitive to detecting visual field loss as compared to automated perimetry.
- Construct validity: not available

Selected References

Kerr NM, Chew SS, Eady EK, Gamble GD, Danesh-Meyer HV. Diagnostic accuracy of confrontation visual field tests. *Neurology.* 2010;74(15):1184–1190.

Shahinfar S, Johnson LN, Madsen RW. Confrontation visual field loss as a function of decibel sensitivity loss on automated static perimetry. Implications on the accuracy of confrontation visual field testing. *Ophthalmology.* Jun 1995;102(6):872–877.

Trobe JD, Acosta PC, Krischer JP, Trick GL. Confrontation visual field techniques in the detection of anterior visual pathway lesions. *Ann Neurol.* 1980;10:28–34.

Administration Protocol

Part 1

Preparation
1. Patch the patient's left eye; patch your right eye.
2. Sit approximately 20 inches opposite the patient; your left eye should be directly opposite the patient's right eye. Optimally, there should be a dark, uniform wall behind the patient.
3. Provide instructions to the patient. Tell the patient that you will show various finger counts with your hand from the side. Ask the patient to report as soon as he or she sees your hand and how many fingers you are holding up, while continuing to look directly at your left eye.

Testing
1. Start at the 12-o'clock position and slowly move your hand (3-finger count) until the patient first reports seeing it (the object should be placed evenly between the therapist and the patient).
2. Compare the patient's response to yours. If the patient cannot see the target as soon as you can, it is an indication of a possible problem.

3. Move clockwise to the 2-, 4-, 6-, 8-, and 10-o'clock positions and repeat procedures 1 and 2.
4. Record approximately where the patient reports seeing the target in each orientation tested.
5. Patch the patient's right eye; patch your left eye.
6. Sit opposite the patient. Your right eye should be directly opposite the patient's left eye.
7. Repeat the testing procedure described in Steps 1-4.
8. Record results (Exhibit 4-6).

Part 2

Preparation
1. Patch the patient's left eye; patch your right eye.
2. Sit approximately 20 inches opposite the patient; your left eye should be directly opposite the patient's right eye. Optimally, there should be a dark, uniform wall behind the patient.

Testing
1. Extend your arms so your hands are in the 3- and 9-o'clock positions. Your fingers should be positioned so that you can see them from your open eye. Instruct the

EXHIBIT 4-6

CONFRONTATION FIELD TEST RESULTS

Part 1

Position	Right Eye		Left Eye	
	Does the patient see the target when expected? (Y/N)	If no, # of approximate degrees from center, patient sees the object	Does the patient see the target when expected? (Y/N)	If no, # of approximate degrees from center, patient sees the object
12				
2				
4				
6				
8				
10				

Part 2

Right Eye	Left Eye
Does the patient see the correct # of fingers? (Y/N)	Does the patient see the correct # of fingers? (Y/N)

patient to tell you how many fingers you are holding up with each hand.

2. Patch the patient's right eye; patch your left eye.
3. Repeat Step 1.
4. Record results (see Exhibit 4-6).

Confrontation Field Test Results

- In Testing Part 1 the patient should be able to see the target at approximately the same point at which you can see it. If there appears to be a significant discrepancy, a visual field deficit may be present and a referral is necessary for a more precise measurement of the patient's visual field.
- In Testing Part 2, you are testing the patient's ability to see two objects simultaneously. Patients with visual neglect will have problems with the task even if they do well with testing Part 1.

STEREO RANDOT TEST

Purpose/Description

The Stereo Randot Test is used to screen for stereopsis (binocular vision). This test requires the patient to identify forms (geometric forms or animals) from random dot backgrounds while wearing polarized 3-D viewing glasses. It may be used to identify problems, provide treatment, and make referrals; it is not intended to replace a comprehensive vision evaluation by an optometrist.

Recommended Instrument Use: Practice Option

This test may be a helpful inclusion in an initial occupational therapy evaluation when:

- the patient has not had a comprehensive visual assessment by an optometrist/ophthalmologist to identify visual impairments, and
- the patient has mild-to-moderate brain injury or c/mTBI and observation of

functional performance suggests the possibility of visual dysfunction in a number of domains.

This test can be used in conjunction with a full vision screen to assess for stereopsis.

Administration Protocol/Equipment/Time

Equipment needs include the Stereo Randot Test kit (available through Bernell VTP. www.stereooptical.com/products/stereotests#randot). Administration time is less than 2 minutes.

Groups Tested With This Measure: not available

Interpretability

- Norms: normal stereo is expected in all adults. The patient should be able to identify all of the simple forms correctly. A patient who has a constant strabismus will be unable to identify any of the forms. Patients with less severe problems, such as intermittent strabismus and heterophoria, will generally have a normal response. It is possible for a patient with acquired brain injury to report double vision on this task, which would suggest that a strabismus is present.
- MDC: not applicable, no expected change in performance
- Responsiveness estimates: not applicable

Reliability and Validity Estimates: not available for adults

Setup

The patient must be able to position his or her head vertically (without tilting) to correctly perform this test. If not, do not use this test.

Administration Protocol

Clinicians are advised to follow the administration protocol specified in the Stereo Randot Test kit's Instruction Manual. In general, this test is administered as follows.

1. Ask the patient to put on the 3-D viewing glasses (over prescription lenses, if need be). Hold the Test upright 16 inches from the patient's eyes. Ask what the patient sees. If the patient has stereopsis, he or she will report seeing geometric forms (depending upon the version of the test selected by the clinician). Give the patient 20 to 30 seconds to try to see the targets.
2. If the patient has difficulty, make sure the head is not tilted to the side.
3. It is helpful to have a drawing available of the test forms (located on the front of the instruction manual). If the patient struggles with the task, you can show the possible forms. Of course, it is more convincing if the patient, without prior knowledge of the forms, is able to identify all correctly (Exhibit 4-7).

Expected Results

Normal performance: The patient should be able to identify forms correctly; however, it should be noted that patients with less severe problems, such as intermittent strabismus and heterophoria, will generally have a normal response.

Abnormal performance: Those with constant strabismus will be unable to identify any of the forms. It is possible for a patient with acquired brain injury to report double vision on this task, suggesting possible strabismus.

BRAIN INJURY VISUAL ASSESSMENT BATTERY FOR ADULTS

Purpose/Description

The Brain Injury Visual Assessment Battery for Adults (biVABA) is a battery of tests used to screen visual processing following brain injury. Results enable therapists to make appropriate referrals and address functional limitations.[35] The biVABA is not intended to replace a comprehensive vision evaluation by an optometrist/ophthalmologist.

EXHIBIT 4-7

STEREO RANDOT TEST RESULTS

Able to identify all forms correctly?

                      Yes _____   No _____

Correct: _____ / 6

Recommended Instrument Use: Practice Option

This test may be a helpful inclusion in an initial occupational therapy evaluation when:

- the patient has not had a comprehensive visual assessment by an optometrist/ophthalmologist to identify visual impairments, and
- the patient has mild-to-moderate brain injury or complicated concussion/mTBI and observation of functional performance suggests the possibility of visual dysfunction.

The biVABA is also appropriate for anyone who has experienced a brain injury from any cause, including cerebrovascular accident, TBI, brain tumor, anoxia, or anyone who has experienced trauma to the eye.[35] The biVABA can be used for patients ages 14 years and above without modification.

Administration Protocol/Equipment/Time

The biVABA is comprised of a battery of subtests that includes a clinical observation checklist and assessments of visual acuity (distance and reading), contrast sensitivity function, visual field, oculomotor function, visual attention, and scanning. Administration takes approximately 60 minutes.

Detailed administration and scoring procedures are available for purchase from the developer (vis-ABILITIIES Rehab Services, Inc; www.visabilities.com) and are not included in this Toolkit. Clinicians should refer to the biVABA's test booklet and manual for additional information regarding psychometric properties and score interpretation.

Groups Tested With This Measure

The biVABA has not been tested on adults with TBI, and only the visual search section of the biVABA has been empirically tested. The seven subtests used to assess visual search have been included in two studies: they were field tested on 25 subjects between ages 16 and 83 to determine usual search patterns and norms[35,36] and to describe the performance and types of search patterns of the subtests in 81 participants.[37]

Interpretability

The manual provides result interpretation, including descriptions of normal testing reactions. For example, for acuity, 1M print is standard-sized print (newspaper); for pupillary responses, the normal pupil shape is described and an approximate size for pupils in a well-illuminated room is given. See manual for interpretations of patient responses.

- Norms: Analysis of norms of descriptive search strategies and cut-off percentiles are given for the seven subtests of the visual scanning section (see full detailed discussion in product manual).
- MDC: not available
- Responsiveness estimates: not available

Reliability and Validity Estimates

Most of the subtests that comprise the biVABA have previously been evaluated for reliability and validity.[36]

- The biVABA includes three standard visual screening tests that are accepted by ophthalmologists as valid and reliable assessment tools (the Lea Numbers Intermediate Acuity test, the Lea Low Contrast Acuity test, and the Damato Campimeter).
- The Warren text card is a modification of the Lighthouse Near Vision Reading Card.
- The screening for oculomotor performance is composed of standard screening tests that are routinely used by ophthalmologists and neurologists.
- The design copy test is adapted from the literature.
- The visual search subtests use a cancellation test format that has been studied and used extensively in research and has very good validity established by research.

SECTION 2: VISUAL INTERVENTIONS

INTRODUCTION

Vision is the most far-reaching of our sensory systems. Changes to this system can affect patients' ability to participate in therapy as well as function in everyday life.[15] Brahm and colleagues[2] suggest that combat troops with blast-related c/mTBI are at risk for visual dysfunction. Occupational therapists are often the first-line clinicians who are able to identify possible visual impairment. The occupational therapist's roles include evaluating vision function through vision screening and functional observations and determining whether and how visual impairment may be affecting the patient's functional performance.

If visual impairment is suspected, the occupational therapist is responsible for:

- referring the patient to a staff optometrist with expertise in vision and TBI for further evaluation and intervention management,
- educating the patient and the rehabilitation team about how the impairment is affecting the patient functionally,
- providing compensatory treatment,
- providing remedial therapy under the supervision of an optometrist with expertise in vision and TBI, and
- providing various activities that will address visual impairments while working on other impairments.

General Instructions for Treating Visual Impairments

Always make sure the patient has the best corrected vision (ie, wearing the correct glasses) for participating in therapy and that the correction fits well (see General Instructions for Vision Assessment for instructions on best fit and use of bifocals and trifocals). Decide what kind of environment is best for the impairment and focus of the treatment (determined by the patient's level of impairment and distractibility). The environment should be:

- well lit with no glare;
- clutter-free, unless the patient is working on more complex visual tasks; and
- quiet, unless the patient is working on more complex tasks.

Determine whether the patient should be seated, standing, or performing a task that involves walking.

Compensatory Approaches to Visual Deficit

- Modify the task or the environment to maximize the patient's ability to participate.
- Educate the patient about the impairment.
- Teach and practice methods to compensate for the deficit.

Grading the Tasks, Activity Analysis

- Density: low density to high density (eg, start with two columns of letters, one on each side of the page, then progress to 10 columns of letters; Figure 4-2)
- Structure: task (ie, start with organized simple structure and move towards random; Figure 4-3)
- Speed: start with slow, deliberate movement; slowly increase speed (use a metronome, if desired)

Other Suggestions for Oculomotor Therapy

- Enable the patient to achieve early success.
- Emphasize accuracy then work on speed (saccadic and pursuit activities).
- For saccades activities, work from large to small eye movements.
- For pursuits activities, progress from small to large eye movements.
- Work on eyes individually until eyes are equal in ability, then work on eyes together.
- Eliminate head movements during pursuit and saccadic eye movements for activities that can be accomplished without head movement.
- Increase the complexity of the tasks to work toward automatic eye movements. Options include adding a metronome, balance board, or cognitive task that incorporates eye movements.

Selected References

Brahm KD, Wilgenburg HM, Kirby J, Ingalla S, Chang CY, Goodrich GL. Visual impairment and dysfunction in combat-injured servicemembers with traumatic brain injury. *Optom Vis Sci.* Jul 2009;86(7):817–825.

Scheiman M. *Understanding and Managing Vision Deficits: A Guide for Occupational Therapists.* 3rd ed. Thorofare, NJ: SLACK Incorporated; 2011.

Warren M. A hierarchal model for evaluation and treatment of visual perception dysfunction in adult acquired brain injury, Part II. *Am J Occup Ther.* 1993;47:55–66.

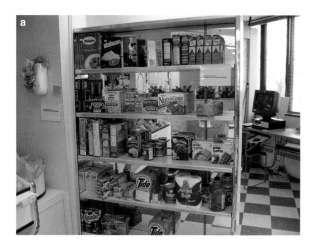 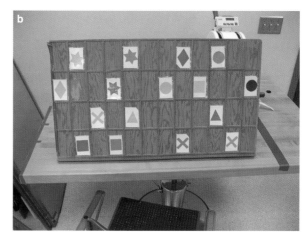

Figure 4-2. Examples of high-density **(a)** and low-density **(b)** visual stimuli.

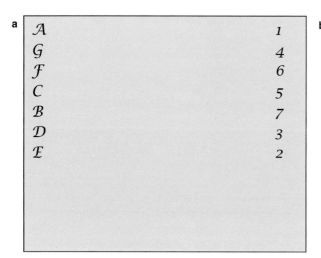 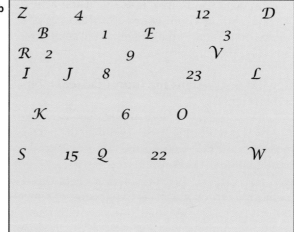

Figure 4-3. Examples of structured **(a)** and unstructured **(b)** visual stimuli.

Other Resources for Occupational Therapy and Vision

Gillen G. *Cognitive and Perceptual Rehabilitation: Optimizing Function*. St Louis, MO: Mosby; 2009.

Zoltan B. *Vision, Perception, and Cognition: A Manual for the Evaluation and Treatment of the Adult With Acquired Brain Injury*. 4th ed. Thorofare, NJ: SLACK Incorporated; 2007.

POOR ACUITY

Purpose/Background

Acuity refers to clarity of vision and the ability to see detail. When acuity is affected, a patient may have difficulty reading, doing fine motor tasks that involve hand-eye coordination, recognizing faces, and the like. Impaired acuity may be connected to reduced central vision and visual field loss. For some patients, treatment may be as simple as wearing glasses correctly or referral to an eye doctor, other patients may have some damage to the eye or eye system that may limit the amount of corrected prescription options available to make a patient functional again.

Visual impairment is acuity less than 20/60 (normal being 20/20).[36] The legal definition of blindness in the United States is visual acuity of 20/200 or worse (or severely restricted peripheral vision). Blindness is defined as visual acuity worse than 20/400.[39]

Strength of Recommendation: Practice Option

Although there are no formal studies that indicate which interventions are best, the interventions that follow are included in textbooks and literature related to low vision.

Interventions

- Refer the patient to an eye specialist (optometrist or ophthalmologist). The patient needs to be evaluated for appropriate prescription to maximize vision clarity.
- If the patient has significant acuity impairment, he or she may need to be referred to a low-vision specialist.
- Educate the patient on proper use of glasses and about impairment.
- Teach the patient compensatory strategies, such as
  - increasing illumination,
  - increasing contrast,
  - increasing size (enlargement or magnification),
  - decreasing background pattern or clutter, and
  - organizing the environment.
- Provide sensory substitution using assistive devices.

Selected References

Answers.com. Visually Impaired webpage. http://www.answers.com/topic/visually-impaired. Accessed June 17, 2013.

Gillen G. *Cognitive and Perceptual Rehabilitation: Optimizing Function.* St Louis, MO: Mosby; 2009.

Scheiman M. *Understanding and Managing Vision Deficits: A Guide for Occupational Therapists.* 3rd ed. Thorofare, NJ: SLACK Incorporated; 2011.

Warren M. Evaluation and treatment of visual deficits. In: Pedretti LW, Early MB, eds. *Occupational Therapy: Practice Skills for Physical Dysfunction.* 5th ed. St Louis, MO: Mosby; 2001: 386–421.

Education

Encourage Proper Use of Glasses

- Patient should wear the appropriate glasses for the task (eg, distance, reading, and computer distance glasses).
- Be sure the patient's glasses fit correctly.
- Be sure the patient uses the appropriate portion and focal distance (working distance) for the glasses. Some people wear progressive lenses, which will not have obvious segments, but placement should be similar (see Figure 4-1).
  - Upper portion is for distance
  - Trifocal for mid-distance (18–24 inches; eg, computer monitor)
  - Near distance
- Some people now wear monovision contacts in which one eye is used for distance and the other for near vision. This will affect how patients use their eyes and how to approach treatment.

Compensatory Techniques and Teaching

The following are compensatory techniques that can be used in the clinic for a patient with poor visual acuity as well as to teach the patient to better function outside the clinic.

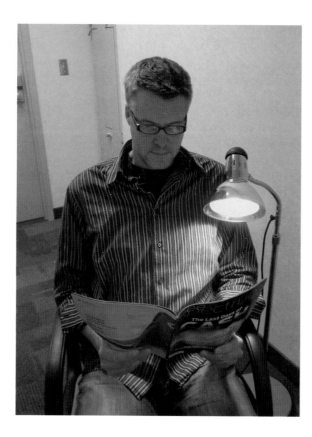

Figure 4-4. Task lamp should be placed below the patient's glasses and directed onto the table, reading material, or task.

Increase Illumination

- Increase the amount of light.
- Determine the best lighting option for the patient that also minimizes glare (eg, incandescent bulbs, halogen, fluorescent [may have flicker effect], and full spectrum).

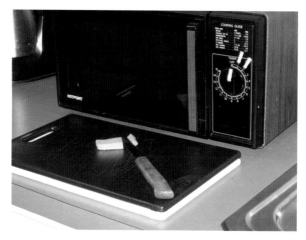

Figure 4-5. Increase contrast for food preparations and put bright tape or textured stickers on dials.

- If possible, place the light below patient's glasses or optical device to prevent glare off the glass (Figure 4-4).
- Sometimes task lamps are better than room lights.

Increase Contrast

Increase contrast by, for example, placing black coffee in a white mug, butter on a dark plate, contrasting colored tape on the edge of steps, colored soap on a white sink (Figures 4-5, 4-6, and 4-7).

Decrease Background Pattern

- Use solid colors for tablecloth or bedspread to more easily find items set on top of it.

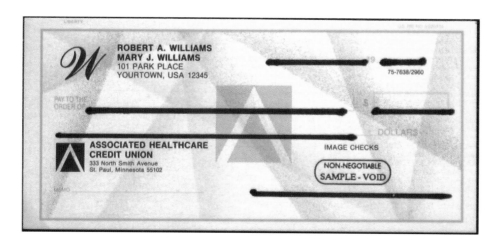

Figure 4-6. Add thick, dark lines to checks and other forms.

- Use plain dishes and solid-colored place-mats.
- Simplify junk drawers.

Decrease Clutter and Organize Environment

- Put items away.
- Organize storage places.

Increase Size

- Enlarge print.
- Use thick markers (see Figure 4-6).
- Enlarge computer font.

Magnify

- Use handheld devices and determine the best focal distance of the device (the distance of the lens from the object or reading material with the best clarity; the light rays converge).
- Teach patient methods to maintain the distance.
- Use hand or finger to stabilize the hand held device
- Use handheld stand magnifier that

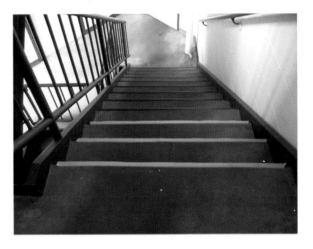

Figure 4-7. Add contrasting colored stripes to edges of stairs.

maintains distance (good for patients with incoordination and ataxia).

Use Visual Markers

- For reading, use a ruler under the line being read.
- For dials on appliances, put bright tape or textured stickers on the most commonly used settings (see Figure 4-5).

IMPAIRED PURSUITS

Purpose/Background

Patients with c/mTBI may demonstrate impairment with pursuits during the occupational therapy vision screen. This could be due to a variety of issues, including (but not limited to) motor control, poor innervation, damage to cranial nerves, and poor visual attention. The occupational therapist's roles are as follows:

- identify the potential impairment and how it is affecting the patient functionally,
- refer the patient to a staff optometrist with expertise in vision and TBI,
- educate the patient about the impairment and its functional implications,
- provide compensatory intervention, and
- provide basic range-of-motion exercises for the eye and opportunities within therapy to address visual pursuits during various activities while addressing other areas of treatment.

It is not recommended that occupational therapists spend more than 5 to 10 minutes doing vision exercises unless more time has been recommended by a staff optometrist with expertise in vision and TBI. Although the exercises will not harm the patient, the optometrist will be able to determine whether the exercises will be beneficial or unnecessary to the diagnosis.

Occupational therapy intervention emphasizes the functional implications of possible vision impairment. Therapists address impairments by grading functional activities and monitoring patients' ability and success.

Strength of Recommendation: Practice Option

There is minimal to no objective research demonstrating that the use of eye exercises will benefit pursuit dysfunction for patients with c/mTBI; however, basic range-of-motion or functional activities that use these skills will not harm a patient and may improve function.

Intervention Methods

- Refer patient to an eye specialist for assessment and treatment.
- Provide education.
  - Provide individualized information to the patient about his or her vision strengths and weaknesses and potential strategies.
  - Provide compensatory strategies to maximize function.
  - Assign basic vision exercises, as appropriate.
  - Introduce therapeutic activities that include visual pursuits while addressing other areas of occupational therapy intervention.

CLINICIAN TIP SHEET: INTERVENTION METHODS FOR PURSUITS

Education

What are Pursuits?

Pursuits are "eye movements that maintain continued fixation on a moving target."[27(p241)] Examples include:

- following a ball with your eyes in sports,
- watching people or animals walk or run,
- following an electrical cord from an appliance to an outlet with just your eyes, and
- watching a pen or pencil while writing.

Examples of visual pursuits when the object is stationary and the person is moving include:

- reading a sign or looking at a house while driving by in a car (on a bike, etc), and
- looking in the mirror while turning your head to fix your hair.

When an eye has impaired pursuits, it is difficult to:

- follow moving objects (eg, you lose sight of the ball while watching sports),
- locate which cord goes to which appliance from a power strip, or
- follow the pen while writing.

Compensatory Options

Compensatory options for pursuits are similar to the techniques used for low vision and poor acuity and include:

- increasing illumination, contrast, and size of print (enlarging);
- decreasing clutter and background pattern; and
- using visual markers (eg, using a guide or finger to assist in looking at different objects).

CLINICIAN TIP SHEET: TREATMENT IDEAS FOR PURSUITS

There is minimal to no objective research demonstrating that eye exercises will benefit visual pursuit impairment for patients with c/mTBI; however, basic eye exercises or functional activities will not harm a patient and may assist in improving function (see Range-of-Motion Exercises). If the patient complains of dizziness or nausea with range-of-motion exercise, stop the exercise and find a less visual task to work on. If the patient has not been referred to an eye specialist already, he or she should be.

Following the exercise is a list of treatment suggestions that use visual pursuit skills while addressing other treatment areas as well (Exhibit 4-8). These activities could be easily incorporated into treatment while addressing other impairments.

General Suggestions

- Start with only one eye at a time (cover the other eye with a patch) until both eyes are doing the exercise equally. Once eyes are able to do the task at the same quality, perform with both eyes.
- Have patient keep his or her head still and focus on moving the eye (or eyes).
- Start with small movements and progress to larger movements.
- This should only take about 5 minutes of session time unless recommended by a staff optometrist with expertise in vision and TBI.

Range-of-Motion Exercises

Using a target (eg, a small ball or object on a dowel or penlight) and an eye patch or occluder, move the target slowly back and forth several times into all directions of view (eg, make a "+" and an "X").

IMPAIRED SACCADES

Purpose/Background

Patients with c/mTBI may demonstrate impairment with saccades during the occupational therapy vision screen. This could be due to a variety of issues, including (but not exclusively) motor control, poor innervation, damage to cranial nerves, and poor visual attention. The occupational therapist's role is as follows:

- identify the potential impairment and how it is affecting the patient functionally,
- refer the patient to an optometrist with expertise in vision and TBI,
- educate the patient about the impairment and its functional implications,
- provide compensatory intervention, and
- provide basic eye exercises and opportunities within therapy to address visual inefficiencies during various activities while also addressing other areas of treatment.

It is not recommended that occupational therapists spend more than 5 to 10 minutes doing vision exercises unless more time has been specifically recommended by a staff optometrist with expertise in vision and TBI. Although the exercises will not harm the patient, the optometrist will be able to determine whether the exercises will be beneficial or unnecessary to the diagnosis.

Occupational therapy intervention emphasizes the functional implications of possible vision impairment. Therapists address impairments by grading functional activities and monitoring patients' abilities and successes.

Strength of Recommendation: Practice Option

There is minimal to no objective research demonstrating that eye exercises will benefit visual saccade impairment for patients with c/mTBI; however, basic eye exercises or functional activities will not harm a patient and may improve oculomotor control and movement (and thus function).

Intervention Methods

- Refer patient to eye specialist for assessment and treatment.
- Education: provide individualized information to the patient about his or her vision strengths and weaknesses and potential strategies.
- Provide compensatory strategies to maximize function.
- Assign basic vision exercises, as appropriate.
- Use therapeutic activities that include visual saccades while also addressing other areas of treatment.

CLINICIAN TIP SHEET: INTERVENTION METHODS FOR SACCADES

Education

What are Saccades?

Saccades are quick eye movements that occur when the eyes fix on various targets in the visual field.[27] Examples include:

- reading (the eye jumps from one group of words and letters to the next);
- looking up information on displays, charts, or phone books;
- looking at photos or paintings; and
- driving (looking from one object or car to the next).

When an eye has impaired saccades, a patient may:

- lose his or her place when reading or searching for information;
- miss or skip words, lines, or letters; and
- not see significant objects when looking for them.

Compensatory Options

- Use a guide or finger to assist in looking at different objects or when reading.
- Increase print size.
- Decrease clutter.

CLINICIAN TIP SHEET: TREATMENT IDEAS FOR SACCADES

Basic Saccade Exercise

General Setup

- Start with only one eye at a time (cover other eye with patch) until both eyes are doing the exercise equally. Once eyes are able to do the task at the same quality, perform the exercise with both eyes together.
- Have the patient keep his or her head still and focus on moving the eye (or eyes).
- Start with large movements and progress to smaller movements.

Procedure

- Use two targets (eg, a small ball or object on a dowel, penlight, or fingers) and an eye patch or occluder. Ask the patient to look back and forth between the two targets.
- Start slowly, holding the gaze for several seconds, and move back and forth between targets. As patient improves, gradually increase speed.
- Move targets so patient moves gaze into different directions of view (eg, have the targets as if at the end points of a plus sign and an X; move side to side, up and down, diagonal).
- This should only take up about 5 minutes.

Alternate Saccadic Exercise

General Setup

- Start with one eye at a time (cover the other eye with a patch) until both eyes are doing the exercise equally. Once eyes are able to do task at the same quality, perform with both eyes together.
- Have patient keep his or her head still and focus on moving the eye (or eyes).
- Start with large movements and progress to smaller movements.

Procedure

- Use columns of numbers or letters on paper (small distance saccades) or on a grease board (larger distance saccades) and an eye patch or occluder.
- Have patient read the two columns left to right, moving from top to bottom.
- As needed, have the patient use fingers or other anchors, progressing to no anchors.
- Use stopwatch to document progress.
- Change speed using a metronome.
- Start with two columns, then increase the number of columns.
- This should only take about 5 minutes.

Incorporate activities that challenge saccadic movement into the therapy recommendations (Exhibit 4-9).

IMPAIRED ACCOMMODATION

Purpose/Background

Patients with c/mTBI may demonstrate impaired accommodation. They may report discomfort and eye strain with near tasks, blurred vision, visual fatigue, or difficulty changing focus from near to far and far to near. The occupational therapist's role is to:

- identify the potential impairment and how it is affecting the patient functionally,
- refer the patient to a staff optometrist or ophthalmologist with expertise in vision and TBI,
- educate the patient about the impairment

and its functional implications,
- provide compensatory intervention if needed, and
- provide basic eye exercises and opportunities within therapy to address the impaired accommodation.

It is not recommended that occupational therapists spend more than 5 to 10 minutes doing vision exercises unless more time has been specifically recommended by an optometrist. Although the exercises will not harm the patient, the optometrist will be able to determine if the exercises will be beneficial or unnecessary to the diagnosis.

EXHIBIT 4-8

FUNCTIONAL ACTIVITIES TO ADDRESS PURSUITS

Paper-and-Pencil Tasks

- Line scrambles
- Mazes
- Computer games (slow-moving objects)
- Remote control car (move through obstacle course)

Also Improves

- Attention span
- Hand-eye coordination
- Problem solving
- Preplanning

Penlight on the Wall

- Trace a shape or movement outlined on the wall
- Identify letters or numbers on the wall

Also Improves

- Hand-eye coordination
- Upper extremity strength and coordination

Ball Games

- Bounce against a wall and catch
- Ball on a string (track and hit)
- Play catch
- Balloon volleyball (tracking and bursting bubbles)
- Beanbag toss

Also Improves

- Hand-eye coordination
- Upper extremity strength and coordination
- Bilateral hand tasks

Dynavision (West Chester, OH; see Clinician Tip Sheet: Dynavision in Supplementary Therapeutic Activity Options section for information about the Dynavision)

- Mode C (outer circle tracking)

Also Improves

- Upper extremity strength and coordination

EXHIBIT 4-9

FUNCTIONAL ACTIVITIES TO ADDRESS SACCADES

Copy Tasks

- Telephone numbers
- Words
- Sudoku
- Write checks from list
- Enter checks in register

Also Improves

- Attention span
- Hand-eye coordination
- Hand writing
- Problem solving
- IADL tasks

Card Games

- Solitaire: table or computer
- War: use metronome to increase speed
- Jigsaw puzzles: begin simple and large and progress
- Computer games: slow

Also Improves

- Hand-eye coordination
- Upper extremity strength and coordination
- Bilateral hand tasks
- Problem solving
- Preplanning

Dynavision (West Chester, OH)

- Mode A
- Mode B
- Mode A with digits

Also Improves

- Hand-eye coordination
- Upper extremity strength and coordination
- Reaction time
- Divided attention (mode A with digits)

IADL: instrumental activities of daily living

Strength of Recommendation: Practice Option

The compensatory interventions included in this section are found in Scheiman, *Understanding and Managing Vision Deficits: A Guide for Occupational Therapists.*[15]

Selected Reference

Scheiman M. *Understanding and Managing Vision Deficits: A Guide for Occupational Therapists.* 3rd ed. Thorofare, NJ: SLACK Incorporated; 2011.

Intervention Methods

Refer patient to eye specialist for assessment and treatment. See Clinician Tip Sheet for education, instructions in compensatory strategies, and exercises.

CLINICIAN TIP SHEET: INTERVENTION METHODS FOR IMPAIRED ACCOMMODATION

Education

What is Impaired Accommodation?

Accommodation is the ability of the eyes to focus at various distances (including shifting from one distance to another). According to Scheiman and Wick, "it also permits the individual to maintain clear focus at the normal reading distance."[40(p697)] There is a natural decline in accommodative ability from childhood through adulthood. This decline reaches a critical level at about the age of 40 to 45 years, which is the age when most adults begin to notice blurred vision with reading.

If someone demonstrates impaired accommodation (as evidenced by discomfort and eye strain with near tasks, blurred vision, visual fatigue with near tasks, or difficulty changing focus from near to far and far to near), he or she may have impaired accommodation. This may occur due to impaired innervation.

Symptoms of Impaired Convergence

- Complaints of discomfort and eye strain with visual tasks
- Complaints of blurriness
- Eye rubbing
- Complaints of visual fatigue with near tasks
- Easy fatigue with visual tasks
- Inattention with visual tasks
- Difficulty concentrating on tasks
- Difficulty with tasks that require sustained close work

Symptoms may occur at different times and intervals (ie, all the time, at different times of day, intermittently, or only when fatigued).

Functional Implications

- Reading or near tasks may be difficult (eg, inability to maintain focus)
- Vision blurriness
- Difficulty adjusting visual distances (eg, while driving, looking at the road then looking at the dashboard)
- Inattention with visual tasks

Compensatory Strategies

Specific Accommodation Compensatory Strategies

- If glasses are prescribed, ensure compliance with wear.
- If bifocals have been prescribed, ensure patient does close work while using the bottom of the bifocal.
- Larger print may help relieve symptoms until treatment is complete.
- Take frequent breaks.[15(p140)]

General Compensatory Strategies

The compensatory options are similar to the techniques used for low vision and poor acuity. Refer to Poor Acuity, Compensatory Techniques and Teaching for further detail. Other options include the following:

- increase illumination, contrast, or print size (enlarge);
- decrease clutter and background pattern;
- use visual markers;
- use a guide or finger to assist in looking at different objects, or rulers or anchors to avoid losing place;
- avoid glare;
- limit time doing visual tasks that take concentration; and
- take frequent breaks.

IMPAIRED CONVERGENCE

Purpose/Background

Patients with c/mTBI may demonstrate impaired convergence. The patient may complain of eye strain, headache, or difficulties with near tasks. The occupational therapist's role is to:

- identify the potential impairment and how it is affecting the patient functionally,
- refer the patient to a staff optometrist with expertise in vision and TBI,
- educate the patient about the impairment and its functional implications,
- provide compensatory intervention if needed, and
- provide basic eye exercises and opportunities within therapy to address the impaired convergence.

It is not recommended that occupational therapists spend more than 5 to 10 minutes doing vision exercises unless more time has been recommended by a staff optometrist with expertise in vision and TBI. Although the exercises will not harm the patient, the optometrist will be able to determine if the exercises will be beneficial or unnecessary to the diagnosis.

Strength of Recommendation: Practice Option

The compensatory interventions included in this section are widely presented in textbooks and literature related to vision deficits. There is minimal to no objective research demonstrating that eye exercises will benefit complaints of impaired convergence for patients with c/mTBI; however, there is strong evidence that intervention improves convergence in children and adults,[41] including one randomized controlled trial that reported success in alleviating symptoms of convergence insufficiency in young adults, as it affected reading and close-up work.[42]

Intervention Methods

Refer patient to an eye specialist for assessment and treatment. See clinician tip sheet for education and instructions in compensatory strategies and basic eye exercises.

Selected References

Lavrich JB. Convergence insufficiency and its current treatment. *Curr Opin Ophthalmol.* 2010;21(5):356–360.

Scheiman M, Mitchell GL, Cotter S, et al. A randomized clinical trial of vision therapy/orthoptics versus pencil pushups for the treatment of convergence insufficiency in young adults. *Optom Vis Sci.* Jul 2005;82(7):583–595.

CLINICIAN TIP SHEET: INTERVENTION METHODS FOR IMPAIRED CONVERGENCE

Education

What is Impaired Convergence?

Normally when eyes are working together they are able to converge and focus (fuse) on a single item or object and maintain the fusion as the object moves closer to the eyes, until it is about 2 to 4 inches from the eye. The eyes should be able to fuse again when the object is moved 4 to 6 inches away. If someone demonstrates impaired convergence (as evidenced by one eye moving laterally away, complaints of double vision, or significant eye strain when bringing the target close to the eyes), he or she may have impaired convergence.

If a patient is able to converge and maintain fusion up close but complains of double vision as an object moves out, the patient may have impaired divergence (difficulty allowing the eyes to maintain fusion with distance tasks). The treatment suggestions in Diplopia (below) will address impaired divergence. Referral to an eye specialist is recommended.

Impaired convergence may be due to poor innervation or motor control, or may result from a longstanding eye muscle problem that becomes decompensated after TBI.

Symptoms

- Double vision or blurriness with up-close tasks
- Headaches or difficulty with near tasks
- Words moving when trying to read
- Eye strain
- Squinting one eye
- Difficulty concentrating on tasks
- Turning the head to see an object clearly

Symptoms may occur at different times and intervals (eg, all the time, at different times of day, intermittently, only when fatigued). Impaired convergence may occur when looking into different fields of vision, as well (eg, straight ahead, to one side or another, in the superior or inferior fields, or any combination or direction).

Functional Implications

- Stationary objects may appear to move.
- Reading may be difficult (eg, skipping over words, losing one's place).
- Headaches and blurriness may occur.

CLINICIAN TIP SHEET: INTERVENTION METHODS FOR IMPAIRED CONVERGENCE

Compensatory Strategies

Patching

Patching is a short-term method to manage impaired convergence so the patient is able to function. If the patient does not complain of the aforementioned symptoms, patching is inappropriate; however, if a patient is having difficulty with reading or near tasks due to double vision, headaches, and the like, this may be a task-specific compensatory technique allowing patients to read or perform other up-close tasks.

To determine which eye is dominant, ask the patient to roll up a standard-sized sheet of paper to create a paper spyglass. Ask the patient to "spy" an object on the other side of the room, then watch which eye the patient automatically uses to do so. The patient will automatically select his or her dominant eye to use with the spyglass.

Patching should only be done during the times when the patient complains of difficulty performing near tasks (eg, intermittently or when fatigued). Unless a patient has poor acuity in one eye or is unable to adequately move one eye, alternate which eye is patched each day. Patches may be translucent or opaque. There are three options for patching (Figure 4-8):

1. Partial patching: nasal field of nondominant eye.
2. Partial patching: central spot patching on nondominant eye.
3. Full occlusion (less frequently recommended): reduces vision to single eye, thereby eliminating double vision. However, patient loses peripheral vision, will sustain eye fatigue, and there are safety concerns due to vision loss.

NOTE: Intervention for impaired convergence that involves patching must be directed/guided by an eye care provider.

General Compensatory Strategies

The compensatory options are similar to the techniques used for low vision or poor acuity, as follows:

- Increase illumination, contrast, or print size (enlarge).
- Decrease clutter and background pattern.
- Use visual markers, such as a guide or finger to assist in looking at different objects, or rulers or anchors to avoid losing place when reading.
- Avoid glare.
- Limit time doing visual tasks that take concentration and take frequent breaks.

CLINICIAN TIP SHEET: INTERVENTION METHODS FOR IMPAIRED CONVERGENCE

Treatment Ideas

Although there is minimal research demonstrating that eye exercises will benefit impairment convergence for patients with c/mTBI, there is strong evidence supporting its effectiveness with children and adults.[41,42] Basic eye exercises or functional activities will not harm a patient and may improve function. If the patient reports dizziness or nausea with this exercise, stop the exercise and find a less visually demanding task to work on.

NOTE: Occupational therapists incorporate eye exercises into their treatment plans in consultation with and under supervision of optometrists with expertise in TBI.

Pencil Pushups

This exercise uses both eyes together. Our eyes must come together smoothly and evenly when we do near activities, such as reading or needlework.

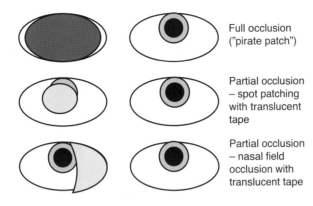

Full occlusion ("pirate patch")

Partial occlusion – spot patching with translucent tape

Partial occlusion – nasal field occlusion with translucent tape

Figure 4-8. Visual occlusion options for diplopia. Full visual occlusion (eg, "pirate patch"; top image) will result in the person seeing one image, but secondary complications include loss of peripheral vision, body image issues, and so on. Partial occlusion can be done with spot patching with translucent tape (middle) and occluding the nasal field of the nondominant eye (bottom image).

1. Hold a target (pen, small ball or object on a dowel, penlight) at arm's length directly in front of the patient's nose. Slowly move the pencil in toward the nose. Stop when two pencils are seen or when one eye moves away.
2. Slowly move the pencil away several inches beyond the point the two images turn into one (or the deviated eye moves back into focus on the target and the eyes are fused on the target together). The goal is to keep the eyes turning in and focusing on the pencil as it is moved closer to the nose. The image of the pencil should stay single as it moves all the way to the nose (within 2 to 4 inches of the eyes).
3. Repeat the exercise 5 times, then rest for 1 to 2 minutes and begin again.

The therapist must be sure the patient's eyes are moving in and converging on the target. If one eye deviates, stop and bring the target back until the eyes are fused on the target again. Do not have a patient do this alone if he or she is not aware of the eyes losing fusion. If the patient complains of double vision throughout the range, this exercise is inappropriate.

DIPLOPIA

Purpose/Background

Patients with c/mTBI may report double vision. The complaints of double vision may be intermittent, located in various locations of the visual field, or come about when doing different kinds of tasks. The occupational therapist's roles are to:

- Identify the potential impairment and how it is affecting the patient functionally.
- Refer the patient to a staff optometrist with expertise in vision and TBI who will be able to tell if it is a monocular or binocular issue.
- Educate the patient about the impairment and its functional implications.
- Provide compensatory intervention.
- Provide basic eye exercises and opportunities within therapy to address the double vision.

It is not recommend that occupational therapists spend more than 5 to 10 minutes doing vision exercises unless more time has been specifically recommended by a staff optometrist with expertise in vision and TBI. Although the exercises will not harm the patient, the optometrist will be able to determine if the exercises will be beneficial or unnecessary to the diagnosis.

Strength of Recommendation: Practice Option

The compensatory interventions included in this section are widely presented in textbooks and literature related to vision deficits. There is minimal to no objective research demonstrating that the use of eye exercises will alleviate complaints of double vision for patients with c/mTBI; however, basic eye exercises or functional activities will not harm a patient and may improve oculomotor control and movement (and thus function).

Intervention Methods

Refer patient to an eye specialist for assessment and treatment. See clinician tip sheet for education and instructions in compensatory strategies and basic range-of-motion exercises.

CLINICIAN TIP SHEET: INTERVENTION METHODS FOR DIPLOPIA

Education

What is Double Vision?

Normally when the eyes are working together, they are able to converge and focus (fuse) on a single item or object. If someone reports double vision that disappears when one eye is closed, the patient most likely has binocular diplopia and may be unable to hold both eyes focused on an item or object at the same time; thus, the brain receives two different images. If the double vision does not disappear with closing one eye, it is monocular; intervention in this realm is outside the occupational therapist's scope of practice. Either way, the patient should be seen by an eye care professional. The most likely cause of double vision is misalignment of the eyes, which may be due to poor innervation of eye muscles, poor oculomotor control, inflammation, muscle adhesions, or obstructions.

Symptoms

- Double vision
- Blurriness

- Difficulty with near tasks
- Words moving when reading
- Headaches with near tasks
- Eye strain
- Squinting one eye
- Difficulty concentrating on tasks
- Turning the head to see an object clearly

Symptoms may occur at varying times and intervals (eg, all the time, at different times of day, intermittently, only when fatigued, only when doing near tasks, only when looking in the distance, or when looking near and far). Double vision also may occur when looking into different fields of vision (eg, straight ahead, to one side or another, in the superior or inferior fields, or any combination or direction).

Functional Implications

- Decreased depth perception.
- Stationary objects may appear to move.
- Reading may be difficult (eg, skipping over words, losing one's place).
- Headaches and blurriness may occur.

CLINICIAN TIP SHEET: INTERVENTION METHODS FOR DIPLOPIA

Compensatory Strategies

Patching

Patching is a short-term method to manage diplopia so the patient is able to function (see Figure 4-8). The three patching options include:

1. Partial patching: nasal field of nondominant eye.
2. Partial patching: central spot patching on nondominant eye.
3. Full occlusion (less frequently recommended): reduces vision to single eye, thereby eliminating double vision. However, patient loses peripheral vision, will sustain eye fatigue, and there are safety concerns due to vision loss.

To determine which eye is dominant, ask the patient to roll up a standard-sized sheet paper to create a paper spyglass. Ask the patient to "spy" an object on the other side of the room and watch which eye the patient automatically uses to do so. The patient will automatically select his or her

dominant eye to use with the spyglass.

Patching can be translucent or opaque and should only be done when the patient reports double vision (may be intermittent or occur when the patient is fatigued) or all the time if one eye is noticeably out of alignment. Unless a patient has poor acuity in one eye or is unable to adequately move one eye, alternate the eye that is patched daily.

General Compensatory Strategies

The compensatory options are similar to the techniques used for low vision or poor acuity, including:

- increase illumination, contrast, or print size (enlarge);
- decrease clutter and background pattern;
- use visual markers, such as a guide or finger, to assist in looking at different objects or rulers or anchors to avoid losing place when reading;
- avoid glare; and
- limit time doing visual tasks that take concentration and take frequent breaks.

VISUAL FIELD LOSS

Purpose/Background

Individuals with TBI may experience visual field loss.[43] Although visual field loss is typically not associated with c/mTBI, clinicians need to understand this issue in case their patients have experienced complicated mTBI or more severe injuries. Loss of vision in the visual field can be disorienting and gives a narrower scope of useable vision. A person may miss details or not see critical information or objects. Once the loss of vision is identified and defined, the occupational therapist's role is to educate the patient and teach compensatory techniques so the patient can participate in therapy and function in his or her everyday life.

Strength of Recommendation: Practice Option

There is little empirical literature to inform practice in this area. Riggs and colleagues[43] did a systematic review of the literature and found only two articles for visual field deficits after stroke met their criteria for inclusion, neither of which had strong recommendations due to lack of functional outcomes and study limitations. A study by Warren and colleagues[37] addressed the types of search strategies used by healthy adults.

Intervention Methods

- Refer patient to eye specialist for assessment (visual field test).
- Educate patient.
- Teach patients to use compensatory techniques for field loss such as:
  - use of anchors and rulers,
  - visual search strategies,
  - large- and small-scale eye movements,
  - increased head turns, and
  - increased attention to detail.
- Employ activities for engaging patients to address visual field loss.

Selected References

Riggs RV, Andrews K, Roberts P, Gilewski M. Visual deficit interventions in adult stroke and brain injury: a systematic review. *Am J Phys Med Rehabil*. Oct 2007;86(10):853–860.

Warren M, Moore JM, Vogtle LK. Search performance of healthy adults on cancellation tests. *Am J Occup Ther*. Sep-Oct 2008;62(5):588–594.

CLINICIAN TIP SHEET: INTERVENTION METHODS FOR VISUAL FIELD LOSS

Education

It is essential that patients with visual field loss understand what has happened to their vision and how it will interfere with various activities.

What is a Visual Field Loss?

Visual fields are the total area visible to an eye that is fixating straight ahead, measured in degrees from fixation.[44] Visual field loss is the loss of vision in a specified area of vision. The area of the injury or lesion along the visual pathway determines the field loss location. Visual field loss can be in any area of the visual field and can be different in each eye.

Functional Implications of Specific Types of Field Loss

- Central field loss: leads to decreased acuity
- Superior field loss: results in difficulty seeing signs, reading, and writing; inability to find higher placed items
- Inferior field loss: causes difficulty with mobility (clearing curbs, steps, rugs, low furniture), slower paced walking with shortened stride, walking behind others, trailing behind others, and poor balance
- Lateral field loss: leads to bumping into things, missing items on the side affected
- Loss in any field: results in difficulty reading and writing, misidentification of details or long words, and difficulty finding or being aware of objects in the affected field.

Compensatory Strategies

Because visual field loss can be disorienting and confusing for patients, it may be necessary to teach patients how to use their vision again with the new impairment (for more on teaching and learning methods, see Chapter 7: Cognitive Assessment and

Intervention, specifically Techniques to Promote Patient Engagement and Learning). For treatment activity ideas see Table 4-4.

Techniques to Teach the Patient

- Visual search strategies (to maximize organization and efficiency), including left-to-right for reading. Start in at the far end of the affected side, use a circular pattern for larger scanning activities.
- Large-scale eye movements for mobility and scanning in the environment.
- Small-scale eye movements for reading and near tasks.
- Increased head turns, especially into the affected area.

Increased Attention to Detail

- Promotes ensuring that patient sees into the area affected.
- Watching the pen or pencil when writing.

Using Anchors and Rulers

- Use a ruler to keep track of each line being read.
- Use a bright colored line or ruler vertically at the edge of the text on the side of the missing field to ensure finding the edge of the text.

Approaching Treatment Tasks

Grading the Tasks Using Activity Analysis

- Density: low density to high density (eg, start with two columns of letters, one on each side of the page, and progress to ten columns of letters)[38]

TABLE 4-4

DIFFERENCES BETWEEN FIELD CUT AND NEGLECT

Field cut	Neglect
- Awareness emerges early - Compensatory strategies observed early, easily taught - Early eye movement to affected side - Organized	- Lack of awareness more persistent - Compensatory strategies are hard to learn, may not be effective - Rightward gaze preference - Random

Data source: Gillen G. *Cognitive and Perceptual Rehabilitation: Optimizing Function.* St Louis, MO: Mosby; 2009.

- Structure: task organization (ie, start with organized, simple structure and move toward random)
- Speed: start with slow, deliberate movement and work toward increasing speed.

Size of Treatment Tasks

- Large tasks (full room and larger, 5 feet or more away)
- Small tasks (paper, pencil, and tabletop)

Scanning Patterns of Healthy Adults

Warren and colleagues[37] found the scanning pattern predominantly used by healthy adults were structured patterns, with a strong tendency for left to right, and top to bottom scanning patterns.

VISUAL NEGLECT AND INATTENTION

Purpose/Background

Individuals with TBI may experience visual neglect or inattention.[45] Although not typically associated with c/mTBI, clinicians need to understand this issue in case their patients have experienced complicated mTBI or more severe injuries.

Neglect is a failure to report, respond, or orient to novel or meaningful stimuli on the contralesional side of a brain lesion that cannot be attributed to sensory or motor dysfunction.[46] A person may bump into doorframes when ambulating, read only partial lines or words, miss details, or not see critical information or objects. Once the neglect or inattention is identified, the occupational therapist's role is to educate the patient and teach compensatory techniques so the patient may participate in therapy and function in everyday life.

Strength of Recommendation: Practice Option

There is little empirical literature to inform practice in this area. Bowen[47] did a systematic review of the literature and only found 12 articles for visual field deficits after stroke that met criteria for inclusion. He found the rehabilitation treatments that targeted neglect demonstrated test improvement (eg, finding visual targets or marking midpoints of lines); however, the functional implications for performing everyday activities or independent living skills were unclear. A study by Warren and colleagues[37] addressed the types of search strategies used by healthy adults.

Selected References

Bowen A, Lincoln N. Cognitive rehabilitation for spatial neglect following stroke. *The Cochrane Library.* 2009;4.

Cherney LR. Unilateral neglect: a disorder of attention. *Semin Speech Lang.* 2002;23(2):117–128.

Cockerham GC, Goodrich GL, Weichel ED, et al. Eye and visual function in traumatic brain injury. *J Rehabil Res Dev.* 2009;46:811–818.

Gillen G. *Cognitive and Perceptual Rehabilitation: Optimizing Function.* St Louis, MO: Mosby; 2009.

Heilman KM, Watson R, Valenstein E. Neglect and related disorders. In: Heilman KM, Valenstein E, eds. *Clinical Neuropsychology.* 3rd ed. New York, NY: Oxford University Press; 1993: 279–336.

Mesulam MM. Attention, confusional states and neglect. In: Mesulam MM, ed. *Principles of Behavioral Neurology.* Hove, England: Erlbaum; 1985: 173–176.

Intervention Methods

- Refer patient to an eye specialist for assessment.
- Provide patient education.
- Teach the patient compensatory strategies, including:
  - use of anchors and rulers,
  - visual search strategies (organized and efficient),
  - large- and small-scale eye movements,
  - increased head turns, and
  - increased attention to detail.
- Employ activities for engaging patients to address neglect and inattention.

CLINICIAN TIP SHEET: INTERVENTION METHODS FOR VISUAL INATTENTION AND NEGLECT

Education

It is essential that patients with visual neglect (with or without a visual field loss) understand what has happened to their vision and how it will interfere with various activities.

The Difference Between Visual Field Loss and Visual Neglect

Inattention/Neglect is a failure to report, respond, or orient to novel or meaningful stimuli on the contralesional side of a brain lesion that cannot be attributed to sensory or motor dysfunction.[46]
Visual Field Deficit is an area visible to the eye when it is fixated straight ahead. It is measured in degrees from fixation.[44] Visual field loss is the loss of vision in a specified area of vision. The area of the injury or lesion along the visual pathway determines the field loss location.

Spatial Domains of Neglect

- Personal body space. Patients tend to ignore the left side (contralesional side) of their body, which can result in a deficit in grooming or dressing.
- Peripersonal space. Neglect is observed with tabletop pencil-and-paper tasks in near space within reach or grasp.
- Extrapersonal space. Neglect is observed with environmental scanning in far space beyond reach.[48]

Categories of Attentional Deficits

- Action-intentional disorders (motor neglect): failure or decreased ability to move into contralesional space
- Inattention (sensory neglect): lack or decreased awareness of sensory stimulation in contralesional space

- Memory and representational deficits: deficit of the internal representation of the contralesional space or limbs[46,49]

Functional Implications of Neglect

- Not paying attention to or "seeing" people and objects on patient's left side (specifically, left neglect)
- Missing the food on the left side of the plate

- Not being aware of the person sitting or standing to patient's left side
- Not being able to find objects to the left side of the sink or counter
- Reading: starting to read in the middle of a line, missing the beginning letters of a word, or losing one's place when reading
- Ambulating: bumping into doorways or furniture, not looking to the left when crossing the street

CLINICIAN TIP SHEET: TREATMENT APPROACH TO VISUAL INATTENTION AND NEGLECT

Insight and awareness are key to a patient's compensation with neglect (which is challenging; patients lack insight and awareness due to the decreased attention).[50]

Response to Treatment and Education

Treatment activities and compensatory strategies are similar to visual field deficits; however, therapists need to adapt treatment approaches to allow for increased treatment duration and frequency of repetition (see Table 4-4). For treatment activity ideas see Table 4-5.

Techniques to Teach the Patient

Visual Search Strategies

To maximize organization and efficiency, teach patients the following techniques:

- reading left to right,
- starting in at the far end of the affected side, and
- using a circular pattern for larger scanning activities.

Large-scale eye movements are useful for mobility and scanning in the environment. Small-scale eye movements help with reading and near tasks. Increasing head turns is helpful especially into affected area.

Increased Attention to Detail

- Promotes ensuring that the patient sees into the area affected.
- Encourage patient to watch the pen or pencil when writing.

Using Anchors and Rulers

- Use a ruler to keep track of each line being read.
- Use a brightly colored line or ruler vertically at the edge of the text on the side of the missing field to ensure finding the edge of the text.

Approaching the Treatment Tasks

Grading the Tasks Using Activity Analysis

- Density: low density to high density (eg, start with two columns of letters, one on each side of the page, and progress to ten columns of letters).
- Structure: organization of the task (ie, start with organized simple structure and move towards random).
- Speed: start with slow, deliberate movement and work toward increasing speed.[38]

Size of Treatment Tasks

- Large tasks (full room and larger, 5 feet or more away)
- Small tasks (paper, pencil, and tabletop)

Scanning Patterns of Healthy Adults

Warren and colleagues[37] found the scanning pattern predominantly used by healthy adults was structured patterns, with a strong tendency for left to right and top to bottom scanning patterns.

TABLE 4-5

ACTIVITIES TO ENGAGE PATIENTS

Visual Scanning Activity	Works On
• Paper-and-pencil activities (cancellation tasks, reading, mazes, word search puzzles, crossword puzzles) • Prereading and writing exercises[*]	Near scanning for return to reading (books, maps, etc)
• Easel or table with card matching • Card and games on a table • Find items on shelf or cupboard • Jigsaw puzzles (spread out on table) • Hitting a ball against a wall turned sideways so the visual field loss is towards the wall • Dynavision[†] • NVT Scanning Device[‡] • Neurovision Rehabilitator[§]	Mid-distance scanning for IADLs (meal preparation, bill paying, shopping, etc)
• Identify all objects in a room • Walk down a hallway and identify what is on the wall (or place sticky notes with numbers or letters on them) • Walk through obstacle course • Do a scavenger hunt of objects in the clinic	Distant activities for looking far and for mobility

IADLs: instrumental activities of daily living
[*] From visABILITIES Rehab Services Inc (Hoover, AL). Includes various paper pencil activities.
[†] From Dynavision (West Chester, OH). All modes.
[‡] From Neuro Vision Technology Systems (Torrensville, SA, Australia).
[§] The Neuro-Vision Rehabilitator (http://nvrvision.com).

GLARE/PHOTOPHOBIA MANAGEMENT

Purpose/Background

Patients with c/mTBI may report photophobia.[51] They can be sensitive to specific kinds of lights (eg, fluorescent lights may cause a flicker effect) or different weather conditions (eg, bright sun or clouds), among other things, which can lead to complaints of headaches, light intolerance, squinting, and frequent eye closing. Occupational therapists can have a role in identifying patients with these complaints and providing options that minimize symptoms and help patients participate in therapy and everyday activities.

Strength of Recommendation: Practice Option

There is no specific evidence to inform intervention for photophobia associated with c/mTBI.

Selected Reference

Jackowski MM, Sturr JF, Taub HA, Turk MA. Photophobia in patients with traumatic brain injury: uses of light filtering lenses to enhance contrast sensitivity and reading rate. *Neurorehabilitation.* 1996;6:194–201.

However, a small study conducted by Jackowski and colleagues[51] demonstrated visual function (reading) improvement with the use of light-filtering lenses for patients following TBI who reported photophobia (N=14). It should be noted that the study was conducted indoors only.

Intervention Methods

- Refer patient to eye specialist for assessment and treatment.
- Educate patient.
- Teach compensatory strategies.

CLINICIAN TIP SHEET: INTERVENTION METHODS FOR GLARE/PHOTOPHOBIA

Education

Photophobia can be a common complaint after TBI. The mechanism is not clear at this time.

Compensatory Strategies

The patient should be referred to an eye specialist; however, an occupational therapist can help the patient be as functional as possible using compensatory strategies. Some options include the following:

- Tinted glasses (color and density need to be tried to determine optimal visual clarity and comfort). For indoors,[51] use three photochromatic filters (Corning Photochromic Filters CPF450, 527-S, and 550-S; Corning, Inc, Avon Cedex, France) which significantly improved (P < 0.01) the reading rates of the TBI subjects with photophobia. Outdoor settings were not tested. These are commercially available at eyeglass stores. Other options include NoIR and UVShield sunglasses (NoIR Medical Technologies, South Lyon, MI).
- Encourage the patient to wean off tinted glasses over time.
- Encourage use of baseball hats and visors; have some available in the clinic for trial or use.
- Limit overhead light use and use task lights.

SUPPLEMENTARY THERAPEUTIC ACTIVITY OPTIONS

Purpose/Background

When working with patients on vision, it is helpful to have a variety of tasks that can be graded in terms of complexity, size, and distance. The tasks selected for the patient should be easy enough to ensure some success, but challenging enough to promote improvement. Once the patient demonstrates some preliminary competence with compensatory techniques, the activities should begin to reflect real-life tasks and situations the patient will encounter in everyday life.

Strength of Recommendation: Practice Options

Intervention Methods

- Dynavision 2000 Light Training Board (West Chester, OH) for visual field deficits.
- Prereading and writing exercises.
- Neuro Vision Technology (NVT) Scanning Device (NVT Systems Pty Ltd, Torrensville, SA).
- Neurovision Rehabilitator (NVR; www.nvrvision.com).

CLINICIAN TIP SHEET: DYNAVISION

General Information

According to the Dynavision (West Chester, OH) Website:

Originally designed as a device to improve the visuomotor skills of athletes, the Dynavision™ 2000 Light Training Board has been adapted to provide the same training benefits to persons whose visual and motor function has been compromised by injury or disease. For persons with visual and visuomotor impairment the apparatus is used to train compensatory search strategies, improve oculomotor skills such as localization, fixation, gaze shift, and tracking, increase peripheral visual awareness, visual attention and anticipation, and improve eye-hand coordination and visuomotor reaction time. For persons with motor impairment it can be used to increase active upper extremity range of motion and coordination, muscular and physical endurance and improve motor planning. It has been successfully used to improve function in children and adults with limitations from stroke, head injury, amputation, spinal cord injury, and orthopedic injury. Currently there are over 400 units in rehabilitation hospitals across the United States.[52]

Applicability to Service Members

According to Mary Warren:

One of the great advantages of the device [Dynavision] as a tool specifically for the rehabilitation of wounded Soldiers is its competitive nature. Dynavision drills are presented as games of skill by instructing the persons to strike as many lighted buttons as possible within the allotted time. This challenges the client to give their best effort each time. The device records and analyzes performance showing the client where deficiencies exist to enable the client to improve performance on the board. Clients can compare their performance and compete with each other. Because the device was designed for athletes, the lights can be programmed to move at very high speeds and it is impossible to beat the board, which draws out the competitive nature of young men.[53]

Dynavision has also been used in vision rehabilitation for individuals with brain injury (primarily stroke).[54–56]

Use and Options

Dynavision can be used for mid-distance scanning skills and is programmable to start with easier to more challenging tasks. The visual impairments it may be used to address include saccades, pursuits, visual field deficits, and visual neglect and inattention.

Dynavision has four modes of operation:

1. Mode A: self-paced task. One button at a time randomly lights up and stays on until it is pushed. Patient tries to locate and push the lit-up button as quickly as possible.
2. Mode B: apparatus paced. A button will randomly light up for a selected period of time (1 second or less) before the next light comes on. Patient tries to locate and push the button before the next one comes on.
3. Mode C: visual tracking task. A single light "moves" around the edges of the ring of lights, periodically changing direction (the speed of the buttons changing light can be selected at 1 second or less). The patient visually tracks the light.
4. Mode A, B, or C with digital flash option. During the task (selected by mode), digits (select from 1 to 7 digits at a time) are flashed on a screen at eye height. Patient calls out the numbers as they are flashed while performing the other tasks (divided attention).

Tasks may be set for a duration of 30, 60, or 240 seconds and may be varied by size and area (eg, select any one or more the four quadrants, select the inner [three rings], middle [four rings], or full [five rings] board). Task results can be printed out (including total hits and reaction time).

Reliability Studies

- Test-retest reliability: tested with Mode B using two apparatus-paced tasks. Moderate reliability with correlation coefficient ranging from 0.71 (for 76 subjects) to 0.73 (for 41 subjects) and paired correlation coefficients ranging from – .75 to 0.93.[57]
- Test-retest reliability: tested reliability of three tasks of difficulty graded extremely high (.88, .92, and .97).[58]

Selected References

Klavora P, Gaskovski P, Forsyth RD. Test-retest reliability of the Dynavision apparatus. *Percept Mot Skills*. Aug 1994;79(1 Pt 2):448–450.

Klavora P, Gaskovski P, Martin K, et al. The effects of Dynavision rehabilitation on behind-the-wheel driving ability and selected psychomotor abilities of persons after stroke. *Am J Occup Ther*. Jun 1995;49(6):534–542.

Traumatic Brain Injury Related Vision Issues: Hearing Before the Subcommittee on Oversight and Investigations of the Committee on Veterans' Affairs, Before the U.S. House of Representatives, 110th Cong, Second Session. Application of the Dynavision 2000 to Rehabilitation of Soldiers With Traumatic Brain Injury. Written testimony of Mary Warren. April 2, 2008.

CLINICIAN TIP SHEET: PREREADING AND WRITING EXERCISES

General Information

According to Mary Warren:

These exercises consist of reproducible worksheet activities designed to provide patients with practice making the precise eye movements needed to accurately identify letters and numbers and to write legibly on line. The exercises are appropriate for persons with scotomas (a blind or partially blind area in the visual field) secondary to neurological impairment (hemianopsia).

The pre-reading drills consist of letter and number combinations printed in four different M unit sizes to accommodate acuities ranging as low as 20/200. The exercises emphasize letters and numbers which are easily misread when not seen clearly such as, V and W and 6 and 8. They are intended to increase accuracy in identifying letters and numbers and to increase confidence in reading ability prior to attempting to read actual text. The pre-writing worksheets consist of tracing exercises to promote reintegration of the eye directing the hand in movement.

The exercises can be incorporated within treatment to improve the visual skills needed for reading performance and also be used as homework to supplement treatment programs. However, no empirical evidence is available about the outcomes associated with these exercises.[59]

Use and Options

These exercises can be used for near scanning. The font size and density of the letters vary to provide simple to complex tasks. The exercises are used to address saccades, visual field deficits, and visual neglect or inattention. Examples of the exercises are available at: www.visabilities.com.

CLINICIAN TIP SHEET: NEURO VISION TECHNOLOGY SCANNING DEVICE

General Information

According to the manufacturer's website:

The NVT Vision Rehabilitation System aims to promote independent living for people with a Neurological Vision Impairment by:

- Assessment of visual and perceptual deficits that impact on activities of daily living.
- Training in compensatory scanning strategies.
- Transfer of scanning skills to Mobility in a dynamic environment.

This is a unique program of interest to all staff working in the area of rehabilitation of Acquired Brain Injury.[60]

Neuro Vision Technology Scanning Device Use: Practice Option

The exercises can be used for mid-distance scanning skills. Various programs differ in complexity. Although research is currently underway (email communication, Allison Hayes, Manager Training and Research, Neuro Vision Technology Pty Ltd, Torrensville, South Australia, Australia, December 16, 2009), no empirical evidence is currently available about the outcomes associated with the NVT Scanning Device. This device and program were developed for research. It addresses visual field deficits and visual neglect and inattention and is available through the developer's website (www.neurovisiontech.com.au).

CLINICIAN TIP SHEET: NEUROVISION REHABILITATOR

General Information

The NVR is a computer-based, instrumented vision therapy system that uses Wii (Nintendo, Kyoto, Japan) hardware to address deficits in visual processing.[61] The system includes a Bluetooth-integrated (Bluetooth, Kirkland, WA) balance board, an infrared head sensor, a controller sensor receiver, a wireless remote controller ("hand shooter"), and NVR software system. Additionally, a computer, projector, and screen are needed.

NVR Use: Practice Option

Using remotes and sensors, the NVR provides interactive, multisystem challenge and feedback that integrates vision with auditory, proprioceptive, balance, and visuomotor control.[62] There are five software treatment modules: (1) visual motor enhancer, (2) ocular vestibular integrator, (3) dynamic ocular motor processing, (4) visuomotor integrator, and (5) fixation anomalies.

Allen Cohen, one of the NVR developers,

created three treatment protocols (which are described in the operations manual). The first phase of treatment aims to enhance the stability of the visual input system. The goal of phase two is to develop fusional sustenance, and the goal of phase three is to develop speed of visual information processing and stability of visual performance.[61] No empirical evidence is currently available about the outcomes associated with the NVR and adults with c/mTBI.

Available through the developer's website (www.nvrvision.com).

Selected Reference

Suchoff IB. New product review: the Neuro-Vision Rehabilitator (NVR). *J Behav Optom.* 2011;22:13–15.

REFERENCES

1. Scheiman M. *Understanding and Managing Vision Deficits*. Thorofare, NJ: SLACK Incorporated; 1997.

2. Brahm KD, Wilgenburg HM, Kirby J, Ingalla S, Chang CY, Goodrich GL. Visual impairment and dysfunction in combat–injured servicemembers with traumatic brain injury. *Optom Vis Sci.* Jul 2009;86(7):817–825.

3. Gillen G. *Cognitive and Perceptual Rehabilitation: Optimizing Function*. St Louis, MO: Mosby; 2009.

4. Maples WC. Test–retest reliability of the college of optometrists in vision development quality of life outcomes assessment short form. *J Optom Vis Develop.* 2002;33:126–134.

5. Maples WC. Test-retest reliability of the College of Optometrists in Vision Development Quality of Life Outcomes Assessment. *Optometry.* Sep 2000;71(9):579–585.

6. Harris P, Gormley L. Changes in scores on the COVD quality of life assessment before and after vision therapy, a multi–office study. *J Behav Optom.* 2007;18:43–47.

7. Shin HS, Park SC, Park CM. Relationship between accommodative and vergence dysfunctions and academic achievement for primary school children. *Ophthalmic Physiol Opt.* Nov 2009;29(6):615–624.

8. Farrar R, Call M, Maples WC. A comparison of the visual symptoms between ADD/ADHD and normal children. *Optometry.* Jul 2001;72(7):441–451.

9. Daugherty KM, Frantz KA, Allison CL, Gabriel HM. Evaluating changes in quality of life after vision therapy using the COVD Quality of Life Outcomes Assessment. *Optom Vis Develop.* 2007;38:75–81.

10. White T, Major A. A comparison of subjects with convergence insufficiency and subjects with normal binocular vision using a quality of life questionnaire. *J Behav Optom.* 2004;15:37–133.

11. Benjamin WJ. *Borish's Clinical Refraction*. Burlington, MA: Butterworth–Heinemann; 2006.

12. Green W, Ciuffreda KJ, Thiagarajan P, Szymanowicz D, Ludlam DP, Kapoor N. Accommodation in mild traumatic brain injury. *J Rehabil Res Dev.* 2010;47(3):183–199.

13. Chen AH, O'Leary DJ. Validity and repeatability of the modified push-up method for measuring the amplitude of accommodation. *Clin Exper Optom.* 1998;81:63–71.

14. Rouse MW, Borsting E, Deland PN. Reliability of binocular vision measurements used in the classification of convergence insufficiency. *Optom Vis Sci.* Apr 2002;79(4):254–264.

15. Scheiman M. *Understanding and Managing Vision Deficits: A Guide for Occupational Therapists*. 3rd ed. Thorofare, NJ: SLACK Incorporated; 2011.

16. Scheiman M, Gallaway M, Frantz KA, et al. Nearpoint of convergence: test procedure, target selection, and normative data. *Optom Vis Sci.* Mar 2003;80(3):214–225.

17. Thiagarajan P, Ciuffreda KJ, Ludlam DP. *Ophthalmic Physiol Opt.* 2011;31:456–467.

18. Goss DA, Moyer BJ, Teske MC. A Comparison of Dissociated Phoria Test Findings with Von Graefe Phorometry & Modified Thorington Testing. *J Behav Optom.* 2008;19(6):145–149.

19. Rainey BB, Schroeder TL, Goss DA, Grosvenor TP. Inter–examiner repeatability of heterophoria tests. *Optom Vis Sci.* Oct 1998;75(10):719–726.

20. Gross DA, Moyer BJ, Teske MC. A Comparison of dissociated phoria test findings with von Graefe phorometry and modified Thorington testing. *J Behav Optom.* 2008;19(6):145–149.

21. Lyon DW, Goss DA, Horner D, Downey JP, Rainey B. Normative data for modified Thorington phorias and prism bar vergences from the Benton–IU study. *Optometry.* Oct 2005;76(10):593–599.

22. Antona B, Gonzalez E, Barrio A, Barra F, Sanchez I, Cebrian JL. Strabometry precision: intra–examiner repeatability and agreement in measuring the magnitude of the angle of latent binocular ocular deviations (heterophorias or latent strabismus). *Binocul Vis Strabolog Q Simms Romano.* 2011;26(2):91–104.

23. Sampedro AG, Richman M, Sanchez Pardo M. The Adult Developmental Eye Movement Test (A–DEM). *J Behav Optom.* 2003;14(4):101–105.

24. Powell JM, Birk K, Cummings EH, Col MA. The Need for Adult Norms on the Developmental Eye Movement Test. *J Behav Optom.* 2005;16(2):38–41.

25. Garzia RP, Richman JE, Nicholson SB, Gaines CS. A new visual-verbal saccade test: the development eye movement test (DEM). *J Am Optom Assoc.* Feb 1990;61(2):124–135.

26. Tassinari JT, DeLand P. Developmental Eye Movement Test: reliability and symptomatology. *Optometry.* Jul 2005;76(7):387–399.

27. Quintana LA. Assessing abilities and capacities: Vision, visual perception and praxis. In: Radomski MV, Trombly Latham CA, eds. *Occupational Therapy for Physical Dysfunction.* Philadelphia, PA: Lippincott Williams & Wilkins; 2008:234–259.

28. Maples WC, Ficklin TW. Inter–rater and test–rater reliability of pursuits and saccades. *J Am Optom Assoc.* 1988;59:549–552.

29. Maples WC, Ficklin TW. A preliminary study of the oculomotor skills of learning–disabled, gifted, and normal children. *J Optom Vis Devel.* 1989;20:9–14.

30. Maples WC, Ficklin TW. Comparison of eye movement skills between above average and below average readers. *J Behav Optom.* 1990;1:87–91.

31. Maples WC, Atchley J, Ficklin TW. Northeastern State University College of Optometry's oculomotor norms. *J Behav Optom.* 1992;3:143–150.

32. Kerr NM, Chew SS, Eady EK, Gamble GD, Danesh–Meyer HV. Diagnostic accuracy of confrontation visual field tests. *Neurology.* Apr 13 2010;74(15):1184–1190.

33. Trobe JD, Acosta PC, Krischer JP, Trick GL. Confrontation visual field techniques in the detection of anterior visual pathway lesions. *Ann Neurol.* 1980;10:28–34.

34. Shahinfar S, Johnson LN, Madsen RW. Confrontation visual field loss as a function of decibel sensitivity loss on automated static perimetry. Implications on the accuracy of confrontation visual field testing. *Ophthalmology.* Jun 1995;102(6):872–877.

35. Warren M. *biVABA: Brain Injury Visual Assessment Battery for Adults.* Lenexa, KS: visABILITIES Rehab Services Inc; 1998.

36. Warren M. *Brain Injury Visual Assessment Battery for Adults: Test Manual*. Birmingham, AL: VisAbilities Rehab Services Inc; 1998.

37. Warren M, Moore JM, Vogtle LK. Search performance of healthy adults on cancellation tests. *Am J Occup Ther*. Sep–Oct 2008;62(5):588–594.

38. Warren M. A hierarchal model for evaluation and treatment of visual perception dysfunction in adult acquired brain injury, Part II. *Am J Occup Ther*. 1993;47:55–66.

39. Answers.com Visually Impaired webpage. http://www.answers.com/topic/visually-impaired. Accessed June 17, 2013.

40. Scheiman M, Wick B. *Binocular Vision: Heterophoric, Accommodative and Eye Movement Disorders*. 3rd ed. Philadelphia, PA: Lippincott Williams & Wilkins; 2008.

41. Lavrich JB. Convergence insufficiency and its current treatment. *Curr Opin Ophthalmol*. 2010;21(5):356–360.

42. Scheiman M, Mitchell GL, Cotter S, et al. A randomized clinical trial of vision therapy/orthoptics versus pencil pushups for the treatment of convergence insufficiency in young adults. *Optom Vis Sci*. Jul 2005;82(7):583–595.

43. Riggs RV, Andrews K, Roberts P, Gilewski M. Visual deficit interventions in adult stroke and brain injury: a systematic review. *Am J Phys Med Rehabil*. Oct 2007;86(10):853–860.

44. Cassin B, Solomon SAB, Rubin ML. *Dictionary of Eye Terminology*. Gainesville, FL: Triad Publishing Co; 1997.

45. Cockerham GC, Goodrich GL, Weichel ED, et al. Eye and visual function in traumatic brain injury. *J Rehabil Res Devel*. 2009;46:811–818.

46. Heilman KM, Watson R, Valenstein E. Neglect and related disorders. In: Heilman KM, Valenstein E, eds. *Clinical Neuropsychology*. 3rd ed. New York, NY: Oxford University Press; 1993: 279–336.

47. Bowen A, Lincoln N. Cognitive rehabilitation for spatial neglect following stroke. *The Cochrane Library*. 2009;4.

48. Cherney LR. Unilateral neglect: a disorder of attention. *Semin Speech Lang*. 2002;23(2):117–128.

49. Mesulam MM. Attention, confusional states and neglect. In: Mesulam MM, ed. *Principles of Behavioral Neurology*. Hove, England: Erlbaum; 1985: 173–176.

50. Warren M. Evaluation and treatment of visual perceptual dysfunction in adult brain injury, Part I. Minneapolis, MN: visABILITIES Rehab Services, Inc.; 1999.

51. Jackowski MM, Sturr JF, Taub HA, Turk MA. Photophobia in patients with traumatic brain injury: Uses of light filtering lenses to enhance contrast sensitivity and reading rate. *NeuroRehabilitation*. 1996;6:194–201.

52. Dynavision website. http://www.dynavisiond2.com/dynavision_in_rehabilitation.php. Accessed June 25, 2013.

53. *Traumatic Brain Injury Related Vision Issues: Hearing Before the Subcommittee on Oversight and Investigations of the Committee on Veterans' Affairs, Before the U.S. House of Representatives,* 110th Cong, Second Session. Application of the Dynavision 2000 to Rehabilitation of Soldiers With Traumatic Brain Injury. Written testimony of Mary Warren. April 2, 2008.

54. Klavora P, Gaskovski P, Heslegrave R, Quinn R, Young M. Rehabilitation of visual skills using the Dynavision: a single case experimental design. *Can J Occup Ther*. 1995;62:37–43.

55. Klavora P, Warren M. Rehabilitation of visuomotor skills in poststroke patients using the Dynavision apparatus. *Percept Mot Skills*. Feb 1998;86(1):23–30.

56. Klavora P, Heslegrave RJ, Young M. Driving skills in elderly persons with stroke: comparison of two new assessment options. *Arch Phys Med Rehabil.* 2000;81:701–705.

57. Klavora P, Gaskovski P, Forsyth RD. Test-retest reliability of the Dynavision apparatus. *Percept Mot Skills.* Aug 1994;79(1 Pt 2):448–450.

58. Klavora P, Gaskovski P, Martin K, et al. The effects of Dynavision rehabilitation on behind-the-wheel driving ability and selected psychomotor abilities of persons after stroke. *Am J Occup Ther.* Jun 1995;49(6):534–542.

59. Suchoff IB. New product review: The Neuro-Vision Rehabilitator (NVR). *J Behav Optom.* 2011;22:13–15.

60. visABILITIES Rehab Services Incorporated. visABILITIES website. http://www.visabilities.com/prereading.html. Accessed June 25, 2013.

61. Neuro Vision Technology Pty Ltd. NVT Scanning Device product website. http://www.nvtsystems.com.au/products_services/nvt_scanning_device/. Accessed June 25, 2013.

62. Neuro-Vision Rehabilitator website. http://nvrvision.com. Accessed June 25, 2013.

Chapter 5

POSTTRAUMATIC HEADACHE ASSESSMENT AND INTERVENTION

MARGARET M. WEIGHTMAN, PhD, PT* AND JANICE P. KEHLER, BPT, MS, MA†

*Clinical Scientist /Physical Therapist, Courage Kenny Research Center, 800 E 28th Street, Mail Stop 12212, Minneapolis, Minnesota 55407-3799
†Physical Therapist, Physical Medicine and Rehabilitation, VA Medical Center, One Veterans Drive, Room 3R141, Minneapolis, Minnesota 55417

INTRODUCTION

Posttraumatic headache (PTH) is defined as a headache that occurs within 1 week after regaining consciousness after an injury or within 1 week of head trauma.[1] It has recently been acknowledged that some new PTHs may have an onset outside the 7-day window required for diagnosis by these guidelines.[2] Most headaches resolve within 6–12 months and are associated with cervical muscle tenderness and postural abnormalities. Lew et al[1] found that many patients with PTH presented clinically with symptoms similar to tension headache (37%), migraine (29%), and cluster headaches (6%–10%). The number of individuals who develop PTH following a concussion/mild traumatic brain injury (c/mTBI) usually ranges from 30% to 50%,[3] though frequency may be underreported.[2] In a recent survey of Army infantry soldiers, 3 to 4 months after return from a yearlong deployment in Iraq, about 30% who had been injured with loss of consciousness also described headache as a disability affecting their overall health.[4] Females and those with a history of headache prior to a head injury are more at risk for PTH.[2] Chronic PTH can lead to poor return-to-duty rates.[5]

Although the type and quality of headache may be different for a service member exposed to blast injury (more often migraine[6]) than other mechanisms of concussive injury, a consistent means to assess pain level and the functional impact of headache is recommended. Clinicians are encouraged to use a standardized approach for a musculoskeletal evaluation. Neck pain, temporomandibular disorders, and shoulder pain are common complaints reported in conjunction with c/mTBI, all of which contribute to PTH. Headache assessment includes both general measures of the frequency, severity, and limitations caused by headache pain (Numeric Pain Rating Scale [NPRS] or visual analog scale and Patient-Specific Functional Scale [PSFS]), and condition-specific measures that are used to determine the disability and severity of that disability related to the neck (Neck Disability Index [NDI]), the jaw (Jaw Functional Limitation Scale), and headache (Headache Disability Inventory [HDI]).[7–10]

Therapeutic interventions with the strongest evidence for treating PTH include a multimodal approach of specific training in exercise and postural retraining, stretching and ergonomic education, and manipulation and/or mobilization in combination with exercise.[11,12] Patient education regarding PTH and appropriate exercise program handouts are effective intervention techniques. Unique to headache is the inclusion of education regarding environmental triggers.[13] Pharmacologic treatment is common for headache; it is also used preventatively.[2] Therapists should work closely with and refer patients to physicians with headache management expertise to handle appropriate pharmacologic interventions.

PTH assessment using a standard musculoskeletal evaluation of the head, cervical spine, and other neck structures in conjunction with a pain scale and the HDI are considered **practice standards**, the therapeutic interventions are **practice options**, though recommended by experts.

SECTION 1: POSTTRAUMATIC HEADACHE ASSESSMENT

INTRODUCTION

In addition to a standard musculoskeletal evaluation of head and neck structures specifically looking for cervicogenic contributions to headache, a basic physical therapy clinical assessment of PTH should involve a standardized approach, including:

- A numeric or visual analog pain scale that assesses two dimensions of pain within a consistent timeframe: (1) pain limitation due to activity during the last 24 hours or last week, etc; and (2) pain intensity in the last 24 hours or last week, etc.
- Recording the number and type of headaches within a consistent timeframe.
- Recording the amount and type of headache-related medications under a standard context, such as within the last 24 hours, or the amount and type of medication needed to complete a work day, or any context associated with pain management.

The PSFS is a unique tool that helps physical therapists develop an individualized approach and should be considered for patients with headache resulting from c/mTBI. It is a patient-specific outcome measure that investigates functional status.[9]

Condition-specific measures should be used to determine disability and severity of disability related to the neck, jaw, and headache. These measures can be administered before and after an episode of care to determine the degree of improvement. Data can be aggregated to inform overall treatment program effectiveness. These condition-specific measures may include the HDI, Jaw Functional Limitation Scale (see Chapter 6, Temporomandibular Dysfunction), and the NDI.

HENRY FORD HEADACHE DISABILITY INVENTORY

Purpose/Description

The HDI is a 25-item patient self-report that measures the impact of headache on daily living. There are two scales, including 12 functional and 13 emotional items that combine for a maximum total score of 100.[8] This self-report questionnaire can be found in Jacobson, et al[8] and is available on multiple external websites.

Recommended Instrument Use

This tool is useful for determining the overall impact of headache on a patient's activities of daily living. It should be used in conjunction with standard measures of impairment to cervical and jaw function and muscle performance (range of motion, strength, etc). Headache pain should also be monitored in terms of type, frequency, duration, and severity.[14]

Administration Protocol/Equipment /Time

This is a paper-and-pencil self-test that may take up to 20 minutes to fill out. Scoring requires about 5 minutes.

Groups Tested With This Measure

Patients of all ages with a variety of headache etiologies are tested with the HDI. The majority of studies appear to be in patients with chronic headache.[8,15]

Interpretability

Norms: A higher score indicates greater disability due to headache.

- Minimum score: 0
- Maximum emotional subscale: 52
- Maximal functional subscale: 48
- Maximum score: 100

Minimal detectable change (MDC): 95% confidence level (based on a mean of 67-day retest on patients with headache[8]):

- 29 point change or greater in the total score
- 18 points for the functional scale
- 15 points for the emotional scale

If the patient's score is less than the MDC value, it is considered indistinguishable from measurement error.

Responsiveness Estimates: not available

Reliability Estimates

Internal consistency: Correlations using Chronbach's alpha between the functional and emotional subscale and total score were both $r = 0.89$[8] tested in a sample of patients that presented to a headache clinic for evaluation of their headache.

Interrater: not applicable (questionnaire)
Intrarater: not applicable (questionnaire)
Test-Retest: Test-retest scores in 77 patients (60 women, 17 men) seen in a diagnostic headache center on two occasions separated by a mean of 67 (standard deviation 27 days) days, $r = .76$ for the functional score, .82 for the emotional score.[8] Reliability coefficients were similar when tested one week apart (.76), showing good test-retest reliability for the total score and the two subscale scores.[15]

Validity Estimates

Content/Face: derived from existing scales for hearing and dizziness disability and from a clinical expert in a headache diagnostic center[8]
Criterion: Patients' spouses generally agreed with patients' ratings.[15] Age and sex or type of headache did not significantly affect the disability ratings.[8]
Construct: 109 patients with a mean age of 38 (standard deviation 11.6) years old, seen in a diagnostic headache center, evaluated their headache frequency and severity on a 3-point scale. This was compared to their ratings on the HDI using an analysis of variance to determine if self–perceived headache disability would increase with number of headaches and the number of severe headaches. A significant effect between headache magnitude and HDI was found for the total score and for both subscales.[8]

Selected References

Jacobson GP, Ramadan NM, Aggarwal SK, Newman CW. The Henry Ford Hospital Headache Disability Inventory (HDI). *Neurology.* 1994;44(5):837–842.

Jacobson GP, Ramadan NM, Norris L, Newman CW. Headache disability inventory (HDI): short-term test-retest reliability and spouse perceptions. *Headache.* 1995;35(9):534–539.

PATIENT-SPECIFIC FUNCTIONAL SCALE

Purpose/Description

The PSFS quantifies the amount of functional limitation for a specific patient (Form 5-1).[9,22] Patients are asked to nominate up to five activities with which they have difficulty due to their condition and, using a 0-to-10 scale, rate the functional limitation associated with these activities. The PSFS is intended to complement global or condition-specific measures.

Recommended Instrument Use

The PSFS is not designed to compare patients or groups of patients. Because each patient selects items that are important to his or her quality of life, it can only be used to follow individual items over time for a specific patient. It has been validated in patients with a variety of musculoskeletal dysfunctions and could be useful in patients with temporomandibular disorders or headaches, although specific studies in these patient populations have not been identified.

The scale includes a pain intensity/pain limitation rating. In pain-focused patients, the PSFS may be useful to redirect questioning toward function and ability rather than pain and disability.

It is important to note that clients are asked to rate their present functional status rather than a change in functional status. Therefore, it is a different construct then scales that rely on patients to remember what their prior level of functioning was and then rate a change in that level.

Administration Protocol/Equipment/Time

The PSFS may be administered verbally or as a pencil-and-paper task. Clients rate their functional limitations with each nominated activity on a scale of 0 to 10, where 0 represents an inability to perform the activity and 10 represents ability to perform the activity at the same level as before the injury or problem. At follow-up assessments, clients are informed of their previous ratings and asked to rate each of their previously nominated activities on the same scale again. The score total is the sum of the activity scores divided by the number of activities. The PSFS takes only 5 to 10 minutes to complete and score.

Some tips for PSFS administration include the following:

- Encourage patients to use a selection of activities they are likely to perform prior to the subsequent assessment so that a comparison may be drawn.
- If treatment is being directed toward a work-related injury, it is important that occupational activities are included to align with the broader goal of return to work.
- Document function specifics, such as chair height and timing variables, so future comparison will be accurate.

Groups Tested With This Measure

The PSFS has been shown to be valid and responsive to change in musculoskeletal conditions such as neck pain, cervical radiculopathy, knee pain, and low back pain.[16–19] When compared to other instruments in which a patient selects from a fixed set of functions, the PSFS has been shown to be more responsive than the NDI,[17] the pain rating index, and the Roland Morris Disability Questionnaire (RMDQ).[18]

In a patient population of workman's compensation patients, the PSFS was associated with timely recovery.[20] Originally the scale had patients list up to five activities; some studies have reduced it to three activities because patients most commonly report three activities.

Interpretability

The PSFS is not designed to compare clients to one another, but rather individual items are followed over time.

FORM 5-1

PATIENT-SPECIFIC FUNCTIONAL SCALE

Clinician to read and fill in. Complete at the end of the history and prior to physical.

Read at baseline assessment:

I'm going to ask you to identify up to three important activities that you are able to do or have difficulty with as a result of your problem. Today are there any activities that you are unable to do or have difficulty with because of your _____ problem? (Show scale.)

Read at follow-up visits:

When I assessed you on (state previous assessment date) *you told me that you had difficulty with* (read 1, 2, and 3 from the list). *Today, do you still have difficulty with 1* (have patient score item), *2* (have patient score item), *and 3* (have patient score item)?

Scoring scheme (show patient scale):

0	1	2	3	4	5	6	7	8	9	10

Unable to perform activity at same level as before injury or problem

Able to perform activity at same level as before injury or problem

Date/score

Activity						
1						
2						
3						
Additional						
Additional						

Reprinted with permission from: Dr. Paul Stratford, 1995.

MDC: The minimal detectable change (90% confidence interval) for an average score from three activities is 1 point, when informed ratings are made (that is, patients are reminded of their original ratings).[19] Note that patients in this study had neck pain.

- MDC for a single activity score was 2 points.
- A rating of pain limitation requires a 1-point change.

- A rating of pain intensity requires 2-point change for patients with neck pain.[19]

If the patient's score is less than the MDC value, it is considered indistinguishable from measurement error.

Responsiveness Estimates

According to Jolles,[21] responsiveness is likely greater for the PSFS when compared to fixed-item

151

instruments because of the patient's selection of areas of functional difficulty that are relevant to their situation. However, change scores may be exaggerated because of regression towards the mean, especially if patients select their most difficult activity. Further, selection of these difficult activities may make it harder to detect deterioration (a type of floor effect where all the scores are at the bottom end of the distribution due to the difficulty of the chosen activities).

Reliability Estimates

Internal consistency: not available
Interrater: not applicable (questionnaire)
Intrarater: not applicable (questionnaire)
Test-Retest: measured by standard error of measurement (SEM) during a period of time that the patient was known to be stable, SEM = .41; intraclass correlation coefficient (ICC) = 0.97 (reported for neck disability)[19]

Validity Estimates

Content/Face: not available
Criterion: moderate to excellent relationship between the PSFS[19] and:

- RMDQ ICC = .53–.74[9]
- NDI ICC = .73–.83[19]

Construct: for patients with neck pain[19]:

- Easier activities have greater ability scores than harder activities (P < .001).
- The amount of change over two measurement intervals was as predicted; that is, greater change was seen for easier activities than harder ones (P < .005).
- Ability to detect change over time was similar to the RMDQ and to a global rating of change evaluated by therapists and patients (P < .006).

ADDITIONAL RESOURCES FOR PATIENT-SPECIFIC FUNCTIONAL SCALE

In addition to Form 5-1, the PSFS can be found in the following:

- Stratford PW, Gill C, Westaway M, Binkley J. Assessing disability and change on individual patients: a report of a patient specific measure. *Physiother Can.* 1995;47(4):258–263.
- Horn KK, Jennings S, Richardson G, Vliet DV, Hefford C, Abbott JH. The Patient-Specific Functional Scale: psychometrics, clinimetrics, and application as a clinical outcome measure. *J Orthop Sports Phys Ther.* 2012;42(1):30–40.
- Rehabilitation Measures Database. http://www.rehabmeasures.org/Lists/RehabMeasures/DispForm.aspx?ID=890. Accessed July 24, 2013.

Selected References

Stratford P, Gill C, Westaway M, Binkley J. Assessing disability and change on individual patients: a report of a patient specific measure. *Physiother Can.* 1995:47(4) 258–263.

Horn K, Jennings S, Richardson G, van Vliet D, Hefford C, Abbott JH. The Patient-Specific Functional Scale: psychometrics, clinimetrics, and application as a clinical outcome measure. *J Orthop Sports Phys Ther.* 2012:42(1)30–40.

NUMERIC PAIN RATING SCALE

Purpose/Description

The NPRS is a subjective measurement of pain intensity administered either by a therapist or used as a self-report tool.[23,24] Clients rate their pain intensity on an 11-point scale (0–10), with 0 indicating no pain and 10 indicating pain as bad as it can be (Exhibit 5-1).

The Visual Analog Scale is a similar measure with a 10-cm (100-mm) straight line anchored by the same 0 and 10 as above, with patients marking their perceived pain level on the line and a clinician measuring the distance from the 0 ("no pain") anchor in millimeters with a ruler.

Recommended Instrument Use

The NPRS is a quick, effective method to measure pain intensity during an episode of care or before and after performance tests. Measuring pain intensity with the NPRS after performance tests, such as the Timed Up and Go and the Six-Minute Walk test, have demonstrated similar psychometric properties as other investigations that only studied the NPRS in diagnostic groups or different health-care settings.[25]

Pain scales associated with disability measures (eg, Patient-Specific Functional Limitation Scale or HDI) may not measure the same understanding of pain intensity as the NPRS.[25]

Administration Protocol/Equipment/Time

- Self-report: Clients are presented with a copy of the NPRS and instructed to circle the number that represents their pain intensity.
- Interview: The clinician describes the scale and its reference points and asks for a verbal rating of clients' perceived pain intensity.
- Scoring is the numbered response given by clients; that is, the score circled or the verbal rating provided by clients.
- When clients rate their "usual pain" after an intervention rather than pain over the previous 24 hours, larger changes have been recorded. Consistent instruction wording should be used so that scores can be compared.

Groups Tested With This Measure

This test has been used on individuals with a variety of orthopedic diagnoses that involve neck, back, upper extremity, and lower extremity dysfunction.[26,27] Studies have also involved acute (emergency department and post surgical) as well as chronic (rheumatoid arthritis) patient populations.[23,28–31]

Interpretability

Norms: not applicable

MDC: +/− 3 points on scale (90% confidence interval).[24] This amount of change reflects over 25% of the scale range, which indicates it may not be sensitive to small changes in pain intensity. If the patient's score is less than the MDC value, it is considered indistinguishable from measurement error.

Responsiveness Estimates

Patients (124 total) with neck, back, upper extremity, or lower extremity problems were tested on two occasions 7 days apart. Patients considered to be stable demonstrated a change of less than 3 points or 27% of the scale range.[24] In 79 new patients with pain complaints treated by chiropractic student interns supervised by clinical tutors, the effect size for NPRS was .77 when patients were asked to rate their current pain level, and 1.34 when instructed to measure their usual pain level.[26]

Reliability Estimates

Internal consistency: not applicable
Interrater: not available
Intrarater: not available
Test-Retest: ICCs reported in patients with orthopedic dysfunction, acute or chronic, ranged from 0.6 to 0.96.[23,24,30,31]

Validity Estimates

Content/Face: not available
Criterion: not available
Construct: assessed in patients in emergency department and immediate postoperative period the NPRS correlated with the visual analogue scale: 0.79 to 0.95.[28,29]

Selected References

Jensen MP, Karoly P, Braver S. The measurement of clinical pain intensity: a comparison of six methods. *Pain.* 1986;27:117–126.

Stratford PW, Spadoni G. The reliability, consistency, and clinical application of a numeric pain rating scale. *Physiother Can.* 2001;53(2):88.

EXHIBIT 5-1

NUMERIC PAIN RATING SCALE

PAIN INTENSITY

Over the past 24 hours, how bad has your pain been?

(Point to one number or circle one number)

Pain as bad as it can be

10

9

8

7

6

5

4

3

2

1

0

No pain

NECK DISABILITY INDEX

Purpose/Description

The NDI is a patient self-report questionnaire that measures clinical change in individuals that have acute or chronic neck pain due to a musculoskeletal or neurogenic origin.[10] Ten items are measured on a 6-point scale from 0 (no disability) to 5 (full disability), with a maximum score of 50 indicating full disability (see Attachment).

Recommended Instrument Use

The NDI can be used to describe levels of disability due to impairments of the cervical spine and neck pain due to musculoskeletal dysfunction, whiplash disorders, and cervical radiculopathy. The NDI should be scored out of 50, as recommended by the developer.[10] Benchmarks, if used, have not been sufficiently validated nor can they predict outcomes for such factors as return to work.[32] Ceiling (score of 40–50) and floor (score of 0–10) effects may be concerning; consider using the PSFS in conjunction with the NDI when scores are less than 10 and greater than 40.

Administration Protocol/Equipment/Time

The NDI is a paper-and-pencil self-test that takes 5 to 10 minutes to administer and 5 minutes to score. It has been translated into several languages. NDI scores vary from 0 to 50, where 0 is considered no activity limitation and 50 is considered complete disability. Some authors suggest that if more than two or three items are missing, the score is not considered valid.[32]

Groups Tested With This Measure

The NDI has been studied in patients with both acute and chronic neck pain (including those with traumatic etiology) and in a variety of settings (hospitals, rural clinics, urban settings, tertiary care).[32]

Interpretability

Norms: A score of 0 indicates no disability and 50 is considered complete disability. MacDermid and colleagues[32] propose three benchmark schemes (described below). Note that these studies involved subjects with whiplash syndrome.

- A "normal" score of between 0 to 20 points represents no to mild disability.[33]
- A score between:
  - 0 and 4: no disability
  - 5 and 14: mild disability
  - 15 and 24: moderate disability
  - 25 and 34: severe disability
  - greater than 35: complete disability[10]
- Individuals who have recovered have an NDI score of 8 or less, those with mild disability have a score of 10 to 28, and those with moderate to severe disability have a score greater than 30.[34]

MDC: The most common estimate for MDC is 5/50, or a 10% change.[35] Other estimates vary from 1.66 to 10.5, depending on diagnosis.[32] If the patient's score is less than the MDC value, it is considered indistinguishable from measurement error.

Responsiveness Estimates: clinically important difference is approximately 5 points[35] to 7 points.[17,32]

Reliability Estimates

Internal consistency: Consistently high Chronbach's alpha (0.70–0.96) was found in multiple studies. More rigorous studies using a highly powered Rasch analysis (n = 521 patients) suggest that the NDI items did not contribute to a single underlying construct. The item on headaches did not fit with other items in the scale. A newer, eight-item version is being developed to further test just one construct.[32,36]

Interrater: not applicable (questionnaire)

Intrarater: not applicable (questionnaire)

Test-Retest: reliability coefficients of 0.94 to 0.99; SEM of 0.64 to 8.4.[32] Others report retest reliability ICCs of 0.50 to 0.68.[17,37]

Validity Estimates

Content/Face: The NDI was developed using the Oswestry Low Back Pain Index as a template,[10] with additional questions based on recommendations of a consulting team.

Criterion: A single pain item and the total score both predicted visual analog pain ratings.[32]

Construct: correlated with Patient-Specific Functional Scale, Northwick Park Neck Pain Questionnaire, Neck Disability and Pain Disability Score, Disability Rating Index.[32]

Selected References

MacDermid JC, Walton DM, Avery S, et al. Measurement properties of the neck disability index: a systematic review. *J Orthop Sports Phys Ther.* 2009;39(5):400–417.

Vernon HT, Mior SA. The Neck Disability Index: a study of reliability and validity. *J Manipulative Physiol Ther.* 1991;14:409–415.

SECTION 2: POSTTRAUMATIC HEADACHE INTERVENTION

BACKGROUND

It may be difficult to distinguish between different types of headache because the clinical presentation of one headache disorder can mimic or co-exist with others. In addition to resulting from trauma to the head, headaches are also reported following trauma to the body that did not involve head or whiplash trauma.[38] High levels of muscle tenderness, as well as postural and mechanical abnormalities, have been reported in patients with tension headaches, migraine, whiplash syndromes, and cervicogenic headaches.[3,11,39] Headaches following exposure to blast appear to occur more frequently than following other types of head injury and often resemble migraines.[6]

Physical therapy appears to have at least a modest impact on outcome in patients experiencing headache.[11] Multimodal approaches that include manual therapy in combination with exercise and postural training are generally more effective. Patient education on medication management, avoidance of headache triggers, and home exercises is considered essential.

STRENGTH OF RECOMMNENDATION: PRACTICE OPTION

A structured review of the literature that examined treatment for headache[11] concluded that physical therapy appears to have a modest impact on outcome in patients experiencing headache of both traumatic and nontraumatic origin with individualized evaluation and intervention considered the best approach.

INTERVENTION METHODS

Address physical deficits (including movement-related disabilities, postural deficits, and muscle tenderness) that result in increased head, neck, and jaw pain. A thorough cervical spine evaluation is appropriate. Movement-related disabilities may additionally include low back pain or dysfunction, poor trunk stability, and poor scapular stability.

Symptom management of head and neck pain includes self-care instruction (practicing cervical range of motion in the pain-free range, using ice, avoiding headache triggers) and education, stretching (without aggravating pain) and strengthening (such as pain-free isometrics, scapular stabilization, and trunk stabilization) exercise, manual therapy, and application of therapeutic modalities.

Pharmacologic interventions are the primary medical approach for the treatment of PTH[2]; therefore, it is important for therapists to monitor patients' medication changes along with their pain levels. Use of pain-relieving medications can impact pain ratings, so the timing of medication use is relevant to pain-level evaluation (ie, patient ratings on a pain rating scale may be impacted by recent ingestion of pain-relieving medications).

Individualized goal setting (as with the PSFS) has shown promise in developing a more positive tone to the physical therapy episode of care, focusing on change in function that is most important to an individual patient. Support service member participation in and refer the service member for interventions for anxiety, depression, posttraumatic stress, and other psychological comorbidities associated with PTH.

REFERENCES

1. Lew HL, Lin PH, Fuh JL, Wang SJ, Clark DJ, Walker WC. Characteristics and treatment of headache after traumatic brain injury: a focused review. *Am J Phys Med Rehabil.* 2006;85(7):619–627.

2. Lucas S. Headache management in concussion and mild traumatic brain injury. *PM R.* Oct 2011;3(10 Suppl 2):S406–S412.

3. Packard RC. Chronic posttraumatic headache: associations with mild traumatic brain injury, concussion, and post-concussive disorder. *Curr Pain Headache Rep.* 2008;12:67–73.

4. Vereeck L, Wuyts F, Truijen S, van de Heyning P. Clinical assessment of balance: normative data, and gender and age effects. *Int J Audiol.* Feb 2008;47(2):67–75.

5. Cohen SP, Plunkett AR, Wilkinson I, et al. Headaches during war: analysis of presentation, treatment, and factors associated with outcome. *Cephalalgia.* Jan 2012;32(2):94–108.

6. Theeler BJ, Erickson JC. Posttraumatic headache in military personnel and veterans of the iraq and afghanistan conflicts. *Curr Treat Options Neurol.* Feb 2012;14(1):36–49.

7. Bijur PE, Silver W, Gallagher EJ. Reliability of the visual analog scale for measurement of acute pain. *Acad Emerg Med.* 2001;8:1153–1157.

8. Jacobson GP, Ramadan NM, Aggarwal SK, Newman CW. The Henry Ford Hospital Headache Disability Inventory (HDI). *Neurology.* 1994;44(5):837–842.

9. Stratford PW, Gill C, Westaway M, Binkley J. Assessing disability and change on individual patients: a report of a patient specific measure. *Physio Canada.* 1995;47(4):258–263.

10. Vernon HT, Mior SA. The Neck Disability Index: a study of reliability and validity. *J Manipulative Physiol Therapy.* 1991;14:409–415.

11. Biondi DM. Physical treatments for headache: a structured review. *Headache.* 2005;45(6):738–746.

12. Pho C, Godges J. Management of whiplash-associated disorder addressing thoracic and cervical spine impairments: a case report. *J Orthop Sports Phys Ther.* 2004;34(9):511–523.

13. Bell KR, Kraus EE, Zasler ND. Medical management of posttraumatic headaches: pharmacological and physical treatment. *J Head Trauma Rehabil.* 1999;14(1):34–48.

14. McDonnell MK, Sahrmann SA, van Dillen L. A specific exercise program and modification of postural alignment for treatment of cervicogenic headache: a case report. *J Orthop Sports Phys Ther.* 2005;35(1):3–15.

15. Jacobson GP, Ramadan NM, Norris L, Newman CW. Headache disability inventory (HDI): short-term test-retest reliability and spouse perceptions. *Headache.* 1995;35(9):534–539.

16. Chatman AB, Hyams SP, Neel JM, et al. The Patient-Specific Functional Scale: measurement properties in patients with knee dysfunction. *Phys Ther.* Aug 1997;77(8):820–829.

17. Cleland JA, Fritz JM, Whitman JM, Palmer JA. The reliability and construct validity of the Neck Disability Index and patient specific functional scale in patients with cervical radiculopathy. *Spine.* 2006;31(5):598–602.

18. Pengel LH, Refshauge KM, Maher CG. Responsiveness of pain, disability, and physical impairment outcomes in patients with low back pain. *Spine.* 2004;29(8):879–883.

19. Westaway MD, Stratford PW, Binkley JM. The patient-specific functional scale: validation of its use in persons with neck dysfunction. *J Orthop Sports Phys Ther.* 1998;27(5):331–338.

20. Gross DP, Battié MC, Asante AK. The Patient-Specific Functional Scale: validity in workers' compensation claimants. *Arch Phys Med Rehabil.* 2008;89(7):1294–1299.

21. Jolles BM, Buchbinder R, Beaton DE. A study compared nine patient-specific indices for musculoskeletal disorders. *J Clini Epidemiol.* 2005;58(8):791–801.

22. Horn KK, Jennings S, Richardson G, Vliet DV, Hefford C, Abbott JH. The patient-specific functional scale: psychometrics, clinimetrics, and application as a clinical outcome measure. *J Orthop Sports Phys Ther.* 2012;42(1):30–40.

23. Jensen MP, Karoly P, Braver S. The measurement of clinical pain intensity: a comparison of six methods. *Pain.* 1986;27:117–126.

24. Stratford PW, Spadoni G. The reliability, consistency, and clinical application of a numeric pain rating scale. *Physiotherapy Canada.* 2001;53(2):88.

25. Halket A, Stratford PW, Kennedy DM, Woodhouse LJ, Spadoni G. Measurement properties of performance-specific pain ratings of patients awaiting total joint arthroplasty as a consequence of osteoarthritis. *Physiother Can.* 2008;60(3):255–263.

26. Bolten JE, Wildson RC. Responsiveness of pain scales: a comparison of three intensity measures in chiropractic patients. *J Manipulative Physiother.* 1998;21:1–7.

27. Stratford PW, Kennedy DM, Woodhouse LJ. Performance measures provide assessments of pain and function in people with advanced osteoarthritis of the hip or knee. *Phys Ther.* Nov 2006;86(11):1489–1496.

28. Berthier F, Potel G, Leconte P, Touze MD, Baron D. Comparative study of methods of measuring acute pain intensity in an ED. *Am J Emerg Med.* Mar 1998;16(2):132–136.

29. DeLoach LJ, Higgins MS, Caplan AB, Stiff JL. The visual analog scale in the immediate postoperative period: intrasubject variability and correlation with a numeric scale. *Anesth Analg.* Jan 1998;86(1):102–106.

30. Ferraz MB, Quaresma MR, Aquino LR, Atra E, Tugwell P, Goldsmith CH. Reliability of pain scales in the assessment of literate and illiterate patients with rheumatoid arthritis. *J Rheumatol.* Aug 1990;17(8):1022–1024.

31. Jensen MP, Turner JA, Romano JM, Fisher LD. Comparative reliability and validity of chronic pain intensity measures. *Pain.* Nov 1999;83(2):157–162.

32. MacDermid JC, Walton DM, Avery S, et al. Measurement properties of the neck disability index: a systematic review. *J Orthop Sports Phys Ther.* 2009;39(5):400–417.

33. Miettinen T, Leino E, Airaksinen O, Lindgren KA. The possibility to use simple validated questionnaires to predict long-term health problems after whiplash injury. *Spine (Phila Pa 1976).* Feb 1 2004;29(3):E47–E51.

34. Sterling M, Jull G, Kenardy J. Physical and psychological factors maintain long-term predictive capacity post-whiplash injury. *Pain.* May 2006;122(1–2):102–108.

35. Stratford PW, Riddle DL, Binkley JM, Spadoni G, Westaway MD, Padfield B. Using the Neck Disability Index to make decisions concerning individual patients. *Physio Canada.* 1999;51:107–112.

36. van der Velde G, Beaton D, Hogg-Johnston S, Hurwitz E, Tennant A. Rasch analysis provides new insights into the measurement properties of the neck disability index. *Arthritis Rheum.* Apr 15 2009;61(4):544–551.

37. Cleland JA, Childs JD, Whitman JM. Psychometric properties of the Neck Disability Index and Numeric Pain Rating Scale in patients with mechanical neck pain. *Arch Phys Med Rehabil.* Jan 2008;89(1):69–74.

38. Haas DC. Traumatic-event headaches. *BMC Neurol.* Oct 29 2004;4(1):17.

39. Packard RC. Epidemiology and pathogenesis of posttraumatic headache. *J Head Trauma Rehabil.* 1999;4:9–21.

ATTACHMENT: THE NECK DISABILITY INDEX

An instrument for measuring self-rated disability due to neck pain or whiplash-associated disorder

Canadian Memorial Chiropractic College
6100 Leslie Street
Toronto, Ontario, Canada
M2H 3J1

1. Introduction

The Neck Disability Index (NDI) was developed in the late 1980s by Dr. Howard Vernon and first published in the Journal of Manipulative and Physiological Therapeutics in 1991.[1] The NDI was modeled on a similar instrument for assessing self-rated disability in low back pain patients: the Oswestry Low Back Pain Disability Questionnaire, which had been in existence for about eight years. Dr. Vernon received permission from the developer of the "Oswestry Index" to modify it for use in neck pain patients.

After selecting some of the original items from the Oswestry Index and then developing new items for neck pain patients, the prototype of the NDI was tested on a group of neck pain patients as well as chiropractors. Several modifications were made until a final version was acceptable. This version was then tested for reliability and validity and the results of these tests were published in the 1991 article. When it was published, the NDI became the first instrument for testing self-rated disability in neck pain patients.

Since 1991, a number of other questionnaires for neck pain patients have been developed, but the NDI remains the oldest and most widely used of these instruments.[2] Here are some more details:

- As of mid-2008, over 350 articles in the scientific literature have cited the NDI
- It has been used in 40 studies related to whiplash injury
- It has been translated into over 20 languages
- It has been used in 103 treatment studies, including 43 surgical studies, 57 studies of non-surgical treatments; 46 of these studies have been randomized clinical trials

2. Primary findings on the NDI

Vernon's review paper of 2008[3] is included in this manual and provides specific data from all of the studies of the psychometric properties of the NDI. The following is a summary of these findings:

The NDI has been shown to be highly reliable on what is called "test-retest" reliability.[1] The individual items have been shown to group together well as a single measure of self-rated physical disability.[4] The NDI has also been shown to be valid by comparing NDI scores to other measures of pain and disability.[1,5]

An important finding was published in the late 1990s by Riddle and Stratford.[6] They found that, for patients with scores in the mild-to-moderate range (where most patients score), there was a certain number of NDI points that could be regarded as "minimally important clinical change" by patients. This number is 5 or 10%. So, if your patient first scores 15 out of 50, and then, two weeks later, scores 12, this would not be regarded as a clinically important change. However, if they scored 10 or less, then this would be regarded as a clinically important change.

3. Scoring the NDI

The NDI consists of ten items, each with a score up to 5, for a total score of 50. The lower the score, the less self-rated disability. Dr. Vernon established the following guide to interpretation of a patient's score [1]:

- 0–4 = No disability
- 5–14 = Mild disability
- 15–24 = Moderate disability
- 25–34 = Severe disability
- 35 or over = Complete disability

4. Item issues

Users should attempt to have all ten items completed at all administrations. Some patients may find 1–2 items not applicable to their lives. This is especially true of "driving." This item may be omitted and the instrument scored out of 45, converted to 100% and then divided by 2.

The other item which may cause some problem is "work." While the term "work" was meant for any circumstance, many people interpret it as "work at my job." Therefore, if they are not employed, they may decline to complete this item. In that case, please re-interpret this item as "housework" for anyone not working out of the house.

For missing items not explained above (simple omissions, etc), only up to two missed items should be allowed. With three or more missed items, the administration would be regarded as unacceptable.

For 1–2 missed items, there are two strategies that amount to the same result:

- take the score out of 45 or 40, convert to 100% and divide by 2
- insert the average item score (total score divided by 9 or 8) into each missing item

5. Using the NDI

The NDI should be an important part of your first assessment of any patient with neck pain, especially due to trauma. The question arises, "when should I repeat the NDI?" Remember that the NDI measures self-rated disability, not just current pain level. This applies to a person's ability to perform their daily activities. A single, composite measure of this ability (the NDI score) is not likely to change over a short period of time. So, we recommend that the NDI be used on <u>two-week intervals</u> over the course of your treatment of a patient with neck pain.

6. Links

- http://www.proqolid.org/
- http://www.pedro.fhs.usyd.edu.au/CEBP/index_cebp.html
- http://www.worksafe.vic.gov.au
- http://www.medigraphsoftware.com
- http://www.painworld.zip.com
- http://medal.org
- http://outcomesassessment.org
- http://www.maa.nsw.gov.au
- http://apa.advsol.com.au/physio_and_health/research/evidence/outcome_measures.cf   m
- http://caretrak-outcomes.com
- http://ccachiro.org
- http://www.unisa.edu.au/cahe/
- http://www.tac.vic.gov.au
- http://clinicaltrials.gov/ct/show/NCT00349544;jsessionid=26CC121CFA39CE943448CF75822 A8C60?order=1
- http://www.cks.library.nhs.uk

7. References

1. Vernon HT, Mior SA. The Neck Disability Index: a study of reliability and validity. *J Manip Physiol Ther*. 1991;14:409–415.

2. Pietrobon B, Coeytaux RB, Carey TS, Richardson WJ, DeVellis RF. Standard scales for measurement of functional outcome for cervical pain or dysfunction—a systematic review. *Spine*. 2002; 27(5):515–522.

3. Vernon H. The Neck Disability Index: state-of-the-art, 1991–2008. *J Manip Physiol Ther*. 2008;31:491–502.

4. Hains F, Waalen J, Mior S. Psychometric properties of the neck disability index. *J Manip Physiol Ther*. 1998; 21(2):75–80.

5. Vernon H. Assessment of self-rated disability, impairment, and sincerity of effort in whiplash-associated disorder. Journal of Musculoskeletal Pain 2000; 8(1-2):155–167.

6. Riddle DL, Stratford PW. Use of generic versus region-specific functional status measures on patients with cervical spine disorders. *Phys Ther*. 1998; 78(9):951–963.

NECK DISABILITY INDEX

This questionnaire is designed to help us better understand how your neck pain affects your ability to manage everyday-life activities. Please mark in each section the one box that applies to you. Although you may consider that two of the statements in any one section relate to you, please mark the box that most closely describes your present-day situation.

SECTION 1–PAIN INTENSITY

❑ I have no neck pain at the moment.

❑ The pain is very mild at the moment.

❑ The pain is moderate at the moment.

❑ The pain is fairly severe at the moment.

❑ The pain is very severe at the moment.

❑ The pain is the worst imaginable at the moment.

SECTION 2–PERSONAL CARE

❑ I can look after myself normally without causing extra neck pain.

❑ I can look after myself normally, but it causes extra neck pain.

❑ It is painful to look after myself, and I am slow and careful.

❑ I need some help but manage most of my personal care.

❑ I need help everyday in most aspects of self-care.

❑ I do not get dressed. I wash with difficulty and stay in bed.

SECTION 3–LIFTING

❑ I can lift heavy weights without causing extra neck pain.

❑ I can lift heavy weights, but it gives me extra neck pain.

❑ Neck pain prevents me from lifting heavy weights off the floor but I can manage if items are conveniently positioned (ie, on a table).

❑ Neck pain prevents me from lifting heavy weights, but I can manage light weights if they are conveniently positioned.

SECTION 4–READING

❑ I can read as much as I want with no neck pain.

❑ I can read as much as I want with slight neck pain.

❑ I can read as much as I want with moderate neck pain.

❑ I can't read as much as I want because of moderate neck pain.

❑ I can't read as much as I want because of severe neck pain.

❑ I can't read at all.

SECTION 5–HEADACHES

❑ I have no headaches at all.

❑ I have slight headaches that come infrequently.

❑ I have moderate headaches that come infrequently.

❑ I have moderate headaches that come frequently.

❑ I have severe headaches that come frequently.

❑ I have headaches almost all the time.

SECTION 6–CONCENTRATION

❑ I can concentrate fully without difficulty.

❑ I can concentrate fully with slight difficulty.

❑ I have a fair degree of difficulty concentrating.

❑ I have a lot of difficulty concentrating.

❑ I have a great deal of difficulty concentrating.

❑ I can't concentrate at all.

SECTION 7–WORK

❑ I can do as much work as I want.

❑ I can only do my usual work, but no more.

❑ I can do most of my work, but no more.

❑ I can't do my usual work.

❑ I can hardly do any work at all.

❑ I can't do any work at all.

SECTION 8–DRIVING

❑ I can drive my car without neck pain.

❑ I can drive my car with only slight neck pain.

❑ I can drive as long as I want with moderate neck pain.

❑ I can't drive as long as I want because of moderate neck pain.

❑ I can hardly drive at all because of severe neck pain.

❑ I can't drive my car at all because of neck pain.

SECTION 9–SLEEPING

❑ I have no trouble sleeping.

❑ My sleep is slightly disturbed for less than 1 hour.

❑ My sleep is mildly disturbed for up to 1–2 hours.

❑ My sleep is moderately disturbed for up to 2–3 hours.

❑ My sleep is greatly disturbed for up to 3–5 hours.

❑ My sleep is completely disturbed for up to 5–7 hours.

SECTION 10–RECREATION

❑ I am able to engage in all my recreational activities with no neck pain at all.

❑ I am able to engage in all my recreational activities with some neck pain.

❑ I am able to engage in most, but not all, of my recreational activities because of neck pain.

❑ I can hardly do recreational activities because of neck pain.

❑ I can't do any recreational activities because of neck pain.

Patient name _____   Date _____

Score _____

Chapter 6

TEMPOROMANDIBULAR DYSFUNCTION ASSESSMENT AND INTERVENTION

MARGARET M. WEIGHTMAN, PhD, PT* AND JANICE P. KEHLER, BPT, MS, MA†

*Clinical Scientist/Physical Therapist, Courage Kenny Research Center, 800 E 28th Street, Mail Stop 12212, Minneapolis, Minnesota 55407-3799
†Physical Therapist, Physical Medicine and Rehabilitation, VA Medical Center, One Veterans Drive, Room 3R141, Minneapolis, Minnesota 55417

INTRODUCTION

Temporomandibular disorders (TMDs) are defined as a subgroup of craniofacial pain problems that involve the temporomandibular joint (TMJ), muscles of mastication, and associated musculoskeletal structures of the head and neck.[1] In addition to pain, limited mandibular motion, and joint sounds, common symptoms can include ear pain and stuffiness, tinnitus, dizziness, neck pain, and headache.

At least one sign of TMD is reported in 40% to 75% of adults in the United States.[1] Although up to 40% of those who experience signs and symptoms of TMD show spontaneous resolution of their symptoms,[1] patients with posttraumatic TMD may differ to a small extent from those with nontraumatic disorders on reaction-time testing, neuropsychological testing, and clinical testing of TMD.[2] TMD may contribute to posttraumatic headache.[3]

A very basic measurement for TMD dysfunction that may be applied by a generalist therapist is a measure of pain-free mouth opening (maximal incisal opening). Typically, a therapist who specializes in TMD uses a complete physical assessment of the TMJ and surrounding musculature, such as the Temporomandibular Index, which combines the functional indices in a total score.[4] Additional measures of pain and of functional limitation brought on by TMD are recommended.[4-6] The Jaw Functional Limitation Scale (JFLS) is a joint-specific patient self-report designed to test a patient's functional level.[6,7] Although it is not yet specifically tested in persons with TMD, the Patient-Specific Functional Scale (see Chapter 5: Posttraumatic Headache Assessment and Intervention), a patient-specific outcome measure that investigates functional status,[8-12] may be considered for use in this population. An option for a quick method of measuring subjective pain intensity that may or may not be context specific is the Numeric Pain Rating Scale (see Chapter 5: Posttraumatic Headache Assessment and Intervention), which can be administered either by a therapist or used as a self-report tool.[13,14]

Although no studies that specifically address interventions for TMD that occur as a result of MTBI were found, several systematic reviews of TMD interventions support symptom management using a multimodal approach.[1,15-17] The majority of individuals with TMD respond to symptom management techniques, but for those who experience chronic pain, referral to and collaboration with dentists, a multidisciplinary chronic pain center, or both may be needed.

This section of the toolkit provides a limited number of assessments for the generalist therapist, along with suggestions for conservative interventions for service members with TMD. Although a specific physical assessment format is not included here, a standardized physical assessment of joint and muscles[4] that is used consistently is recommended. The other assessments included here are considered **practice options** and are focused on functional limitations and pain that may occur in those with TMD issues. Initial conservative intervention suggestions are considered **practice standards** based on a number of systematic reviews.[15,16]

SECTION 1: ASSESSMENT

INTRODUCTION

A complete evaluation of TMD involves a physical assessment of the TMJ as well as of the surrounding musculature. A TMD specialist may use a valid and reliable assessment tool, such as the Temporomandibular Index.[4] The generalist therapist may begin by using a measure of maximal voluntary mandibular opening, which is obtained by measuring between the maxillary and mandibular incisal edges with a ruler scaled in millimeters. According to Higbie et al, the "internationally accepted norms for vertical mandibular opening in healthy adults 18 to 60 years of age have been reported to be between 36 and 68 mm of opening at the incisal edge."[18] Head position is an important factor in the amount of vertical mandibular opening available[18] and should be tested consistently. Some complete assessment tools consider the range of motion for vertical mandibular opening as normal if it is greater than or equal to 40 mm.[4] Additional measures of functional limitation and pain are used to assess and follow change over time in individuals with TMD.

THE JAW FUNCTIONAL LIMITATION SCALE

Purpose/Description

The JFLS is a patient self-report questionnaire designed to assess a patient's functional level that is both joint-specific and separate from pain-related disability (Form 6-1).[6,7] It has a total of 20 items that address three levels of functional limitation including mastication (6 items), jaw mobility (4 items), and verbal and emotional expression (10 items). There is also an eight-item version that measures global functional limitation of the jaw. Each item is rated on a numerical rating scale of 0 to 10 (0 indicates no limitation; 10 indicates severe limitation).

Recommended Instrument Use

The eight-item scale has been shown to be sensitive to change following short-term interventions, but the developers assume that the 20-item scale will also be sensitive to change because it contains more focused items that correlated with the eight-item version.[6] The developers recommend that the 20-item scale be used to evaluate the effects of interventions on individual clients. These scales should be used in conjunction with a standard physical therapy evaluation of jaw mobility and muscle performance.

Administration Protocol/Equipment/Time

This is a pencil-and-paper test that the client can fill out in less than 5 minutes. The eight-item version is a global scale; the 20-item version is better for individual assessment.

Groups Tested With This Measure

Five diagnostic groups were included in research studies, including TMD, primary Sjogren's syndrome, burning mouth syndrome, skeletal malocclusion, and healthy controls.[6,7] Items from two other self-report measures were studied to develop a new scale related to jaw-specific limitations that were separate from disability and pain behaviors. Most of the subjects were females with an age range from 10–93 years.

Interpretability

Norms: not available
Minimal Detectable Change (MDC): not available.

If the patient's score is less than the MDC value, it is considered indistinguishable from measurement error.

Responsiveness Estimates

Sensitivity to change in a pre-post test population (subjects tested both before and after intervention) of subjects diagnosed with TMD has moderate effect size (mean change divided by the standard deviation) of 0.41.[6] Note that only the original eight-item version has been tested for sensitivity to change.

Reliability Estimates

Internal consistency: determined in a sample of patients (72% female; ages 10–93). Chronbach's alpha (α) for mastication (0.83–0.89), for vertical mobility (0.69–0.97), and for verbal and emotional expression (0.83–0.95).[6,7]
Interrater: not applicable (questionnaire)
Intrarater: not applicable (questionnaire)
Test-Retest: Subjects with TMD disorders test-retest over 2 weeks Chronbach's rho for eight-item version 0.81; for 20-item version 0.87.[6]

Validity Estimates

Content/Face: Draft self-report instrument was constructed using the initial eight-item JFLS with 44 other items added by a consensus panel of five expert clinicians and researchers in the dental fields of orofacial pain, oral medicine, and prosthodontics. Rasch methodology was used for item reduction and assessment of model fit. Qualitative interviews of patients determined that the final items were understandable, sufficient, and clinically relevant.[6,7]
Criterion: not available
Construct: The eight-item JFLS was tested to determine whether it measured functional limitation separate from personal disability. As hypothesized, low correlations (0.02–0.26) were found between the JFLS-8 as compared to depression, anxiety, somatization, pain interference, pain-free opening, and palpation sensitivity. Moderate correlations (0.49–0.57) were found with pain and jaw symptoms. Correlations between the eight-item version and 20-item version on all items and individual constructs ranged from 0.80–0.96.[6]

FORM 6-1

JAW FUNCTIONAL LIMITATION SCALE

For each of the items below, please indicate the level of limitation **during the last month**. If the activity has been completely avoided because it is too difficult, circle "10." If you avoid an activity for reasons other than pain or difficulty, leave the item blank.

	No limitation										Severe limitation
1. Chew tough food	0	1	2	3	4	5	6	7	8	9	10
2. Chew hard bread	0	1	2	3	4	5	6	7	8	9	10
3. Chew chicken (for example, prepared in oven)	0	1	2	3	4	5	6	7	8	9	10
4. Chew crackers	0	1	2	3	4	5	6	7	8	9	10
5. Chew soft food (for example, macaroni, canned or soft fruits, cooked vegetables, fish)	0	1	2	3	4	5	6	7	8	9	10
6. Eat soft food requiring no chewing (for example, mashed potatoes, applesauce, pudding, pureed food)	0	1	2	3	4	5	6	7	8	9	10
7. Open wide enough to bite from a whole apple	0	1	2	3	4	5	6	7	8	9	10
8. Open wide enough to bite into a sandwich	0	1	2	3	4	5	6	7	8	9	10
9. Open wide enough to talk	0	1	2	3	4	5	6	7	8	9	10
10. Open wide enough to drink from a cup	0	1	2	3	4	5	6	7	8	9	10
11. Swallow	0	1	2	3	4	5	6	7	8	9	10
12. Yawn	0	1	2	3	4	5	6	7	8	9	10
13. Talk	0	1	2	3	4	5	6	7	8	9	10
14. Sing	0	1	2	3	4	5	6	7	8	9	10
15. Putting on a happy face	0	1	2	3	4	5	6	7	8	9	10
16. Putting on an angry face	0	1	2	3	4	5	6	7	8	9	10
17. Frown	0	1	2	3	4	5	6	7	8	9	10
18. Kiss	0	1	2	3	4	5	6	7	8	9	10
19. Smile	0	1	2	3	4	5	6	7	8	9	10
20. Laugh	0	1	2	3	4	5	6	7	8	9	10

Reproduced with permission from: Richard Ohrbach, DDS, PhD; Associate Professor, Department of Oral Diagnostic Sciences, University of Buffalo, 355 Squire Hall, Buffalo, New York.

Selected References

Ohrbach R, Larsson P, List T. The Jaw Functional Limitation Scale: development, reliability, and validity of 8-item and 20-item versions. *J Orofac Pain.* 2008;22(3):219–230.

Ohrbach R, Granger C, List T, Dworkin S. Preliminary development and validation of the Jaw Functional Limitation Scale. *Community Dent Oral Epidemiol.* 2008;36(3):228–236.

SECTION 2: INTERVENTION

INTRODUCTION

Treatment for TMD should begin with conservative management techniques including application of heat or cold, instruction in postural and relaxation exercises, instruction in self-care and activities to avoid, and the use of over-the-counter pain-reducing medication or other medication as prescribed by the patient's physician.[15,16] Those who fail to respond to conservative management should be referred for dental and additional specialty evaluation.

BACKGROUND

No studies were found that specifically address intervention for TMJ disorders that occur as a result of mild traumatic brain injury; however, systematic reviews suggest TMD symptoms are best managed using a multimodal approach.[1,15–17] The majority of those with TMD respond to symptom management techniques, but for those who experience chronic pain, referral and collaboration with dentists, a multidisciplinary chronic pain center, or both may be needed.

STRENGTH OF RECOMMENDATION: PRACTICE STANDARD

Systematic reviews of the literature indicate that the majority of TMDs can be treated with noninvasive, conservative interventions.[1,15] In randomized studies that have controlled for severity, patients with mostly physical limitations have shown improvement with patient education on self-care, including use of heat or cold packs, jaw exercises, guidance in activities to avoid (ie, chewing gum, eating hard candy), and progressive muscle relaxation.[17]

Intervention Methods

- Provide educational material regarding precautions and activities to avoid for persons with TMD.
- TMD symptoms are best managed using a multimodal approach that includes self-care instruction, stretching exercise, manual therapy, and application of therapeutic modalities.[15,16]
- Treatment should also include instruction in postural exercises for the neck and upper back.[19]
  - Recommended exercises include stretching that is done slowly, gradually, and in a pain-free manner. Recommendations are to have the patient move to the point of mild tension and hold.
  - Exercises recommended by Wright et al[19] include:

  i. chin tucks done hourly;
  ii. chest stretches done in a doorway or corner, several times daily;
  iii. wall stretches with back against wall, elbows and back of hands against wall, stretching arms overhead, several times daily;
  iv. supine chest stretches with hands behind head extending elbows to floor, done each evening; and
  v. prone/face down arm lifts with arms at 90 degrees and arms overhead, done daily.

- The majority of TMDs respond to symptom management techniques, but for those who develop a chronic pain situation, referral to and collaboration with dentists (occlusal splints, evaluation of intracranial sources of pain) or referral to a multidisciplinary chronic pain center (or both) may be needed.

Intervention Resources

- Medline Plus: patient education including an interactive tutorial on TMD disorders, found at: www.nlm.nih.gov/medlineplus/temporomandibularjointdysfunction.html
- National Institute of Dental Craniofacial Research, found at: www.nidcr.nih.gov/OralHealth/Topics/TMJ

JOINT PROTECTION AND SELF-CARE FOR TEMPOROMANDIBULAR DYSFUNCTION

- Relax your jaw muscles. Avoid clenching or grinding your teeth. In your jaw's resting posture, your tongue should rest lightly on the top of your mouth wherever it is most comfortable, while allowing the teeth to come apart and the jaw muscles to relax. Avoid biting on objects like pens or pencils.
- Eat a "pain-free" diet. Avoid chewing gum or eating hard foods, such as bagels, crusty bread, carrot sticks, chewy candy, and tough meat. Eat a softer diet.
- Cut up your food into small pieces. Chew on both sides of your mouth at the same time.
- Avoid resting your jaw on your hand. Do not sleep on your stomach. Sleeping on your side is okay as long as you do not put force on your jaw. Sleeping on your back is best.
- Avoid activities that involve wide opening of the jaw, such as yawning. When you feel like yawning, put your tongue hard against the top of your mouth and let your mouth open as far as it can without letting your tongue off the top of your mouth.

- Avoid or limit caffeine. Caffeine is a "muscle-tensing" drug that can make muscles feel tighter. Caffeine or caffeine-like drugs are in coffee, tea, soda, energy drinks, chocolate, and some aspirins. Decaffeinated coffee typically has half as much caffeine as regular.
- Follow your doctors' suggestions regarding the use of antiinflammatory and pain-reducing medications like ibuprofen, acetaminophen, and aspirin (without caffeine) to reduce joint and muscle pain.
- Use hot packs or ice on the painful area, whatever you find most comfortable.
  ○ Apply a moist hot pack to the painful area for 15 to 20 minutes, two to four times each day.
  ○ You can wrap a towel around a gel pack that has been heated according to instructions or a hot water bottle and put it on both sides of your jaw. This should be very warm but comfortable.
  ○ Try using ice wrapped in a very thin cloth for 5 to 10 minutes, two to four times per day. Keep the ice on the painful area **only** until you first sense some numbness, then remove it.[20]

REFERENCES

1. Scrivani SJ, Keith DA, Kaban LB. Temporomandibular disorders. *N Eng J Med.* 2008;359(25):2693–2705.

2. Goldberg MB, Mock D, Ichise M, et al. Neuropsychologic deficits and clinical features of posttraumatic temporomandibular disorders. *J Orofac Pain.* 1996;10(2):126–140.

3. Packard RC. Epidemiology and pathogenesis of posttraumatic headache. *J Head Trauma Rehabil.* 1999;14(1):9–21.

4. Pehling J, Schiffman E, Look J, Shaefer J, Lenton P, Fricton J. Interexaminer reliability and clinical validity of the Temporomandibular Index: a new outcome measure for temporomandibular disorders. *J Orofac Pain.* 2002;16(4):296–304.

5. Dworkin SF, Turner JA, Mancl L, et al. A randomized clinical trial of a tailored comprehensive care treatment program for temporomandibular disorders. *J Orofac Pain.* 2002;16(4):259–276.

6. Ohrbach R, Larsson P, List T. The Jaw Functional Limitation Scale: Development, reliability, and validity of 8-item and 20-item versions. *J Orofac Pain.* 2008;22(3):219–230.

7. Ohrbach R, Granger C, List T, Dworkin S. Preliminary development and validation of the Jaw Functional Limitation Scale. *Community Dent Oral Epidemiol.* 2008;36(3):228–236.

8. Abernethy B. Dual-task methodology and motor skills research: some applications and methodological constraints. *J Human Movement Studies.* 1988;14:101–132.

9. Cleland JA, Fritz JM, Whitman JM, Palmer JA. The reliability and construct validity of the Neck Disability Index and patient specific functional scale in patients with cervical radiculopathy. *Spine.* 2006;31(5):598–602.

10. Stratford P. Assessing disability and change on individual patients: a report of a patient specific measure. *Physio Canada.* 1995;47:258–263.

11. Westaway MD, Stratford PW, Binkley JM. The patient-specific functional scale: validation of its use in persons with neck dysfunction. *J Orthop Sports Phys Ther.* 1998;27(5):331–338.

12. Pengel LH, Refshauge KM, Maher CG. Responsiveness of pain, disability, and physical impairment outcomes in patients with low back pain. *Spine.* 2004;29(8):879–883.

13. Jensen MP, Karoly P, Braver S. The measurement of clinical pain intensity: a comparison of six methods. *Pain.* 1986;27:117–126.

14. Stratford PW, Spadoni G. The reliability, consistency, and clinical application of a numeric pain rating scale. *Physiother Can.* 2001;53(2):88.

15. McNeely ML, Armijo Olivo S, Magee DJ. A systematic review of the effectiveness of physical therapy interventions for temporomandibular disorders. *Phys Ther.* 2006;86(5):710–725.

16. Medlicott MS, Harris SR. A systematic review of the effectiveness of exercise, manual therapy, electrotherapy, relaxation training, and biofeedback in the management of temporomandibular disorder. *Phys Ther.* 2006;86(7):955–973.

17. Truelove E, Huggins KH, Mancl L, Dworkin SF. The efficacy of traditional, low-cost and nonsplint therapies for temporomandibular disorder: a randomized controlled trial. *J Am Dent Assoc.* 2006;137(8):1099–1107; quiz 1169.

18. Higbie EJ, Seidel-Cobb D, Taylor LF, Cummings GS. Effect of head position on vertical mandibular opening. *J Orthop Sports Phys Ther.* Feb 1999;29(2):127–130.

19. Wright EF, Domenech MA, Fischer JR, Jr. Usefulness of posture training for patients with temporomandibular disorders. *J Am Dent Assoc.* 2000;131(2):202–210.

20. Wright EF, Schiffman EL. Treatment alternatives for patients with masticatory myofascial pain. *J Am Dent Assoc.* 1995;126:1030–1039.

Chapter 7

COGNITION ASSESSMENT AND INTERVENTION

MARY VINING RADOMSKI, PhD, OTR/L*; SHARI GOO-YOSHINO, MS[†]; CAROL SMITH HAMMOND, PhD, CCC/SLP[‡]; EMI ISAKI, PhD[§]; DON MACLENNAN, MA[¥]; R. KEVIN MANNING, PhD[¶]; PAULINE MASHIMA, PhD, CCC/SLP[**]; LINDA M. PICON, MCD, CCC/SLP[††]; CAROLE R. ROTH, PhD, BC-ANCDS[‡‡]; AND JOETTE ZOLA, BS, OT[§§]

PATIENT HANDOUTS

REFERENCES

Clinical Scientist, Courage Kenny Research Center, 800 East 28th Street, Mail Stop 12212, Minneapolis, Minnesota 55407-3799

†*Staff, Speech-Language Pathologist, Otolaryngology Service, Department of Surgery, Tripler Army Medical Center, 1 Jarrett White Road, Tripler Army Medical Center, Honolulu, Hawaii 96859-5000*

‡*Research Speech Pathologist, Audiology/Speech Pathology, Durham VA Medical Center, #126, 508 Fulton Street, Durham, North Carolina 27705*

§*Assistant Professor, Communication Sciences & Disorders, Northern Arizona University, Department of Communication Sciences & Disorders, Building 66, PO Box 15045, Flagstaff, Arizona 86011-5045*

¥*Chief, Speech Pathology Section, Minneapolis VA Health Care System, One Veterans' Drive 127A, Minneapolis, Minnesota 55417*

¶*Speech Pathologist, Traumatic Brain Injury Service, San Antonio Military Medical Center–North, 3551 Roger Brooke Drive, Joint-Base Fort Sam Houston, Texas 78234-6500*

**Chief, Speech Pathology Section, Department of Surgery, Otolaryngology Service, Tripler Army Medical Center, 1 Jarrett White Road, Tripler Army Medical Center, Honolulu, Hawaii 96859-5000*

††*Speech-Language Pathologist, Veterans' Health Administration, James A. Haley Veterans' Hospital, Audiology and Speech Pathology (ASP 126), 13000 Bruce B. Downs Boulevard, Tampa, FL 33612; and 4202 East Fowler Avenue, PCD1017, Tampa, Florida 33620-8200*

‡‡*Division Head, Speech Pathology, Naval Medical Center San Diego, 34800 Bob Wilson Drive, Building 2/2, 2K-11R5, San Diego, California 92134-6200*

§§*Occupational Therapist, Brain Injury Clinic, Courage Kenny Rehabilitation Institute, Allina Health, 800 East 28th Street, Mail Stop 12210, Minneapolis, Minnesota 55407-3799*

INTRODUCTION

Cognitive complaints that follow concussion/mild traumatic brain injury (c/mTBI), especially those resulting from blasts or other injuries sustained in a combat zone, are multifactorial and not well understood. Clinicians serving service members (SMs) with persistent cognitive complaints that impact daily functions, including communication, must recognize potential contributing factors, such as comorbid pain, fatigue, stress, sleep deprivation, drug effects, and psychological concerns (eg, posttraumatic stress disorder [PTSD], depression, anxiety).[1] For a more extensive discussion of these comorbid factors, as well as for literature reviews of the evidence for the recommended assessments and interventions, clinicians are referred to *Occupational and Physical Therapy Mild Traumatic Brain Injury Clinical Management Guidance*[2] and the *Speech-Language Pathology Clinical Management Guidance: Cognitive-Communication Rehabilitation for Concussion/Mild Traumatic Brain Injury.*[3]

This section of the Toolkit was developed by an interdisciplinary group of clinicians, including occupational therapists (OTs) and speech-language pathologists (SLPs). The Toolkit and guidance documents were written to provide practical assistance for generalist clinicians working with SMs with c/mTBI, including those clinicians with limited experience in cognitive rehabilitation. SMs and veterans presenting with c/mTBI and persistent cognitive symptoms often have complex comorbid conditions that may also undermine cognitive abilities and complicate the treatment process. Therefore, it is imperative that clinicians recognize when to refer SMs with complex issues to specialists. Additionally, clinicians are encouraged to move beyond the basics provided in this Toolkit to acquire knowledge and develop skills necessary to manage the challenges and complexities of assessing and providing cognitive rehabilitation for this patient population.

Experts recommend that cognitive assessment after c/mTBI consist of a thorough neurobehavioral and cognitive evaluation using standardized performance measures, self-report measures, and measures of effort.[4] OTs and SLPs often contribute to this process with the use of multiple assessment tools to fully characterize the extent of cognitive and communication concerns. While it is a **practice standard** to assess cognition and cognitive-communication complaints following c/mTBI, the choice of which assessment tools to use is determined by the individual clinician (**practice option**) based on the needs of the SM and the specifics of the environment of care. Although the Toolkit includes the best available options, clinicians are advised that many of the assessments have not been validated on adults with c/mTBI.

Similarly, most cognitive rehabilitation interventions were developed for civilians with moderate to severe traumatic brain injury. The efficacy and effectiveness of these interventions have largely been evaluated on more severely injured populations or subject groups consisting of a range of injury severity levels. Despite this ambiguity of evidence, an expert panel convened by the Defense Centers of Excellence (DCoE) for Psychological Health and Traumatic Brain Injury recommended cognitive rehabilitation for SMs with c/mTBI who describe persistent cognitive symptoms at 3 months or more after concussion.[4] Therefore, those interventions that are either supported by empirical evidence involving studies of adults with c/mTBI or endorsed by the DCoE expert panel are characterized as **practice standards** in the Toolkit. Findings from future studies that are specific to SMs with c/mTBI may lead to further modifications of these recommendations.

The approach and focus of cognitive and cognitive-communication assessment and intervention will vary by discipline and potentially by site. Clinicians are referred to the Toolkit introductions and to the companion guidance documents for a more in-depth discussion of the discipline-specific rationales for recommended rehabilitation practices for c/mTBI.

SECTION 1: ASSESSMENT

INTRODUCTION

Cognitive assessment in acute c/mTBI focuses on tracking the resolution of symptoms to make return-to-activity decisions.[5] OTs and SLPs may screen patients with c/mTBI within the first 90 days following concussion to determine the presence or absence of cognitive changes as perceived by the patient, family members, or members of the patient's command. Interaction with the injured individual allows an opportunity to provide education about the relationship between his or her symptoms and the concussion, recommendations to facilitate recovery during the acute phase after injury, and reassurance about expectation of positive recovery. The screening activity and education have been shown to prevent or reduce the development of persistent symptoms.[6]

Because most acute cognitive changes resolve within 90 days following trauma,[4,7] comprehensive evaluation is typically deferred until after that time. Cognitive assessment for those with persisting postconcussive symptoms is typically used to guide treatment. This evaluation may be conducted by any combination of rehabilitation professionals, including OTs, SLPs, and neuropsychologists. Specific roles in evaluating cognitive deficits may vary by site and rehabilitation team availability. Evaluating persistent cognitive symptoms following c/mTBI, especially when the injury occurred in a combat zone, should account for the fact that symptoms are likely to be multifactorial in presentation and etiology.

Occupational Therapist Evaluation

OTs assess cognition for several reasons, including to measure baseline, progress, or outcome status; to understand patients' cognitive strengths, weaknesses, and capacity for using strategies to plan intervention; and to estimate the patient's ability to safely perform everyday activities.[8] Cognitive assessment in occupational therapy involves three elements: (1) evaluating everyday functioning to make inferences about cognition (real-world observation and dynamic assessment), (2) evaluating cognitive processes to make inferences about functioning (standardized tests),[9] and (3) patient and family interview and self-report.

Interpreting findings is as important to OTs as test administration. Because cognitive assessment involves more than observation checklists and score assignment, OTs consider and document the possible impact of personal and situational factors on performance, including pain, fatigue, stress, and environmental distracters. In fact, many experts suggest that it is impossible to obtain a true picture of SMs' cognitive functioning until these other factors are resolved.[1]

In general, cognitive assessment in occupational therapy complements but does not duplicate cognitive assessment provided by other disciplines (including speech-language pathology and neuropsychology). For example, OTs make an effort to avoid using tests or components of tests that comprise a neuropsychological battery to minimize the likelihood that patients will pre-learn tests and thereby bias findings of a more comprehensive cognitive evaluation. The methods that OTs use to assess cognition vary by site, clinician expertise, and available resources.

Speech-Language Pathologist Evaluation

Assessing cognitive-communication disorders resulting from combat-acquired c/mTBI can be challenging. The Academy of Neurologic Communication Disorders and Sciences Practice Guidelines Group dedicated a specific committee to address this topic. Experts from this group recommended administering a combination of cognitive and language tests, acknowledging the many psychometric problems with using standardized tests for assessing functional performance outside clinical settings, especially tests that have not been designed or validated for individuals with c/mTBI.[10]

SLPs assess cognitive-communication impairments that result from c/mTBI for a variety of purposes. Speech-language pathology assessment is conducted to identify and describe the following:

- the nature and severity of the cognitive-communication impairments;
- other factors that may be contributing to these impairments;
- whether the history and physical are consistent with the diagnosis of c/mTBI;
- the underlying strengths and weaknesses related to attention and concentration, retention and memory, information processing, executive function and self-regulation, and linguistic factors, including social skills that affect communication performance;
- the effects of cognitive-communication impairments on the individual's activities (capacity and performance in everyday communication contexts) and participation; and
- contextual factors that serve as barriers to or facilitators of successful communication and participation for individuals with cognitive-communication impairment.[11]

These functions help clinicians determine the need for behavioral intervention or referral to other healthcare providers, define a therapeutic plan (including goals), and determine prognosis. Initial assessment measures of cognitive-communication performance may also be used following intervention to provide measures of treatment outcome.

Summary

Specific roles for OTs and SLPs and the methods used to assess cognition vary by site, clinician expertise, availability of members of the rehabilitation team, and available resources. This Toolkit includes assessment options determined to be appropriate in the c/mTBI population and available to generalist clinicians. Some assess-

ments may be more appropriate for occupational therapy interests and goals; other instruments may be more appropriate for communication deficits resulting from cognitive impairments. The ultimate choice for assessment is determined by the clinician's clinical judgment and experience and is based on the needs of the individual SM. Clinicians are advised to select assessments based on what is necessary to determine current status and to plan treatment for a specific SM. More specific information on the assessment tools and their recommended uses are found on the "face sheet" describing each assessment.

BRIEF COGNITIVE ASSESSMENT

Cognistat

Purpose/Description

The Cognistat (Cognistat, Inc, Fairfax, CA; Exhibit 7-1), also known as the Neurobehavioral Cognitive Status Examination, is administered to quantify and characterize possible impairment in a number of cognitive domains when clinical observation or patient self-report suggests concern. It is a microbattery of ten subtests for screening five major areas of cognitive functioning: (1) language, (2) constructions, (3) memory, (4) calculations, and (5) reasoning. It may be used to identify problems, provide treatment, and make referrals. It is **not** intended to replace neuropsychological assessment.

Recommended Instrument Use: Practice Option

This test may be a helpful inclusion in an initial evaluation when:

- the patient has not had or will not have a comprehensive cognitive assessment (eg, neuropsychological assessment or cognitive-communication assessment performed by an SLP) to identify cognitive impairments, and
- the patient has mild to moderate brain injury or complicated mTBI and observation of functional performance suggests the possibility of cognitive dysfunction in a number of domains.

Caution: The Cognistat may not be sensitive enough to detect subtle problems among high-functioning, community-dwelling individuals after TBI.[12] It may not have adequate specificity when

used with adults with psychiatric problems (ie, performance on the Cognistat may suggest cognitive disability when, in fact, there is none).[13]

Administration Protocol/Equipment/Time

The Cognistat is comprised of the test kit (including equipment such as the stimulus book and tokens), the manual (which specifies the step-by-step administration protocol), and the profile form.

For each area of the test other than memory, the patient is first presented with a screening item. Ability is assumed to be normal if the patient passes the screen and no further testing is done in that area. If the patient does not pass the area screen, the clinician administers all the items in the respective subtest. Therefore, it takes approximately 5 minutes to administer the Cognistat to individuals with normal cognition, and about 30 minutes to administer to those with cognitive impairments. The results of each Cognistat subtest are plotted on the profile form.

Detailed administration and scoring procedures are available for purchase from the developer and are not included in this Toolkit. Clinicians should

---

EXHIBIT 7-1

COGNISTAT RESOURCE INFORMATION

Available from:
    Cognistat, Inc
    PO Box 460
    Fairfax, CA 94978
    www.cognistat.com

---

refer to the test booklet and manual for additional information regarding psychometric properties and score interpretation, particularly for the most recent edition of the test.[14]

Groups Tested With This Measure

The Cognistat has been tested on a number of populations, such as those with stroke,[15] TBI[12] (including c/mTBI during initial trauma hospitalization[16]), and older adults (with and without dementia or disability).[17,18]

Interpretability

A clinician plots the patient's scores for each subtest, which may be within the average range or reflecting mild, moderate, or severe dysfunction in the following areas: orientation, attention, comprehension, repetition, naming, constructions, memory, calculations, similarities, and judgment.

The Cognistat manual discusses cautions in interpreting test data. For example, the Cognistat may be insensitive to those with superior premorbid intelligence and to patients with frontal lobe injuries who are able to correctly provide a verbal response to practical judgment questions but who may not be able to execute the described performance in real life. The manual also describes the potential influence of medications, pain, and fatigue or sleep deprivation on test performance.

The test was standardized on 60 normal, nongeriatric volunteers, 59 nonmedically or psychiatrically ill geriatric subjects, and 30 neurosurgical patients with documented lesions.

- Minimal detectable change (MDC): No information on MDC was provided. Because

the test is designed to focus on the degree of disability, it does not discriminate between average and superior performance. This ceiling effect limits the relevance of test-retest reliability.[19]

- Responsiveness estimates: not applicable. The purpose of this test is not to measure change over time.

Reliability and Validity Estimates

- Reliability: There is no published literature that describes interrater or intrarater reliability of the English version of the Cognistat. However, Chan and colleagues describe earlier work in establishing high levels of interrater reliability (with intraclass correlations of 0.85–0.99) in the Chinese version of the Cognistat.[20]
- Concurrent validity: In a retrospective study involving adults with TBI admitted to a tertiary care rehabilitation, the results of the Cognistat were compared to that of other neuropsychological tests.[21] Forty-seven percent of the 45 participants had c/mTBI. There were statistically significant correlations with the neuropsychological test for the following subtests: Cognistat attention with Trail Making Test ($r = -.33$, $P < .05$); Cognistat comprehension with the Token Test ($r = .30$, $P < .05$); Cognistat memory with the California Verbal Learning Test ($r = .68$, $P < .001$) and the Logical Memory II from the Weschler Memory Scale—Revised ($r = .43$, $P < .005$); Cognistat Construction with the Wechsler Adult Intelligence Scale—Revised Block Design ($r = .54$, $P < .005$).

Selected Reference

Kiernan RJ, Mueller J, Langston JW, Van Dyke C. The Neurobehavioral Cognitive Status Examination: a brief but differentiated approach to cognitive assessment. *Ann Intern Med.*1987;107:481–485.

Repeatable Battery for the Assessment of Neuropsychological Status

Purpose/Description

The Repeatable Battery for the Assessment of Neuropsychological Status (RBANS; Psychological Assessment Resources Inc, Lutz, FL; Exhibit 7-2) is a screening measure of cognitive functioning.

Twelve subtests comprise the five domain-specific index scores in addition to a combined total-scale index score.[22] The domain-specific areas include:

- immediate memory (word list and story recall),
- visuospatial/constructional (complex figure copying and line orientation judgment),
- language (confrontation naming and gen-

erative naming),

- attention (digit span and coding), and
- delayed memory (delayed free recall of a word list, story, and complex figure, in addition to recognition trial of the word list).

Recommended Instrument Use: Practice Option

The RBANS is a useful cognitive screening tool to measure general performance level.[23] Because the RBANS is a screening measure, it should be given in conjunction with other cognitive tests. The RBANS can be used for repeated screenings.[22,24] It was designed as a brief measure to characterize mild deficits and has been demonstrated to be sensitive to concussion.[25,26]

Administration Protocol/Equipment/Time

The RBANS[22] includes manuals, record forms, two equivalent alternate test forms (for repeated testing or tracking neurological status over time), and scoring templates. This test is usually administered in less than 30 minutes.[22,24,27]

Groups Tested With This Measure

The test manual contains additional clinical data for 404 individuals diagnosed with Alzheimer's disease, vascular dementia, human immunodeficiency virus dementia, Huntington's disease, Parkinson's disease, depression, schizophrenia, and mild to severe TBI.[22,24]

Interpretability

- Norms: The RBANS has been standardized on 540 individuals between the ages of 20 to 89 years.[22,24] Norms are available in the test manual.
- Scoring: RBANS scores are interval data with a normative mean of 100 and a standard deviation of 15.[22,24]
- MDC: not available
- Responsiveness estimates: not available

Reliability Estimates

- Internal consistency: Cronbach's alphas were calculated for the RBANS and showed strong internal consistency (0.84) for the total scale score for patients with

---

EXHIBIT 7-2

REPEATABLE BATTERY FOR THE ASSESSMENT OF NEUROPSYCHOLOGICAL STATUS RESOURCE INFORMATION

Available from:
 Psychological Assessment Resources Inc.
 16204 North Florida Avenue
 Lutz, FL 33549
 www4.parinc.com
 Phone: 800-331-8378
 Fax: 800-727-9329

---

moderate to severe TBI.[28] Strong internal reliability was also shown for the immediate memory, delayed memory, and visuospatial/constructional index scores, while weak reliability was shown for the language and attention index scores.[28]

- Interrater: not available
- Intrarater: not available
- Test-Retest: Forms A and B of the RBANS allow for retesting patients without content-related practice effects.[24] Specific information was available for comparisons between patients with schizophrenia and a normal control group. Test-retest intervals using forms A and B ranged from 1 to 134 days, and there was no effect of time on the retest performance.[29]

Validity Estimates

- Content/Face: not available
- Criterion: not available
- Construct: The RBANS has been validated as a useful and sensitive instrument for a variety of populations, including those with TBI, dementia, stroke, schizophrenia, substance abuse, and multiple sclerosis.[24,27]

In another study that included patients with mild to severe TBI and a control group, significantly lower scores were found for the total scale, attention, and delayed memory indexes for patients with TBI, followed by the immediate memory, language, and visuospatial/construction index scores.[30]

Selected References

McKay C, Casey JE, Wertheimer JC, Fichtenberg NL. Reliability and validity of the RBANS in a traumatic brain injured sample. *Arch Clin Neuropsychol.* 2007;22:91–98.

Randolph C. *Repeatable Battery for the Assessment of Neuropsychological Status: Manual.* San Antonio, TX: Psychological Corporation; 1998.

Randolph C. *Repeatable Battery for the Assessment of Neuropsychological Status (RBANS) Supplement 1.* Upper Saddle River, NJ: Pearson Education, Inc; 2008.

Cognitive Linguistic Quick Test

Purpose/Description

The Cognitive-Linguistic Quick Test (CLQT; Pearson/PsychCorp, San Antonio, TX; Exhibit 7-3) was designed to enable a quick assessment of strengths and weaknesses in five cognitive domains in adults with known or suspected neurological dysfunction: (1) attention, (2) memory, (3) language, (4) executive functions, and (5) visuospatial skills. The test is composed of ten tasks, with five tasks created specifically with minimal language demands to assist in evaluating the cognitive functions of those with language disorders. The ten tasks of the CLQT are:

1. personal facts,
2. symbol cancellation,
3. confrontation naming,
4. clock design,
5. story retelling,
6. symbol trails,
7. generative naming,
8. design memory,
9. mazes, and
10. design generation.

The CLQT is useful for screening a full range of cognitive processes in patients who may have decreased language skills.

Recommended Instrument Use: Practice Option

The CLQT may be used to target areas for direct treatment or everyday management of impaired skills, to identify the need for more in-depth testing, or to help determine a differential diagnosis. The test was developed as a broad cognitive screening instrument to provide the examiner direction for further observation or administration of more in-depth formal and informal measures in the specific areas where the examinee has difficulty. The CLQT was not developed as a comprehensive tool for

---

EXHIBIT 7-3

COGNITIVE LINGUISTIC QUICK TEST RESOURCE INFORMATION

Helm-Estabrooks N. *Cognitive Linguistic Quick Test (CLQT).* San Antonio, TX: The Psychological Corporation; 2001.

Available from:
Pearson/PsychCorp
Pearson, Attn: Inbound Sales & Customer Support
19500 Bulverde Road
San Antonio, TX 78259-3701
Phone: 800-627-7271
Fax: 800-232-1223
Clinical Customer Support@Pearson.com

---

determining differential diagnosis. The CLQT may be given by professionals experienced in administering cognitive assessment instruments to adults with acquired neurological dysfunction.

Administration Protocol/Equipment/Time

- Administration time: 15 to 30 minutes
- Scoring time: 10 to 15 minutes (cut scores, no normative data)
- Can be administered at a table or bedside (as long as the patient can sit up and use a pen)
- Test components: examiner's manual, stimulus manual, record form, response booklet, and scoring transparencies
- Additional materials: pen and stopwatch or a watch that can measure seconds
- Available in both English and Spanish

Groups Tested With This Measure

The CLQT has been administered to individuals who sustained right, left, and bilateral hemisphere strokes, TBI, and Alzheimer's disease.[31] In a study comparing the cognitive-communication results from the Cognistat and the CLQT in participants with mTBI, the CLQT identified more individuals with high-level cognitive-communication deficits than the Cognistat in the acute setting.[32]

Interpretability

The CLQT is a criterion-referenced test with severity ratings for two age categories (ages 18–69 and 70–89). Severity ratings of mild, moderate, severe, and within normal limits are established for each of five cognitive domains: (1) attention, (2) memory, (3) executive functions, (4) language, and (5) visuospatial skills. A total composite severity rating and a clock-drawing severity rating are also derived. Criterion cut scores are available for each task for both age categories.[31]

The author's clinical expertise, informed by the data from the CLQT Nonclinical Research Sample and the CLQT Clinical Research Sample, guided the development of age categories, task criterion cut scores, and cognitive domain severity ratings.[31]

- Norms: none
- MDC: not available
- Responsiveness estimates: not available

Reliability and Validity Estimates

- Reliability: Test-retest stability coefficients ranged between 0.03 and 0.81 for the tasks. The test-retest stability coefficients ranged between 0.61 and 0.90 for the cognitive domains.
  Measures were based on a nonclinical sample, where there was little difference in performance between test and retest as the examinees received a perfect score on most tasks, resulting in attenuation.[31]
- Validity: The manual provides descriptive evidence to support test validity or "the appropriateness of proposed interpretations and uses of the test," including test content, internal structure, and relations to other variables.[31]

In a study of persons with Parkinson's disease, the CLQT correlated well with the Mini-Mental State Examination.[33] The CLQT was judged to be superior to the Mini-Mental State Examination because it also provides domain-specific information.

Selected References

Helm-Estabrooks N. *Cognitive Linguistic Quick Test (CLQT)*. San Antonio, TX: The Psychological Corporation; 2001.

Parashos SA, Johnson ML, Erickson-Davis C, Wielinski CL. Assessing cognition in Parkinson disease: use of the Cognitive Linguistic Quick Test. *J Geriatr Psychiatry Neurol*.2009; 22(4):228–234.

BROAD ASSESSMENT OF COGNITIVE-LINGUISTIC ABILITIES

Woodcock-Johnson III Tests of Cognitive Abilities

Purpose/Description

The Woodcock-Johnson III Tests of Cognitive Abilities (WJ III COG; The Riverside Publishing Company, Rolling Meadows, IL; Exhibit 7-4) is an assessment instrument that provides a comprehensive set of individually administered, norm-referenced tests for measuring intellectual abilities.[34] The test results provide standard scores and percentiles for general intellectual ability, broad cognitive subdomains referred to as "clusters," and specific cognitive subtests. Certain clusters represent broad categories of cognitive abilities related to cognitive performance. The clusters include verbal ability (standard and extended scales), thinking ability (standard and extended scales), and cognitive efficiency (standard and extended scales). The WJ III COG provides a strong normative reference against which to compare the c/mTBI population.[35] The standard battery contains the following subtests:

1. Verbal Comprehension: picture vocabulary, synonyms, antonyms, and verbal analogies.
2. Visual-Auditory Learning: long-term storage and retrieval of visual and auditory association.
3. Special Relations: identifying pieces that complete a target shape.
4. Sound Blending: auditory processing of blending sounds into a word.

EXHIBIT 7-4

WOODCOCK-JOHNSON III TESTS OF
COGNITIVE ABILITIES RESOURCE
INFORMATION

Available from:
The Riverside Publishing Company
3800 Golf Road, Suite 200
Rolling Meadows, IL 60008
www.riversidepublishing.com
Phone: 800-323-9540
Fax: 630-467-7192

5. Concept Formation: categorical reasoning based on inductive logic.
6. Visual Matching: perceptual speed.
7. Numbers Reversed: short-term memory span.
8. Incomplete Words: auditory analysis and closure.
9. Auditory Working Memory: working memory for digits and words.
10. Visual-Auditory Learning-Delayed: recall of information for subset (visual-auditory learning) after a delay.

Recommended Instrument Use: Practice Option

The WJ III COG has not been normed on patients with brain injury; however, it has been used extensively to evaluate cognitive-communication abilities across an age span.[35] Clinicians using the WJ III COG need to follow the guidelines specified in the examiner's manual for training prior to administering and scoring the tests. Competent interpretation of the WJ III COG requires a higher degree of knowledge and experience than is required for test administration and scoring.[34(p7)] Graduate-level training in the areas of cognitive assessment and diagnostic decision-making is suggested.

Administration Protocol/Equipment/Time

The WJ III COG[34] contains two easel test books, an examiner's manual, a technical manual, a computer scoring program, test records, subject response booklets, a CD recording, scoring guides, and an optional carrying case. The standard battery contains subtests 1 through 10 and takes approximately 45 to 50 minutes to administer by an experienced examiner. The extended battery contains subtests 11 through 20 and takes approximately 1.5 to 1.75 hours to complete.

Groups Tested With This Measure

The WJ III COG can be used for educational, clinical, or research purposes in individuals from preschool to geriatric age.[34] The test can identify the client's strengths and weaknesses to determine the nature and extent of impairment and to aid in classification and diagnosis. The WJ III COG was used in the validation of the Automated Neurological Assessment Metric, a library of computer-based assessments of cognitive domains developed and implemented by the Department of Defense as a pre- and postcombat measure of neurocognitive performance.[36] In its earlier version (Woodcock-Johnson Psycho-Educational Battery-Revised) the test was shown to differentiate between patients with and without confirmed brain damage, and between closed head injury cases and psychiatric diagnoses.[37] In a study of 117 SMs who sustained blast-related mTBI, Parrish and colleagues[35] found that the WJ III COG consistently highlighted deficits in cognitive efficiency, while patients scored higher on verbal performance measures.

Interpretability

- Norms: Normative data has been obtained on over 8,800 subjects from 2 to 90 years of age with demographic characteristics that closely match the general population of the United States.[34] Normative data can be found in the WJ III COG test manual.
- Parrish, Roth, Roberts, and Davie[35] reported that the majority of SMs with c/mTBI scored within normal limits on the subtests, but measures of cognitive efficiency were consistently below the mean when compared to the normative sample. The standard score across subtests for SMs was 92; that was below the normative mean of 100. More than 25% of patients scored below one standard deviation on 8 of 11 subtests and clusters.
- Scoring: Specific instructions for scoring subtests are provided in the manual.[34] Raw scores and birthdate can be entered in the Compuscore and profiles program to calculate derived scores and discrepancies. The program also provides a summary narrative report, age and grade profiles, and standard score and percentile rank profiles.

- MDC: not available
- Responsiveness estimates: not available

Reliability Estimates

- Internal consistency: not available
- Interrater: Of the median cluster reliabilities, most are 0.90 or higher. Of the median test reliabilities, most are 0.80 or higher and several are 0.90 or higher.[34] The full-scale score reliability (general intellectual ability) is .97.
- Intrarater: not available
- Test-Retest: Across the 29 reliabilities for the subtests of the WJ III COG and tests of achievements for all ages, the median retest reliability was 0.94. Test-retest correlations by age and length of retest intervals ranged from 0.60 to 0.96 on the subtests.[34]

Validity Estimates

- Content/Face: not available

- Criterion: The WJ III COG items were developed based on a complex array of statistical measures, including Rasch single-parameter logistic test model, multiple regression, and factor analyses for item calibration, scaling, cluster composition, and validation. Coverage of content, including tables, can be found in the technical manual.[34]
- Construct: Woodcock, McGrew, and Mather[34] state that all of the WJ III COG tests conform to the areas of narrow ability, broad ability, and general intellectual ability derived from the Cattell-Horn-Carroll theory of cognitive abilities. Confirmatory factor analyses patterns indicated that all tests for the W III COG have minimal influence of construct-irrelevant variance. The cognitive cluster intercorrelations are low to moderate (0.20–0.60), suggesting that the broad cognitive abilities are related to, yet distinct from, one another.[34]

Selected References

Jones WP, Loe SA, Krach SK, Rager RY, Jones HM. Automated Neuropsychological Assessment Metrics (ANAM) and Woodcock-Johnson III Tests of Cognitive Ability: a concurrent validity study. *Clin Neuropsychol.* 2008;22(2):305–320.

Parrish C, Roth C, Roberts B, Davie G. Assessment of cognitive-communication disorders of mild traumatic brain injury sustained in combat. *Perspect Neurophysiol Neurogenic Speech Lang Disord.* 2009;19:47–57.

Woodcock RW, McGrew KS, Mather N. *Woodcock-Johnson III Tests of Cognitive Abilities Examiner and Technical Manuals.* Itasca, Il: Riverside Publishing; 2001.

DOMAIN-SPECIFIC ASSESSMENTS

Attention

Test of Everyday Attention

Purpose/Description. The Test of Everyday Attention (TEA; Thames Valley Test Company, Suffolk, England; Exhibit 7-5) is administered during initial evaluation to quantify and specify difficulties with attention if they have been reported by the patient or family member or observed by the clinician. The TEA is premised on the theoretical assumption that attention is comprised of at least three separate systems: selective attention, sustained attention, and attentional switching. The test is based on the imaginary scenario of a vacation to Philadelphia and involves the following eight ecologically plausible subtests.

1. **Map Search** (selective attention). Patients try to locate as many symbols as possible (eg, knife-and-fork sign representing an eating facility) on a colored map of Philadelphia in 2 minutes.
2. **Elevator Counting** (sustained attention). Patients pretend they are in an elevator and the visual floor indicator is not working. They figure out what floor they are on by counting a series of tape-presented tones.
3. **Elevator Counting With Distraction** (selective attention). Patients follow the same procedure as number 2, except they count low tones while ignoring high tones.
4. **Visual Elevator** (attentional switching). Patients perform a reversal (attentional

shifting/cognitive flexibility) task as they count up and down to follow a series of visually presented "floors" in the elevator.

5. **Auditory Elevator With Reversal** (attentional switching). As with subtest 4, patients perform a reversal task involving counting "floors," but the stimuli are presented via audiotape.

6. **Telephone Search** (selective attention). Patients look for key symbols indicating plumbers (or restaurants or hotels in versions B and C) in a simulated telephone directory.

7. **Telephone Search Dual Task** (divided attention). Participants search the telephone directory while counting strings of auditory tones. The difference between scores for subtests 6 and 7 represents a "dual task decrement."

8. **Lottery** (sustained attention). Patients listen for their winning number (such as BC155) in this 1-minute test, writing down the two letters preceding all numbers ending in "55."

Recommended Instrument Use: Practice Option. This test may be a helpful inclusion in an initial occupational therapy evaluation when:

- the patient has not had and will not have a comprehensive cognitive assessment (eg, neuropsychological assessment or cognitive communication assessment performed by an SLP) to identify cognitive impairments **or** if the results of aforementioned testing do not specify attentional performance, and

- the patient has c/mTBI and self-report or observation of functional performance suggests possible attention deficits.

Note: Because of the level of challenge associated with some of the subtests, the TEA may not be appropriate for individuals who are sensitive to auditory stimuli (as in some cases of PTSD) or those with hearing or vision limitations.[38]

Administration Protocol/Equipment/Time. The TEA is comprised of the test kit (including stimulus cards and maps, cue book, three audiotapes, and one videotape), the administration and scoring manual (which specifies the step-by-step administration protocol), and procedural guide scoring sheets. It takes 45 to 60 minutes to administer. Detailed administration and scoring procedures are available for purchase from the developer and are not included in this Toolkit.

Groups Tested With This Measure

The TEA has been tested on or used with a variety of diagnostic groups who are at risk for having attentional deficits, including mild,[39] moderate, and severe TBI; mild Alzheimer's disease; and stroke.[38] It is sensitive to age effects in the normal population.[39]

Interpretability

- Norms: TEA scores of 154 healthy volunteers (ages 18–80 years) were used to establish normative values. Scores were stratified by four age bands and two levels of educational attainment.[38]
- Scoring: Rather than a single summary score, the TEA results are plotted as scaled-scores for each subtest on the scoring sheet's summary plot. Cut-off scores (signifying abnormal performance) and detailed scoring and interpretation procedures are described in the administration manual.
- MDC: Although three versions of the test are provided, there are practical and time limitations to readministering the test solely to quantify progress or impact of treatment. Test developers recommend against readministering only portions of the test.
- Minimal clinically important differences: not available
- Responsiveness estimates: not available

Reliability Estimates

- Internal consistency: not available
- Interrater: not available
- Intrarater: not available
- Test-Retest: One week after taking version A of the TEA, 118 normal volunteers performed version B; a subsample who were given version B were tested with version C after 1 week. Correlation coefficients (Pearson product-moment) ranged from .59 to .87, not including the elevator counting and lottery tasks, for which there was a ceiling effect.[38] Decreased reliability was noted with the dual-task decrement due to learning effects.

Validity Estimates

- Content/Face: Test developers suggest that the imaginary scenario associated with the TEA (that of visiting Philadelphia as a tourist) adds to the face validity of the subtests.
- Construct: TEA subtest scores are moderately to strongly correlated with existing tests of attention (Pearson product-moment correlations ranging from 0.49–0.63).[38]
- Discriminative: Robertson and colleagues reported statistically significant differences in most subtest scores for healthy controls and stroke survivors.[38] Chan[40] reported similar findings for TBI.
- Criterion: not available

Selected References

Chan RC, Lai MK. Latent structure of the Test of Everyday Attention: convergent evidence from patients with traumatic brain injury. *Brain Inj.* Jun 2006;20(6):653–659.

Robertson IH, Ward T, Ridgeway V, Nimmo-Smith I. The structure of normal human attention: The Test of Everyday Attention. *J Int Neuropsychol Soc.* 1996;2(6):525–534.

Information Processing Speed

Speed and Capacity of Language Processing

Purpose/Description. The Speed and Capacity of Language Processing (SCOLP; Pearson/PsychCorp Support San Antonio, TX; Exhibit 7-6) provides a measure of slowing in the rate of information processing, particularly with regard to language comprehension.[41] It consists of two tasks: the speed of comprehension test (silly sentences, or SST), which measures rate of information processing, and the spot-the-word (STW) test, which estimates premorbid verbal ability. The clinician can determine whether poor performance on the SST represents a decrement secondary to brain injury or to an individual's premorbid low-verbal functioning.

Recommended Instrument Use: Practice Option. The SCOLP may be informative during an initial speech-language pathology assessment of an individual's cognitive abilities, especially when the examiner is interested in capturing a measure of verbal processing speed. In addition, this instrument may be used as a broad estimate of premorbid ability. The test may be given when a patient has not had and will not have a comprehensive neuropsychological assessment.

Consider using the SCOLP when the patient has

c/mTBI and self-report or observation of functional performance suggests possible deficits of information processing speed. This test may be used as an outcome measure following a period of focused intervention for information processing speed. The SCOLP offers multiple parallel versions for repeat testing.

Administration Protocol/Equipment/Time. The approximate time required for each task (SST and STW) is about 5 minutes. The SST requires individuals to verify simple sentences, half of which are true

---

EXHIBIT 7-6

SPEED AND CAPACITY OF LANGUAGE PROCESSING RESOURCE INFORMATION

Developed by Alan Baddeley, Hazel Emslie, Ian Nimmo-Smith, the SCOLP is available from:
Pearson/PsychCorp Support
19500 Bulverde Road
San Antonio, TX 78259-3701
ClinicalCustomerSupport@Pearson.com
Phone: 800-627-7271
Fax: 800-232-1223

(eg, "Rats have teeth."), and half of which are false (eg, "Nuns are sold in pairs."). The individual has 2 minutes to evaluate as many of the 100 sentences as possible. Four parallel forms of the test (versions A, B, C, and D) are available for repeat testing. Each set of 100 sentences has an instruction page with a brief explanation of the test, together with six practice items.

For the STW, the patient is instructed to place a checkmark beside the real word in each pair. Guessing is encouraged when the person is uncertain about a word pair. The test is untimed. For each subtest, raw scores are converted into an age-based scaled score or percentile score by means of tables provided in the test manual.

Groups Tested With This Measure. The SCOLP has been tested on a number of populations, including older Americans who are living in the community[42,43]; individuals with mTBI[44,45] or schizophrenia[46]; juvenile offenders[47]; persons using a range of drugs, including alcohol and benzodiazapines; those who have experienced intense stressors, such as individuals with high-pressure nervous syndrome[41]; and as an indicator for dysexecutive syndrome.[48]

Interpretability.
- Norms: Normative data was collected on a stratified sample of 224 subjects, with approximately equal numbers sampled from six socioeconomic classes, and from four age bands (16–31, 32–47, 48–64, and 65–80). The age group above 65 was considered insufficient to provide robust norms. Norms are available for three age groups: 16 to 31, 32 to 47, and 48 to 64 in the test manual[41] to assess the speed-capacity discrepancy (the extent to which comprehension speed deviates from that predicted by vocabulary). This provides an indication of the probable degree of cognitive impairment.
- MDC: not available
- Responsiveness estimates: The SST is sensitive to information-processing deficits associated with mTBI in the early postinjury phases. Ponsford et al[49] investigated the outcome of adults with c/mTBI at 1 week and 3 months postinjury to identify factors associated with persisting problems. By 3 months postinjury, the symptoms present at 1 week postinjury were resolved and no impairments were evident on neuropsychological measures, including the SCOLP.

Reliability Estimates.
- Internal consistency:
  - SST: Based on a sample of 25 people tested with the SST on two occasions, performing two different versions on day one and day two, and timed over the first 25 and second 25 sentences on each occasion, correlation between performance on these two halves was 0.84 for the first session and 0.87 for the second, suggesting good split-half reliability for these abbreviated versions.[41]
  - STW: Internal reliability was 0.78 for version A and 0.83 for version B.[41]
- Interrater: not available
- Intrarater: not available
- Test-Retest reliability, alternate-form reliability, and practice effects:
  - SST: Parallel form reliability (versions A and B) was 0.93. Test-retest reliability of the performance of rugby players was 0.78.[44] The performance of normal and head-injured people across 20 successive test sessions, tested on 10 different forms with each used twice, showed an improvement in both groups over the 20 occasions.[50]
  - STW: Parallel form reliability (versions A and B) was 0.78.[41,51] Test-retest reliability of rugby players after a 1- to 2-week interval was 0.64. There was no effect of practice on the number of words correctly identified.[44]

Validity Estimates.
- Content/Face: not available
- Criterion: not available
- Construct validity:
  - SST: The SST correlates highly with measures of general language processing capacity (category generation: 0.52; color naming: 0.56; semantic categorization: 0.55; grammatical reasoning: 0.60; vocabulary: 0.51; and the STW: 0.57[41]). Correlations with nonsemantic speeded tasks (eg, digit symbol: 0.44; symbol digit: 0.44; letter-matching: 0.34–0.39) and fluid reasoning (Raven's Matrices: 0.20) were lower.[41,44] Clinically, the SST has been shown to be sensitive to information-processing deficits associated with c/mTBI in the early postinjury phase.[44,45,52] Deficits tended to resolve 3 months postinjury.[45]

○ STW: The STW has shown adequate convergent validity with other measures of crystallized intelligence and premorbid function. Moderately high correlations have been reported between the STW and the Mill Hill Vocabulary Scale (0.60–0.71)[41,51] Wechsler Verbal Intelligence Quotient (r = 0.61) and Full Scale Intelligence Quotient (r = 0.58).[53]

Selected References

Baddeley AD, Emslie H, Nimmo-Smith I. *The Speed and Capacity of Language Processing (SCOLP) Test*. Bury St. Edmunds, ENG: Thames Valley Test Company; 1992.

Hinton-Bayre AD, Geffen G, McFarland K. Mild head injury and speed of information processing: a prospective study of professional rugby league players. *J Clin Exp Neuropsychol.* Apr 1997;19(2):275–289.

Papagno C, Baddeley AD. Confabulation in a dysexecutive patient: implication for models of retrieval. *Cortex.* Dec 1997;33(4):743–752.

Ponsford J, Willmott C, Rothwell A, et al. Impact of early intervention on outcome following head injury in adults. *J Neurol Neurosurg Psychiatry.* 2002;73(3):330–332.

Executive Functions

Behavior Rating Inventory of Executive Function-Adult

Purpose/Description. The Behavior Rating Inventory of Executive Function-Adult (BRIEF-A; Psychological Assessment Resources Inc, Lutz, FL; Exhibit 7-7) is a standardized measure of an adult's executive functions or self-regulation skills in his or her everyday environment.[54] The BRIEF-A includes a self-report that is completed by the patient and an informant report from a person familiar with the patient. The informant report can be used alone if the patient has limited awareness of his or her deficits. There are a total of 75 items that are scored using a 3-point rating scale. Five of the items are validation items, resulting in a total of 70 items separated into the behavior rating index (BRI; 30 items) and the metacognitive index (MI; 40 items). The BRI and MI are further divided into non-overlapping clinical scales that measure various aspects of executive function. These areas include:

1. Inhibit
2. Self-Monitor
3. Plan/Organize
4. Shift
5. Initiate
6. Task Monitor
7. Emotional Control
8. Working Memory
9. Organization of Materials

Recommended Instrument Use: Practice Option. The BRIEF-A was designed for a broad range of individuals with developmental, neurological, psychiatric, and medical conditions. It may be administered in research and clinical settings by neuropsychologists, psychologists, and rehabilitation professionals, and is available in over 20 different languages (see product detail at www4.parinc.com). Executive functions are not often evident in a structured, quiet, one-on-one testing environment. This instrument provides an option for measuring the presence of executive deficits as observed by family members in everyday functioning. It can be used alone when the rated individual is unable to complete the self-report form or has limited awareness of his or her own difficulties, or in addition to the self-report form to gain multiple perspectives on the individual's functioning. Data from

---

EXHIBIT 7-7

BEHAVIOR RATING INVENTORY OF EXECUTIVE FUNCTION-ADULT VERSION RESOURCE INFORMATION

This tool, developed by Roth, Isquith, and Gioia, is available from:
   Psychological Assessment Resources
     Incorporated
   16204 North Florida Avenue
   Lutz, FL 33549
   www4.parinc.com
   Phone: 800-331-8378
   Fax: 800-727-9329

the BRIEF-A can help the clinician identify areas requiring further assessment as well as suggest specific problems for targeting treatment goals and strategies.

Administration Protocol/Equipment/Time. The BRIEF-A[54] contains a professional manual, self-report forms, self-report scoring summary/profile form, and informant report scoring summary/profile form. It takes approximately 10 to 15 minutes to administer and 15 to 20 minutes to score.

Groups Tested With This Measure. The BRIEF-A was standardized on men and women 18 to 90 years of age and validated on mixed clinical, healthy samples of 223 subjects with a variety of developmental, systemic, neurological, and psychiatric disorders, such as attention disorders, learning disabilities, autism spectrum disorders, TBI, multiple sclerosis, depression, mild cognitive impairment, dementia, and schizophrenia.[54] Brown et al[55] demonstrated a positive effect of atomoxetine treatment on the BRIEF-Adult Version Self-Report (BRIEF-A) compared to a placebo in young adults with attention deficit hyperactivity disorder. In a study of 98 11- to 16-year-old adolescents with TBI compared to 97 neuropsychologically healthy controls, the BRIEF-A demonstrated significantly greater parent-adolescent discrepancies on ratings of executive dysfunction in the TBI group than in the control group.

Interpretability.
- Norms: Normative data for the BRIEF-A was obtained on 1,050 men and women between 18 to 90 years of age from a wide range of racial, ethnic, and educational backgrounds and geographic regions.[54]
- Scoring: Roth, Isquith, and Gioia[54] report that computer software is available for scoring test items. Scale scores are converted into T-scores, which can be graphed, and also into percentiles. T-scores have a mean of 50 and standard-deviation of 10 for all nine scale scores, the BRI index score, the MI index score, and the global executive

composite (GEC) score. There are also three validity scales (negativity, inconsistency, and infrequency) used in the BRIEF-A.
- MDC: not available
- Responsiveness estimates: not available

Reliability Estimates.
- Internal consistency: Internal consistency was moderate to high for the self-report normative sample (alpha coefficients ranged from 0.73–0.90 for clinical scales and 0.93–0.96 for indices and GEC score) and high for the informant report normative sample (0.80–0.93 for clinical scales and 0.95–0.98 for indices and GEC score). For the mixed clinical/healthy adult sample, the self-report alpha coefficients ranged from 0.80–0.94 for clinical scales and 0.96–0.98 for indices and GEC.[54]
- Interrater agreement: The manual states that the self-report-to-informant-report correlations ranged from 0.44–0.68 for the scales, 0.63 for the BRI, 0.61 for the MI, and 0.63 for the GEC.[54] General disagreement between patients and informants should be taken into consideration.
- Intrarater agreement: not available
- Test-retest: Test-retest correlations ranged from 0.82 to 0.94 over an average interval of 4.2 weeks for the self-report form (n = 50), and ranged from 0.91 to 0.96 over an average interval of 4.2 weeks for the informant report form (n = 44).[54]

Validity Estimates.
- Content/Face: not available
- Criterion: not available
- Construct: Roth, Isquith, and Gioia[54] state that validity was demonstrated via profiles of the BRIEF-A scores in clinical populations, such as individuals with attention deficit hyperactivity disorder, multiple sclerosis, and TBI.

Selected References

Roth R, Isquith P, Gioia G. *Behavior Rating Inventory of Executive Function-Adult Version (BRIEF-A)*. Lutz, FL: Psychological Assessment Resources, Inc; 2005.

Behavioural Assessment of Dysexecutive Syndrome

Purpose/Description. The Behavioural Assessment of Dysexecutive Syndrome (BADS; Thames

Valley Test Company, Suffolk, England; Exhibit 7-8)[56] was designed to assess the effects of dysexecutive syndrome, impairments associated with damage to the frontal lobes of the brain.[57] These

EXHIBIT 7-8

BEHAVIOURAL ASSESSMENT OF DYSEXECUTIVE SYNDROME RESOURCE INFORMATION

Developed by Thames Valley Test Company, Suffolk, England, the Behavioural Assessment of Dysexecutive Syndrome is available from:

Northern Speech Services & National Rehabilitation Services
117 North Elm Street
PO Box 1247
Gaylord, MI 49734
www.nss-nrs.com
Phone: 888-337-3866
Fax: 989-732-6164

impairments lead to difficulties with planning, organizing, initiating, and self-monitoring. The battery is comprised of six tests that replicate real-life, complex tasks, and the dysexecutive questionnaire (a 20-item self-report of how dysexecutive syndrome impacts daily functioning). The six tests include:

1. Temporal Judgment: involves the patient's ability to estimate how long various events last.
2. Rule Shift Cards: tests the patient's ability to change an established pattern of responding.
3. Action Program: tests practical problem solving in which a cork has to be extracted from a tall tube.
4. Key Search: tests strategy formation in which patients demonstrate how they would search for lost keys.
5. Zoo Map: tests the patient's ability to develop a plan to visit 6 of 12 possible locations in a zoo.
6. Modified Six Elements: tests planning, task scheduling, and performance monitoring.

Recommended Instrument Use: Practice Option. The BADS is to be administered by OTs, SLPs, or psychologists (see product detail at www.nss-nrs.com).

- This test may be a helpful inclusion in an initial occupational therapy evaluation when dysexecutive syndrome is the primary barrier to functioning.

- Administration of the BADS may also provide valuable information at various decision-making junctures (eg, discharge to independent living, return to work, etc).

Because of its length and time involved in administration, the BADS is **not** recommended for repeat administration as an outcome measure of treatment.

Administration Protocol/Equipment/Time. The BADS is comprised of the test kit (including all materials and supplies), the administration and scoring manual (which specifies the step-by-step administration protocol), and procedural guide scoring sheets. It takes 45 to 60 minutes to administer. Detailed administration and scoring procedures are available for purchase from the developer and are not included in this Toolkit.

Groups Tested With This Measure. The BADS has been tested on individuals with brain injury, healthy controls, and those with schizophrenia,[56] including those with c/mTBI.[58]

Interpretability.
- Norms: The BADS was normed on 216 non-brain-injured individuals with a range of abilities and ages (16–87 years of age). Age-stratified norms are provided (up to 40 years, 41–65, and 65–87).
- Scoring: The patient is assigned a profile score for each test (0–4), and these are summed to calculate an overall profile score. Profile scores can be converted to a standard score, from impaired, low average, average, and high average to superior.
- MDC: Not calculated. As mentioned earlier, because of its length and time involved in administration, it is **not** recommended for repeat administration as an outcome measure of treatment.

Reliability Estimates.
- Interrater: Twenty-five healthy controls were tested with a second tester present. Interrater reliability was high, ranging from 0.88 to 10.00.[56]
- Test-Retest: Twenty-nine healthy controls repeated the BADS 6 to 12 months after they took it the first time.[56] None of the differences in means between first and second testing were statistically significant.

Correlation coefficients ranged from −0.08 (rule shift cards) to 0.71 (key search).

Validity Estimate. Construct: The BADS discriminated between groups with and without brain injury.[56]

Selected Reference

Wilson BA, Evans JJ, Alderman N, Burgess P. The development of an ecologically valid test for assessing patients with a dysexecutive syndrome. *Neuropsychol Rehabil.* 1998;8:213–228.

Functional Assessment of Verbal Reasoning and Executive Strategies

Purpose/Description. The Functional Assessment of Verbal Reasoning and Executive Strategies (FAVRES; CCD Publishing, Guelph, ON, Canada; Exhibit 7-9) is designed to assess subtle cognitive-communication difficulties in adults with acquired brain injuries. This functional measure targets aspects of complex communication, verbal reasoning, and executive functioning. It was designed to detect deficits that may not be apparent on typical standardized tasks.

The FAVRES tasks challenge the examinee's language and executive functions through timed reading (under pressure), comprehending complex material, reasoning, and problem solving. The level of comprehension assessed includes discriminating relevant versus irrelevant information, detecting the speaker's purpose, discriminating between statements of fact and opinion, distinguishing between emotional and logical arguments, and evaluating the speaker's bias, prejudice, and attitude.

The FAVRES consists of four verbal reasoning tasks. Each task provides a meaningful context one might encounter at work or in family or social situations. Each task presents a situation novel to the examinee. All the information needed is provided within the task. The four tasks address planning an event, scheduling, making a decision, and building a case.

Recommended Instrument Use: Practice Option. This instrument was designed for adults with acquired brain injury with suspected impairment of cognitive-communication functions, practical reasoning, or executive functions. It was designed to be administered by SLPs to provide further analysis of complex communication. According to the developer, Sheila MacDonald, "Education at the master's and Ph.D. level is recommended as well as registration or certification in a regulated profession."[59(p23)] Examinees that were tested originally were 18 years of age and over. A preliminary study suggested that the FAVRES tasks may be useful in predicting readiness for return to work.[60]

Administration Protocol/Equipment/Time. Administration takes about 50 to 60 minutes for all 4 tasks. Tasks can be administered separately over several sessions if required. A 5-point scoring system captures the degree of accuracy. There are four types of scoring: (1) time score, (2) accuracy score, (3) rationale score, and (4) strengths and weaknesses checklist. After the examinee completes the reasoning task, a post hoc analysis of reasoning subskills is conducted. Equipment needed for the test includes a stopwatch, two pens, the examiner's scoring booklet, response booklet, stimulus pages for task 1, and stimulus page for task 3.

Groups Tested With This Measure. Groups tested with this measure include adults ages 18 to 79 with mild to moderate acquired brain injury; pregroup therapy and postgroup therapy to assess for therapy outcome and return to duty; and participants with TBI who are at the community reintegration phase of intervention. It was not designed for severely or acutely impaired patients.[59]

Interpretability.
- Norms: control group of 101 adults aged 18 to 79 years without a history of acquired brain injury, learning disability, or psychiatric

---

EXHIBIT 7-9

FUNCTIONAL ASSESSMENT OF VERBAL REASONING AND EXECUTIVE STRATEGIES RESOURCE INFORMATION

The Functional Assessment of Verbal Reasoning and Executive Strategies was developed by Sheila MacDonald in 2005 and is available from:
    CCD Publishing
    Suite 26
    5420 Highway 6 North
    Guelph, ON, Canada, N1H612

disorder. The normative sample was compared to that of 52 individuals with acquired brain injury who ranged in age from 19 to 64 years old. The individuals with brain injury functioned at or above Rancho Level 6 (confused appropriate) on the Rancho Levels of Cognitive Functioning[61]; could tolerate at least 1 hour of assessment; and were able to read at least one page of text.

- MDC: not available
- Responsiveness estimates: not available

Reliability and Validity Estimates.

- Interrater reliability: for the accuracy and reasons scores of the four tasks across 20 participants, kappa coefficients were 0.81 and 0.85, respectively. A second interrater reliability analysis compared the accuracy scoring of two different examiners on one task for all 153 subjects. The kappa coefficient was 0.86 for this comparison.[59]
- Parallel-form reliability: not available
- Construct validity: to differentiate individuals with acquired brain injury from those without: t-test P < 0.0001.[59]
- Predictive validity: sensitivity and specificity demonstrated when FAVRES total accuracy and/or total rationale scores were used to classify subjects as brain injured.
- Concurrent validity: FAVRES scores were compared with the Scales of Cognitive Ability for TBI (SCATBI,[62] preliminary data only; further research is warranted).

Selected References

Isaki E, Turkstra L. Communication abilities and work re-entry following traumatic brain injury. *Brain Inj.* May 2000;14(5):441–453.

MacDonald S. *Functional Assessment of Verbal Reasoning and Executive Strategies.* London, UK: CCD Publishing; 2005.

Memory

Rivermead Behavioral Memory Test

Purpose/Description. The Rivermead Behavioral Memory Test (RBMT; Thames Valley Test Company, Suffolk, England; Exhibit 7-10) is administered to quantify and characterize impairment of everyday memory functioning when clinical observation or patient self-report suggests concerns in this area. The subtests simulate everyday memory challenges experienced by individuals with c/mTBI (eg, remembering names, faces, routes, appointments) and results are used to inform treatment focusing on memory compensation. An extended version (RBMT–E) was designed to detect subtle decrements in memory performance.[63]

The first version of the test was published in 1991. RBMT–E was published in 1999 and RBMT–II was published in 2003. In 2008, the RBMT-3 was released, incorporating elements of the RBMT and RBMT-E and a new subtest (novel task) was added. Clinicians should refer to the *RBMT Administration and Scoring Manual*[64] for additional information regarding psychometric properties and interpretation of scores specific to the version of the test they are administering.

The discussion of the RBMT in this document is not specific to any particular version of the test unless otherwise indicated.

Recommended Instrument Use: Practice Option. This test may be a helpful inclusion in an initial evaluation when:

- the patient has not had and will not have a comprehensive cognitive assessment (eg, neuropsychological assessment or cognitive-communication assessment performed by an SLP) to identify cognitive impairments or if the results of aforementioned testing do not specify memory performance; and

---

EXHIBIT 7-10

RIVERMEAD BEHAVIORAL MEMORY TEST RESOURCE INFORMATION

The Rivermead Behavioral Memory Test was developed by the Thames Valley Test Company, Suffolk, England and is available from:
  Northern Speech Services & National
    Rehabilitation Services
  117 North Elm Street, PO Box 1247
  Gaylord, MI 49734
  www.nss-nrs.com
  Phone: 888-337-3866
  Fax: 989-732-6164

- the patient has c/mTBI and self-report or observation of functional performance suggests the possible memory dysfunction.

This test is not recommended as an outcome measure. Cognitive rehabilitation for memory inefficiencies associated with c/mTBI involves instruction in compensatory memory strategies, not remediation of memory impairments. Because the RBMT administration and scoring procedures do not incorporate use of memory aids, repeated administrations of the test do not measure the impact or nature of intervention.

Administration Protocol/Equipment/Time. The RBMT is comprised of the test kit (including stimulus books and assessment materials), the administration and scoring manual (which specifies the step-by-step administration protocol), and procedural guide scoring sheets. As indicated above, the test includes remembering the following: names and faces, location of a hidden object, an appointment, details about a story, and a route. The RBMT-3 also includes performance of a novel task. It takes approximately 30 minutes to administer.

There are two types of scoring: a screening score and a standardized profile score. The screening score is obtained by pass or fail scoring and ranges from 0 to 12. Raw scores vary by subtest (eg, up to 21 points for story [immediate] versus up to 5 points for route [delayed]). Therefore, raw scores are standardized to equate the weight of each subtest by giving it a maximum weighting of 2, resulting in a standardized profile score ranging from 0 to 24. Use of the profile score is recommended because it is believed to give the more reliable estimate of patients' memory capabilities.[65]

Groups Tested With This Measure. The RBMT has been tested on a number of populations, including community-dwelling older adults with mild cognitive impairment,[66] veterans with combat-related PTSD,[67] adults hospitalized for unipolar depression,[68] and individuals with TBI,[65] including those with mild cognitive impairment.[69]

Interpretability.
- Norms: RBMT has been standardized on healthy people ages 16 to 69 and on people with brain injury ages 14 to 69.[65] Normative

data has been expanded for subsequent versions of the test; clinicians should rely on normative data provided in the manual specific to the RBMT version used.
- MDC: not applicable (repeat administration is not recommended)
- Responsiveness estimates: Not applicable (repeat administration is not recommended)

To interpret the score, the clinician locates the patient's RBMT score in one of the four memory impairment categories based on cut-off scores described in the administration manual. Because the RBMT and RBMT-II may not be sensitive enough to identify subtle memory deficits,[70] it is possible that individuals with c/mTBI may obtain a "normal" score on the RBMT and still have memory impairment.

Reliability and Validity Estimates. Reliability and validity of the RBMT were evaluated in a study involving 176 adults with brain injury.[65]

- Interrater reliability: In the aforementioned study, interrater reliability was established by having 40 subjects scored separately but simultaneously by two raters. Ten raters participated in the study and there was 100% agreement between raters for all 40 subjects.
- Parallel-form reliability: There are four parallel versions of the RBMT within the test kit. Parallel-form reliability was evaluated by administering two versions of the test to 118 people with brain injury. Overall, the correlation between the two scores was .78 for the screening score, and .85 for the profile score.
- Concurrent validity: RBMT profile scores had moderate to substantial correlation with the Warrington Recognition Test (0.63 with the Recognition Memory Test for Words, 0.43 with the Recognition Memory Test for Faces).[65]
- Construct validity: Wilson and colleagues[65] found statistically significant differences between RBMT subtest scores (P < .001) for patients with brain injury as compared to healthy controls (n = 118).

Selected References

Makatura TJ, Lam CS, Leahy BJ, Castillo MT, Kalpakjian CZ. Standardized memory tests and the appraisal of everyday memory. *Brain Injury*. 1999;5:355–367.

Wilson BA, Cockburn J, Baddeley AD, Hiorns R. The development and validation of a test battery for detecting and monitoring everyday memory problems. *J Clin Exp Neuropsychol*. Dec 1989;11(6):855–870.

Contextual Memory Test

Purpose/Description. The Contextual Memory Test (CMT; Harcourt Assessment, Inc, San Antonio, TX; Exhibit 7-11)[71] was developed to assess awareness of memory performance, strategy initiation, and recall of visual information in adults with memory dysfunction. It is comprised of a memory questionnaire and a memory task.

Recommended Instrument Use: Practice Option. This test may be a helpful inclusion in an initial evaluation when:

- the patient has not had and will not have a comprehensive cognitive assessment (eg, neuropsychological assessment and/or cognitive communication assessment performed by an SLP) to identify cognitive impairments **or** if the results of aforementioned testing do not specify memory performance, and
- the patient has c/mTBI and self-report or observation of functional performance suggests possible memory dysfunction.

Administration Protocol/Equipment/Time. Detailed administration procedures are specified in the manual, which, along with score sheets and pictures, is available for purchase. Test administration takes 5 to 10 minutes (plus a 15- to 20-minute interference task). The patient is instructed to study a picture card comprised of objects associated with either a morning routine or restaurant for 90 seconds. Immediate, delayed, and total recall scores are recorded. The questionnaire is used to examine performance awareness and strategy use.

EXHIBIT 7-11

CONTEXTUAL MEMORY TEST RESOURCE INFORMATION

The Contextual Memory Test is available from:
Harcourt Assessment, Inc
19500 Bulverde Road
San Antonio, TX 78259
www.harcourtassessment.com

Groups Tested With This Measure. Groups tested with this measure include adults 18 years and older with memory impairment secondary to multiple pathologies, as reported by Gillen.[72] No studies have been conducted using this measure with large groups of individuals with c/mTBI.

Interpretability.
- Norms: The normative sample is based on 375 adults, ages 17 to 86, as reported by Asher.[73]
- Scoring: The test yields immediate, delayed, and total recall scores that are compared to norms and analyzed for patterns using the summary of findings worksheet.[73]

Reliability and Validity Estimates.
- Parallel forms: Reliability of the two versions (restaurant picture card, morning routine picture card) ranges from 0.73 to 0.81.[72]
- Test-retest: Reliability ranges from 0.85 to 0.94.[72]
- Concurrent validity: established based on comparisons with the Rivermead Behavioral Memory Test (correlations ranging from 0.80 to 0.84).[72]

Selected References

Gillen G. *Cognitive and Perceptual Rehabilitation: Optimizing Function.* St. Louis, MO: Mosby, Inc; 2009.

Toglia JP. *The Contextual Memory Test.* San Antonio, TX: Harcourt Assessments; 1993.

Social Communication

Boston Naming Test

Purpose/Description. The Boston Naming Test (BNT) is used to evaluate visual confrontation naming ability.[74] The test consists of 60 black-and-white line drawings of objects, ranging from simple, high-frequency vocabulary to rare words. The test is a measure of confrontation naming based on findings that dysnomia results in greater difficulties with the naming of low-frequency objects. Naming difficulties may be rank-ordered along a continuum. Items on the BNT are ordered according to their ability to be named, which is thought to be correlated with their frequency.

Recommended Instrument Use: Practice Option. Word-finding difficulties can occur with neurological impairment resulting from many different etiologies, including c/mTBI. This instrument may be used by an SLP to further evaluate suspected word-finding difficulties after a more comprehensive language assessment has been administered or when a patient complains of word retrieval difficulties.

Administration Protocol/Equipment/Time. Equipment needed for testing is the test stimulus booklet, the response booklet, a stopwatch or watch or clock with a seconds hand, and a pen or pencil for recording responses. The complete test takes 10 to 20 minutes to administer. Detailed administration and scoring procedures are available with test materials.[74]

Groups Tested With This Measure. The BNT has been used extensively in adults and children. This type of picture-naming vocabulary test is useful when examining children with learning disabilities and evaluating adults with brain injury or dysfunction.[74] The BNT has been adapted and translated for use in at least a dozen languages, including a 30-item adaptation for Spanish-speaking people in the United States.[75] The test is commonly administered by neuropsychologists as well as speech pathologists and other clinicians to assess naming ability. Patients with TBI have been tested with this instrument; however, there is a paucity of literature describing the performance of individuals with c/mTBI. The BNT was included in a test battery administered to 11 individuals who sustained c/mTBI.[76] No significant differences in performance between patients and controls were found on the BNT.

Interpretability.
- Norms: The norms available in the test booklet are limited to small groups of adults ranging in age between 18 and 79 (N = 178), who were of above average education (mean = about 14 years), and children ranging in age between 0 and 5 years old and 5 to 12 years (N = 356). Information about geographical region, ethnicity, or time reference for this normative data is not provided.

Additional normative reports for English speakers are found in the literature. Heaton et al[77] compiled data from studies conducted over a period of 25 years and presented norms separately for two ethnicity groups, Caucasians and African Americans, organized by age, gender, and education.[78–80]

The mean number of items correct for 1,000 adults (ages 20 to 85) was 53.3 for males and 47.7 for females[77]; for 78 adults,[81] 54.31; and for 60 adults,[82] 54.50 (standard deviation 3.52, range 40 to 59 years). Cross-sectional studies suggest that age[77,80] and verbal intelligence affect the BNT scores.[83] Gender has been reported to be unrelated to BNT performance.[78,79,84,85]

- MDC: Based on a study of 541 "normal" elderly (ages 50 to 99 years old), reliable change index scores indicated that an annual decline of four points on the BNT is needed for a statistically reliable decline in an individual.[86]
- Responsiveness estimates: not available

Reliability Estimates.
- Internal consistency: coefficient alpha for the 60-item form has been reported to range from 0.78 and 0.96.[87-90]
- Interrater reliability: For the 60-item form, interrater reliability has been reported to range between 0.78 and 0.96, with an average of 0.89.
- Intrarater reliability: 0.98[82]
- Test-retest reliability was high over short intervals. For longer time intervals, such as 11 to 12 months, test-retest reliability was marginal to high; for example, in a healthy, elderly Caucasian adult population, test-retest reliability ranged between 0.62 and 0.89[91]; and high retest reliability (0.92) was measured in a normal or neurologically stable adult population.[92]

Validity Estimates. The BNT has been shown to correlate highly with other language-related measures, including the Visual Naming Test of the Multilingual Aphasia Examination,[93,94] as well as with measures of intelligence, including the Verbal Comprehension Factor of the Wechsler Adult Intelligence Scale–Revised. Poor performance on the BNT has been described in subjects with neurologic disease, including left hemisphere and brainstem strokes,[95] anoxia,[96] multiple sclerosis and Parkinson's disease,[97–99] Alzheimer's disease,[98,100] and closed head injuries.[10,101,102]

Selected References

Goodglass H, Kaplan E, Barresi B. *The Assessment of Aphasia and Related Disorders.* 3rd ed. Philadelphia, PA: Lea & Febiger; 2000.

Graves RE, Bezeau SC, Fogarty J, Blair R. Boston Naming Test short forms: a comparison of previous forms with new item response theory based forms. *J Clin Exp Neuropsychol.* Oct 2004;26(7):891–902.

Henderson LW, Frank EW, Pigatt T, Abramson RK, Houston M. Race, gender and educational level effects on Boston Naming Test scores. *Aphasiology.* 1998;12:901–911.

Kaplan EF, Goodglass H, Weintraub S. *The Boston Naming Test.* 2nd ed. Philadelphia, PA: Lippincott Williams & Wilkins; 2001.

Nicholas LE, Brookshire RH, MacLennan DL, Schumacher JG, Porrazzo S. The Boston Naming Test: Revised administration and scoring procedures and normative information for non-brain-damaged adults. *Clinical Aphasiology.* 1988;18:103–115.

Saxton JA, Ratcliff G, Munro CA, et al. Normative data on the Boston Naming Test and two equivalent 30-item short forms. *Clin Neuropsychol.* Nov 2000;14(4):526–534.

The Awareness of Social Inference Test

Purpose/Description. The Awareness of Social Inference Test (TASIT; Pearson/PsychCorp, San Antonio, TX; Exhibit 7-12) provides a systematic examination of social perception (ie, the ability to identify emotions and to make mental state inferences or to understand the meaning of conversational remarks meant nonliterally and to differentiate between these and literally intended remarks). It was designed as a criterion referenced test (ie, to have strong ceiling effects and low variability for individuals with a normal range of social perception skills) to assess whether individuals meet a criterion of adequate social perception ability and clearly differentiate neurologically normal individuals and those with significant deficits in social perception.

The test is comprised of videotaped vignettes of everyday social interactions and response probes. Based on recent theoretical accounts of how social cues contribute meaning in conversations, it assesses poor understanding of emotional expressions and difficulty integrating the contextual information that is part of normal social encounters.

TASIT has three sections assessing different components of social perception:

1. Part 1: The Emotion Evaluation Test (EET) is an ecologically valid test of emotion recognition.
2. Parts 2 and 3: Social Inference–Minimal and Social Inference–Enriched assess the ability to interpret conversational remarks meant literally or nonliterally as well as the ability to make judgments about the thoughts, intentions, and feelings of speakers.

Statistically equivalent alternate forms are available for retesting.

Recommended Instrument Use: Practice Option. The test may be a helpful component of an evaluation when there is a history of brain injury and the observation of functional performance suggests the possibility of cognitive dysfunction in a number of domains, including social communication.

EXHIBIT 7-12

THE AWARENESS OF SOCIAL INFERENCE TEST RESOURCE INFORMATION

The Awareness of Social Inference Test is available from:
Pearson/PsychCorp
Pearson, Attn: Inbound Sales & Customer Support
19500 Bulverde Road
San Antonio, TX 78259-3701
Phone: 800-627-7271
Fax: 800-232-1223
ClinicalCustomerSupport@Pearson.com

Administration Protocol/Equipment/Time. The complete TASIT test kit includes: a manual, record forms A and B, a DVD, and stimulus books.[103] The DVD contains 28 video-recorded vignettes of professional actors enacting ambiguous scripts representing 7 basic emotions. The stimuli are dynamic; portray naturalistic, complex expressions; and provide intonation and gestural cues. Respondents choose the perceived emotion from the following descriptors: happy, surprised, sad, angry, anxious, revolted, neutral.

On Part 1, the EET, the ability to correctly recognize emotional expression is assessed by asking subjects to decide which of the basic seven categories each emotional expression represented. On Part 2, Social Inference–Minimal, after viewing each vignette, participants are required to answer questions regarding the speaker's feelings, beliefs, intentions, and meaning. On Part 3, Social Inference–Enriched, 16 vignettes are presented that provide additional information before or after the dialogue of interest to "set the scene." The ability to interpret the vignettes correctly is assessed via a set of four questions for each vignette.

The TASIT requires between 75 and 90 minutes to administer and score. More severely involved patients requires more time for viewing and responding to questions.

Groups Tested With This Measure. This test has been administered to neurologically normal, English-speaking, Australian adults, ages 14 to 60 years old, including some from the police training academy and the navy. All subjects had secondary school education or higher (average 13 years; standard deviation 2 years of education).[103]

The test has also been administered to adults with severe traumatic brain injuries,[104–107] schizophrenia,[108,109] and progressive degenerative diseases, including frontotemporal dementia, progressive nonfluent aphasia, Alzheimer's disease, corticobasal degeneration, and progressive supranuclear palsy.[110] No published studies to date have specifically used this measure in individuals with c/mTBI.

Interpretability.
- Norms: The test was administered to 275 young adults who scored 84% accuracy or above on all facets. The mean performance of the group with TBI, for both first and second administration of Form A and Form B, showed significant differences from the normal population.[104]

- TASIT Part 1:
  - Normative means: Form A, 24.86 (standard deviation 2.11); Form B, 24.15 (standard deviation 2.53)
  - TBI means: Form A, 19.22 (standard deviation 5.06); Form B, 19.53 (standard deviation 4.72)
- TASIT Part 2:
  - Normative means: Form A, 54.11 (standard deviation 4.29); Form B, 52.88 (standard deviation 5.30)
  - TBI means: Form A, 44.13 (standard deviation 8.66); Form B, 40.59 (standard deviation 8.62)
- TASIT Part 3:
  - Normative means: Form A, 55.64 (standard deviation 4.82); Form B, 55.11 (standard deviation 5.28)
  - TBI means: Form A, 44.47 (standard deviation 7.38); Form B, 42.44 (standard deviation 8.09)

For the TBI group, poor scores on sarcasm and lies reflected difficulty answering questions concerning the thoughts, feelings, and intentions of the speakers.

- MDC: not reported
- Responsiveness estimates: not available

Reliability and Validity Estimates.
- Test-retest reliability: ranged from 0.74 to 0.88. On alternate forms, reliability ranged from 0.62 to 0.83. There was no significant difference between total scores on Forms A and B. TASIT is not overly prone to practice effects and is reliable for repeat administrations.[104]
- Interrater: There is no published literature that describes interrater or intrarater reliability of the TASIT.[104]
- Validity: Concurrent validity was examined in subsets of a sample of 116 adults with TBI by relating TASIT performance to standard tests of neuropsychological function and specific social perception measures. TASIT was associated with face perception, information processing speed, and working memory. Socially relevant new learning and executive tasks were significantly associated with TASIT performance. Nonsocial tasks showed little association. Ekman photos and theory of mind stories were also associated.[104]

- Construct validity: For Part 1, 12 adults with severe TBI were significantly worse than controls, especially on fear and neutral items. For Part 2, speakers with severe TBI performed normally on sincere exchanges but were poor on sarcastic exchanges. For Part 3, speakers with TBI were poorer than normal speakers on sarcasm but not on lies.

Ecological validity: 21 people with severe TBI were assessed on TASIT as well as rated for their social competence in a spontaneous encounter. Poor TASIT performance predicted social interaction skills. Persons with TBI displayed especially insensitive use of humor.[105]

Selected References

McDonald S, Bornhofen C, Shum D, Long E, Saunders C, Neulinger K. Reliability and validity of The Awareness of Social Inference Test (TASIT): a clinical test of social perception. *Disabil Rehabil.* Dec 30 2006;28(24):1529–1542.

McDonald S, Flanagan S. Social perception deficits after traumatic brain injury: interaction between emotion recognition, mentalizing ability, and social communication. *Neuropsychology.* Jul 2004;18(3):572–579.

McDonald S, Flanagan S, Rollins J. *The Awareness of Social Inference Test.* Bury St. Edmonds, UK: Thames Valley Test Company; 2002.

McDonald S, Flanagan S, Rollins J, Kinch J. TASIT: a new clinical tool for assessing social perception after traumatic brain injury. *J Head Trauma Rehabil.* May–Jun 2003;18(3):219–238.

McDonald S, Tate R, Togher L, et al. Social skills treatment for people with severe, chronic acquired brain injuries: a multicenter trial. *Arch Phys Med Rehabil.* 2007;89(9):1648–1659.

The La Trobe Communication Questionnaire

Purpose/Description. The La Trobe Communication Questionnaire (LCQ; may be obtained from J.Douglas@latrobe.edu.au) measures perceived social communication ability from multiple sources, including self and others (eg, friends, family, and clinicians) who regularly converse with the individual.[111] The LCQ is derived from the four conversational maxims of Grice's Co-operative Principle,[112] including: 1) quantity (amount of information), 2) quality (accuracy of contribution), 3) relation (relevance of contribution), and 4) manner (how the information is said). The LCQ includes two forms: Form S, to be administered to the primary subject, and Form O, for the subject's nominated "close other" (a person who knows the patient well). Both forms are identical in content and contain 30 items that were initially developed and psychometrically evaluated on young adults and healthy close others. A variation of Form O is available for use with rehabilitation workers when data are collected on clinical populations.[111]

Recommended Instrument Use: Practice Option. The LCQ is to be administered for clinical and research use by SLPs and other rehabilitation professionals.[111] This instrument is recommended for use by a single person or in a group context to assess each individual's self-perception of communication competence. It is designed for persons with diagnoses of TBI, stroke, or dementia. The instrument may also be administered by a close other. It is recommended that the LCQ be administered "interview-style" to people with TBI so assistance can be provided if needed.[113]

Administration Protocol/Equipment/Time. The LCQ consists of Form S, Form O, and a variation of Form O.[110] Administration time with informants is approximately 15 minutes, and interview format with individuals with TBI takes approximately 30 minutes.

Groups Tested With This Measure. The LCQ was evaluated with young healthy adults, individuals with severe TBI, and close others (relatives or friends).[111,113] Although the LCQ has been evaluated with young healthy adults, it has not been formally studied with the c/mTBI population.

Interpretability.
- Norms: The LCQ was psychometrically evaluated on 147 young adults and 109 close others; all were healthy and had no history of psychiatric or neurological dis-

order.[111] Further psychometric evaluation was conducted on 88 adults with severe TBI and 71 close others.[113] Norms are as follows:

- Control group (mean age 21.2; range 16 to 39 years): 88% completed high school: LCQ score 52.47 (standard deviation 9.62)[111]
- Informants group (mean age 32.76): LCQ score 47.17 (standard deviation 9.93)[111]
- In a clinical group with severe TBI[113] with a mean age of 32.26 years (standard deviation 12.12): LCQ score 54.94 (standard deviation 14.08)
- Informants group of close others: LCQ score 59.35 (standard deviation 14.94)

- Scoring: Modified Likert-type scales with 1 (never or rarely) to 4 (usually or always) are used to score responses. Six items on the LCQ require reverse scoring (ie, lowest frequency rating represents the highest perceived difficulty) distributed randomly to serve as internal response bias checks.[111]
- MDC: not available
- Responsiveness estimates: not available

Reliability Estimates.
- Internal consistency: This was found to be high for the LCQ (Cronbach's alpha for primary respondents was 0.85; for close others, it was 0.86; for those with severe TBI was 0.91 and close others was 0.92).[110,112]
- Interrater and intrarater: not applicable (patient and familiar others fill out questionnaires)
- Test-retest: Test-retest reliability was acceptable at 8 weeks for the self-report (r = 0.76).[111] For 18 participants with severe TBI, greater than 5 years after injury, test-retest Pearson r coefficients across a 2-week interval were acceptable (in individuals with TBI, r = 0.81; in close others, r = 0.87).[113]

Validity Estimates.
- Content/Face validity: not available
- Criterion: not available
- Construct validity: A principal-component factor analytic procedure was completed on the self-report data (n = 147). A six-factor solution was produced with all factors, including items from at least two Gricean maxims, and the cognitive construct used to guide the original item selection.[113]

Selected References

Douglas JM, Bracy CA, Snow PC. Measuring perceived communicative ability after traumatic brain injury: reliability and validity of the La Trobe Communication Questionnaire. *J Head Trauma Rehabil.* Jan–Feb 2007;22(1):31–38.

Douglas JM, O'Flaherty CA, Snow P. Measuring perception of communicative ability: the development and evaluation of the La Trobe Communication Questionnaire. *Aphasiology.* 2000;14:251–268.

Discourse Comprehension Test

Purpose/Description. The Discourse Comprehension Test (DCT; Exhibit 7-13) was designed to assess comprehension and retention of spoken narrative discourse by adults with aphasia, right-hemisphere brain damage, or TBI. The test consists of 10 stories and a set of yes-or-no questions for each story. The stories are controlled for length, grammatical complexity, listening difficulty, and reading level. The questions systematically assess a listener's comprehension and retention of directly stated and implied main ideas and details from a homogeneous set of stories. The stories are presented in two versions:

1. Listening comprehension version: to assess comprehension and retention of spoken narrative discourse.
2. Silent reading comprehension version: to assess comprehension and retention of written narrative discourse.

EXHIBIT 7-13

DISCOURSE COMPREHENSION TEST RESOURCE INFORMATION

The Discourse Comprehension Test, developed by Brookshire and Nicholas, is available from:
BRK Publishers
Minneapolis, MN 55438
Phone: 612-835-2940

Recommended Instrument Use: Practice Option. This test is intended to supplement the information gained from standard multimodality language tests and from tests that assess comprehension and retention of single words and isolated sentences. The DCT is designed to provide a more complete picture of how the individual performs in more natural communication interactions.

The DCT can be used to:

- identify deficits that may affect daily-life communication,
- guide the selection of treatment tasks,
- monitor changes in performance with treatment, and
- counsel communication partners.

The test is appropriate for brain-injured adults who have:

- adequate hearing for the test conditions,
- intelligible and reliable "yes" and "no" responses (either spoken, by head nods, or by pointing to response cards), or
- correct responses to at least half of the question pairs in the listening version of the sentence comprehension test, or the subject should respond correctly to at least half of the 20 yes-or-no questions in the auditory verbal comprehension subtest of the Western Aphasia Battery.[114]

Administration Protocol/Equipment/Time. Administration time is approximately 20 minutes. Materials include the listening comprehension version (stories and questions), stimulus tape, audiocassette player, story cards, silent reading comprehension version, question sheets, response record form, test report forms, and a stopwatch.

Detailed administration and scoring procedures are available with test materials.

Groups Tested With This Measure. Non-brain-damaged adults, aphasic adults with left-hemisphere brain damage, nonaphasic adults with right-hemisphere brain damage, and adults with TBI,[115] including c/mTBI,[116] have been tested with this measure. The test was designed to assess comprehension and retention of spoken narrative discourse by adults with aphasia with right-hemisphere brain injury; it was not designed to differentiate non-brain-damaged from brain-damaged adults, nor was it designed to differentiate between brain-damaged adults with different etiologies or sites of brain injury.[117] However, no published studies have specifically used this measure on individuals with c/mTBI.

Interpretability.
- Norms: Forty non-brain-damaged adults, 20 aphasic adults with left-hemisphere brain damage, 20 nonaphasic adults with right-hemisphere brain damage, and 20 adults with TBI were tested with the listening version of the DCT.[115]
- MDC: not available
- Responsiveness estimates: not available

Reliability Estimates.
- Internal consistency: not available
- Test-Retest: The test-retest reliability of performance was measured for the aphasic subjects and the right-brain-damaged subjects (r = .87 for aphasic subjects, r = .95 for right-brain-damaged).[115]

Validity Estimates.
- Content: The stories in the DCT were constructed to evaluate comprehension and retention of main ideas, details, and directly stated and implied information. The eight questions for each story test four main ideas (two stated and two implied) and four details (two stated and two implied). The validity of the DCT's classification of questions is supported by the performances of non-brain-damaged adults and the three groups of brain-damaged adults.[117]
- Construct and criterion-related validity: There are no standardized tests for assessing brain-damaged adults' comprehension of spoken discourse. Therefore, DCT performance cannot be compared to performance on other measures of discourse comprehension. DCT has been compared to auditory comprehension subtests of other assessments, including the Boston Diagnostic Aphasia Exam (.76),[118] a shortened version of the Porch Index of Communicative Ability (.64),[119] and the Sentence Comprehension Test (.53).[120]

EXHIBIT 7-14

MORTERA-COGNITIVE SCREENING MEASURE ADDITIONAL INFORMATION

The test author wishes to provide free access to the Mortera-Cognitive Screening Measure (M-CSM). In return, the author requests that the user of the M-CSM send her the results. In addition, the author requests that the following information be included:

- the population (age, diagnosis, or disability) assessed with the M-CSM;
- the clinical setting in which the M-CSM was used;
- the user's background related to profession, years of experience, and area of practice; and
- any questions or specific comments on the M-CSM regarding ease of use, content, format, levels of scores, or any other areas of concern.

Any information submitted to the author that is related to results or feedback must not contain any identifying or personal information. All results and feedback must be anonymous and reported in aggregate.

At the request of the author, please send the above information in either paper or electronic format to:
Marianne Mortera, PhD, OTR/L
Columbia University—Programs in Occupational Therapy
710 West 168th Street, Neurological Institute, 8th Floor
New York, NY 10032
mhm2101@columbia.edu

Selected References

Brookshire RH, Nicholas LR. *Discourse Comprehension Test*. Minneapolis, MN: BRK Publishers; 1997.

Duff MC, Proctor A, Haley K. Mild traumatic brain injury (MTBI): assessment and treatment procedures used by speech-language pathologists (SLPs). *Brain Inj*. Sep 2002;16(9):773–787.

Nicholas LE, Brookshire RH. Consistency of the effects of rate of speech on brain-damaged adults' comprehension of narrative discourse. *J Speech Hear Res*. Dec 1986;29(4):462–470.

Nicholas LE, Brookshire RH. Comprehension of spoken narrative discourse by adults with aphasia, right-hemisphere-brain damage, or traumatic brain injury. *Am J Speech-Lang Path*. 1995;4:69–81.

FUNCTIONAL PERFORMANCE ASSESSMENTS

Mortera-Cognitive Screening Measure

Purpose/Description

The Mortera-Cognitive Screening Measure (M-CSM; academiccommons.columbia.edu/catalog/ac:123173; Exhibit 7-14) is a structured observational tool that involves two functional tasks associated with preparing a light meal (soup and sandwich). The clinician rates patient behaviors during task performance based on the cognitive dimensions of each subtask. The cognitive dimensions included in the M-CSM are often problematic after brain injury (shifting and sustaining attention, visual-attention scanning, awareness of disability, judgment relative to safety, recall, planning and problem solving).[121,122]

Recommended Instrument Use: Practice Option

This functional assessment may be used to identify ways in which possible cognitive inefficiencies or impairments manifest themselves in the performance of everyday tasks. While the M-CSM may not be sensitive to cognitive inefficiencies typical of c/mTBI, it may be particularly useful in observing kitchen performance and competence for service members who lack experience in meal preparation.

Administration Protocol/Equipment/Time

A kitchen setting (including a stovetop) is required to administer the M-CSM along with food ingredients and cooking supplies. The M-CSM takes 20 to 60 minutes to administer, depending upon the patient's meal preparation skills and background, and his or her familiarity with the testing environment (eg, location of supplies; Form 7-1).

Groups Tested With This Measure

The M-CSM was designed for use on patients with brain injury. However, no published studies have specifically used this measure on individuals with c/mTBI.

Interpretability

- Norms: No norms have been developed for this instrument.
- Scoring: The clinician rates patient behaviors.

(0 = no problem, 1 = potential problem, 2 = problem) during task performance based on the cognitive dimensions of each subtask.

- MDC: not available

Reliability and Validity Estimates

- Interrater reliability: Two groups of therapists rated videotaped task performance with intraclass correlation coefficients ranging from 0.71 to 0.93 (videotape 1) and 0.54 to 0.68 (videotape 2).[123]
- Content validity: Two groups of five occupational therapists with clinical expertise in brain injury and cognitive rehabilitation examined the M-CSM by using the content validity rating form, which comprised three parts (cognitive processes and the theoretical foundation, cognitive processes and their necessity with the CSM functional tasks, and adequacy of the cognitive descriptors).[123]

Selected References

Mortera MH. Instrument development in brain injury rehabilitation: Part I. *Phys Disabilities Special Interest Section Q.* 2006a;29(3):1–4.

Mortera MH. Instrument development in brain injury rehabilitation: Part II. *Phys Disabilities Special Interest Section Q.* 2006b;29(4):1–2.

Dynamic Assessment of Functional Performance

Purpose/Description

Functional task observation is a critical component of a comprehensive cognitive and visual assessment. Because they are highly structured, many standardized tests do not challenge patients' ability to utilize their executive skills in unstructured tasks or environments. Therefore, systematic observation of functional task performance provides unique opportunities to further understand patients' challenges and strengths. By observing patients as they perform everyday tasks, OTs assess the extent to which task, environment, and personal characteristics interact to impact performance. Furthermore, therapists modify task and environmental variables to just-right challenges specific to an individual's goals and to determine under which circumstances the patient's performance is optimized.

OTs design patient-relevant functional tasks and use an observation worksheet, like the Sister Kenny Dynamic Functional Task Observation Checklist (Form 7-2), to analyze task and environmental characteristics and to catalog the associated personal characteristics and overall performance.

Recommended Instrument Use

The Dynamic Functional Task Observation Checklist may be used to structure patient performance observations during the assessment phase and throughout the episode of care.

Administration Protocol/Equipment/Time

These dimensions vary depending on the task that is developed by the clinician. The sample tasks that follow take 15 to 25 minutes to perform and involve various office supplies.

Groups Tested With This Measure

These methods have not been formally tested on any groups. This description is an effort to propose methods by which OTs can standardize observational tasks for their own use.

Patient name:_____

Date:_____

FORM 7-1

OBSERVATION SCHEDULE FOR THE MORTERA-COGNITIVE SCREENING MEASURE

Directions: For each cognitive process observed, mark one of the three levels that best indicates the individual's level of performance.

Soup

A. Gathering items: saucepan, can of soup, bowl, spoon/ladle, manual or electric can opener

1) Sustained attention	Score
(2) Unable to sustain focus on gathering all items even with visual, verbal, or tactile cues (1) Requires 1–2 visual, verbal, or tactile cues to sustain focus on gathering all items (0) Sustains focus on gathering all items	
2) Shifting attention	**Score**
(2) Unable to resume retrieval of items if interrupted, even with visual, verbal, or tactile cues (1) Requires 1–2 visual, verbal, or tactile cues to resume retrieval of items (0) Able to resume retrieval of items if interrupted from task	
3) Visual-attention scanning	**Score**
(2) Unable to locate items within visual fields even with visual, verbal, or tactile cues (1) Requires 1–2 visual, verbal, or tactile cues to locate items within visual fields (0) Locates all items within visual fields	
4) Judgment relative to safety	**Score**
(2) Intervention by other required to avoid a problem (1) Requires 1–2 visual, verbal, or tactile cues to incorporate safety strategy if item(s) out of reach	

(0) Retrieves items in a safe manner	
5) Recall	**Score**
(2) Unable to retrieve all necessary items even with visual, verbal, or tactile cues (1) Requires 1–2 visual, verbal, or tactile cues to retrieve necessary items (0) Retrieves all necessary items	

B. Reads and/or follows directions on soup can

6) Sustained attention	**Score**
(2) If refers to directions, unable to sustain focus on reading directions even with visual, verbal, or tactile cues (1) If refers to directions, requires 1–2 visual, verbal, or tactile cues to sustain focus on reading directions (0) If refers to directions, sustains focus on reading directions	
7) Visual-attention scanning	**Score**
(2) If refers to directions, unable to locate/read directions in all visual fields (1) If refers to directions, requires 1–2 visual, verbal, or tactile cues to locate/read directions in all visual fields (0) If refers to directions, able to locate/read directions in all visual fields	
8) Awareness of disability	**Score**
(2) Unable to indicate difficulty locating/reading directions (1) Requires 1–2 visual, verbal, or tactile cues to indicate difficulty locating/reading directions (0) Not applicable or indicates if having difficulty locating/reading directions	
9) Recall	**Score**
(2) Checks directions repeatedly yet unable to initiate steps (1) Checks directions repeatedly but able to initiate steps	

	Score
(0) Indicates no need for directions and is able to initiate steps	
10) Planning/problem solving	**Score**
(2) Unable to complete steps in an orderly sequence even with visual, verbal, or tactile cues (1) Requires 1–2 visual, verbal, or tactile cues to complete steps in an orderly sequence with or without following directions (0) Completes steps in an orderly sequence with or without following directions	

C. Opens can with can opener

	Score
11) Sustained attention	**Score**
(2) Internal/external distractions interfere even with visual, verbal, or tactile cues (1) Requires 1–2 visual, verbal, or tactile cues to sustain focus on task (0) Opens can without internal/external distractions within appropriate timeframe	
12) Visual-attention scanning	**Score**
(2) Can is partially opened even with visual, verbal, or tactile cues (1) Requires 1–2 visual, verbal, or tactile cues to completely open can (0) Can opened completely	
13) Awareness of disability	**Score**
(2) Unable to acknowledge difficulty with can opener even with visual, verbal, or tactile cues (1) Requires 1–2 visual, verbal, or tactile cues to acknowledge difficulty with can opener (0) Not applicable or acknowledges difficulty with can opener	
14) Judgment relative to safety	**Score**
(2) Requires immediate visual, verbal, or tactile cues to avoid possible injury from sharp edges (1) Requires 1–2 visual, verbal, or tactile cues to stabilize can and carefully handle sharp edges (0) Safely stabilizes can and carefully handles sharp edges	

D. Pours soup and/or liquid into saucepan

15) Sustained attention	Score
(2) Internal/external distractions interfere even with visual, verbal, or tactile cues (1) Requires 1–2 visual, verbal, or tactile cues in order to refocus on task (0) Pours soup without internal/external distractions within appropriate timeframe	
16) Visual-attention scanning	Score
(2) Pours soup over edge of saucepan (1) Requires 1–2 visual, verbal, or tactile cues to prevent pouring soup over the edge of saucepan (0) Pours soup toward center of saucepan	
17) Awareness of disability	Score
(2) Unable to indicate difficulty pouring soup/liquids (1) Requires 1–2 visual, verbal, or tactile cues to indicate difficulty pouring soup/liquids (0) Not applicable or indicates difficulty pouring soup/liquids	
18) Judgment relative to safety	Score
(2) Unable to pour liquids slowly and carefully even with visual, verbal, or tactile cues (1) Requires 1–2 visual, verbal, or tactile cues to pour liquids slowly and carefully (0) Pours liquids slowly and carefully	

E. Heats soup

19) Visual-attention scanning	Score
(2) Unable to check for signs that soup heats and/or adjusts correct dial even with visual, verbal, or tactile cues	

(1) Requires 1–2 visual, verbal, or tactile cues to check that soup heats and/or adjusts correct dial	
(0) Checks for signs that soup heats and/or adjusts correct dial accordingly	
20) Judgment relative to safety	**Score**
(2) Requires immediate cues/intervention to avoid contact with heat	
(1) Requires 1–2 visual, verbal, or tactile cues to note temperature of soup or avoids contact with heat	
(0) Vigilance noted regarding temperature of soup and avoids contact with heat	
21) Planning/problem solving	**Score**
(2) Unable to adjust dial sequentially with heating soup even with visual, verbal, or tactile cues	
(1) Requires 1–2 visual, verbal, or tactile cues to adjust dial sequentially with heating soup	
(0) Not applicable or adjusts sequentially with heating soup	

F. Turns off burner

22) Visual-attention scanning	**Score**
(2) Unable to locate correct dial for burner	
(1) Requires 1–2 visual, verbal, or tactile cues to locate correct dial for burner	
(0) Locates correct dial for burner	
23) Judgment relative to safety	**Score**
(2) Unable to note if dial is in "off" position with visual, verbal, or tactile cues	
(1) Requires 1–2 visual, verbal, or tactile cues to note if dial is in "off" position	
(0) Able to note if dial is in "off" position	

G. Pours soup into bowl or uses ladle

24) Sustained attention	Score
(2) Distractions interfere, causing spilling of soup (1) Requires 1–2 visual, verbal, or tactile cues to avoid spilling soup (0) Pours or ladles soup without distractions interfering	
25) Visual-attention scanning	**Score**
(2) Pours or ladles soup outside bowl (1) Requires 1–2 visual, verbal, or tactile cues to pour or ladle soup into center of bowl (0) Pours or ladles soup toward center of bowl	
26) Awareness of disability	**Score**
(2) Unable to indicate difficulty pouring or ladling soup (1) Requires 1–2 visual, verbal, or tactile cues to indicate difficulty pouring or ladling soup (0) Not applicable or indicates having difficulty pouring or ladling soup	
27) Judgment relative to safety	**Score**
(2) Requires immediate cues/intervention to make contact with hot soup (1) Requires 1–2 visual, verbal, or tactile cues to safely and slowly ladle soup into bowl (0) Safely and slowly pours or ladles soup into bowl	

Sandwich

A. Gathering items: can of tuna, condiments, bread, can opener, bowl, plate, utensils

28) Sustained attention	Score
(2) Internal/external distractions interfere even with visual, verbal, or tactile cues (1) Requires 1–2 visual, verbal, or tactile cues to refocus on task (0) Pours soup without internal/external distractions within appropriate timeframe	

29) Shifting attention	Score
(2) Unable to retrieve items from various locations even with visual, verbal, or tactile cues	
(1) Requires 1–2 visual, verbal, or tactile cues to retrieve items from various locations	
(0) Able to retrieve all necessary items from various locations	
30) Visual-attention scanning	Score
(2) Unable to locate items within visual fields even with visual, verbal, or tactile cues	
(1) Requires 1–2 visual, verbal, or tactile cues to locate items within visual fields	
(0) Locates all items within visual fields	
31) Awareness of disability	
(2) Unable to indicate difficulty with retrieving	
(1) Requires 1–2 visual, verbal, tactile cues to indicate difficulty retrieving items	
(0) Not applicable or indicates difficulty retrieving items	
32) Judgment relative to safety	Score
(2) Intervention by other required to avoid a problem	
(1) Retrieves items without thought to safety when item out of reach	
(0) Retrieves items in a safe manner	
33) Recall	Score
(2) Unable to retrieve all necessary items even with visual, verbal, or tactile cues	
(1) Requires 1–2 visual, verbal, or tactile cues to retrieve necessary items	
(0) Retrieves all necessary items	

B. Opens cans with can opener

34) Sustained attention	Score
(2) Internal/external distractions interfere even with visual, verbal, or tactile cues	
(1) Requires 1–2 visual, verbal, or tactile cues to sustain focus on task	

(0) Opens can without internal/external distractions interfering with task performance	
35) Visual-attention scanning	Score
(2) Can is partially opened even with visual, verbal, or tactile cues (1) Requires 1–2 visual, verbal, or tactile cues to completely open can (0) Can opened completely	
36) Awareness of disability	Score
(2) Unable to indicate difficulty using can opener (1) Requires 1–2 visual, verbal, or tactile cues to indicate difficulty using can opener (0) Not applicable or indicates difficulty using can opener	
37) Judgment relative to safety	Score
(2) Requires immediate intervention to avoid possible injury (1) Requires 1–2 verbal or tactile cues to stabilize can or avoid sharp edges (0) Safely stabilizes can and avoids sharp edges	

C. Drains liquid from can

38) Shifting attention	Score
(2) Unable to resume focus on draining liquid even with visual, verbal, or tactile cues (1) Requires 1–2 visual, verbal, or tactile cues to sustain focus on task (0) Able to empty can of liquid	
39) Judgment relative to safety	Score
(2) Requires immediate cues/intervention required to avoid contact with sharp edges (1) Requires 1–2 verbal or tactile cues to stabilize can or avoid sharp edges (0) Safely and carefully avoids sharp edges	

D. Places tuna in bowl

40) Visual attention-scanning	Score
(2) Tuna placed outside bowl (1) Requires 1–2 visual, verbal, or tactile cues to place tuna in bowl (0) Places tuna in bowl	

E. Adds condiments

41) Visual attention-scanning	Score
(2) Condiments placed outside bowl (1) Requires 1–2 visual, verbal, or tactile cues to place condiments in bowl (0) Places condiments in bowl	

F. Spreads tuna mixture on bread

42) Visual attention-scanning	Score
(2) Unable to spread tuna over bread even with visual, verbal, or tactile cues (1) Requires 1–2 visual, verbal, or tactile cues to spread tuna mixture evenly over bread (0) Spreads tuna mixture evenly over bread	

Reproduced with permission from: Mortera MH: *Mortera-Cognitive Screening Measure*. http://academiccommons.columbia.edu/catalog/ac:123173. New York, NY: Programs in Occupational Therapy, Columbia University; 2004. Accessed August 21, 2013.

FORM 7-2

SISTER KENNY DYNAMIC FUNCTIONAL TASK OBSERVATION CHECKLIST

Component		Descriptions of Characteristics		Notes
Task	Perceived degree of difficulty	□ Easy □ Moderate □ Difficult		
	Perceived degree of familiarity	□ Familiar □ Familiar with new challenges □ Unfamiliar		
	Type of instruction provided	□ Verbal □ Written □ Demonstrated □ Pictorial		
	Physical demands	□ Sedentary □ Active □ Gross motor □ Fine motor □ Other: □ Other:		
	Cognitive Demands	Attention	□ Sustained □ Divided □ Alternating	
		Memory	□ Processing new info □ Retrieving info	

	Cognitive Demands	Executive functioning	□ Planning	
			□ Prioritizing	
			□ Self-monitoring	
			□ Problem solving	
Task (cont)		Visual demands	□ Visual acuity	
			□ Scanning	
			□ Visual attention	
			□ Other:	
Environment		Performance setting	□ Clinic	
			□ Community	
		Stimulus-arousal properties	□ Little to no distracters	
			□ Auditory distracters	
			□ Visual distracters	
Person		Physical considerations	□ None	
			□ Pain	
			□ Decreased endurance	
			□ U/E limitations	
			□ L/E limitations	
			□ Decreased balance	
		Emotional considerations	□ None	
			□ Seems anxious	
			□ Seems depressed	
			□ Other	
		Visual/auditory considerations	□ Lighting needs	
			□ Glasses, patches	
			□ Hearing device	

Person	Self-awareness associated with the task at-hand	□ Anticipatory □ Emergent □ Intellectual □ Little to none	
Performance	Task completion	□ Task completion □ Task partially completed □ Could not complete	
	Task accuracy	□ Totally accurate □ Somewhat accurate □ Not accurate	
	Activity tolerance	□ Functional with no breaks □ Functional with self-initiated breaks □ Impaired, needed breaks and cues to take them □ Lethargic/unable	
	Problem-solving approach	□ Logical/systematic □ Trial and error □ Unable to initiate	
	Self-prediction-reflection	□ Able to accurately predict performance □ Able to reflect on performance □ Needed cues to predict performance □ Needed cues to reflect on performance	
	Response to feedback	□ Responsive to feedback: uses feedback □ Defensive and reluctant □ Refusal to listen/argues	

Component	Descriptions of characteristics		Notes
Performance (cont)	Strategy use (specify)	Strategy: □ Independently initiated □ Cues required Strategy: □ Independently initiated □ Cues required Strategy: □ Independently initiated □ Cues required Strategy: □ Independently initiated □ Cues required	

Interpretability

- Norms: There are no norms for this process, but as individual clinicians craft and frequently use a core set of observational tasks, they will readily identify abnormalities, errors, or discrepancies in performance.
- MDC: not established
- Responsiveness estimates: not established
- Reliability and validity estimates: not established

Selected References: none

Protocol

The following sample tasks provide opportunities for clinicians to observe a patient's ability to initiate memory compensation strategies (task instructions are too detailed to be easily remembered) and ability to stay on task during an activity of some duration. Adding time pressure may further challenge the patient's organizational skills.

Sample Functional Tasks

I. Filing Task
  A. Items needed:
    i. Eight file folders: four files labeled with capital letters (A–F, G–L, M–R, S–Z) and four labeled with lowercase letters (a–g, h–m, n–s, t–z)
    ii. 26 index cards with letters of the alphabet, all capitalized
    iii. 26 index cards with letters of the alphabet, all lowercase
    iv. 25 index cards with random first and last names (eg, John Smith)
    v. A yellow piece of paper
    vi. One business envelope
    vii. Red and black pens
  B. Give the patient the following directions:
    i. Ask for filing supplies. File for 5 minutes. Place the uppercase letters in the uppercase folders, the lowercase letters in the lowercase folders. File the name cards in the uppercase folders according to the first letter of the first name.
    ii. Ask for a yellow piece of paper. Draw a stick figure and make sure the figure is wearing a hat and one shoe. Fold the paper in thirds. Place it in the envelope and seal the envelope.
    iii. Using a black pen, write your mailing address on the envelope and draw a stamp in the corner.
    iv. Tell me when you are done.
  C. The patient is asked to predict:
    i. How long the task will take
    ii. How many errors he or she will have
    iii. How difficult it will be (easy, average, difficult)
    iv. Which aspects will be easy and which will present a challenge

II. Envelope Task
  A. Items needed:
    i. 20 business envelopes addressed with random names and addresses in six different cities with six different zip codes
    ii. A deck of cards, with 10 cards from 3 of the suits removed
    iii. Pen and paper
  B. Give the patient the following instructions:
    i. Sort the envelopes into zip codes.
    ii. Within each zip code, alphabetize the names by the first letter of the last name.
    iii. Sort for 5 minutes.
    iv. Ask for a deck of cards.
    v. Identify the missing cards.
    vi. Verbally describe another method you could have used to identify the missing cards.
    vii. Identify which method would be most efficient.
    viii. Draw a picture of a clock with the hands at 2:15.
    ix. Tell me when you are done.
  C. The patient is asked to predict as described above.

American Speech Language and Hearing Association Functional Assessment of Communication Skills for Adults

Purpose/Description

The American Speech Language and Hearing Association Functional Assessment of Communication Skills for Adults (ASHA-FACS; Exhibit 7-15) is a quick and easy-to-administer measure of functional communication behaviors at the level of disability, based on direct observations of typical communication performance across the following domains: social communication; communication of basic needs; reading, writing, and number concepts; and daily planning. Within each domain, specific functional behaviors are rated on a seven-point scale of independence, ranging from ability to perform the activity fully independently, through five levels of "does with" varying degrees of assistance, to unable to perform the activity at all.

Recommended Instrument Use: Practice Option

ASHA-FACS was designed for clinicians to rate functional communication behaviors of adults with speech, language, and cognitive-communication disorders resulting from left hemisphere stroke and from TBI. It is designed to measure at the level of disability, consistent with the World Health Organization's international classification scheme. The design of the ASHA-FACS was based on a definition of functional communication formulated in 1990 by an ASHA advisory group, stated as "the ability to receive or to convey a message, regardless of the mode, to communicate effectively and independently in natural environments."[124(p2)]

In a review of the evidence leading to recommended best practices for assessing individuals with cognitive-communication disorders after TBI (including c/mTBI), the ASHA-FACS was one of a few standardized, norm-referenced tests that met most established criteria for validity and reliability for use with this clinical population.[10] It was 1 of only 4 of the 31 tests reviewed that evaluated performance outside clinical settings. It was unique in that it was based on research about daily communication needs in the target population and incorporated consumer feedback about ecological validity into the design.

EXHIBIT 7-15

AMERICAN SPEECH LANGUAGE AND HEARING ASSOCIATION FUNCTIONAL ASSESSMENT OF COMMUNICATION SKILLS FOR ADULTS RESOURCE INFORMATION

Developed by Carol Frattali, Audrey Holland, Cynthia Thompson, Cheryl Wohl, and Michelle Ferketic, the American Speech Language and Hearing Association Functional Assessment of Communication Skills for Adults is available from:

> American Speech-Language and Hearing Association
> ASHA Product Sales 426, PO Box 1160
> Rockville, MD 20849
> Phone: 301-296-8590, 888-498-6699
> www.asha.org/shop

Administration Protocol/Equipment/Time

The ASHA-FACS includes a 117-page manual and a CD version, allowing automatic tabulation of incremental client assessments in Microsoft Excel (Microsoft Corporation, Redmond, WA).[124] Also included are a paper-and-pencil version with score summary and profile forms that purchasers can copy, a rating key on a 5-by-7-inch card, and an electronic index of *The International Classification of Diseases, Ninth Revision, Clinical Modification* (ICD-9-CM) codes. The ASHA-FACS requires approximately 20 minutes to administer.

Refer to the test manual for specific descriptions of the domains of communication. Each domain is rated globally on the basis of a scale of qualitative dimensions: adequacy, appropriateness, promptness, and communication sharing. The measure yields domain and dimension mean scores, overall scores, and profiles of both communication independence and qualitative dimensions.

Groups Tested With This Measure

Field-testing included 185 adults: 131 with aphasia from left cerebrovascular accident, 54 with cognitive-communication impairment resulting from TBI. Subjects from three severity groups were tested: mild, moderate, and severe, based on Western Aphasia Battery scores. Ages ranged from 16 to 89 years (133 males, 52 females).[124]

Interpretability

- Norms: Communication independence mean scores by impairment group are available for persons with aphasia and with cognitive-communication impairments. No test norms are available.[124]
- MDC: not available
- Responsiveness estimates: not available

Reliability and Validity Estimates

The usability, sensitivity, reliability, and validity of the ASHA-FACS were demonstrated through two separate pilot tests and one field test.[124]

- Sensitivity and specificity: The ASHA-FACS scale showed good sensitivity (75%) and specificity (82.4%) values.[124]
- Internal consistency: Cronbach's alpha was 0.955; internal consistency indicated that most item scores covered the full seven-point rating scale, showed high cor-

relations between items within assessment domains, were internally consistent with respect to assessment domain, and that all items were measuring the same underlying construct. The data indicated that all domain scores correlated with overall ASHA-FACS scores.[124]

- Interrater reliability: Interrater reliability correlations on the seven assessment domain scores ranged from 0.72 to 0.92. Overall communication independence scores had high interrater agreement (mean correlation was 0.95), as did overall scores (mean correlation was 0.90).[124]
- Intrarater reliability: Intrarater reliability for communication independence mean scores by assessment domain ranged from 0.95 to 0.99, and intrarater reliability of overall communication independence scores was 0.99. Intrarater reliability of qualitative dimension mean scores ranged from 0.94 to 0.99, and 0.99 for the overall qualitative dimension scores.[124]
- Test-Retest reliability: Interclass correlation coefficient was 0.995 (P < 0.001).[124]

Validity Estimates

- Criterion: The ASHA-FACS was moderately correlated with other measures of language and cognitive function, as demonstrated by external criterion measures used with subjects with aphasia and cognitive-communication impairments from TBI. Correlations that were significant at the 0.05 level were as follows:
  - 0.76 between Western Aphasia Battery,[114] Aphasia Quotients, and ASHA-FACS overall scores.
  - 0.82 between the ASHA-FACS and the Functional Independence Measure scales[125]
  - 0.84 between the ASHA-FACS overall scores with the SCATBI[62] severity scores.
  - Nonsignificant correlations were obtained from SCATBI subtest scores and ASHA-FACS domain scores obtained from the mild to moderately impaired TBI group.
- Social validity: Evaluation of social validity indicated high positive correlations between ASHA-FACS overall scores and ratings of overall communication effectiveness by clinicians (r = 0.81).[124]

Selected References

Frattali CM, Thompson CK, Holland AL, Wohl CB, Ferketic MM. *The American Speech-Language-Hearing Association Functional Assessment of Communication Skills for Adults (ASHA FACS)*. Rockville, MD: ASHA; 1995.

Mitrushina MM, Boone KB, Razani J, D'Elia LF. *Handbook of Normative Data for Neuropsychological Assessment*. 2nd ed. New York, NY: Oxford University Press; 2005.

Turkstra LS, Coelho C, Ylvisaker M. The use of standardized tests for individuals with cognitive-communication disorders. *Semin Speech Lang.* Nov 2005;26(4):215–222.

SECTION 2: INTERVENTION

INTRODUCTION

Cognitive rehabilitation is a systematic, functionally oriented therapy program based on assessment and an understanding of a patient's brain-behavioral deficits.[126] The goals of therapeutic interventions for cognitive sequelae of c/mTBI are to enhance the individual's capacity to process and interpret information, foster independence, and improve the individual's ability to function in all aspects of family, work, and community life.[126–129]

A review of the cognitive rehabilitation literature[130] yielded substantial evidence to support interventions for attention, memory, executive function, and social communication skills. Only a few of these interventions have been evaluated empirically for persons with c/mTBI. In fact, few studies have addressed cognitive treatment for individuals with mild injuries.[131] However, severity-of-injury classification does not always correspond to the severity of the deficit requiring rehabilitation, and "a mild TBI can result in mild but very disabling cognitive impairments that interfere with one's ability to participate in society."[131(p261)] While acknowledging the methodological shortcomings of existing studies on the efficacy and effectiveness of cognitive intervention with the c/mTBI population, this should not be interpreted as evidence for the lack of potential meaningful benefit of such treatments.[131,132] Because evidence on combat-related c/mTBI is still emerging, recommendations for cognitive interventions in this section evolved from several sources, including literature reviews that encompassed mild as well as moderate TBI in persons with injuries incurred in civilian and military settings, and through a consensus process of experienced clinicians working with civilian patients seen in rehabilitation centers as well as SMs and veterans with c/mTBI seen in military treatment facilities, Veterans Administration medical centers, and academic settings.

Cognitive intervention in the Department of Defense and the US Department of Veterans Affairs should address the unique needs of military and veteran populations with reference to returning to duty, school, or work; balancing military and family relationships; and readjusting to civilian life (see Chapter 9, Performance and Self-Management, Work, Social, and School Roles), and should consider the risk for posttraumatic stress and other comorbidities, including pain, headache, irritability, sleep disturbances, and poor anger management.[132] The overwhelming majority of people who sustain c/mTBI recover fully in a matter of days to months.[133–135] Some, however, may develop chronic neuropsychological problems and functional disability and require intervention.[4,136] The presence of comorbidities, such as PTSD, is a significant predictor of physical, cognitive, and emotional symptoms following deployment, including symptoms associated with c/mTBI.[137,138] Pain and sleep disorders may also challenge an individual's cognitive abilities and complicate the treatment process; therefore, caution must be exercised when attributing cognitive difficulties to a specific etiology, such as c/mTBI.

An interdisciplinary team approach reduces the risk of missing potential complicating factors that may negatively influence rehabilitation outcomes. Members of the team, including OTs, SLPs, and neuropsychologists, have complementary roles in cognitive intervention,[4] and many professional disciplines contribute to the cognitive rehabilitation literature. Consistent with the interdisciplinary nature of cognitive rehabilitation, clinicians from different disciplines will likely develop common strategies with the patients they serve and reinforce the use of those strategies in their own practices. In general, cognitive rehabilitation helps patients with c/mTBI develop improved understanding of the factors contributing to their performance problems, along with strategies and life-management skills necessary to optimize execution of everyday activities. Cognitive rehabilitation comprises these components:

- **Patient education**. Important components include instruction in the core concepts related to thinking skills. SMs with cognitive complaints benefit from an understanding of their own thinking strategies, situations where breakdowns or inefficiencies occur, and ways to emphasize and use personal strengths.
- **Strategy identification and skill development**. As patients begin to understand their personal cognitive vulnerabilities, opportunities are provided to collaborate with a clinician to identify compensatory strategies compatible with their roles and responsibilities, personality, and preferences. SMs then learn how to use these strategies in personally relevant activities.
- **Skill transfer and habit formation**. Once patients are proficient with the strategies and skills necessary to compensate for cognitive inefficiencies, the clinician encourages and reinforces their use to create habits that support productivity and optimal quality of life.

OVERVIEW OF COGNITIVE REHABILITATION

Cognitive rehabilitation may focus on attention, concentration, speed of processing, perception, memory, auditory and reading comprehension, communication, reasoning, problem solving, judgment, initiation, planning, and self-monitoring. Specific interventions may be directed at the following:

- reinforcing, strengthening, or reestablishing previously learned patterns of behavior,
- establishing new patterns of cognition

through compensatory mechanisms for impaired neurologic systems, and
- enabling patients to adapt to their cognitive disability to improve their overall functioning and quality of life.[126]

A paradigm shift has occurred in cognitive therapy. Traditionally, exercises and mass learning trials were used to restore cognitive processes. The focus has now shifted to a contextualized paradigm with patient-centered needs that allows evaluation and therapy to be functional and naturalistic. This paradigm examines the support available in the patient's personal interactions and communication environments.[139]

Training and education in the use of compensatory strategies has been shown to be effective in decreasing the functional impact of cognitive impairments.[128,140] Metacognitive strategy instruction involves systematic, step-by-step procedures that focus on formulating goals, self-monitoring and comparing performance with goals or outcomes, making strategy decisions based on the performance–goal comparison (ie, adjusting the plan based on feedback to achieve the desired goal), and implementing the change in behavior (ie, executing alternative solution).[141]

Although directly aimed at improving cognitive and psychosocial functioning, cognitive rehabilitation may indirectly result in enhanced overall functioning. For example, improvement in memory may facilitate compliance with a medication regimen, improvement in attention and auditory and reading comprehension may increase understanding of instructions from healthcare providers, and improvement in executive function may foster better decision-making with respect to treatment options.[129]

INTERVENTION METHODS

Cognitive rehabilitation is grounded in scientific evidence, including theoretical foundations of brain-behavior relationships, cognition, communication, neuroplasticity, learning theories, behavioral modification, and counseling. Neuroplasticity refers to the adaptive capacity of the nervous system and the mechanism by which the brain encodes experience and learns new behavior, and relearns lost behavior in response to environmental demands and rehabilitation.[142] Instructional practices that enhance neuroplasticity include providing intensive, repetitive practice of functional targets with careful consideration of salience, potential for generalization, and personal factors.[143]

At present, there are no empirically supported cognitive rehabilitation practices specific to c/mTBI. The cognitive rehabilitation practices described herein are based on the broader cognitive rehabilitation literature derived from research on individuals with moderate to severe TBI.

CLINICIAN TIP SHEET: PRINCIPLES OF COGNITIVE REHABILITATION

The following is a practice summary for cognitive rehabilitation.

- Positive expectations for recovery should be emphasized by providing education regarding the natural course of c/mTBI and using risk-communication strategies that highlight the patient's strengths and abilities and demonstrate the improvements that occur during the treatment course.[144]

- During the intervention process, clinicians help patients better understand and manage the influence of various factors on their cognitive performance. The term "awareness" in this context refers to self-understanding; it does **not** describe impaired self-awareness that is associated with brain impairment found in moderate to severe TBI.

- Intervention programs should be based on results of thorough individualized assessments to identify cognitive strengths and weaknesses and changes in cognitive function following c/mTBI.[126,143,144]

- Rehabilitation plans should be developed with consideration for the timeframe available, realistic discharge criteria, and skills and abilities that the patient brings to the rehabilitation process.

- Therapeutic intervention should focus on retraining previously learned skills, reinforcing strengths, teaching compensatory strategies, developing functional skills, modifying the environment, and increasing self-awareness to facilitate successful adaptation or adjustment.[126,143]

- Rehabilitation of cognitive processes and functional skills should be combined to facilitate application of compensatory strategies to real-life situations.[145] Treatment should be embedded in meaningful contexts and individualized to fulfill the unique needs of each patient and ensure ecological validity and generalizability from controlled situations in therapy to natural environments in daily routines.[127,143]

- Clinicians should be systematic in their treatment planning and should realize that every patient learns differently and requires individually tailored instructions or strategies.[146] Methods involved in selecting instructional targets and presenting and reinforcing target information can facilitate learning and directly influence learner outcomes.[143]
- Group intervention should be considered throughout the rehabilitation process when appropriate and available.[4]
- Involvement of significant others is highly encouraged, and community activities and vocational trials should be incorporated when appropriate to promote generalization.[4,127,129]
- Comorbidities should be addressed, as appropriate, to optimize recovery and rehabilitation.[4,132,134]

COGNITIVE INTERVENTION TECHNIQUES TO PROMOTE PATIENT ENGAGEMENT, AWARENESS, AND LEARNING

Purpose/Background

Cognitive intervention after c/mTBI largely involves helping the patient understand his or her cognitive vulnerabilities, then learn and employ appropriate and effective strategies for managing information in everyday life. The extent to which patients actually learn new approaches and adhere to recommendations will be determined, in part, by clinicians' effectiveness as teachers and in engaging patients in the process of learning and behavior change. Intervention will be optimally effective if:

- patients decide to make changes, such as using a memory aid, because they believe that doing so will enable them to meet their own goals; and
- patients understand why a cognitive strategy is being recommended, how to use the strategy correctly, develop effective skills in employing the strategy, and have ample opportunity and reinforcement to repeatedly practice the new skill or strategy in the context of personally relevant, real-life tasks.

Strength of Recommendation: Practice Option

Use of motivational interviewing and experiential learning methods have not been empirically evaluated in patients who have c/mTBI. However, these methods are recommended by clinicians with expertise in cognitive rehabilitation after c/mTBI.

Intervention Methods (Select From the Following Options as Relevant to the Patient)

- Use motivational interviewing[147] so the patient assumes responsibility for the learning and change process. See the clinician tip sheet on motivational interviewing for information about how to use this technique to promote patient engagement in behavior change.
- Provide education about the role of self-awareness in the therapy process, using the awareness hierarchy proposed by Crosson and colleagues.[148] Awareness in this context refers to having an understanding of factors that influence cognitive performance (rather than awareness deficits associated with brain impairment in moderate or severe TBI; see Patient Handout: Change Begins with Awareness).
- Incorporate self-reflection into intervention when patients are practicing newly learned compensatory cognitive strategies (see Clinician Tip Sheet: AAA Self-Reflection).
- Employ training methods in therapy so the patient has both factual and experiential knowledge regarding when and how to use cognitive compensatory strategies (see Clinician Tip Sheet: Methods to Promote Compensatory Cognitive Strategy Learning).
- Help patients identify core cognitive compensatory strategies that improve performance in an array of everyday activities (see Clinician Tip Sheet: Core Cognitive Strategy Recommendations Grid).

CLINICIAN TIP SHEET: MOTIVATIONAL INTERVIEWING

Motivational interviewing refers to the therapeutic style of interacting with patients that has a clear goal of eliciting self-motivating statements and behavioral changes. The clinician provides nonconfrontational feedback about the degree and type of inefficiency that has been noted from interview, structured assessment, and objective observation (Exhibit 7-16).

223

EXHIBIT 7-16

MOTIVATIONAL INTERVIEWING

Using motivational interviewing during therapy sessions enables the clinician to work **with** a patient rather than work **on** a patient. By guiding patients and helping them identify the areas they wish to change and the methods that work for them, the ideas become their own and change becomes more readily accepted.

Background

This approach was developed for individuals with chemical dependency issues. There is a complete guide available free of charge, Treatment Improvement Protocols #35 (order by calling the National Clearing House for Alcohol and Drug Information at 800-729-6686 or 301-468-2600).

The clinician who uses these techniques is able to:

- express empathy through reflective listening;
- communicate acceptance and respect for the patient's perspective;
- establish a nonjudgmental collaborative relationship;
- be a supportive and knowledgeable consultant;
- compliment rather than denigrate;
- listen rather than tell;
- gently persuade, understanding that change is up to the patient;
- provide support through the process of change;
- develop discrepancy between patient goals and values and current behavior;
- help patients recognize the discrepancy between current abilities and future goals;
- avoid arguments or direct confrontation;
- adjust to rather than oppose resistance; and
- support self-efficacy and focus on strengths and hope.

Six strategies that help achieve these goals include:

1. **Ask open-ended questions** (questions that cannot be answered with one word or single phrases). For example: "Tell me about some strategies you are currently using or have tried in the past to help you deal with the memory changes you are describing," rather than: "Are you using a calendar system?"
2. **Listen reflectively**. Demonstrate that you have heard and understood the patient by reflecting what the patient said. For example: "It sounds like the calendar system you are using has helped you avoid missing appointments."
3. **Summarize**. It is useful to periodically summarize what has transpired up to a certain point in treatment. For example: "It sounds to me like your memory errors are really frustrating for you. It also sounds like you have found some ways to decrease that frustration by using your calendar."
4. **Affirm**. Support and comment on the patient's strengths, motivation, intentions, and progress. For example: "The self-discipline you are using to write up a plan each day in your calendar before you leave home is really going to serve you well as you continue to recover and adjust."
5. **Elicit self-motivational statements**. Have the patient voice personal concerns and intentions, rather than try to persuade the patient that change is necessary. For example:

Clinician: "Describe for me the biggest frustration or concern that you are encountering with your memory."
Patient: "I am often late for things because I look at my book in the morning but can lose track of time or forget about my afternoon appointments.

EXHIBIT 7-17

FRAMES ACRONYM FOR MOTIVATIONAL INTERVIEWING

Feedback: Reflect your observations of inefficiency in a respectful manner.

Responsibility: Place responsibility for change squarely on the patient. Help the patient identify areas for change and investigate the methods that could help with that process.

Advice: Give advice in a non-judgmental manner.

Menus: Provide self-directed change options.

Empathy: Show genuine warmth and respect for each patient.

Self-Efficacy: Help the patient develop optimistic empowerment.

I was never late before this injury."
Clinician: "It sounds like being late for things is really frustrating for you."
Patient: "It is embarrassing. It makes me look irresponsible."
Clinician: "I can understand how looking irresponsible is frustrating."

6. **Ask permission to share your observations and or ideas.** This simple step really creates trust and respect. For example:

"Are you interested in exploring some strategies that could help you manage time and avoid being late?" If the patient indicates that he or she is not interested in your ideas, you may need to move on to other areas of concern that are not as intimidating to the patient.

Use the **FRAMES** acronym to remember how to use motivational interviewing during all therapy assessment and intervention sessions (Exhibit 7-17).

CLINICIAN TIP SHEET: AAA SELF-REFLECTION FORM

Once the patient has identified compensatory cognitive strategies that appear workable, he or she practices using the strategies to perform clinic or real-life tasks. The patient uses the AAA worksheet to reflect on performance, which is the primary benefit of performing the practice tasks (see Patient Handout: AAA Self-Reflection).

"AAA" refers to the three parts of the worksheet:

1. **Anticipation.** The patient fills out the anticipation section **before** he or she performs the task. The patient is

asked to predict performance time, anticipate number of errors, and outline the strategies that he or she intends to use or practice.
2. **Action.** The patient fills out the action section **while** performing the task.
3. **Analysis.** The patient fills out the analysis section **after** performing the task. The patient compares predicted performance to actual performance and generates his or her own feedback, which is more potent than receiving feedback from others.

CLINICIAN TIP SHEET: METHODS TO PROMOTE COMPENSATORY COGNITIVE STRATEGY LEARNING

Background

To learn compensatory cognitive strategies and use them in everyday life, patients need ample opportunities for strategy practice and application. Rather than simply talking with patients about recommended strategies, clinicians should allocate over 60% of the patient's learning and training time to actual practice using the newly learned strategy in the context of real-life tasks.[147] The learning process proceeds as follows:

1. The patient learns factual knowledge about the recommended compensatory cognitive strategy and how to use it (Table 7-1).
2. The patient gains experience using the compensatory cognitive strategy while receiving assistance to use it in increasingly complex and personally relevant activities within therapy sessions and as therapy homework (Exhibit 7-18).

CLINICIAN TIP SHEET: CORE COGNITIVE STRATEGY RECOMMENDATIONS GRID AND WORKING LOG

Purpose/Background

It is imperative that clinicians help patients develop habitual use of a select number of core strategies that can be employed in a variety of life areas, rather than a separate strategy for each unique situation or challenge. If the latter approach is used, the patient becomes overwhelmed and often does not use any compensatory strategies at all. There-

fore, developing an individualized core cognitive strategy recommendations grid is one central goal of a therapy episode of care (see Patient Handout: Core Cognitive Strategy Recommendations Grid). A core cognitive strategy recommendations grid is an individualized summary sheet that lists the primary cognitive compensatory strategies that the patient has selected and successfully employed to address his or her problems of greatest concern.

TABLE 7-1

USING DECLARATIVE AND PROCEDURAL KNOWLEDGE IN STRATEGY TRAINING

Type of Knowledge	Teaching Methods	Clinical Examples
Patient learns **what** to do via interactive discussions with the clinician (declarative knowledge)	Discussion, provision of written materials	Patient and clinician review a handout that describes various internal memory strategies. Patient and clinician discuss ways in which the patient could use an alarm watch for appointment reminders.
Patient learns **how** to do it via supervised practice (procedural knowledge)	Demonstration-return demonstration of strategy procedures	Patient practices using PQRST (a memory strategy to recall reading material) during a therapy session. Patient practices setting alarm prompts on the alarm watch.

PQRST: preview, question, read, summary, test

Developing a Core Cognitive Strategies Recommendations Grid

1. During the assessment process, the patient identifies his or her most concerning areas of functioning; the clinician and patient jointly determine which problem area to tackle first in therapy. The top areas of concern are listed in the "problem area" column of the working log (see Patient Handout: Working Log).
2. The clinician keeps track of the specific compensatory strategies that the patient employs to address the problem areas he or she has identified. Additionally, the clinician indicates whether or not, once employed, the strategy effectively helped improve the patient's performance. The recommended strategy is listed adjoining the related problem area. Once the patient has actually used the strategy (either in the clinical or home setting), its effectiveness is rated. Less-than-optimal strategies are refined, logged, and again evaluated for effectiveness.
3. The clinician refers to the lists of compensatory cognitive strategies described in the Attention, Memory, and Executive Function sections of the Toolkit for ideas about what to recommend to the patient.
4. The clinician will initially use the working log to track the areas addressed in treatment and the strategies being considered.
5. Over the episode of care, patterns of key compensatory cognitive strategies (core strategies) will be evident; these are the strategies that the patient has successfully employed to improve performance associated with a number of problem areas.

EXHIBIT 7-18

USING CONTEXTUAL KNOWLEDGE IN STRATEGY TRAINING

Type of Knowledge	Teaching Method	Clinical Examples
Patient learns **when** to use the strategy in real-life situations (contextual knowledge)	Strategy refinement and practice in the context of work simulations, personally relevant tasks	• Patient uses the PQRST every day when reading the newspaper. • Patient sets up alarm prompts on an alarm watch specific to his/her medication regimen. • Patient practices using note-taking strategies to learn a new task at work.

PQRST: preview, question, read, summary, test

6. As the therapy midpoint approaches, the patient and clinician collaborate to create the core cognitive strategy recommendations grid. The grid is finalized at discharge from therapy.

Benefits of the Core Strategies Grid

The process of developing a core strategies grid advances patient ownership of the strategies during treatment and at the discharge session. For successful use after intervention, it is very important that patients take the thinking options and strategies that have been covered in treatment and make them their own. The working log can be completed at multiple junctures in treatment to reinforce the importance of these strategies; the core recommendations form should be assembled with the patient at his or her last session.

Patients can refer to the grid when they need to get back on track. It is not uncommon for patients to quit using strategies when their lives become easier to manage. However, at times when personal factors are no longer being managed and a patient's situational demands have changed, he or she may need to review the list and reestablish strategy use. Sometimes previous strategies may not be adequate due to promotion or family changes, and the patient can be counseled to come back for another episode of care.

If patients return for follow-up care, the grid helps remind clinicians of what was effective for specific individuals. If patients contact the clinician with questions or are scheduled to come back for a follow-up session, the grid is an excellent tool to determine what strategies should be reemployed and what areas need further exploration. This tool can result in more effective follow-ups.

COGNITION EDUCATION

Purpose/Background

Experts recommend the provision of verbal and written educational information about c/mTBI symptoms (eg, headache, difficulties with memory or attention) as well as reassurance that these are likely to recover over a period of weeks or a few months.[149–151] As people are helped to understand their symptoms, they are less likely to overreact to them or misattribute them to significant brain damage.[151] By explaining normal cognition and the impact of c/mTBI on cognition, clinicians help patients understand why errors occur and thus help them avoid declines in self-efficacy that can be caused by misattributing errors to significant brain damage. Also, postconcussion syndrome may be averted or ameliorated because people with c/mTBI learn to appreciate how personal and situational factors may interact with typically transient symptoms of brain injury[152] and implement cognitive compensatory strategies that optimize effectiveness.

As well, information provided to the individual's support system (eg, spouse, family members, friends) is a critical aspect of intervention.[153] Although some patients may respond to self-guided education and access to the correct information about c/mTBI recovery, others will require a structured educational program that is clinician-guided and individualized, particularly those patients with prolonged exposure to untreated cognitive and emotional symptoms.

Intervention will be optimally effective in this realm if education efforts involve a two-way discussion rather than a formal lecture and topics are discussed if and when relevant to patients. Components of a structured patient education program about c/mTBI and its effect on cognition include discussion of:

- common specific and nonspecific symptoms and potential effects on social, work, school, and family interactions;
- common comorbidities and related disorders, such as anxiety, pain, PTSD, sleep difficulties, and depression;
- the overlap in symptoms between c/mTBI and other problems (eg, irritability, anxiety, attention deficit disorder, sleep disturbances); and
- the normal recovery pattern from c/mTBI and the expectation of full recovery within 3 months for most individuals.[150,151]

Strength of Recommendation: Practice Standard

Although there is no specific protocol for cognition education that has been studied empirically, the practice of providing education after c/mTBI is supported by evidence.[150,151,154]

Intervention Methods

- Provide information about c/mTBI educational resources, including websites.
- Provide education regarding human

information processing (see Clinician Tip Sheet: How to Explain Human Information Processing).

- Provide information about the multifactor model to explain performance declines after c/mTBI (see clinician tip sheet and related patient handout).

Educational Resources

Recognized and reputable websites should be provided to direct the patient to accurate information about c/mTBI. Appropriate resources can guide the individual away from inaccurate or alarming information about moderate to severe TBI, and can provide an excellent framework for education, access to interactive brain anatomy videos, and additional handouts and personal success stories that reinforce the expectation of recovery.

Support and educational groups developed specifically for those recovering from c/mTBI can also provide an excellent setting for education in a peer-supported environment. These groups may help remove the focus on self and the individual experience of impairments while reinforcing the concepts of normalization and that "you are not alone."

National Resources

- Department of Veterans Affairs/Department of Defense Evidence-Based Guideline: Evaluation and Management of Concussion/mTBI—Subacute/Chronic: http://www.healthquality.va.gov/mtbi/concussion_mtbi_full_1_0.pdf
- DCoE Summary Fact Sheets: http://www.dcoe.health.mil/ForHealthPros.aspx.

- Defense and Veterans Brain Injury Center patient education materials, which include topics such as mood changes, headache management, healthy sleep, improving memory, c/mTBI information at the time of injury (acute), c/mTBI information for use more than 1 month after injury or at postdeployment health assessment (not for acute period concussion), 10 ways to improve your memory, TBI and mood changes, rehabilitation for healthy sleep, headache and neck pain, and head injury and dizziness: www.dvbic.org.
- Brain Injury Association: www.biausa.org.
- American Veterans With Brain Injury: www.avbi.org.
- Department of Veterans Affairs, National Center for PTSD: www.ptsd.va.gov.
- The Journey Home–the CEMM Traumatic Brain Injury website: www.traumaticbrain-injuryatoz.org.
- Rehabilitation and Reintegration Division, Office of the Surgeon General, US Army: www.armymedicine.army.mil/prr/edtraining.html.
- Michigan TBI Services and Prevention Council: www.michigan.gov/documents/mdch/TBI_Recovery_Guide_10.8.08_252053_7.pdf.

Local Resources

Local resources include area support groups and organizations. The National Brain Injury Association website provides links to local resources by state. Regional, state, and city-specific organizations and healthcare facilities may provide additional information regarding available local resources.

CLINICIAN TIP SHEET: HOW TO EXPLAIN HUMAN INFORMATION PROCESSING

Purpose/Description

This information helps the patient understand normal cognition and how cognitive compensatory strategies may improve performance after c/mTBI (see Patient Handout: How to Explain Human Information Processing). Although some aspects of how people remember new information remain unknown, it is generally believed to be a multistage process referred to as "human information processing." One explanation as to how this takes place is based on the work of Atkinson and Shiffrin.[155]

Human information processing is thought to

involve three components: (1) short-term sensory register, (2) short-term (working) memory, and (3) long-term memory. Information from the environment comes into the human information processing system through the senses (seeing, hearing, smelling, etc). Sensory data are held briefly in a series of short-term registers associated with the sensory systems involved in the incoming information. Short-term sensory registers have a large capacity; data are automatically advanced to short-term memory storage after a few seconds without any effort or awareness on our part. It is important to note that people's ability to remember information is in part based on accurate information coming in through the senses; therefore, people can optimize memory performance by wearing glasses or using hearing aids, if needed.

From the sensory registers, data are held in short-term memory, which is sometimes referred to as "working memory." This component is associated with concentration, paying attention, and conscious mental effort. Whereas the short-term sensory registers can hold large amounts of data, people can concentrate on or pay attention to only a finite number of things at once; on average and under normal circumstances, people can simultaneously pay attention to between five and nine things at a conscious or semiconscious level (imagine pots on stovetop burners; see handout).[156] To remember new input (ie, get it stored in long-term memory), a person needs to consciously "simmer" or attend to the idea, name, or action item for 15 to 30 seconds. If that does not occur or if all the available "burners" are full with other thoughts, the input falls out of the system and is not stored in long-term memory.

To remember new information, a person has to be awake, alert, and ready to pay attention. Therefore, patients can optimize their memory by managing sleep, fatigue, and pain; avoiding alcohol; and working with their doctor to optimize medications. Additionally, for an individual to remember new or incoming information, he or she must focus attention on the thought for approximately half a minute for it to "stick" (ie, be encoded and move from working memory to long-term memory for storage and retrieval).

People may use internal memory strategies to help them actively encode the new, incoming information. Anything that a person is paying attention to (pain, distractions in the environment, worries, intrusive thoughts, hypervigilance) takes up space in working memory. If people have a lot on their minds, they will be vulnerable to forgetting new, incoming information. Most memory failures or inefficiencies (such as forgetting appointments, forgetting things to do, coming into a room and forgetting why, forgetting what was said in a conversation) can be explained by problems associated with working memory; that is, people do not pay attention long enough for the information to get stored in long-term memory.

Most experts believe all the information we have learned is stored in our long-term memory. This includes something as recent as the name of a person you just met to the name of your third grade teacher. Long-term memory storage has an infinite capacity and stores newly learned information (ie, what we learned moments ago) as well as what we learned in the distant past. Information is thought to be stored in related groups that are linked in a network to other groups of information.

Here's a snapshot of how working memory and long-term memory work together. Imagine you are fixing a leaky pipe at home. As you are planning your approach, you think about how you handled the problem the last time. In doing so, working memory sends a request to long-term memory, which kick-starts a search process to locate the needed information. Once found, long-term memory storage sends the information to working memory, where it takes space on a "burner" as you think about it and plan your next steps. Most people with c/mTBI do not have difficulty with long-term memory; once the information is stored, they are able to retrieve it as well as everybody else.

Many people use external memory aids, such as planners or smartphones, to help them manage information. Doing so allows them to offload incoming information from working memory (including appointments, chores, and errands), remain confident that they have a back-up, and keep limited-capacity working memory resources available for attending to other incoming information or to the task at hand.

Implications for Concussion/Mild Traumatic Brain Injury

After c/mTBI, people may have a variety of distracting physical symptoms (eg, dizziness, headache, musculoskeletal pain, hearing and visual problems). These distractions take up space in the thinking process, using up some of their five to nine "burners." As a result, people with c/mTBI have difficulty remembering information, concentrating, and even problem solving. Stress and worry can have the same effect, taking up mental space that could otherwise be used in the process of remembering information.

Compensatory strategies, like writing things down or placing the information in an electronic device (eg, smartphone) can help patients keep track of necessary information if the burners are full of symptom-related distractions or worries and remain in control of their lives.

IMPROVING ATTENTION AND SPEED OF PROCESSING

Purpose/Background

After c/mTBI, many patients describe difficulty paying attention during tasks and handling all of the distracters in the environment. Many patients also complain of difficulty dividing their attention between tasks. Attention problems may be in part due to slowed information processing speed associated with diffuse axonal injury.[157,158] Sohlberg and Mateer's[159] model of attention includes a hierarchy of subsystems, with divided attention requiring the most mental effort. The integrity of each attention component is dependent on the integrity of those below it. The attention hierarchy is as follows:

- **Divided**: the ability to respond concurrently to multiple tasks or demands.
- **Alternating**: the capacity for mental flexibility to shift attention focus and move between tasks with different cognitive requirements.
- **Selective**: the ability to maintain a behavioral or cognitive set in the context of distracting or competing stimuli.
- **Sustained**: the ability to maintain a consistent response during a continuous and repetitive activity.
- **Focused**: the ability to respond to specific stimuli (auditory, visual, or tactile).

Speed of information processing is the ability to perceive, attend to, organize, analyze, integrate, retain, and apply information in an efficient manner. Slowing of information processing capacity has been shown to have a major impact on various attentional and linguistic processes, such as encoding, verbal comprehension, and adaptive responding to novel situations.[160] The overarching goal of intervention specific to attention and speed of processing is to help patients become more aware of their attentional and processing skills and expand the repertoire of strategies available to manage personal and situational factors. Intervention in this realm takes the patient through the "TEST" process:

- **T**hinking options. Clinicians provide patient education regarding the hierarchy of attentional skills and the impact of personal and situational factors. This information helps patients understand and reframe attention and problems related to speed-of-processing performance and identify options to better manage demands.
- **E**xperiencing attention demands. After providing education about the attention hierarchy and the influence of personal and situational factors, clinicians structure activities in which the patients can experience increasing attentional demands. Experiencing the demands of each level of the hierarchy with clinician feedback helps patients make a personal connection to the education.
- **S**trategy choice. Once areas of inefficiency are observed (via assessment or structured attentional tasks), the clinician helps patients choose individual strategies that will optimize their ability to manage attentional and speed-of-processing demands.
- **T**ransferring strategy use to the real world. Through a combination of clinical tasks and real-world experiences, the clinician helps patients develop habitual use of the strategies they have learned.

Strength of Recommendation: Practice Standard

Evidence-based reviews conducted by the Brain Injury Interdisciplinary Special Interest Group of the American Congress of Rehabilitation Medicine recommends attention treatment with direct and metacognitive training to promote compensatory strategy development and foster generalization to real-world tasks during the post-acute recovery from mild or moderate TBI. Repeated use of computer-based tasks without intervention by a clinician is not recommended.[130]

Intervention Methods

- Provide patient education regarding attention (see Patient Handout: Understanding Hierarchy of Attention Levels). Help the patient describe his or her cognitive difficulties and realize related demands (see Clinician Tip Sheet: Inventory of Attention/Speed-of-Processing Difficulties).
- Help the patient experience and assess performance associated with various levels of attentional demand (see Clinician Tip Sheet: Experiencing Attention Levels).
- Help the patient identify strategies that pertain to his or her key tasks and preferences (see Clinician Tip Sheet: Menu of Strategies to Cope With Attention and Speed-of-Processing Difficulties).
- Create opportunities for the patient to practice strategies and employ training methods in therapy.

CLINICIAN TIP SHEET: INVENTORY OF ATTENTION/SPEED-OF-PROCESSING DIFFICULTIES

Purpose/Description

- Provides a structured and systematic method for gathering information concerning the patient's cognitive difficulties and related demands to gain an understanding of his or her needs, challenges, and awareness of personal and situational factors (see Patient Handout: Inventory of Attention/ Speed of Processing Difficulties).
- Records baseline data to develop functional goals and assess patient's progress.
- Serves as a reference for metacognitive strategy training. Clinician guides discussion to help the patient identify personal and situational factors that can increase or decrease challenges to attention and speed of processing.

Protocol

- Review Patient Handout: Change Begins with Awareness. Have the patient fill out the worksheet considering the following information (assist patient as needed).

- Use motivational interviewing during a guided discussion to help the patient focus on the symptoms and problems, and describe his or her difficulties in specific settings, such as home, work, or school.
- Probe for information, particularly factors that can enhance or interfere with performance, for example:
  - task length;
  - other tasks involved that require shifting or sharing attention;
  - personal factors, such as energy level, stress, mood, comfort, interest, intrusive thoughts, and vigilance;
  - environmental factors (ie, noise, lighting, crowds);
  - rate of incoming information and urgency to process and respond to information (for example, the patient may judge self-paced reading as slow or average, or note-taking in a college course as fast); and
  - strategies that the patient may already be using to cope with difficulties.

CLINICIAN TIP SHEET: EXPERIENCING ATTENTION LEVELS

Purpose/Description

The experiential attention activities are designed to help patients understand firsthand the hierarchical levels of attention. Use the following:

- Patient Handout: Experiencing Attention Levels–Focused and Sustained
- Patient Handout: Experiencing Attention Levels–Selective Attention (Visual and Auditory)
- Patient Handout: Experiencing Attention Levels–Alternating and Divided

This knowledge is geared toward helping patients identify compensatory strategies that optimize their ability to manage various attentional demands and to help them appreciate the importance of managing personal and situational factors.

The attentional activities also provide the clinician with opportunities to observe how the patient manages different levels of attention-based demands, including the following:

- The extent to which the patient modified his or her speed of work to assure accuracy based on the attentional demands of the task.
- The extent to which the patient organized his or her approach to the task, especially those tasks that require systematic scanning.
- The extent to which the patient appeared to employ strategies to optimize his or her ability to attend to the task.

Instructions to Give Patients

- Remind patients that part of your job is to help them increase their awareness, not only of their skill level but of how that interacts with their management of factors that affect their attention (such as fatigue, pain, stress, and negative thoughts).
- Ask permission to share your observations of their performance on the tasks.

Using the Hierarchical Attention Tasks

- Each attention level has an experiential component.
- All the tasks contain self-prediction and self-reflection questions; each takes between 5 to 15 minutes to complete.
- For the patient to experience all attention

levels, you will need the patient worksheet, a radio, a deck of cards, and a pen.

These activities offer the most potential benefit when combined with clinician observation and reflective postperformance dialogue between clinician and patient. However, the activities could be assigned as homework, with patient-therapist reflection on performance at a subsequent session.

CLINICIAN TIP SHEET: OVERVIEW OF STRATEGIES TO COPE WITH ATTENTION AND SPEED-OF-PROCESSING DIFFICULTIES

Purpose/Description

The primary aim of therapy is to help patients identify and implement strategies that relate to areas of weakness, capitalize on preferences and strengths, and are efficient and effective in real-life contexts (eg, environment, people, situations). The strategies presented in this section serve as a springboard and guide for selecting, modifying, and adding strategies to suit patients' individual needs. The strategies include the following:

- optimizing personal factors,
- managing high- and low-demand tasks,
- effectively allocating cognitive resources,
- managing interruptions and multiple tasks, and
- providing strategies for using auditory and visual systems.

Optimizing Personal Factors

Personal factors that may contribute to cognitive performance are identified during review of patient's medical and social history, observed during experiential tasks, or reported by the patient. Help the patient learn to manage these factors to optimize function (see Patient Handout: Understanding the Multifactor Model of Functioning After Concussion). Patients should be advised to talk to their physicians about persistent problems with pain, energy, or sleep and work with a psychologist or psychiatrist to manage stress and negative thoughts. Patients should check with their physicians or psychiatrists regarding current medications that may be sedating. While it may not be possible to substitute or avoid sedating medications, discussing their effects with the patient can reduce misattribution of cognitive symptoms to c/mTBI. Refer to *Co-occurring Conditions Toolkit: Mild Traumatic Brain Injury and Psychological Health,* available from the DCoE website, for a list of medications and their

effects.[161] Clinical experience in treating patients suggests that a comprehensive, holistic approach that integrates treatment of cognitive, emotional, and interpersonal skills is a best-practice model for the rehabilitation of c/mTBI sequelae.

Managing High- and Low-Demand Tasks

Patients will be most successful at managing attention limitations if they can decide which tasks to perform at any given time, based on the demands of the environment and circumstances (see Clinician Tip Sheet: Strategies to Improve Attention).

Effectively Allocating Cognitive Resources

Many theories support the notion that attention is a limited resource.[162,163] One relatively simple strategy is to eliminate or reduce demands that compete for attentional resources and compromise goal-oriented behaviors (see Patient Handout: Modifying Your Approach and Work Space).

Select a task identified by the patient as difficult on the Inventory of Attention and Speed-of-Processing Difficulties handout. Engage the patient in guided discussion and metacognitive training to select appropriate strategies that:

- relate to specific weakness. The patient's postperformance reflections on the Experiencing Attention Levels handout and activities may be used to steer the patient in strategy selection based on demands that be counterproductive.
- can be realistically eliminated or reduced in real-life settings.

Managing Interruptions and Multiple Tasks

Refer to Patient Handout: Strategies to Improve Attention–Managing Interruptions and Multiple Tasks.

Providing Strategies for Using Auditory and Visual Systems

Intervention should focus on reducing the presence of functional limitations caused by difficulties with informational processing to reduce the severity and duration of the symptom as well as any associated anxiety (see the handouts Coping with Slower Speed of Processing–Using the Auditory System, and Coping with Slower Speed of Processing–Using the Visual System).

CLINICIAN TIP SHEET: STRATEGIES TO IMPROVE ATTENTION–IDENTIFYING HIGH- AND LOW-DEMAND TASKS

Purpose/Description

Patients will be most successful at managing attention limitations if they can decide which tasks to perform at any given time, based on the demands of the environment and circumstances. The associated Strategies to Improve Attention–Identifying High- and Low-Demand Tasks, is designed to help patients analyze their everyday tasks and their own abilities to identify high- and low-demand tasks.

Step 1: Task Analysis

Patient lists the key tasks for which he or she is responsible. The patient then rates the consequence level of these tasks.

Step 2: Self-Analysis

Patient rates how easy or difficult these tasks are to perform at present. Tasks may be deemed difficult because of a cognitive or physical challenge.

Step 3: Identifying High- and Low-Demand Tasks

Patient reviews his or her self-ratings and lists those tasks that are rated as high consequence and difficult (high-demand tasks) and those that are low consequence and easy (low-demand tasks).

The clinician's job is to help patients understand that they can enhance their skill level and productivity by choosing the time of day, environments, and tasks they are engaging in. This strategy improves consistency of performance and, therefore, self-confidence.

High-demand tasks:
- should be performed at the patient's best time of day,
- should be performed in the quietest possible environment possible, and
- should be performed when there will be minimal interruption (eg, completing financial reports at work before others arrive or setting up medication boxes for the week when rested and while family members are in another room).

Low-demand tasks:
- may be performed when the patient is fatigued,
- may be performed when the patient is not able to control the environment, and
- may be performed when the patient anticipates lots of interruptions (eg, folding laundry while watching television; sorting and recycling papers, cans, bottles; shoveling, weeding, sweeping; performing aerobic exercises, like walking or jogging; and vacuuming or loading the dishwasher).

CLINICIAN TIP SHEET: MENU OF STRATEGIES BASED ON ATTENTION HIERARCHY

The primary aim of therapy is to help the patient identify and implement three to five attentional strategies that match his or her problematic tasks and preferences. Using the patient handouts and Table 7-2, the clinician guides the patient toward the specific strategies that hold the most promise in improving performance.

CLINICIAN TIP SHEET: PRACTICE TASKS FOR ATTENTION STRATEGY REHEARSAL AND TRANSFER

Purpose/Background

Once patients understand the factors that influence their attentional abilities and have identified cognitive compensatory strategies, they need to practice preferred compensatory cognitive strategies in the context of clinic and real-life tasks. As discussed earlier, simply talking about a potentially

TABLE 7-2

POSSIBLE STRATEGIES BASED ON PATIENTS' VULNERABILITIES ASSOCIATED WITH SPECIFIC LEVELS OF ATTENTION

Level of Attention	Strategy Options
Focused attention	Check with physician or psychologist on current medications, and: • avoid sedating medications, • consider stimulants such as coffee, colas, or tea, if not contraindicated. Take frequent breaks. Schedule higher consequence tasks when most alert. Use external cues to stay on task, such as: • alarms on cell phones or other devices to initiate a task, and • timers set for certain durations to stay on task. Use pause cues.
Sustained attention	Take frequent breaks. Schedule higher consequence tasks when most alert. Use external cues to stay on task, such as: • alarms on cell phones or other devices to initiate a task, and • timers set for certain durations to stay on task. Use pause cues. Allow extra time for tasks.
Selective attention	Control environmental distractions when able; for example: • run errands or tend to social activities at nonpeak hours, • choose to sit in an area with the least number of distractions (corner booth by the wall, etc), • use a personal music player to cancel out background noises, when appropriate. Rest prior to demanding situations. Take frequent breaks. Politely ask others not to visit with you while you are working.
Alternating attention	Control environmental distractions. Take frequent breaks. Use stop notes, including: • cues in your environment that show you where you left off, and • notes that indicate what you did last and what your next thought or action was or would be. Alternate attention between tasks that are high-consequence or difficult and those that are not. Allow phone calls to go to voicemail and address them later. Do not answer people until you have reached a stop point in your work. Politely ask others not to visit with you while you are working. Rest prior to demanding situations. Take frequent breaks. Use alarms to decrease the need to watch the clock.
Divided attention	Do not divide attention on high consequence and difficult tasks. Limit divided attention on high consequence tasks that are easy. Do not talk on a cell phone while driving. Limit conversation while driving. Take frequent breaks. Rest prior to situations that require divided attention. Use alarms to decrease the need to watch the clock.

TABLE 7-3

EXAMPLES OF ATTENTION-RELATED PRACTICE TASKS

Tasks	Description	Vendor/Location
Games for the Brain	Free website that includes 20 games that place various demands on attention.	http://www.gamesforthebrain.com/
Captain's Log	Commercial product that includes 50 multilevel programs and provides more than 2,000 hours of game-like activities.	http://www.braintrain.com/home_users/homeusershome.htm
Mavis Beacon	Software tool that teaches typing skills. It allows the user to build custom lessons, play special typing games, and check the ergonomics.	http://download.cnet.com/Mavis-Beacon-Teaches-Typing-17-Deluxe/3000-2051_4-10441764.html
Brain Bashers	Free website with a collection of brainteasers, puzzles, riddles, games, and optical illusions. BrainBashers is updated with optical illusions and games regularly and has five new puzzles added every other week.	http://www.brainbashers.com/
Freetypinggame.net	30 different typing lessons progressively teach the keyboard. Printable certificates provided on completion. The tests and games have 40 lessons; 10 are based on classic stories to make the typing test more natural. Timed tests of different lengths are available.	http://www.freetypinggame.net/

Technology Tasks	Description	Vendor/Location
Dynavision	Light-training reaction device, developed to train sensory motor integration through the visual system. Challenges individual's ability to take in visual stimuli, process the information, then react to it with a motor response. Originally designed for high-performance athletics and police-military training, it has been used as a rehabilitation training tool for head injuries, visual field deficits, post-stroke recovery, and driver training.	http://www.dynavisiond2.com

Pencil-Paper Tasks	Description	Vendor/Location
Attention-processing training	This comprehensive program helps retrain attention and concentration deficits in adolescents and adults with brain injury. Treatment materials and tasks address five levels of the attention process. Hierarchically organized auditory and visual tasks. Appropriate for patients with attention deficits from mild to severe.	http://www.pearsonassessments.com/HAIWEB/Cultures/en-us/Productdetail
APT-II (also APT-III)	A library of auditory attention compact discs and attention exercises	http://www.pearsonassessments.com/HAIWEB/Cultures/en-us/Productdetail
Brainwave-R	BrainwaveR is a comprehensive pen-and-paper-based cognitive rehabilitation program that is divided into five hierarchically graded modules: attention, visual processing, memory, information processing, and executive functions. The program comprises three components:	http://www.braintreemanagement.co.uk/braintreetraining/bwr.htm

*(**Table 7-3** continues)*

235

Table 7-3 *continued*

1) education—an overview of current theories relevant to rehabilitation that is designed to be used by the clinician with the client and family to ensure good awareness and understanding of the problem area;
2) clinician instructions—rating scales, clinical guidelines, suggestions for how to involve the family, a performance summary chart, and questions to encourage the client to determine the functional relevance of each exercise; and
3) client exercises.

useful strategy does little to improve functioning. Patients need many opportunities for practice during clinic sessions and as part of their therapy homework.

How to Use Attention-Strategy Practice Tasks in Therapy

Use the Patient Handout: AAA Self-Reflection Worksheet for Attention and Speed of Processing.

1. Patient and clinician select a functional, meaningful task based on the attention and speed-of-processing strategies that the patient needs to practice.
2. Anticipation
   - Before the task, the patient completes the "Anticipation" section.
   - The patient is asked to expressly predict performance time, anticipate accuracy, and outline the strategies that he or she intends to use or practice.
3. Action
   - During the activity, the patient fills out the "Action" section.
   - Patient performs the assigned task and self-monitors performance.
   - Clinician observes and assesses performance to provide feedback.
4. Analysis
   - After the activity, the patient fills out the "Analysis" section.
   - The patient and clinician compare predicted performance to actual performance. Through guided discussion, the patient generates his or her own feedback to reinforce strengths and successes and for problem-solving to improve performance, as needed.

Repeat this procedure for other tasks and in different settings to facilitate and assess transfer to everyday and novel activities. Remember that any task can be structured to require attention-strategy practice (Table 7-3); it is the patient's self-reflections and the clinician's guidance and observations that make the task therapeutic. A clinician selects and sets up a practice task to observe all or some of the following:

- How long can the patient sustain his or her attention?
- Does the patient self-initiate breaks?
- Does the patient handle the distracters in the work area?
- Does the patient initiate changing the environmental distracters?
- If the clinician creates interruptions, can the patient manage alternating attention?
- If the clinician creates interruptions, does the patient initiate strategy use?
- If the task requires divided attention, does the patient initiate a strategy to optimize performance?
- How well does the patient use strategies to modify or compensate for slowed speed of processing to optimize accuracy?

Also consider the following activities of daily living (ADLs) and instrumental activities of daily living tasks (IADLs) as practice:

- checkbook (create a checklist of steps),
- medication set-up (creating a grid with name, dosage, description of appearance, reason taken),
- household assembly tasks, and
- driving simulator.

COMPENSATING FOR MEMORY INEFFICIENCIES

Purpose/Background

Decline in memory function is common after c/mTBI and is also associated with postcombat mental health conditions.[164,165] Some people describe decrements in their memory and information processing speed for 3 months or more after c/mTBI.[165] These cognitive symptoms may in part be explained by the brain's limited processing capacity as a person attempts to manage distractions associated with symptom management.[151] Furthermore, multiple concussions can prolong cognitive problems.[166] Before providing intervention for c/mTBI-related memory concerns, clinicians must be well versed in key concepts and terms.

A simple definition for memory is "the ability to take in, store, and retrieve information."[167(p1)] Memory is a complex process that involves perception and attention as well as multiple memory subsystems.[143]

- **Short-term memory** allows people to hold a limited amount of information for a brief length of time. The average person can hold approximately five to seven items in short-term memory in the absence of distractions or interruption.[143,162]
- **Working memory** is similar to short-term memory and allows people to hold information in conscious thought and manipulate that information for storage or retrieval (eg, planning, organizing, sequencing). Working memory provides the mental workspace for temporarily holding onto information while applying strategies during complex activities, such as learning, reasoning, comprehension, and metacognition (ie, reflecting on one's own thinking and making adjustments in the process).
- **Long-term memory** allows people to hold information in a permanent store (ie, minutes to years after initial exposure) and has an unlimited capacity.[143,162] Long-term memory is a more durable system and is typically intact after concussion; however, people with concussion that have problems with short-term memory have difficulty holding information in mind long enough to prepare it for storage into long-term memory.[143] Long-term memory can be divided into two components that differ with regard to types of information stored

and how that information is learned and retrieved: declarative and nondeclarative memory.[143,162]

1. **Declarative memory** encompasses a knowledge base of information and implies conscious awareness and the ability to report something explicitly. It includes two subsystems: episodic and semantic memory. *Episodic memory* is comprised of a person's autobiographical memory or the recall of personal experiences associated with events (eg, birth of a child, wedding anniversary, college graduation). *Semantic memory* is comprised of a person's mental encyclopedia or knowledge base (eg, word meanings, classes of information, facts, ideas). Episodic memory and semantic memory are interdependent when learning and recalling information.[168]

2. **Nondeclarative memory** encompasses the "learning how" portion of skills and is context dependent. It reflects implicit learning through repeated stimulus-response associations and allows a person to learn without having conscious awareness of learning. Nondeclarative memory includes subsystems such as priming and procedural learning. *Priming* refers to the increased probability of producing a response because of previous exposure to or past experiences in producing the response. *Procedural learning* refers to the acquisition of perceptual motor skills or action patterns or sequences (eg, tying shoelaces, learning to program an appointment in an alarm watch).[168]

- **Retrospective memory** refers to memory for the past, including past experiences, actions, and information that we have learned.
- **Prospective memory** refers to memory for things we intend to do in the future, including remembering what we need to do, say to others, or learn.[143]

Memory problems are inconvenient, and they may cause frustration and anxiety. They significantly affect independence, employment, and education.[143] Patients may be unaware of the influence of situational factors on their memory and be unfamiliar with the compensatory strategies that might help.

The overarching goal of therapy specific to memory inefficiencies is to help patients expand their repertoire of strategies in this realm through the TEST process (see above, Cognitive Intervention: Improving Attention and Speed of Processing).

Strength of Recommendation: Practice Standard

Training in the use of memory compensation strategies as applied to real-life tasks is supported by empirical evidence.[126,169] According to the DCoE expert panel, "efficacy has been demonstrated for memory training techniques derived from cognitive neuroscience,"[4(p245)] particularly for patients with c/mTBI and mild memory impairment. Memory strategy training that assists patients in developing techniques to enhance registration and encoding of information and to improve memory retrieval has been shown to be successful. External memory aids in combination with strategy training resulted in improvement that extended into patients' everyday memory function, while repetitive memory drills (eg, memorizing word lists, faces, designs without explicit strategy training) have been shown to have little or no efficacy.[4]

Intervention Methods

Provide patient education regarding human information processing (see Education about Cognition section of the Toolkit).

- Help the patient identify strategies that pertain to his or her key tasks and his or her preferences (see Patient Handout: Compensatory Memory Strategies: Internal and External Options).
- Establish goals and methods for learning new memory strategies (see Clinician Tip sheets: Intervention for Memory Impairment and Training Hierarchy for Memory Strategies, and Defense and Veterans Brain Injury Center Handout, "10 Ways to Improve Your Memory").
- Help patients establish daily and weekly routines for using memory aids (see Patient Handout: Daily and Weekly Planning).
- Help patients keep track of what they read (see Patient Handout: Intentional Reading).
- Create opportunities for the patient to practice strategies in clinic sessions and as homework (see Defense and Veterans Brain Injury Center handout, "10 Ways to Improve Your Memory," and Clinician Tip Sheet: Practice Tasks for Memory Strategy Rehearsal and Transfer).

CLINICIAN TIP SHEET: INTERVENTION FOR MEMORY IMPAIRMENT

The goal of intervention is to decrease demand on impaired memory processes and improve memory function for everyday activities. The following are cognitive rehabilitation principles formulated by Sohlberg and Turkstra[143] applied to memory training:

- During the acquisition phase of training, stimuli and contexts should be as similar as possible to the new behavior, strategy, or task that is being established.
- Do not overload the client with multiple target strategies when initiating training.
- Provide the client with multiple practice sessions with a high number of repetitions of practice trials of a new strategy.
- After initial acquisition, target memory strategies should be practiced with distracters similar to those found in the client's real-life situation.
- Use distributed practice by gradually

lengthening time between probes for new memory strategies.

- Take data to determine the response to intervention and periodically question the client to determine if memory strategies are consistently used in "real-life" situations over time. The client should keep data on the number of times and situations when he or she remembered or forgot to use memory strategies.
- The clinician should help the client develop metacognitive strategies by encouraging self-monitoring and reflection about performance of memory strategies.

Instructional practices that have been experimentally validated and are key to promoting learning for individuals with memory impairments include[146]:

- Provide a clear delineation of targets and

employ task analyses when training multistep procedures.

- Constrain errors and control output while the patient is acquiring new information and procedures.
- Provide sufficient and distributed practice with multiple exemplars and ecologically valid targets.
- Use strategies, such as verbal elaboration and visual imagery, to support more effortful processing.

Structuring or modifying the individual's environment and generating management strategies can be helpful in reducing the load on attention, memory, and organizational abilities. Strategies include[159]:

- organizing and labeling storage cabinets,
- setting up filing systems,
- creating message centers,
- establishing bill payment systems,
- reducing clutter,
- eliminating distractions, and
- posting signs to inform others in the environment about management strategies.

CLINICIAN TIP SHEET: TRAINING HIERARCHY FOR MEMORY STRATEGIES

Learning to use a memory aid (whether low-tech, such as a day planner, or high-tech, such as a personal digital assistant) involves three aspects of training or learning[37]:

- acquisition: learning the skills necessary for using the memory aid (adding appointments, setting alarms, note-taking techniques);

- application: using these skills to perform clinical or practice tasks; and
- adaptation: using skills to perform personally relevant home, work, and community tasks.

These three aspects of learning should be considered in guiding the patient towards his or her ultimate objectives of memory aid use (Tables 7-4 and 7-5).[9]

CLINICIAN TIP SHEET: ELECTRONIC MEMORY AND ORGANIZATION AIDS

Smartphone and Mobile Applications

The use of assistive technology is recommended to compensate for cognitive deficits, including problems with attention, memory, and executive functions that may be associated with c/mTBI and related comorbidities. Smartphones and tablet computers are replacing the calendar and notebook to enhance organizational skills and provide reminders for things such as important events, appointments, tasks, and medications for persons with cognitive impairments. These types of devices are relatively low cost and they are considered fashionable and do not carry a stigma or association with disability, potentially improving compliance for use as a compensatory cognitive aid.

SMs with more moderate to severe memory and cognitive difficulties as well as those with mild deficits and significant comorbid physical deficits that limit dexterity may require a full needs assessment prior to the recommendation for use of a specific assistive technology device. Clinicians are referred to Sohlberg and Turkstra[143] or to Brainline.org[170] for further information on

assessment and evaluation of assistive technology in SMs with more complex conditions.

Assessment should include a systematic process that matches an individual's ability and current and future needs with available devices and strategies.[171] Aspects of current and expected cognitive functioning, and the settings in which the device will assist the individual now and in the future, should be assessed. Comorbid conditions, such as low vision, upper limb amputations or paresis/paralysis, and hearing loss must be taken into account to ensure that the selected device will be effective. Prior experience with assistive devices should also be considered to take full advantage of preinjury familiarity and exposure to electronic systems.

Smartphones and similar devices may require training in the use of a computer interface and in techniques for seeking out and downloading appropriate applications from the Internet. Even individuals who are familiar with devices will need training in the effective use of a smartphone or computer as a cognitive aid to optimize function in daily living. This training may be implemented simultaneously with other cognitive therapies or

TABLE 7-4

LEARNING OBJECTIVES OF MEMORY AID TRAINING

Training Sequence	Specific Skills/Objectives
Information entry/retrieval	• Writing appointment information in the appropriate section of a day planner • Inputting appointment information in a smartphone or personal digital assistant • Setting alarm prompts (via cell phone, personal digital assistant, alarm watch) • Establishing routine times of day to refer to planner
Daily and weekly planning	• Establishing a consistent sequence of steps for reviewing tasks and appointments each day • Establishing a consistent sequence of steps for planning the week ahead
Note taking	• Taking notes in order to perform novel, multistep tasks • Taking notes in order to keep track of conversations • Taking notes on reference information

as part of an educationally oriented program to support functional activity and promote successful return to duty and community reentry. Applications created for entertainment purposes, such as games and social networks, can encourage the SM to explore the full potential of an assistive device and support socialization. SMs who often misplace items should also be guided to set up a back-up system in case they lose their electronic devices.

The technology and applications for these electronic devices are constantly changing. The younger, tech-savvy members of the armed forces and veteran communities are familiar with the constant upgrades for these devices and the myriad useful applications. A comprehensive list of applications for specific devices would be outdated before publication; however, a sample of the types of categories of applications that may be appropriate for SMs with c/mTBI residual complaints is included in Exhibit 7-19.

The Making Positive Connections AppReviews site (http://id4theweb.com/appreviews.php) provides updates on new applications and useful clinical reviews of existing applications. Additional applications may be of particular importance to SMs

TABLE 7-5

LEARNING TO USE PROMPTS FROM AN ALARM WATCH (EXAMPLE)

Component	Task
Acquisition	During a therapy session, the clinician demonstrates how to set an alarm watch. The patient and clinician set up written instructions as to how to set an alarm watch. The patient sets alarm watch for the next day's appointments.
Application	The patient uses an alarm prompt as a reminder to switch tasks during the therapy session.
Adaptation	The patient is assigned to demonstrate alarm use to spouse. The patient sets the alarm watch to sound as a prompt for morning and evening medications.

involved in an education program (see Chapter 9, Performance and Self-Management, Work, Social and School Roles for suggestions on applications for note-taking, reading, and other school-related tasks).

National Center for Telehealth and Technology

A new genre of smartphone programs specifically designed for troops and healthcare providers has been developed by the National Center for

---

EXHIBIT 7-19

SMARTPHONE APPLICATIONS

Calendar/Schedule manager
Task manager/To do/Reminders
Shopping/notes
Home management/Lifestyle
Headache tracking
Medication management
Sleep management
Fitness
PTSD/Stress
Financial management
Cognitive training
Cognitive games
Password manager

PTSD: posttraumatic stress syndrome

Telehealth and Technology (T2), a component of the DCoE for Psychological Health and Traumatic Brain Injury (www.t2health.org/mobile-apps). These applications address psychological health and TBI for SMs and may also be used by civilians with similar conditions. Some examples include:

- Breathe2Relax: guides users through diaphragmatic breathing exercises.
- PTSD Coach: a collaboration between T2 and the Department of Veterans Affairs National Center for PTSD that offers selections such as self-assessment, manage symptoms, find support, and learn about PTSD to assist individuals experiencing PTSD symptoms.
- T2 Mood Tracker: allows users to record and track their emotional states over time, using a visual analog rating scale.
- Tactical Breather: guides users through tactical breathing exercises to help them control physiological and psychological responses to stress.
- Co-Occurring Conditions Toolkit: an electronic version of the DCoE's Co-Occurring Conditions Toolkit, this application can help healthcare providers assess and treat patients with multiple symptoms that may stem from closed head injury or a number of psychological conditions.
- mTBI Pocket Guide: intended for clinicians, this application is a comprehensive quick-reference guide on improving care for c/mTBI patients that emphasizes current clinical standards of care.

PRACTICE TASKS FOR MEMORY STRATEGY REHEARSAL AND TRANSFER

Purpose/Background

Once patients understand the factors that influence their memory abilities, they need to practice preferred compensatory cognitive strategies in the context of clinic and everyday tasks. Simply talking about a potentially useful strategy does little to improve functioning (see Techniques to Improve Learning and Patient Engagement). Patients need many opportunities to practice during clinic sessions and as part of their therapy homework. Practice tasks specific to memory strategies involve using compensatory cognitive strategies to keep track of instructions to novel tasks (Table 7-6).

Procedure for Using Memory-Strategy Practice Tasks in Therapy

1. Patient and clinician collaborate to select a clinic or homework task based on the memory strategies the patient needs to practice.
2. After receiving instructions for the task, the patient completes the Anticipation part of the AAA worksheet (see form in the Techniques to Improve Learning and Patient Engagement section.)
3. Patient performs the assigned task, with clinician observing performance (Exhibit 7-20; some practice should occur in the clinical setting so the patient benefits from this feedback.) During the task, the patient self-observes performance and completes the "Action" section of the AAA worksheet.
4. Upon completing the task, the patient fills out the "Analysis" section of the AAA worksheet.
5. Patient and clinician share their observations and analyses of the performance.

Activities of Daily Living and Instrumental Activities of Daily Living Tasks

Any task can be set up to require memory strategy practice. The patient's self-reflections and the clinician's guidance and observation are what make the task therapeutic. Some ideas for daily activities practice are the following:

- checkbook (create a checklist of steps),
- medication set-up (creating a grid with name, dosage, description of appearance, reason taken),
- kitchen tasks,
- home projects, and
- creating phone lists or address books.

TABLE 7-6

SAMPLE MEMORY STRATEGY PRACTICE TASKS

Computer Tasks*	Description	Vendor/Location
Games for the Brain	Free website includes 20 games that place various demands on memory	http://www.gamesforthebrain.com/
Captain's Log	50 multilevel programs that provide more than 2,000 hours of game-like activities	http://www.braintrain.com/ homeusers/homeusershome.htm
Lumosity	Website with a free 5-day trial (requires membership for a small monthly fee after that) that provides a variety of brain engagement challenges, tracks progress, and adjusts the difficulty level to match the user	http://www.lumosity.com/

Technology Tasks	Description	
Global positioning system smartphones	Developing checklists helps patient manage new learning and procedural memory.	

Clinic Tasks	Description	Vendor/Location
Brainwave-R	Brainwave-R is a comprehensive pen-and-paper-based cognitive rehabilitation program that is divided into five hierarchically graded modules: 1) attention, 2) visual processing, 3) memory, 4) information processing, and 5) executive functions. The program comprises three components: 1) education: an overview of current theories relevant to rehabilitation designed to be used by the clinician with the client and family to ensure good awareness and understanding of the problem area 2) clinician instructions: rating scales, clinical guidelines, suggestions for how to involve the family, a performance summary chart, and questions to encourage the client to determine the functional relevance of each exercise 3) client exercises	http://www.braintreemanagement.co.uk/braintreetraining/bwr.htm
Practice tasks for specific aspects of memory function	Prospective memory: "At 10:30, call your cell and leave a message for yourself listing four items to pick up at the store."	N/A
	Procedural memory: "Develop a daily planning checklist that you can use each morning to plan your day." **OR** "Develop a checklist that gives step-by-step instructions for setting the alarm on your cell phone."	N/A
Card games	Remember or take notes on rules Rehearsal of internal compensatory strategies to optimize recall. Solitaire, cribbage, poker, etc N-factor(requires a deck of cards). Clinician flips the cards and patient must recall:	1 card back, just number; 1 card back, number and suite; 2 cards back; just number; and 2 cards back, number and suite
Reading assignments	Magazine, newspaper, books	N/A

*Logging on, accessing a site, and using different features all require procedural memory. Clinician can have patient create checklists for use as a therapy task. Patients may need to be reminded that the purpose of these tasks is to rehearse compensatory strategy use, not to "fix" memory functioning.

EXHIBIT 7-20

CLINICIAN OBSERVATIONS DURING PRACTICE TASKS

The clinician selects and sets up the practice task to observe all or some of the following:

- Does the patient self-initiate strategy use?
- If the task requires note taking:
  - Are patient notes legible?
  - Are patient notes detailed enough to be useful?
  - Does the patient refer to them during the task?
  - Does he or she use clarification skills to control the pace of the directions?
- If the patient is using a voice recorder:
  - Does the patient remember to turn it off?
  - Does the patient organize the information for efficient retrieval?
  - Does the patient set alarms or use timers if needed?
  - Does the patient put appointments in planner system?
  - Does the patient make to-do lists and include homework assignments?

IMPROVING EXECUTIVE FUNCTIONS

Purpose/Background

The term "executive functions" refers to a set of processes and functions that allow individuals to self-regulate their behavior and solve problems. Executive functions guide purposeful behavior throughout the day and are critical to almost every aspect of everyday activities. Problem solving is required "in any situation that involves decision making."[172(p157)] Despite the structure that active duty military service provides, it is estimated that SMs make approximately 3,000 decisions in their daily routine.[173] When SMs transition to the less-structured context of civilian life, demands may increase to 9,000 decisions a day.[173]

After c/mTBI, many patients report difficulty with high-level executive functions (planning, organization, self-regulation, problem solving), which affects their ability to consistently and safely manage higher-level ADL/IADL roles. The overarching goal of therapy specific to executive dysfunction is to help patients expand their repertoire of strategies in this realm through the TEST process (see above, Cognitive Intervention: Improving Attention and Speed of Processing).[174]

Strength of Recommendation: Practice Standard

Training in the use of problem-solving and organization strategies as applied to real-life tasks is supported by empirical evidence.[126,171] Though not specific to persons with c/mTBI, according to the DCoE expert panel, "a robust literature supports the use of metacognitive strategy training as an intervention for executive function impairments due to TBI."[4(p246)] Strategy training that yielded positive outcomes in executive function included the use of multiple-step strategies, strategic thinking, multitasking, problem identification, weighing pros and cons of solutions, monitoring performance, and improving emotional self-regulation. Evidence is sufficient for a recommendation of this type of cognitive remediation as a **practice standard.**

Intervention Methods

1. Improve executive functions. Educate the patient about executive functions (see Clinician Tip Sheets: Treatment of Executive Dysfunction and Understanding Executive Functions, and Patient Handout: Rating Your Executive Function Skills).
2. Help the patient increase self-awareness and self-regulation to support good decision-making in difficult situations (see Clinician Tip Sheets: Improving Emotional Self-Management and Strategies to Improve Self-Regulation–Pausing, and Patient Handouts: Emotional Self-Management Worksheet and Strategies to Improve Self-Regulation–Pausing).
3. Help the patient identify strategies that pertain to his or her key tasks and

preferences (see Patient Handouts: Strategies for Problem Identification, Strategies to Improve Initiation, Building Habits and Routines, Generative Thinking Strategies, Problem Solving Process, Strategy–Prioritization; and Clinician Tip Sheets: Strategies to Improve Initiation, Building Habits and Project Planning Strategy–Divide and Conquer, Routines, Genera-

tive Thinking Strategies, Problem-Solving Process, and Strategy–Prioritization).

4. Create opportunities for the patient to practice strategies in clinic sessions and as homework (see Clinician Tip Sheets: Menu of Strategies to Manage Executive Function Inefficiencies and Practice Tasks for Executive Functions Strategy Rehearsal and Transfer).

CLINICIAN TIP SHEET: TREATING EXECUTIVE DYSFUNCTION

Although there is no universal definition or agreement as to what constitutes executive functions,[175] treatment for deficits in executive functions may be based on three premises[176]:

1. Difficulties with problem solving are at the core of executive dysfunction.
2. Problem solving is "supported or thwarted" by emotional states.
3. Attentional processing serves as a foundation for executive functions, emotional regulation, and learning.

The following treatment model for executive function deficits is based on the work of Kennedy and Coelho[177] and Gordon et al.[176] Also note that treatments and strategies that improve attention will also improve executive functions (see Improving Attention and Speed of Processing).

Provide Education

Educate patients about executive functions to give them an informational basis for treatment (see Patient Handout: Understanding Executive Functions). Assess the patient's initial awareness of strengths and weaknesses within the area of executive functions (see Patient Handout: Rating Your Executive Function Skills).

Problem-Solving Process and Strategies

- **Problem identification.** Before the problem-solving process can begin, problems need to be recognized and identified. Teach patients to recognize the following cues that indicate when problems exist (see Patient Handout: Strategies for Problem Identification).
  - Emotional cues: recognize signs of frustration, anxiety, irritation, and anger as indications of problem areas that

need to be addressed.
  - Social cues: pay attention to others' facial cues, tone of voice, and body language that may indicate a problem is occurring.
  - Outcome cues: repeated failure to solve a problem or reach a goal is a clear indication that the current approach to the problem is flawed or that the problem has not been fully understood.
- **Self-monitoring.** Self-monitoring can facilitate early identification of problems. Pause strategies (see Patient Handout and Clinician Tip Sheet: Strategies to Improve Self-Regulation–Pausing) and prediction strategies can enhance self-monitoring (see Patient Handout and Clinician Tip Sheet: AAA Self-Reflection Form). Employing a structured problem-solving framework that includes comparisons of expected and actual outcomes may help identify specific difficulties a patient has to approaching a problem (see Patient Handout and Clinician Tip Sheet: Problem-Solving Process).
- **Goal setting.** The problem-solving process is driven by a specific intention or goal. Teach goal development because patients who set their own goals, rather than have them created for them as part of the rehabilitation process, are more likely to attain them. Refer to references on developing clearly stated goals using the SMART (specific, measurable, achievable, realistic and time-targeted) goal process.
- **Strategy selection.** Strategies should be selected based on a clear description of the goal to be accomplished and clear awareness of the strengths and weaknesses a person brings to solve a problem. Although self-awareness tends to be spared after concussion, if there is a mismatch between perceived abilities and actual abilities,

teach self-awareness (see Patient Handout: Change Begins with Awareness).

- **Strategy planning**. Teach techniques to generate strategies for problem solving (see Patient Handout and Clinician Tip Sheet: Generative Thinking Strategies).
  - Impulsivity may result in selecting an inefficient or ineffective strategy. Teach patients to stop and reflect on a range of approaches, evaluate the pros and cons of each approach, and select the one most likely to achieve the desired goal.
  - Strategies often require multiple steps that need to be performed in a specific order and may require specific materials for successful completion. A structured problem-solving framework can facilitate this complex process (see Patient Handout and Clinician Tip Sheet: Problem Solving Process).
  - Prioritization strategies allow patients to divide larger projects into a series of smaller tasks that can be managed more effectively (see Patient Handout and Clinician Tip Sheet: Project Planning Strategy–Divide and Conquer).
- **Strategy implementation**. No strategy will work if it is not acted upon. Difficulty with initiation can occur for different reasons, including lack of motivation, anxiety, fear of failure, problems with memory, and organically related lack of initiation

resulting from the injury itself. Teach techniques that support initiation and strategy follow-through in everyday activities (see Patient Handout and Clinician Tip Sheet: Strategies to Improve Initiation).

- **Self-monitoring and evaluation of goal attainment**. Poor self-monitoring of performance can result in undetected errors in strategy implementation that can cause a well-developed plan to fail. A number of techniques have been used to facilitate self-monitoring, including pausing strategies (see Patient Handout and Clinician Tip Sheet: Strategies to Improve Self-Regulation–Pausing) and systematic comparison of predicted with actual performance that may be supplemented with verbal mediation of behavior using techniques, such as self-talk (see Patient Handout and Clinician Tip Sheet: AAA Self-Reflection Form).

When faced with a multitude of tasks, people often feel overwhelmed. Prioritization strategies may be used to systematically evaluate the urgency and importance of each task to guide decision making (see Patient Handout and Clinician Tip Sheet: Prioritization). In addition, developing a routine with habitual daily and weekly activities reduces demands on decision making and planning (see Patient Handout and Clinician Tip Sheet: Building Habits and Routines).

CLINICIAN TIP SHEET: IMPROVING EMOTIONAL SELF-MANAGEMENT

Purpose/Background

Headaches, insomnia, depression, and emotional dysregulation may occur after c/mTBI. A crucial, yet often omitted, component of c/mTBI management is the provision of education regarding symptoms such as fatigue, irritability, and mood lability that may be experienced during c/mTBI recovery.[7] People who regularly experience significant irritability, anger, anxiety, or fear often make poor decisions and struggle to solve problems.[178] Emotional self-management provides a foundation for each phase of the problem-solving process. Treatment aims to reduce the "emotional noise" and negative self-talk that undermine decision making and work to overcome the tendency to react impulsively or to do nothing.[172] The process of improving emotional regulation involves a three-part strategy:

1. Recognize early warning signs of emotional dysregulation (eg, thoughts and physiologic responses, escalation in mood) that can serve as cues to engage in self-regulation strategies to support good decision making (see Patient Handout: Emotional Self-Management Worksheet and Clinician Tip Sheet: Improving Emotional Self-Management).

2. Review and reflect on antecedent conditions (eg, physiologic symptoms, contexts, and people) that are associated with emotional dysregulation to increase awareness of triggers and allow implementation of self-regulation strategies before emotional dysregulation undermines decision making (see Patient Handout: Emotional Self-Management Worksheet and Clinician Tip Sheet: Improving Emotional Self-Management).

3. Develop strategies that can be used to maintain good emotional regulation (eg, relaxation breathing or positive self-talk) to facilitate a sense of calm in difficult situations, or to disengage from a situation before doing or saying something that will be regretted later (see Clinician Tip Sheet: Improving Emotional Self-Management).

CLINICIAN TIP SHEET: UNDERSTANDING EXECUTIVE FUNCTIONS

Purpose/Background

Patients who understand the nature of problems related to executive functions will be best able to learn new strategies to optimize their performance. The Patient Handout: Understanding Executive Functions can be used to guide a discussion about executive functions between the clinician, the patient, and the patient's significant other.

- Ask patients to complete the self-rating form (see Patient Handout: Rating Your Executive Function Skills) to identify their perceived areas of strengths and weaknesses. Encourage significant others, if present, to share their observations.
- Identifying strengths and weaknesses informs the selection and training of compensatory cognitive strategies described in the Toolkit.

It may be necessary to review this handout again after patients perform clinical tasks that enlist executive functions. Clinicians should ask permission to share their observations of consistency and effectiveness of patients' performance to facilitate understanding of the connection between strategy use and life-management skills. Strategies should be explored to address areas deemed as inefficient.

Self-Regulation

Self-regulation involves:

- Self-awareness (see Techniques to Promote Patient Engagement and Learning)
- Inhibition (regulating emotional responses; see information on emotional self-management and self-regulation in this chapter)
- Resisting distractions and paying attention, learning to focus (see section on Improving Attention Management)
- Appreciating obstacles and problems (see information on problem solving in this chapter)

- Mental flexibility (knowing when and how to change course; see information on generative thinking strategies in this chapter)

Problem Solving

Problem solving involves:

- Understanding the problem itself (see Strategies for Problem Identification in this chapter)
- Generating possible ideas and solutions (see Problem-Solving Process in this chapter)
- Appreciating the limits and restrictions of various solutions
- Prioritizing (see Prioritization in this chapter)
- Flexibility of thinking (see Generative Thinking Strategies in this chapter)
- Making decisions (see Prioritization, Divide and Conquer, and Problem-Solving Process in this chapter)
- Setting goals (see reference materials for information on SMART Goals)
- Anticipating outcomes of a plan (see Problem-Solving Process in this chapter and AAA Self-Reflection Form)

Emotional Self-Management

Emotional self-management involves:

- Identifying early antecedent conditions and signs of emotional dyscontrol
- Identifying strategies to maintain emotional control in difficult situations
- Evaluating strategies to maintain emotional control (see Emotional Regulation Worksheet)

Note that limited self-awareness can undermine any aspect of the problem-solving process. Limited use of self-awareness training is recommended to address specific issues related to self-awareness (see section on Techniques to Promote Engagement and Learning).

CLINICIAN TIP SHEET: STRATEGIES TO IMPROVE SELF-REGULATION–PAUSING

Purpose/Background

Under normal circumstances, most people periodically and unconsciously monitor themselves throughout the day to reflect on how closely their current situation (what they are doing at the moment) matches their goals and intentions. Intact functioning of the frontal lobes and good mental health are essential for such self-reflection. People who experience brain injury, stress, and depression may be less likely to automatically engage in self-regulation and self-monitoring. Therefore, relearning a deliberate pausing strategy may be helpful in reestablishing this important habit of mind (see Patient Handout: Strategies to Improve Self-Regulation–Pausing).

Pausing is a simple concept that relies heavily on executive skills. Patients are continuously counseled to pause and take a moment to reflect. In the beginning phase of treatment, patients use the pausing strategy as a cue to reflect on their current task choices and next steps. As their self-awareness improves and acceptance of strategy use increases, the pause strategy can be expanded to provide a deeper and more enriching form of self-reflection. It is a difficult habit to develop and requires persistence and initiation.

The Basic Steps of Pausing

The patient associates the verbal cues with fingers on his or her hand. He or she is challenged to stop, take a moment, and check-in by considering the following questions:

- What am I doing now?
- Is this what I should be doing?
- If I'm going somewhere, do I have what I need?
- What should I do next?
- Go.

The pause strategy is adapted as patients progress and can be used to meet a variety of treatment areas, such as:

- reminding them to use a compensatory strategy (ie, when leaving a location such as home or work, use checklists, refer to a planner or schedule, ensure they have all belongings and materials);
- managing fatigue or pain via reflection on their body for tension or pain, and the need to take remedial steps; and
- considering the quality of their performance and the presence of a personal or situational factor that is having an effect and might be altered.

Practice

The patient is given a homework assignment and asked to pause at every daily transition (eg, leaving for work, going to lunch, etc) and go through the pause sequence. Patients should be ready to discuss the experience at their next session. Have extra handouts available for them to take home and post in key locations.

CLINICIAN TIP SHEET: STRATEGIES TO IMPROVE INITIATION

Lack of initiation presents a challenge for both patients and clinicians; a team approach is imperative. It is important that the reasons for lack of initiation be explored because the treatments and strategies chosen can vary greatly.

Use the associated patient handout to guide discussion. Patients are asked to highlight reasons that explain their difficulties with initiation. They are encouraged to add any other reasons to the handout. Discuss with the patient each area of concern and strategies that might help (Table 7-7).

REMEMBER: The goal of therapy is to help patients become aware of the barriers to optimal performance and the strategies to help them overcome the problem. It is important to continually highlight patients' role in their own recovery.

TABLE 7-7

INITIATION CONCERNS AND POSSIBLE COMPENSATORY STRATEGIES

Reasons for Lack of Initiation	Helpful Strategies
Decreased awareness of what needs to be done	Develop a weekly/daily activity list that can be kept in the day planner or posted at home. Instruct patient to check off the tasks when completed on the assigned day. Note: It is easier to add a task to an existing daily routine than adding a task when a person has no such structure (a concern for those who have not yet returned to work).
Lack of energy needed to start or see things through	See fatigue discussion in Toolkit. Common strategies include pacing, prioritizing, planning, taking breaks, and exercise.
Inability to break tasks down into achievable steps	See Divide and Conquer handout
Difficulty with prioritization	See Prioritization handout
Difficulty knowing when to do what	Develop a weekly/daily activity list that can be kept in the day planner or posted at home. Instruct patient to check off the tasks when completed on the assigned day.
Fear of being interrupted	Use "stop notes" and distracter management (see Attention section of Toolkit)
Lack of desire	Refer back to physician or psychologist
Inability to generate ideas of things to do	Use a weekly activity list or brainstorm with significant other
Difficulty tracking time	Use cell phone alarms, alarm watches, timers
Difficulty staying on task/attending	Use timers, control distracters (see Attention section of Toolkit)
Procrastination	Use strategies related to planning, prioritization, alarms and times
Different priorities	Have honest conversation with significant others; adjust responsibility lists
Inability to function under pressure	Use planning, prioritizing, and time-management strategies
Pain	Use pacing, taking breaks, ergonomics; refer to doctor

CLINICIAN TIP SHEET: BUILDING HABITS AND ROUTINES

Purpose/Background

The Patient Handout: Building Habits and Routines is a good discussion point for patients who indicate not knowing what to do as a reason for decreases initiation It can prompt a meaningful discussion related to the importance of having things to do during the day. Routines and habits help decrease the cognitive energy required to get through the day. They can also help with memory and fatigue management (see Patient Handout: Building Habits and Routines).

Explore these strategies with patients as a means to add structure to their daily life:

- Get up at the same time every day.
- Reestablish personal care routines.
- Use a calendar and a daily planning checklist.
- Be responsible for creating and maintaining your own schedule.

- Carve out time in your day for a balanced life (scheduled appointments, regular home management tasks, hobbies, and social engagements).
- If work is not yet a reasonable goal, consider volunteering. Set up regular times and expectations.
- Create reasonable expectations; set goals for yourself and ask someone you trust to help hold you accountable.
- Set up a recurring task schedule for tasks of priority (see example below). Schedule tasks of importance for certain days of the week and make an effort to adhere to the new regimen.

Suggested Homework Assignment

Assign the patient to fill out a sample week of recurring activities. Make sure activities include personal tasks (exercise, social outings) as well as home management tasks, work, and the like. Have them report what they find, including answers to the following:

- Is the week well-balanced, or do you tend to do everything on one day and then need time to recover?

- Is the schedule over- or under booked?
- What opportunities do you see for change?

Have them place the grid (Table 7-8) in their information management system or hang it in a prominent place in their home.

CLINICIAN TIP SHEET: GENERATIVE THINKING STRATEGIES

Purpose/Background

For a variety of reasons (including brain injury), people sometimes experience inflexibility in their thinking that leads to feeling "cognitively stuck," resulting in situations such as the following:

- repeatedly employing the same maladaptive or ineffective approach to tasks, even when it is evident that the approach is not working;
- difficulty formulating more than one solution to a complex problem; and
- inefficient or even ineffectual task performance because they are not evaluating and selecting the best alternative.

Even individuals who typically have no cognitive impairments may occasionally experience difficulties with generative thinking, especially when fatigued, anxious, or stressed.

How to Address Problems With Generative Thinking

The primary way of addressing limitations in generative thinking, regardless of cause, is to increase the patient's awareness of this vulnerability so that he or she can employ some or all of the compensatory strategies listed on the Patient Handout: Generative Thinking Strategies. The clinician can assign or observe various experiential tasks to:

- assess the patient's performance in this realm,
- increase the patient's awareness of this inefficiency, and
- provide opportunities for the patient to practice compensatory strategies.

Examples of Experiential Tasks

Sorting Task

1. Get a container and gather approximately 15 random items.

2. Ask the patient to group those items into five categories and verbally describe what they are (function, color, shape, material, etc). Do not cue the patient unless he or she is unable to categorize the items.
3. Give feedback on appropriateness of choices and descriptions.
4. Ask the patient to create three new categories without repeating any of the categories from the first trial. Give feedback on appropriateness of choices.
5. Ask the patient to create two new categories without repeating any of the previous categories from the first two trials. Give feedback on appropriateness of choices.

Games

- Chess
- Connect 4
- Checkers
- Poker

Pencil-and-Paper Tasks

Generate the following:

- ten similarities or differences on topic of choice (Batman versus Spiderman; country versus city living, etc)
- five to ten reasons something occurred (global warming, Steelers winning the Super Bowl in 2009, financial crisis)
- five to ten possible outcomes (global warming, universal healthcare)
- safety questions with two or three possible answers
- a week of meals and grocery lists
- three different approaches to a home improvement project

TABLE 7-8

GRID OR CHECKLIST TO HELP PATIENTS DEVELOP NEW HABITS AND ROUTINES

Tasks	M	T	W	Th	F	Sa	Su

CLINICIAN TIP SHEET: PROJECT PLANNING STRATEGY–DIVIDE AND CONQUER

Purpose/Background

Many patients find themselves easily overwhelmed at the prospect of performing a complex or multistep project. This undertaking is made more difficult when patients embark on the task before first planning their approach, or if they plan without writing things down. Many individuals respond to this challenge by procrastinating or simply not initiating work at all.

The Divide and Conquer worksheet is presented as a strategy to help patients develop a work plan (see Patient Handout: Project Planning Strategy–Divide and Conquer). This process helps with information management, fatigue and pain management, initiation, and attention.

How to Use The Form

1. List the major task components in the shaded rows (they do not need to be put in order).
2. List specific action items under each major task component (again, list them as they come to mind; they do not need to be in order).
3. Put all the action items in order once you have listed them on the worksheet.
4. Assign yourself deadlines for key steps, if desired.

5. Add to-dos to your planner.
6. Review the example of the completed Divide and Conquer worksheet with the patient.

Examples of Experiential Tasks for Clinic Observation or Homework

1. Ask the patient to use the Divide and Conquer worksheet to organize an unstructured, multistep project that is personally relevant. Review the work plan, offer feedback (as necessary), and assign completion as homework.
2. Assign the patient to instruct a family member in the divide-and-conquer process, completing a work plan for another project.
3. Create an unstructured, simulated work task in the clinical setting. This might include a multicomponent clerical task (such as assembling patient education packets) or a sorting and organizing task (such as reorganizing a storage cabinet). Ask the patient to organize his or her approach beforehand using the Divide and Conquer worksheet. Incorporate use of the AAA form as well (see Techniques for Promoting Engagement and Learning).

REMEMBER: Using this process allows the patients to "clear the burners" in their heads, which can lead to better generative thinking and clearer plan development. This, in turn, can lead to better initiation and follow through. Project completion can be a confidence boost to patients and often results in increased activity level.

CLINICIAN TIP SHEET: PROBLEM-SOLVING PROCESS

The ability to solve problems can be compromised by stress, mood changes, and after effects of c/mTBI. Therefore, patients may be helped by learning a structured approach to problem solving to ensure they are making informed choices instead of relying on trial and error.

How to Use the Patient Handout: Problem-Solving Process

As the patient's skill level progresses, the form may be eliminated and the patient able to self-talk through the process.

1. The clinician and patient identify a current problem that the patient is trying to solve.
2. The patient is asked to define the problem. This step is important; often the patient has several concerns and it is important to tease out the main one.
3. The patient is asked to define the desired outcome or his or her main goal. This step is also very important; if the outcome is vague, it is much harder to make choices.

4. The patient needs to determine if there is only one solution to the problem.
   - If the answer is "yes," the patient is instructed to "divide and conquer" the task to develop a project plan.
   - Typically, the answer is "no." The patient is then challenged to come up with three or four alternate solutions and list the pros and cons of each.
5. The patient is instructed to choose a solution, then use the divide-and-conquer strategy to organize the project.
6. Finally, the patient is asked to reflect back on his or her choices or plan. Was he or she pleased with the outcome? The process? What was learned? What, if anything, could be done differently next time?

This structured approach to problem solving:

- slows the patient down,
- structures his or her efforts,
- avoids trial and error,
- allows the patient to walk away and come back later without fear of forgetting, and
- helps the patient address one step at a time.

CLINICIAN TIP SHEET: STRATEGY–PRIORITIZATION

People burdened by stress, mood changes, and after-effects of c/mTBI can easily become overwhelmed with myriad daily tasks; establishing a formal process for prioritizing may be helpful (see Patient Handout: Strategy–Prioritization). People have varying skills with regard to developing a daily "to-do" list. Some lists are too long; others involve too few tasks. It is the clinician's role to ensure that patients are able to make daily lists using the planning checklists that were discussed earlier.

Many patients benefit from a structured process for logically determining how to allocate their energy and time. The four categories associated with importance and urgency, as defined by Covey,[179] are discussed below. The clinician provides examples and encourages the patient to give examples of tasks in his or her life that fit in each category.

- **Urgent and important.** This category includes tasks such as taking medications, paying bills, picking up children, and meeting a higher-ranking officer. They have time deadlines and consequences if not completed. These tasks are usually due that day and at a certain time. Patients may have to set alarms to remember them.

- **Not urgent but important.** This includes tasks such as preparing for a work project at the end of the month, planning a birthday party for a family member, or planning a vacation. These are not due today but will have consequences if they are not worked on. Patients should plan time for these in the week.

- **Urgent but not important.** These tasks must be done by a certain time, but they are not imperative. For example, the garbage truck comes at 8:00 am, but the bins are not full and it is cold outside, or a movie you want to see is at the theater for one more day. Both of these scenarios have deadlines, but there is little or no consequence to you if they are not completed. Patients should only do these tasks if they have extra time and energy.

- **Not urgent and not important.** These are tasks that could easily be completed or deleted with no real cost to you. For example, you want to go to the mall and see what is new for the season, your buddy wants to go fishing but you are not really interested, or you are craving a good cup of coffee. None of these tasks is necessary. Patients should only do these tasks if they have extra time and energy, and the rest of their list is complete.

CLINICIAN TIP SHEET: MENU OF STRATEGIES TO MANAGE EXECUTIVE FUNCTION INEFFICIENCIES

The primary aim of therapy is to help the patient identify and implement core strategies that match his or her problematic tasks and preferences. Using the patient handouts and the list that follows, the clinician guides the patient toward the specific strategies that hold the most promise in improving performance (Table 7-9).

TABLE 7-9

POSSIBLE STRATEGIES TO ADDRESS SPECIFIC EXECUTIVE DYSFUNCTIONS

Executive Inefficiency	Strategy	Practical Application

Self-regulation
  Initiation
  Persisting
  Stopping
  Emotional control
Self-reflection and adaption
	Develop routines/structure
	Weekly activity tracker
	Information management systems
	Checklists
	Timer use (to persist or stop)
		Sit down each morning and plan your day, add
		  activities from your weekly tracker list
		Set a timer and clean the kitchen until it goes off
		Set a timer and get off the computer when it
		  goes off

Problem solving
Understands the problem
  itself
Generates possible ideas
  and solutions
Appreciates limits and
  restrictions of various
  solutions
    Prioritizes
    Anticipates
      consequences
    Makes decisions
	Generative thinking strategies
	Problem-solving grid
	Divide and conquer
	Prioritizing grid
		Identify a home improvement you want to
		  make, go through the problem-solving process,
		  choose your best option and use divide and
		  conquer to create a realistic to-do list

Self-awareness	Self-prediction/reflection forms	Talk with significant other before an event,
		  identify possible concerns and strategies you
		  will use
		Talk with significant other after the event
		  and review successes and opportunities for
		  improvement

CLINICIAN TIP SHEET: PRACTICE TASKS FOR EXECUTIVE FUNCTIONS
STRATEGY REHEARSAL AND TRANSFER

Purpose/Background

Once patients understand the factors that influence their executive function abilities, they need to practice preferred compensatory cognitive strategies in the context of clinic and everyday tasks. As discussed earlier (see Techniques to Improve Learning and Patient Engagement), simply talking about a potentially useful strategy does little to actually improve functioning. Patients need many opportunities for practice during clinic sessions and as part of their therapy homework. Practice tasks for executive functions tend to be unstructured. The clinician describes the end product to the patient, then the patient is instructed to organize an efficient process by which to get the work accomplished.

Procedure for Using Executive Function-Strategy Practice Tasks in Therapy

1. The patient and clinician select a clinic or homework task based on the executive function strategies that the patient needs to practice (Table 7-10).
2. After receiving instructions to the task, the patient completes the "Anticipation" part of the AAA worksheet (see Techniques to Improve Learning and Patient Engagement).
3. The patient performs the assigned task, with the clinician observing performance (some practice should occur in the clinical setting so the patient benefits from this feedback). During the task, the

TABLE 7-10

SAMPLE EXECUTIVE FUNCTION STRATEGY PRACTICE TASKS

Computer Tasks	Description	Vendor/Location
Games for the Brain	Free website that includes 20 games placing various demands on attention	http://www.gamesforthebrain.com/
Captain's Log	50 multilevel programs that provide more than 2,000 hours of game-like activities	http://www.braintrain.com
Brain Bashers	Free website with a collection of brainteasers, puzzles, riddles, games and optical illusions. BrainBashers is regularly updated with optical illusions and games and five new puzzles are added every other week	http://www.brainbashers.com
Lumosity	Website with a free 5-day trial (then requires membership for a small monthly fee) that provides a variety of brain engagement challenges, tracks progress, and adjusts the difficulty level to match the user	http://www.lumosity.com/
Microsoft Excel	Software can be used to have patients set up tables and budgets (can require high-level problem solving)	Microsoft Corporation (Redmond, WA)
Microsoft Word document	Software can be used to have patients create letters, slide shows, and essays on topics of interest	Microsoft Corporation (Redmond, WA)
Internet	Can be used to assign systematic internet searches (eg, plan a trip to a designated city, include flight, hotel, car rental, three tourist activities, three restaurants on a budget of $2,000)	Any

Technology Tasks	Description	Vendor/Location
Driving simulators	Can provide opportunities to observe problem solving, reaction time, higher-level attention skills, and activity tolerance	N/A
GPS units/cell phones	Patient can organize and write directions on how to use the gadgets and applications that they may need for daily use	N/A

Clinic Tasks	Description	Vendor/Location
Snap Circuits board	Varies in number of parts and possible projects. The patient follows visual and written directions to construct different electrical projects using snap-on circuit parts. This task can be used to look at ability to follow directions. The clinician can set up the projects with errors and have the patient repair the circuit.	Elenco Electronics Inc (Wheeling, IL) http://www.acsupplyco.com/elenco1/htm_files/snapcircuits.htm

(**Table 7-10** *continues*)

Table 7-10 *continued*

Brainwave-R	A comprehensive pen-and-paper-based cognitive rehabilitation program that is divided into five hierarchically graded modules: 1) attention, 2) visual processing, 3) memory, 4) information processing, and 5) executive functions. The program comprises three components: 1) education (an overview of current theories relevant to rehabilitation designed to be used by the clinician with the client and family to ensure good awareness and understanding of the problem area); 2) clinician instructions (rating scales, clinical guidelines, suggestions for how to involve the family, a performance summary chart, and questions to encourage the client to determine the functional relevance of each exercise); 3) client exercises.	ProEd Inc (Austin, TX) http://www.braintreetraining.co.uk/bwr.htm
TipOver	Game requiring deductive reasoning and visual spatial skills	ThinkFun, Inc (Alexandria, VA) http://www.thinkfun.com/tipover/Bonus.htm
Rush Hour Traffic Jam	Game requiring deductive reasoning and visual spatial skills	ThinkFun, Inc (Alexandria, VA) http://www.thinkfun.com/shop/product/rush-hour,29,0.htm
SET	Visual perceptual game that requires the patient to attend to a variety of properties simultaneously	SET Enterprises Inc (Fountain Hills, AZ) http://www.setgame.com/
Tower of Hanoi	Strategy game requiring patients to generate a solution and persist. Can be made from wood or played on line.	MathIsFun http://www.mathsisfun.com/games/towerofhanoi.html
Models	Any variety. Motorized parts increase complexity.	
Clerical tasks	Patient can practice filing letters, envelopes, copying papers or projects of varying complexity, word processing tasks, schedule creation and maintenance tasks for self or others	N/A
Editing tasks	Patient can practice editing papers, advertisements, budgets, Microsoft Power Point projects	N/A
Assembly tasks	Patient can assemble storage cubes, shoe racks, small tables or stools	Retail stores
Tasks constructed by the clinician	See what is readily available in the clinic and understand the needs of your patients. Develop a task that has designated components (see sample below)	

Clinic Tasks	Description
Executive tasks created by clinicians should contain:	Information processing demands: • Decide the format in which to give the directions (written, verbal, diagrams, combination)

(**Table 7-10** *continues*)

Table 7-10 *continued*

	• Decide how conclusion or outcome should be communicated (verbal or written summary of status, showing clinician the completed task) More than one project or one project with multiple components: • Determine the number (requires prioritization and alternating or divided attention) • Requires time management Problem-solving requirements: • Organization • Generative thinking • Deductive reasoning Decision making
Executive task example:	Mail sorting task: Task objective (as described to patient): "Sort the mail into five categories, using the most organized and efficient process possible. Once the material is organized into five categories, ask me for the next set of instructions." Task supplies/materials: • Fake mail consisting of bills to be paid, personal correspondence, advertisements and coupons, articles or potentially interesting information to read later, junk mail that can be immediately recycled • Paper clips, sticky notes, pen/pencil, wastebasket After sorting, the patient is instructed to locate the following information and report it to clinician: • Company/date bills are due and the amount • Advertisements for three items that are found in two separate ads • Choose two more details from two sources of the mail (eg, ask patient to find out the phone number at the March of Dimes for donating cell phones and the letter their child was working on for a school newsletter); any information in the pile can be used • Use AAA form throughout the task

AAA: Anticipation, Action, Analysis
GPS: global positioning system

patient self-observes performance and completes the "Action" section of the AAA worksheet.

4. Upon completing the task, the patient fills out the "Analysis" section of the AAA worksheet. Patient and clinician share their observations and analyses of the performance.

ADL and IADL Tasks

- checkbook
- medication set-up
- household assembly tasks
- driving simulator
- kitchen tasks
- schedule creation and maintenance
- planning activities or events

REMEMBER: Any task can be set up to require executive function strategy practice. The patient's self reflections and the clinician's set-up and observation are what make the task therapeutic.

SOCIAL COMMUNICATION

Purpose/Background

Social communication involves a complex interaction of cognitive abilities, awareness of social rules and boundaries, and emotional control.[142] Impairments in social communication may lead to depression, isolation, negative self concept, anxiety, low academic achievement, a reduction in social interaction,[180] or frustrating or embarrassing experiences, and may interfere with relationships or employment.[131,142] After c/mTBI, cognitive inefficiencies may interfere with language and communication.[181]

In addition, changes in behavior, such as irritability, anger, and physical aggression that may be associated with c/mTBI and PTSD can negatively affect social communication.[182] For SMs returning from combat, the "battle" mindset that sustained survival in the combat zone may interfere with social communication when transitioning and reintegrating in the home zone. For example, although controlling emotions during combat is critical for mission success, failing to display and discuss emotions after returning home may be perceived negatively (eg, detached and uncaring) and could potentially impair relationships.[175,183,184]

Evidence-based studies in social communication have generally focused on the moderate to severe TBI population.[143,180,183,185] However, studies investigating social communication and c/mTBI are beginning to emerge in the literature.[143,186,187] Social pragmatic skills are commonly impaired by TBI, and social skills training, typically within a group format, has been shown to be effective in improving these skills.[4]

Struchen et al[187] investigated the use of various self-rating measures of social communication to determine overall social integration outcomes of participants with mild to severe TBI. Results indicated that "reduced social skills can have a major impact on participant restriction for individuals with TBI."[187(p38)] The authors recommended that social communication be evaluated as part of the overall clinical assessment because the information would prove valuable for community reintegration.

Tucker and Hanlon[185] found that cognitive difficulties associated with c/mTBI affect the formulation or expression of descriptive information as assessed on narrative discourse measures. These deficits could negatively affect storytelling during social interactions. Struchen[188] described therapy techniques for social communication that have been used in patients with moderate to severe TBI, such as incorporating structured feedback, videotaping and analyzing interactions, modeling, rehearsing, and training in self-monitoring. Although these techniques have yet to be objectively studied in the c/mTBI population, clinical experience with SMs, particularly in group contexts, have demonstrated their usefulness.

Dahlberg et al[143] investigated the use of social communication group therapy for participants with mild to severe TBI. Four key components to the therapy program included the following:

1. the use of group co-leaders from different disciplines (eg, social work and speech-language pathology) for evaluation and to serve as role models,
2. an emphasis on self-awareness and self-assessment for individual participant goal setting,
3. use of the group format for interaction, feedback, problem solving, and social support, and
4. generalization of skills.[143]

Sessions followed a consistent format that included homework review, brief topic introduction, guided discussions, small group practice, group problem solving and feedback, and homework. Results indicated that this treatment approach was effective in improving social communication.

Based on the literature and clinical experience with SMs with c/mTBI, a comprehensive holistic approach to social communication therapy is recommended that:

1. involves family and friends in individual and group contexts;
2. incorporates self-awareness, emotional, and behavioral self-regulation and executive functions; and
3. uses techniques of direct instruction, modeling, role-playing/simulations, videotaped interactions, feedback, and self-monitoring.

Strength of Recommendation: Practice Option

Despite the lack of robust, evidence-based research in the area of social communication

and TBI,[143] individual and group interventions that improve pragmatic conversational skills appear to be beneficial based on several small clinical studies with TBI participants.[130] Clinical experience with the military c/mTBI population has supported the need to address impairment in social communication, particularly in light of co-morbidities such as PTSD. According to guidance provided by members of the DCoE and Defense and Veterans Brain Injury Center Consensus Conference on Cognitive Rehabilitation for Military Personnel With c/mTBI and Chronic Postconcussional Disorder,[4] social skills training has shown effectiveness in improving problems in comprehending and responding to nonverbal social cues.

Intervention Methods

Treat social communication problems (see Clinician Tip Sheet: Assessment and Treatment of Social Communication Problems).

CLINICIAN TIP SHEET: ASSESSMENT AND TREATMENT OF SOCIAL COMMUNICATION PROBLEMS

Assessment of Social Communication

Competency in social communication should be evaluated through observation and assessment in varied contexts, social functions, activities, and interactions. The evaluation process can include videotaping communicative interactions and incorporating role-play activities to analyze social communication skills.[188]

For participation in social roles, functional outcome measures can be used to identify areas of success and areas that continue to limit quality of life. Other areas for analysis include environmental factors (opportunities for the SM to participate in social communication) and personal factors (how the social communication deficits affect the SM). Family members and friends can provide additional information about the SM's performance in daily interactions. Deficits identified in the evaluation can be selected for treatment, depending on the communication needs and social roles of the SM.[144]

Commonly Observed Deficits in Social Communication

Expert clinicians have identified problems with social communication skills in SMs with c/mTBI, including:

- unawareness of social communication deficits,
- verbosity (ie, production of excessive amounts of unrelated or tangential information during conversation),
- production of limited amounts of information during conversation,
- inability to identify conversational breakdowns,
- inability to repair conversational breakdowns,
- inability to comprehend nonverbal communication, and
- unawareness of actions, verbal and nonverbal language, postures, and proximity, which can appear aggressive, rude, or indifferent to others.

Treatment Progression

Initially, therapy may consist of individual sessions to increase awareness of the problems affecting social interactions and teach and establish compensatory strategies for social communication skills. As the SM progresses, group therapy can be implemented to allow increased practice in using the compensatory strategies.[143]

Reviewing and analyzing video recordings can be helpful in assessing the adequacy and use of compensatory strategies and techniques within group therapy. Treatment should include family members, friends, and other support individuals to facilitate generalizing improvements in social communication to real-life situations.

Intervention Methods

Based on expert clinical experience, the following are therapy suggestions to increase awareness of social communication skills and teach the use of compensatory strategies:

- Highlights from movies or television programs can be used to assist the SM in identifying pragmatic communication deficits. Examples of social communication breakdown in the program highlights should be similar to the problems demonstrated by the SM.
- Identification of social communication problems should be followed by discussion and education about why the deficits are problematic in social interactions.
- Video recordings of conversations between the SM and various communication partners can then be evaluated for problems in social communication skills.
- Discussion and education should follow the analysis of the videotaped interactions.
- Compensatory strategies to improve the SM's social communication skills can be taught and practiced in individual and group therapy, and in the home environment.
- Self-evaluation should be encouraged on the use of compensatory strategies in various settings.
- Generalization of compensatory strategies and self-evaluation in the use and effectiveness of strategies should be facilitated in community settings.

CLINICIAN TIP SHEET: TREATMENT SUGGESTIONS FOR SPECIFIC PROBLEMS IN SOCIAL COMMUNICATION

Tangential Comments and Topic Maintenance

Definition: difficulty maintaining the topic of conversation because of poor sustained attention and auditory working memory skills.

Therapy Suggestions: Incorporate compensatory strategies of using written notes during conversation to identify and track topics or asking for clarification of the topic when uncertain.

Conversational Breakdown and Turn-Taking Repair and Revision

Definition: unawareness that there is confusion or a breakdown in the conversation, difficulty repairing or asking for assistance during conversational breakdown because of decreased awareness or poor insight into the needs of the conversational partner, and poor problem solving and judgment.

Therapy Suggestions: Teach the patient to ask for clarification if there is any confusion during the conversation (eg, "I'm not sure about this," "I don't quite understand"), or teach the patient to identify nonverbal cues of the conversational partner (eg, facial expressions of confusion or uncertainty) to determine whether additional information is needed or information clarification is required.

Verbosity Versus Limited Amounts of Information/Turn-Taking/Quantity/Conciseness

Definition: providing too much or too little information during conversation because of lack of inhibition or awareness, deficits in working memory, or poor problem solving and judgment skills.

Therapy Suggestions: For verbosity or excessive quantity of information, teach the SM to identify the conversational partner's nonverbal cues (eg, facial expression of boredom, conversational partners looking at a watch, looking elsewhere, or shuffling papers). Another suggestion is to provide the SM with a specified number of question cards, tokens, or visual tally marks to use during brief conversations, which will allow the conversational partner to have a turn (eg, "These five cards represent five questions. When you ask the other person questions, it will give him or her the opportunity to talk. We want everyone to take turns during the conversation. Now, try to use all of the cards during the next 5 minutes").

If the patient is providing a limited quantity of information or if the information is vague, teach him or her to identify nonverbal cues (similar to those seen during conversational breakdown) and facial expressions of anticipation for more information. Cards, tokens, or visual tally marks can also be used to specify a number of sentences to produce during a conversational turn (eg, "The cards represent sentences. Try to say at least three sentences per turn").

Anomia, Lexical Selection, Use, Specificity, Accuracy

Definition: difficulty being specific or choosing the correct words in conversation because of deficits in working memory, slow processing speed, or disorganization.

Therapy Suggestions: Teach the patient to use compensatory strategies for anomia (eg, semantic descriptors of a target word) that can aid the listener in determining the intent of the message. Additionally, teach the patient to identify nonverbal cues

related to confusion of the conversational partner so additional descriptions of the target word can be produced. Provide education about the negative effects of using pauses and fillers when anomia occurs.

Anxiety and Anger Management

Definition: an interdisciplinary approach with professionals from medicine, psychology, social work, occupational therapy, and the like is beneficial to address the psychosocial issues of anxiety and anger. Behavioral and medical management may assist in reducing these feelings.

Therapy Suggestions: Educate the patient about how actions, nonverbal and verbal communication, postures, and proximity related to emotions can negatively impact social communication and the conversational partner. For example, the patient's affect (outward appearance) can be judged as aggressive, nervous, unfriendly, rude, or distant, yet this may not match the SM's actual emotions. Additionally, if certain actions related to emotions, such as anger, are not inhibited, the patient may become socially isolated.

ACQUIRED STUTTERING AND OTHER SPEECH DYSFLUENCIES

Purpose/Background

Acquired stuttering may occur in individuals returning from combat with c/mTBI.[33,35,51,117,186] Neurogenic stuttering is generally diagnosed when the onset of stutter-like dysfluencies occurs following a neurological event, such as a head trauma that disrupts normal brain function. In the absence of disruption to neurological function, adult-onset stuttering is often considered to be of psychogenic origin.[189] The differentiation is not always straightforward. The relatively sudden onset of stuttering-like speech can be due to one or a combination of neurological factors, psychological trauma, or medication effects. Trauma can also cause stuttering to recur in adults who previously recovered from developmental stuttering.[190] Fluency disorders may also result from word finding or word retrieval problems associated with cognitive impairments of attention and information processing speed resulting from TBI.[26] A fluency disorder, regardless of etiology, presents a serious communication problem that affects an individual's ability to interact with others. Therefore, it is important to acknowledge and validate the presence of stuttering and to address this communication disorder through evaluation of its nature

and severity. Following the evaluation, therapeutic interventions that focus on symptomatic remediation can be successful with limited intervention. Medication adjustments may be effective in eliminating stuttering symptoms due to medication effects.[33]

Strength of Recommendation: Practice Option

Acquired stuttering due to TBI has been widely discussed through case descriptions in the literature.[28,189–192] The majority of the cases described refer to individuals who sustained moderate to severe brain injuries. An early case description of combat-related acquired stuttering involved an individual diagnosed with combat psychoneuroses.[59] In recent years, SMs and veterans returning from combat have described acquired stuttering in the presence of TBI and PTSD. Some of these case studies can be found in the literature and many more have been described at conferences.[33,35,51,117,186]

Intervention Methods

See Clinician Tip Sheet: Acquired Stuttering and Other Speech Dysfluencies Assessment for cases of acquired stuttering.

CLINICIAN TIP SHEET: ACQUIRED STUTTERING AND OTHER SPEECH DYSFLUENCIES ASSESSMENT

Background

Acquired stuttering occurs primarily in adults; thus it is differentiated from developmental stuttering. Adult-onset of dysfluent speech can be due to:

- neurogenic etiology in people with psychosocial-emotional stress,[193]
- psychogenic etiology in the presence of neurologic symptoms,[194]
- stuttering associated with acquired neurological disorders,[190]
- drug effects,[103] and
- cognitive-linguistic deficits effects.[26]

Evaluation

Components of the evaluation of adult-onset dysfluency include:

- background information and case history;
- cognitive, language, and motor speech assessment;
- observation during a variety of speaking conditions, including:
  - reading (single words, short sentences, paragraphs),
  - spontaneous speech (monologue, conversation [minimum 200 syllables]), and
  - more automatic speech (counting, days, months, singing);
- speech situation checklist;
- stuttering severity (Stuttering Severity Instrument[195]);
- self-assessment of attitudes (S-24,[51] Locus of Control and Behavior[193]);
- analysis of symptom congruity; and
- trials of fluency enhancing techniques (slowed speech, masking and delayed auditory feedback, pacing) to the following:
  - determine the effects on frequency and severity of dysfluencies, and
  - assess for symptom reversibility that will confirm the diagnosis.

Differential diagnosis begins with a comparison of acquired symptoms with developmental stuttering symptoms. It is difficult based on speech characteristics alone. Clues can be found by integrating the history of onset, course of symptoms, speech characteristics, and consideration of the following behavior patterns:

- variability of symptoms across tasks and conditions;
- bizarre or unrelated secondary behaviors;
- psychosocial emotional factors;
- other neurologic symptoms, including speech and language disorders;
- performance on fluency-enhancing tasks; and
- intermittent periods of fluency.

Adult-Onset Stuttering

The following are descriptors to guide differential diagnosis of adult-onset stuttering.

Neurogenic Stuttering

Neurogenic stuttering

- usually co-occurs with other neurologic symptoms, including other speech-language or swallowing symptoms;
- elicits an individual reaction of concern when stuttering is present; and
- improves when demands on speech control are reduced, such as when speaking with whispered voice, or in a paced or rhythmic speech pattern.

Psychogenic Stuttering

Psychogenic stuttering is characterized by:

- a history of stuttering symptoms that resolved with stress resolution;
- symptoms that are variable across different speech tasks;
- "bizarre" or atypical accessory behaviors, struggle, or other secondary behaviors during motor speech examination; and it is
- the only communication complaint in the presence of multiple somatic complaints.

Rapid recovery or marked reduction of symptoms can occur with brief symptomatic intervention.

Because acquired stuttering occurs primarily in adults, diagnosis begins with a differentiation of symptoms from developmental stuttering (Exhibit 7-21).

CLINICIAN TIP SHEET: INTERVENTION FOR ACQUIRED STUTTERING AND OTHER SPEECH DYSFLUENCIES

Interventions and prognosis for acquired stuttering will vary depending on whether the etiology is neurogenic or psychogenic. When the etiology is undetermined, the patient response to intervention often contributes to differential diagnosis. For example, psychogenic stuttering responds to fluency-inducing conditions, whereas neurogenic stuttering will not. Neurogenic stuttering is consistent across speech stimuli and tasks and responds best to intervention focused on reducing demands on speech. Resolution of speech symptoms co-occurs with resolution of the neurologic symptoms.

Neurogenic Stuttering Treatment

Neurogenic stuttering treatment can be addressed using behavioral fluency treatment techniques, such as:

- focusing on breath stream, easy onset, gliding, and other strategies often used with developmental stuttering;
- rate reduction;
- self-monitoring;
- biofeedback and relaxation;
- speech pacing techniques to slow rate (eg, tapping as speaking or using a pacing board);

EXHIBIT 7-21

DIFFERENTIAL DIAGNOSIS OF ADULT-ONSET STUTTERING

Developmental Stuttering	Neurogenic Stuttering	Psychogenic Stuttering
• Gradual onset, usually between 2–4 years of age during rapid period of speech and language development • Can occur with developmental speech and language delay and disorders • Repetition, prolongations, and blocks of initial sounds and syllables; differs from cluttering • Occurs on context words • Adaptation effect • Responds to fluency-inducing conditions • Awareness, anxiety, fear and avoidance, tension, struggle increase over time	• Sudden onset in adults, due to neurologic event (eg, stroke, TBI, medication effect [tardive dyskinesia]) • Can occur with aphasia, apraxia, dysarthria; may occur in isolation • Similar core behaviors but not restricted to initial sounds and syllables • May occur on function words as well as content words; consistent across speech tasks • No adaptation effect • Does not respond to fluency-inducing conditions • Awareness, even annoyance, without anxiety, fear, avoidance, struggle; no secondary behaviors	• Sudden onset, in adults; triggered by somatization, prolonged stress or trauma, conversion disorder • Can occur with neurologic disease or present with suspected neurologic disease • Similar core behaviors but not restricted to initial syllables; excessive repetitions on every phoneme • Can occur anywhere in speech; with unusual secondary behaviors that are independent of core behaviors; unusual grammatical constructions (telegraphic) • No adaptation effect • May respond to fluency-inducing conditions • Awareness with variable anxiety, fear, avoidance and struggle; inconsistent relative to severity of symptoms

TBI: traumatic brain injury

- delayed auditory feedback[189,197]; and
- pharmacological management,[198] including anxiety medications.[192,196]

Psychogenic Stuttering Treatment

Psychogenic stuttering can be treated with symptomatic therapy.

- Observe speech for musculoskeletal tension.
- Palpate the thyrohyoid space for musculoskeletal tension.
- Educate patient about the association between tension and blocking of airflow.
- Teach patient to identify the locus of their musculoskeletal tension relative to stuttering episodes, to contrast feelings of musculoskeletal tension with muscular relaxation, and to modify and reduce tension.
- Select a high-frequency behavior to modify (eg, eye blinking, laryngeal blocking) or reduce musculoskeletal tension, laying your hands on the problem area if necessary.[33]
- Practice speech without musculoskeletal tension, beginning at single word or sound level, depending on severity:
  - Single consonant and vowel syllable prolongation with airflow and easy onset or gliding
  - Single words: change type of dysfluencies (hesitation or repetition and try prolonged rate or synthesized speaking pattern)
  - Present frequent reminders of success with reduced musculoskeletal tension
- Vary speaking patterns after dysfluencies are reduced or eliminated, moving toward natural speech prosody.[33]
- Implement techniques used with developmental stuttering, including prolonged speech, fluency shaping, easy onset, light contact, easy repetitions, and diminishing extra motor (secondary) behaviors.
- Reduce excess musculoskeletal tension associated with efforts to speak.
- Provide education and counseling to minimize frustration and other emotional reactions to speech symptoms.
- Provide frequent reassurance and positive feedback for successes.
- Follow a hierarchy of easy to difficult situations to transfer learned skills outside of therapy.[193,197,199]

PATIENT HANDOUT: CHANGE BEGINS WITH AWARENESS

After c/mTBI, many people are confused and surprised by errors they make on tasks that were easy for them in the past. Progress begins as people become aware of the factors that interfere with their performance. This awareness motivates them to learn and use compensatory cognitive strategies to prevent performance problems before they occur.

AWARENESS = POWER

Becoming aware of inefficiencies, cognitive vulnerabilities, and other factors that sometimes accompany c/mTBI is a learning process in which people move up the awareness hierarchy (Figure 7-1).

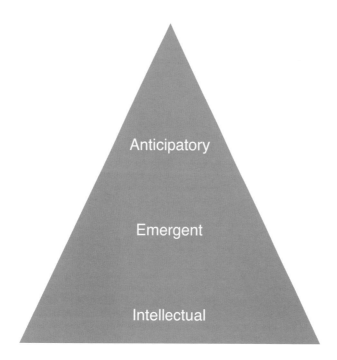

Figure 7-1. Levels of awareness.

TYPES OF AWARENESS

Intellectual awareness: Knowing there is a problem but being unable to recognize it when it is occurring (eg, "People tell me I repeat myself a lot during conversations.").

Emergent awareness: Recognizing a problem when it is occurring (eg, "As soon as I started my story, I saw people look at me funny, I think I was repeating myself again.").

Anticipatory awareness: Anticipating a potential problem and having a strategy in mind (eg, "Because I know that I tend to repeat myself, I always ask people if I've told them one of my stories before I launch in.").

One goal of therapy is to help you improve your awareness of the factors that interfere with your performance and of those strategies that help.

PATIENT HANDOUT: CORE COGNITIVE STRATEGY RECOMMENDATIONS GRID

This grid represents a summary of the core cognitive strategies that have been tested and proven effective for you during your therapy program.

Area of Cognitive Inefficiency	Recommended Core Strategy	Real-World Application

PATIENT HANDOUT: WORKING LOG
CORE COGNITIVE STRATEGY RECOMMENDATIONS GRID

| | | | | Strategy Evaluation | | |
| | | | | Effective | | |
Problem Area	Cognitive Domain(s)	Date	Strategy Recommended	Yes	No	Maybe

PATIENT HANDOUT: "AAA" SELF-REFLECTION

ANTICIPATION (fill this section out before performing the task)

Task Description

Anticipated time (how long it will take to complete the task):

Anticipated accuracy (# of errors likely to make):

Cognitive challenges associated with this task (check all that apply)	Strategies I plan to implement to optimize my effectiveness in performing this task
Attention/concentration	
Memory	
Planning	
Problem solving	

ACTION (fill this section out while performing the task)

Start time: _____ End time: _____

Number of breaks during task performance: _____

ANALYSIS (fill this section out after performing the task)

Actual performance time: _____

- If it took you more time than predicted, why?

- If it took you less time than predicted, why?

Actual accuracy level: _____

- If you made more errors than predicted, why?

- If you made fewer errors than predicted, why?

What factors interfered with your performance?

What strategies **did** you use that helped you perform this task?

In hindsight, what strategies **should** you have used to improve your performance?

List two everyday tasks that pose similar challenges and require similar strategies:

    1.

    2.

PATIENT HANDOUT: UNDERSTANDING HUMAN INFORMATION PROCESSING

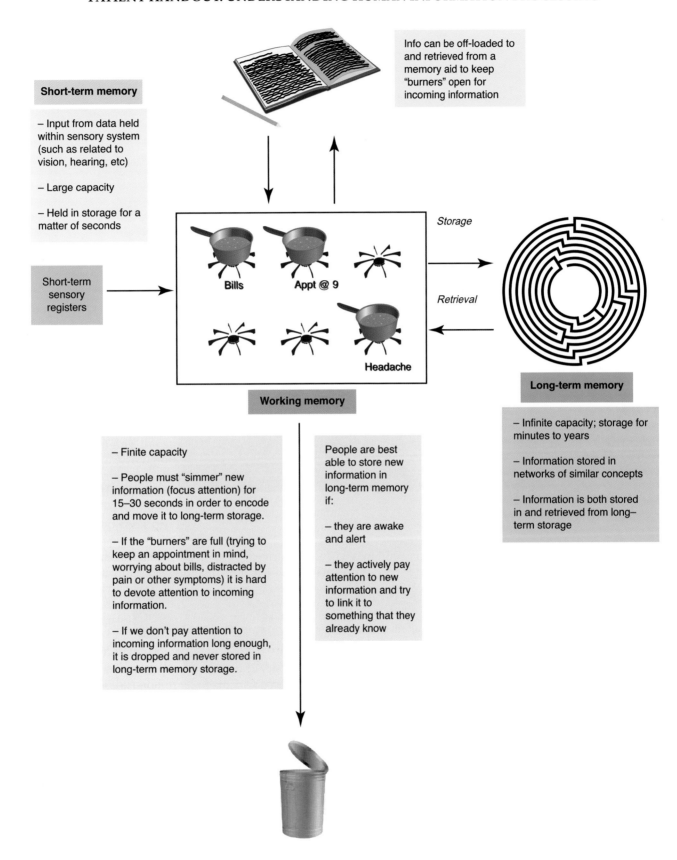

Info can be off-loaded to and retrieved from a memory aid to keep "burners" open for incoming information

Short-term memory

– Input from data held within sensory system (such as related to vision, hearing, etc)

– Large capacity

– Held in storage for a matter of seconds

Short-term sensory registers

Bills

Appt @ 9

Headache

Storage

Retrieval

Working memory

Long-term memory

– Infinite capacity; storage for minutes to years

– Information stored in networks of similar concepts

– Information is both stored in and retrieved from long–term storage

– Finite capacity

– People must "simmer" new information (focus attention) for 15–30 seconds in order to encode and move it to long-term storage.

– If the "burners" are full (trying to keep an appointment in mind, worrying about bills, distracted by pain or other symptoms) it is hard to devote attention to incoming information.

– If we don't pay attention to incoming information long enough, it is dropped and never stored in long-term memory storage.

People are best able to store new information in long-term memory if:

– they are awake and alert

– they actively pay attention to new information and try to link it to something that they already know

Figure 7-2. Human information processing diagram.

PATIENT HANDOUT: UNDERSTANDING THE MULTIFACTOR MODEL
OF FUNCTIONING AFTER CONCUSSION

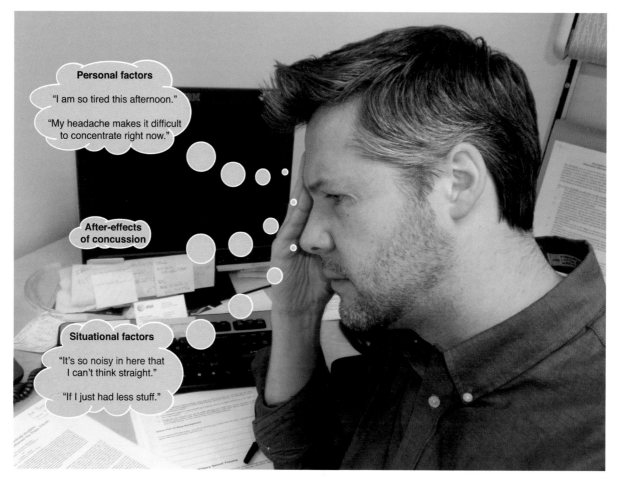

Figure 7-3. Multifactor model of functioning.

After concussion, an individual's injury combines with other factors to impact performance of everyday activities, social interactions, and ability to cope with stress.[1] These factors include:

- **personal factors:** internal distracters (such as fatigue, stress, physical symptoms, and negative thoughts), and
- **situational factors:** external distracters (such as noise, visual stimuli in the environment), multitasking, speed of processing, and information processing demands of the task at hand.

Fluctuations in performance from one day or situation to the next can often be explained by the presence of one or more of these complicating factors. Therapy enables patients to learn how to use various strategies to address and minimize the influence of personal or situational factors that interfere with their performance.

You may be able to improve your functioning after c/mTBI by managing various personal and situational factors. Here are some examples.

Personal Factors

Fatigue

- Perform tasks requiring high levels of concentration during times of the day when you are alert and energized. Save easy or routine tasks for times of the day when you tend to be tired. With this adjustment, you can remain active throughout the day.

- Institute good sleep hygiene practices.

Stress and Negative Thoughts

- Recognize when you are distracted by worries, stress, and negative thoughts.
- Work with mental health providers to identify strategies to manage your worries, stress, and intrusive thoughts.

Pain

- Perform tasks requiring high levels of concentration during times of the day when pain levels are lower. Save easy or routine tasks for times of the day when pain levels are greater. With this adjustment, you can remain active throughout the day.

Situational Factors

Noisy or Visually Distracting Environment

- Recognize when the environment is making it difficult to concentrate and make changes (modify the environment to minimize these factors or move to a different environment to eliminate distracters).
- Consider using "white noise" to buffer distracting sounds and noise.
- Remember that if you have difficulty filtering out noises, you may fatigue more quickly.

Multitasking

- Remember it is generally easier to do one task at a time. To optimize efficiency, avoid dividing or shifting attention among multiple tasks.
- Use strategies that slow down the rate at which you process new information. For example, ask people to repeat information, if necessary. Employ a "pause" strategy to give yourself a moment to stop and focus your attention on what's going on around you and how you can best manage the new information.

PATIENT HANDOUT: UNDERSTANDING HIERARCHY OF ATTENTION LEVELS

Paying attention involves different levels of mental effort (Figure 7-4). We go back and forth between these attention levels all day. The higher the attention demands of the task or situation, the harder a person has to concentrate, and the more effort or energy is required to complete the activity.

- **Some tasks require lower levels of attention; others require higher levels of attention.**
  - ◦ Focused attention: I say your name and you turn and look at me.
  - ◦ Sustained attention: You listen to the news.
  - ◦ Selective attention: You filter out the music on the radio while balancing your checkbook.
  - ◦ Alternating attention: You are conversing with a friend at a coffee shop when your cell phone rings. After speaking to the caller, you hang up and continue the conversation with your friend.
  - ◦ Divided attention: You drive the car while talking with your passenger.
- **In addition to the task itself, personal and situational factors place demands on your attention.**
  - ◦ Personal factors: Being tired or worried makes it harder to pay attention.
  - ◦ Situational factors: Working in a noisy environment makes it harder to pay attention.
- **Remember, you optimize your ability to perform everyday tasks when you…**
  - ◦ understand your strengths and weaknesses specific to paying attention.
  - ◦ manage personal and situational factors that decrease your ability to pay attention.
  - ◦ choose the times of day or circumstances under which you can best handle tasks that demand the highest levels of attention.

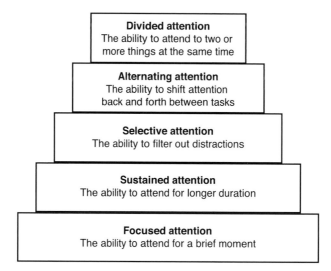

Figure 7-4. Hierarchy of attention levels.

PATIENT HANDOUT
INVENTORY OF ATTENTION/SPEED-OF-PROCESSING DIFFICULTIES

NAME _____ DATE _____

DEMANDS

Task/Setting	Frequency of Problem	Length of Task	Alternate with Another Task	Same Time as Another Task	Personal Factors	Environmental Factors	Rate of Processing
	Times per week	Minutes /hours					Slow / Average / Fast
Strategies:							
	Times per week	Minutes /hours					Slow / Average / Fast
Strategies:							
	Times per week	Minutes /hours					Slow / Average / Fast
Strategies:							
	Times per week	Minutes /hours					Slow / Average / Fast
Strategies:							

PATIENT HANDOUT: EXPERIENCING ATTENTION LEVELS–FOCUSED AND SUSTAINED

Instructions

- Read the activity description for each attention level.
- Before you start the activity, fill in the Self-Prediction chart.
- Perform the activity, then fill in the Self-Reflection chart.
- Be prepared to discuss your impressions with your clinician.

Sustained Attention Activity

Scan the rows of letters and cross out only the vowels. Work as quickly and as accurately as possible.

Self-Prediction: Hard / Average / Easy	No. of Errors:	Energy Cost: Low / Average / High

```
A T U R F G V I E S Q N B V M A O I P L K M P O R T D E V C X W A
S E R U J N M V C X D J U I P K H G R E W Q C S X S Z S D V K L O L
O E I J H G R W Q X C G B V G E D K J N B E I U T Y P K O L C X Z D S
D T F E Q U T Y O P N M G F G V X C S D H J I P L I U T R W S X Z X
V F D U J G I J H N G E R I U Y H L O I U H B G V F D X Z A E R D V O
T U R F G V I Q S Q N B V M A O I P T K M P O R T D E V C X W A T Q
S E R U J N M V C X D J U I P K H G R E W Q C S X S Z S D V K L O L
O E I J H T W Q X C G B V G E Q K J N B E I U T Y P K O L C X Z D S
D T F E Q U T Y O P N M T F G V X C S Q H J I P L I U T R Q S X Z X T
V F T Q J G I J H N G E R I U Y H L O I Q B G V F D X Z A E R D V O R
T U R F G V I Q S Q N B V M A O I P T K M P O R T D E V C X W A T Q
S E R U J N M V C X D J U I P K H G R E W Q C S X S Z S D V K L O L
O E I J H T W Q X C G B V G E Q K J N B E I U T Y P K O L C X Z D S Q
D T F E Q U T Y O P N M T F G V X C S Q H J I P L I U T R Q S X Z X T
V F T Q J G I J H N G E R I U Y H L O I Q B G V F D X Z A E R D V O R
```

Self-Reflection: Hard / Average / Easy	No. of Errors:	Energy Cost: Low / Average / High

CLINICIAN ANSWER KEY

<u>Correct answers</u>: 115 vowels on the sheet
Row #1: 10
Row #2: 6
Row #3: 8
Row #4: 6
Row #5: 11
Row #6: 8
Row #7: 6
Row #8: 8
Row #9: 6
Row #10: 9
Row #11: 8
Row #12: 6
Row #13: 8
Row #14: 6
Row #15: 9

PATIENT HANDOUT: EXPERIENCING ATTENTION LEVELS–SELECTIVE ATTENTION (VISUAL AND AUDITORY)

Instructions

- Read the activity description for each attention level.
- Before you start the activity, fill in the Self-Prediction chart.
- Perform the activity, then fill in the Self-Reflections chart.
- Be prepared to discuss your impressions with your clinician.

Selective Attention (Visual Distracter) Activity

Scan the rows of letters and cross out only the letters T and Q. Work as quickly and accurately as possible.

Self-Prediction: Hard / Average / Easy	No. of Errors:	Energy Cost: Low / Average / High

```
T U R F G V I Q S Q N B V M A O I P T K M P O R T D E V C X W A T
S E R U J N M V C X D J U I P K H G R E W Q C S X S Z S D V K L
O E I J H T W Q X C G B V G E Q K J N B E I U T Y P K O L C X Z D
D T F E Q U T Y O P N M T F G V X C S Q H J I P L I U T R Q S X Z X
V F T Q J G I J H N G E R I U Y H L O I Q B G V F D X Z A E R D V O
T U R F G V I Q S Q N B V M A O I P T K M P O R T D E V C X W A T
S E R U J N M V C X D J U I P K H G R E W Q C S X S Z S D V K L
O E I J H T W Q X C G B V G E Q K J N B E I U T Y P K O L C X Z D
D T F E Q U T Y O P N M T F G V X C S Q H J I P L I U T R Q S X Z X
S O R K W G E A O W G H U S P R G Y H H F D W S F G J U E K Q F I B
M Y D R A E F G H I W J X H U W J K Q O P W I L O W H E A P F
D W T Y U S A G W O P F H W Q I H J K L S E F G M Q D Y S H J X
```

Self-Reflection: Hard / Average / Easy	No. of Errors:	Energy Cost: Low / Average / High

Selective Attention (Auditory Distracters) Activity

Scan the rows of letters and cross out the Fs and Cs; ignore anything you hear.

Self-Prediction: Hard / Average / Easy	No. of Errors:	Energy Cost: Low / Average / High

```
T U R F G V I Q S Q N B V M A O I P T K M P O R T D E V C X W A T
S E R U J N M V C X D J U I P K H G R E W Q C S X S Z S D V K L
O E I J H T W Q X C G B V G E Q K J N B E I U T Y P K O L C X Z D
D T F E Q U T Y O P N M T F G V X C S Q H J I P L I U T R Q S X Z X
V F T Q J G I J H N G E R I U Y H L O I Q B G V F D X Z A E R D V O
T U R F G V I Q S Q N B V M A O I P T K M P O R T D E V C X W A T
S E R U J N M V C X D J U I P K H G R E W Q C S X S Z S D V K L
O E I J H T W Q X C G B V G E Q K J N B E I U T Y P K O L C X Z D
D T F E Q U T Y O P N M T F G V X C S Q H J I P L I U T R Q S X Z X
S O R K W G E A O W G H U S P R G Y H H F D W S F G J U E K Q F I B
M Y D R A E F G H I W J X H U W J K Q O P W I L O W H E A P F
D W T Y U S A G W O P F H W Q I H J K L S E F G M Q D Y S H J X
```

Self-Reflection: Hard / Average / Easy	No. of Errors:	Energy Cost: Low / Average / High

CLINICIAN INSTRUCTIONS AND ANSWER KEY

Alternating Attention Activity 1

Clinician Instructions

Patients begin by adding the numbers in the row. At the first asterisk (*), ask them to switch to subtraction; at the second asterisk, switch to multiplication; at the third asterisk, switch back to addition; at the fourth asterisk, switch back to subtraction; and at the fifth asterisk, switch back to multiplication.

Correct Answers

(+) 4 = 9 = 11 = 15 = 20 = 28 = 29 = 31 = 34 = 35/
(−) 30 = 24 = 20 = 12 = 9 = 5 = 1/
(×) 5 = 1 0 = 10 = 30 = 60/
(+) 65 = 69 = 70 = 79 = 80 = 85 = 86 = 90/
(−) 81 = 80 = 72 = 70 = 61 = 60 = 56 = 50 = 45 = 40 = 32 = 30 = 29 = 20 = 13 = 11/
(×) 22 = 22 = 44 = 0 = 0 = 0/
(+) 2 = 6 = 7 = 12 = 15 = 17 = 18 = 22/
(−) 16 = 12 = 7 = 4 = 3/
(×) 6 = 18 = 18 = 36 = 72 = 72 = 0/
(+) 5 = 12 = 20 = 26 = 28 = 31 = 35 = 42 = 47 = 49 = 55 = 58/
(−) 51 = 47 = 43 = 37 = 31 = 29 = 28 = 20 = 13 = 8 = END

Divided Attention

Clues:
 Outdoors
 Alive
 1 to 2 feet tall
 Has roots
 Has leaves
 Fragrant
 Green
 Colorful
 Pedals
 Needs water
 Answer: flower

CLINICIAN INSTRUCTIONS AND ANSWER KEY

Selective Attention (Visual Distracter)	**Selective Attention (Auditory Distracters)**
Scribble over all the letters to create a visual distracter before giving patient worksheet.	*Turn on a radio; after patient completes two lines, start talking about random subjects.*

Correct answers: 43 Ts and Qs
Row #1: 6
Row #2: 1
Row #3: 4
Row #4: 7
Row #5: 3
Row #6: 5
Row #7: 1
Row #8: 4
Row #9: 7
Row #10: 1
Row #11: 1
Row #12: 3

Correct answers: 26 Fs and Cs
Row #1: 2
Row #2: 2
Row #3: 2
Row #4: 3
Row #5: 2
Row #6: 2
Row #7: 2
Row #8: 2
Row #9: 2
Row #10: 3
Row #11: 2
Row #12: 2

PATIENT HANDOUT: EXPERIENCING ATTENTION LEVELS–ALTERNATING AND DIVIDED

Alternating Attention Activity 1

This is a calculation task. Beginning with the first number, add each number to the one that follows, keeping the sum in mind. When you get to the asterisk (*), report your answer and the clinician will tell you which mathematical operation to do next.

Self-Prediction: Hard / Average / Easy	No. of Errors:	Energy Cost: Low / Average / High

```
1 3 5 2 4 5 8 1 2 3 1 * 5 6 4 8 3 4 4 * 5 2 1 3 2 * 5 4 1 9 1 5 1 4 * 9
1 8 2 9 1 4 6 5 5 8 2 1 9 7 2 * 2 1 2 0 5 8 * 2 4 1 5 3 2 1 4 * 6 4 5 3
1 * 2 3 1 2 2 1 0 * 5 7 8 6 2 3 4 7 5 2 6 3 * 7 4 4 6 6 2 1 8 7 5 END
```

Self-Reflection: Hard / Average / Easy	No. of Errors:	Energy Cost: Low / Average / High

Alternating Attention Activity 2

Your clinician will give you a deck of cards; you are to sort the deck into two piles. Start by putting the red cards in one pile and the black cards in the second pile. In 15 to 20 seconds, the clinician will direct you to sort them into piles of even and odd numbers.

Self-Prediction: Hard / Average / Easy	No. of Errors:	Energy Cost: Low / Average / High

Self-Reflection: Hard / Average / Easy	No. of Errors:	Energy Cost: Low / Average / High

Divided Attention Activity

This task involves doing two things at once. Sort a deck of cards into suits and put them in numerical order, with the aces acting as low cards. At the same time, your clinician will give you a clue every 15 to 30 seconds. Using these clues, you are to figure out what word the clinician is thinking of while you continue to sort the deck of cards.

Self-Prediction: Hard / Average / Easy	No. of Errors:	Energy Cost: Low / Average / High

**PATIENT HANDOUT: STRATEGIES TO IMPROVE ATTENTION–
IDENTIFYING YOUR HIGH- AND LOW-DEMAND TASKS**

Key Attention Management Strategy: Match the Task to Your Attentional Abilities:

- Perform easy or low-consequence (low demand) tasks at times of the day or under circumstances in which your ability to pay close attention is limited.
- Perform easy or low-consequence tasks when the work environment is not something you can control.
- Perform high-consequence or difficult (high demand) tasks at a time in your day when you are well-rested, mentally alert, and when your symptoms (pain, headache) are under control.
- Perform high-consequence or difficult tasks in a quiet environment.

Before you can implement the above strategies, you must identify your high- and low-demand tasks.

1. List the key tasks that you are responsible for in everyday life. Consider work, home, personal, family responsibilities.
2. Rate the consequence level of each task.
   - high-consequence tasks: no tolerance for error (eg, bill paying, data entry, internet stock trading)
   - low-consequence tasks: errors do not really matter (eg, folding laundry, recycling, tooth brushing)
3. Rate the difficulty level of each task.
4. Review the chart and identify the tasks you rated as high consequence or difficult and those you rated as low consequence or easy.

I am responsible for these key tasks:	Consequence Level		Difficulty Level	
	High	**Low**	**Tough**	**Easy**
Personal				
Family				

I am responsible for these key tasks:	Consequence Level		Difficulty Level	
	High	**Low**	**Tough**	**Easy**
Work				
Household				

MY HIGH-DEMAND TASKS:

*Perform in quiet environments or when well rested, when symptoms are under control.

MY LOW-DEMAND TASKS:

*Perform in more distracting environments or when symptoms are present but not debilitating.

PATIENT HANDOUT: STRATEGIES TO IMPROVE ATTENTION–MODIFYING YOUR APPROACH AND WORKSPACE

Optimizing your attention begins with awareness of your vulnerabilities and the strategies that can help. You can make it easier to perform most tasks if you optimize your approach and work environment by reducing demands at this time. Here are some suggestions that may work for you and in your workspace.

Reduce Length of Task

- Set a timer to help you focus for a specific amount of time before taking a break.
- Take a brief quiet break every 30 to 60 minutes or more (get a drink of water, stretch, etc) to optimize your alertness.
- Use an alarm to remind you to take a break and to return to a task or initiate another task.
- Plan ahead so you schedule tasks that require high levels of attention at high-energy times of the day or when you are least likely to be distracted by pain or fatigue. Schedule easy tasks at times you are likely to be tired and less able to pay attention; be assured that these tasks do not require high levels of energy or attention.
- Allow extra time to complete tasks with scheduled breaks.

Reduce Competing Tasks

- Apply the above strategies to reduce demand on focused or sustained attention.
- Do one task at a time if possible, or alternate with another tasks that is not high consequence or difficult.
- Do not divide attention on high consequence and difficult tasks.
- Set an alarm to remind you to initiate another task.
- Organize your space and your work task (eg, keep all things needed for a task in one drawer, categorize and file orders for a task in a binder) so that you can shift from one assignment to another easily.
- Do not talk on a cell phone while driving or operating other equipment.
- Limit conversations while driving.

Reduce Personal and Environmental Factors That Can be Distractions

- Apply the above strategies for focused/sustained and alternating/divided attention.
- Rest prior to demanding situations.
- Set the room temperature so it is cool enough to keep you alert yet comfortable.
- Dim lights, close curtains, wear dark glasses, or face your back to light if glare or bright lights are uncomfortable. On the other hand, increase light or magnitude of what you are seeing or reading if you have low vision to reduce strain.
- Close the door or go to a quiet room or quieter part of a room.
- Choose to sit in an area with the least number of distractions (eg, corner booth by the wall).
- Turn off unnecessary noise in the environment. No television or radio if you find them distracting.
- Create "white noise" to block ambient noises around you that are hard to ignore (eg, turn on a small fan so that the hum of the fan blocks distracting noise from nearby conversations, use music to block out background noise).
- Situate yourself as you work so that visual distractions are minimized (avoid positioning yourself in front of a door or window if outside activities make it hard to concentrate).
- Temporarily move objects out of your sight that draw your attention away from the task at hand.
- Try to refrain from conversation or interruptions during a task or until you have reached a "stop point." Develop a script to politely explain to family members or coworkers that you work most efficiently in quiet without diversions. To maintain relationships, develop another script to invite visits from them or engage in conversation at other times when it will not compete with your work.
- Run errands or attend social activities at nonpeak hours.

**PATIENT HANDOUT: STRATEGIES TO IMPROVE ATTENTION–MANAGING
INTERRUPTIONS AND MULTIPLE TASKS**

Optimizing your attention begins with awareness of your vulnerabilities and the strategies that can help. Minimize the cost of interruptions and best handle multitasking by planning your strategy in advance. Here are some strategies that might work for you.

- If you know you are going to be interrupted, select a highly familiar, mundane task to perform (such as folding laundry, cleaning counter surfaces) rather than a task that requires high levels of accuracy and demands your undivided attention (such as bill paying, computer data entry).
- Knowing that a conversation may cause distractions (and errors) while you work, find a polite way to discontinue the conversation. Come up with some polite phrases ahead of time, such as "I have to concentrate on this right now, so can I get back to you later to hear more?"
- If interrupted, finish your thought or attempt to reach a breakpoint before stopping what you are doing. You may need to hold up your hand to signal the person that you will be right with him or her in a moment.
- Use "stop notes" to pick back up after an interruption (Figure 7-5). Stop notes are a way to capture your thoughts about what you were doing or thinking at the time you stopped work. Here are some examples:
  - If interrupted while reading, write down a few notes and place a "sticky" note at the place you stopped.
  - If interrupted on a project, create a stop note that includes what you last completed and where to restart the task (later in the day, tomorrow, or next week).
- Plan for interruptions before you get started on a project that will take many days (weeks or months) to complete by creating a "divide-and-conquer" project game plan. Developing a step-by-step plan before you begin work enables you to place a checkmark by the last step completed when interrupted and to pick right back up on the next step when you get back to the project. The same strategy may help you juggle two projects at the same time.
- If you know that you need to be interrupted mid-task (to go to an appointment, for example), set an alarm to remind you at the appropriate time. That way you can fully attend to what you are doing without worrying that you will forget to stop.
- Implement strategies aimed at modifying your approach to the task and structuring your environment.

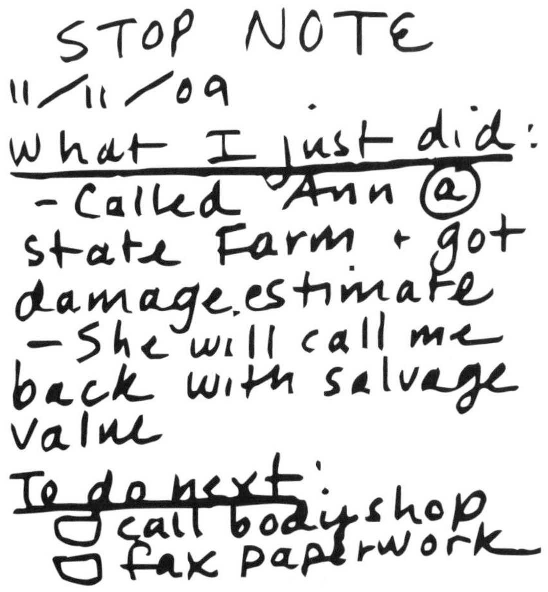

Figure 7-5. Example of a stop note.

**PATIENT HANDOUT: COPING WITH SLOWER SPEED OF
PROCESSING–USING THE AUDITORY SYSTEM**

Background

At times you may not be able to control or change the complexity and rate of incoming information. Under these conditions, you can still be proactive and make it easier to perform most tasks with strategies to enhance your ability to hear, the quality of the listening conditions, and processing of information through optimal use of the auditory system.

Step 1: Recognize adverse listening conditions or demands to predict potential difficulty. This level of awareness allows you to select and use an appropriate strategy.

Step 2: Your clinician will guide you through the process of selecting, trialing, and implementing an appropriate strategy that works for you when you need it. Some examples include:

- Turn off appliances (television, radio) and close doors and windows to reduce extraneous information and noise that can compete with what you really want or need to hear and understand.
- Ask for or seek preferential seating (up front, away from machinery). This will allow you to see the speaker, and possibly even lip read if necessary.
- Do not pretend to understand: clarify! Ask questions to make sure you understand instructions and assignments.
- Retell, restate, or paraphrase directions and instructions to confirm your understanding.
- Use technology (eg, digital recorders, smart pens) to record lectures and lessons for playback at home during study and homework sessions.
- Record meetings, briefings, and appointments for playback at a later time or during daily review.
- Use an assistive listening device to improve your hearing in challenging situations, such as in large meeting rooms and lecture halls.

PATIENT HANDOUT: COPING WITH SLOWER SPEED OF PROCESSING–USING THE VISUAL SYSTEM

Background

At times you may not be able to control or modify the demands or the complexity and rate of incoming information. Under these conditions, you can still be proactive and make it easier to perform most tasks with strategies to enhance ability to hear and to process the information you hear through optimal use of the visual system.

Step 1: Recognize adverse listening conditions or demands that can be helped by adding a visually mediated strategy. This level of awareness allows you to select and use an appropriate strategy.

Step 2: Your clinician will guide you through the process of selecting, trialing, and implementing an appropriate strategy that works for you when you need it. Here are some examples:

- Choose face-to-face interactions and make frequent eye contact with the speaker to keep engaged in an interaction and benefit from verbal and nonverbal cues.
- Make liberal use of visual models, pictures, videos, and computer-generated models, or any other means available.
- Use organizers, like agendas and smartphone applications, create to-do lists, or use calendar applications in cellular phones to store and review information.
- Use your visual reasoning skills to understand materials and to express your own understanding.
- Have tasks demonstrated when possible.
- Select closed-caption (subtitles) option when watching television or videos.
- Send or request texts to clarify information after a conversation.
- Read notes, book chapters, or manuals or do internet searches ahead of time (for example, before a lecture) to cue into and anticipate new terms, words, and concepts.
- Create a study guide that includes key vocabulary with definitions, guiding questions, and a clear statement of learning goals for the task. Prepare for what you are going to hear.
- Ask for assignments and directions in writing, in e-mails, or as a summary after a discussion.

PATIENT HANDOUT: AAA SELF-REFLECTION WORKSHEET FOR ATTENTION AND SPEED OF PROCESSING

Anticipation (complete this section before performing the task)
Task description:

Anticipated time (how long it will take to complete the task):

Challenges associated with this task	Strategies I plan to implement to optimize my effectiveness in performing this task
Sustained attention	
Selective attention	
Alternating attention	
Divided attention	
Speed of processing	

Anticipated accuracy (number correct/errors):

Action (complete this section out while performing the task)
Start time: _____ End time: _____

Number of breaks during task performance:

Analysis (fill this section out after performing the task)
Actual performance time: _____
If it took you more time than predicted, why?

If it took you less time than predicted, why?

Actual accuracy level: _____
If you made more errors than predicted, why?

If you made fewer errors than predicted, why?

What factors interfered with your performance?

What strategies did you use that helped you perform this task?

In hindsight, what strategies should you use to improve your performance?

List two everyday tasks that pose similar challenges and require similar strategies:
1.

2.

PATIENT HANDOUT: COMPENSATORY MEMORY STRATEGIES–INTERNAL AND EXTERNAL OPTIONS

Background

People use a number of strategies to make sure they consistently and effectively keep track of information. After c/mTBI, these strategies become important in assuring ongoing competent performance of daily tasks. In therapy, you will identify and learn to use the memory strategies that help you function at your best.

There are two categories of memory strategies:
1. Internal strategies (those that involve thinking techniques to help you encode new information into memory).
2. External strategies (those that involve physical aids, such as using notes, planners, devices, or alarms to help you keep track of information without relying on your memory).

You will likely find both categories of memory strategies helpful. Here are some examples of strategies to explore with your clinician.

Internal Strategies

- Helpful in situations when it is impractical or inappropriate to take notes (such as remembering information while driving).
- Helpful to remember information for which a written note might be insecure (such as remembering one's personal identification number or password).

Strategy Example	Description	Real-life Application
Visual imagery[1,2]	Making a mental picture of to-be-remembered information	Imagining items to be purchased while sitting around in your living room
First letter mnemonics[2]	Using the first letter of each to-be-remembered item to create a word	To help remember names: **N**: notice (facial features) **A**: associate the person's face with something familiar to you or an image that the name suggests **M**: mention the name in conversation **E**: Exaggerate some aspect of the name or face to hold it in memory
Mental retracing[3]	Reviewing activities from the recent past to help trigger recollection of what they need to do	Can be used when people forget their current intention (eg, walking into a room and forgetting why or what was needed from the room)
Alphabetic searching[3,4]	Word retrieval strategy	When having trouble retrieving a name or concept, individual systematically reviews the letters of the alphabet that may serve as a first letter cue to trigger recall of the desired information
Elaborated encoding of information[5,6]	Strategies are used to hold and manipulate information in short-term memory in ways that will facilitate stronger encoding and storage of the information in long-term memory	When learning definitions for concepts in school, mentally 1) review the definition, 2) rephrase the definition in your own words, 3) match the word to synonyms or antonyms, and, 4) use the word in self-generated sentences

(table *continues***)**

table *continued*

Peg mnemonics[4,7]	An associative memory strategy in which a person memorizes a "peg-set" of imaginable words (eg, one is a bun, two is a shoe, three is a tree, four is a door, five is a hive, six is sticks, seven is heaven, eight is a gate, nine is a line, ten is a hen)	Once the "peg-set" is memorized, additional items that need to be remembered can be associated with items on the list and an image created that incorporates both items. The visual association of new items to those on the memorized list facilitates retrieval of the desired information
Spaced retrieval[8]	Learning is most effective when the learning episodes are spread out over time (distributed learning) rather than all at once (massed practice). Spaced retrieval is a specialized form of distributed learning in which a small amount of information is learned and then retrieved at a very short interval (eg, 1 minute). The length of the interval is systematically increased (eg, 2 minutes, 4 minutes, 8 minutes, etc)	This is a powerful learning strategy that has been used successfully to train people with dementia with new skills

External Strategies

- Helpful in situations when keeping track of information would be effortful or unreliable.
- Helpful in situations when you want to focus your attention fully on the task at hand (rather than worrying about potentially forgetting something important).
- Assistive technology for cognition provides a means of recording important information for later review. Devices that serve this purpose include smart pens, smartphones, and voice recorders as well as low-tech options such as a notepad and pencil or wipe-off board.

Strategy Example	Description	Real-life Application
Day planner/calendar	Low technology Paper-and-pencil planner Dry-erase board	Using a daily planner to keep track of medical appointments, therapy assignments, and family activities
Cellular phone, other smartphone, or computer	Calendar with alarm Task applications Alarm clock Stopwatch	Using calendar or scheduler function to set alarms for time-specific prompts
Environmental cues	Organizing and structuring the environment to facilitate efficient retrieval of personal items, compliance with due dates or medication schedules, recall of information; includes use of sticky notes, checklists, labels, key holders, mail sorters, pill boxes	Organizing and labeling storage cabinets, setting up filing systems, creating message centers, establishing bill payment systems, reducing clutter

(table *continues*)

table *continued*

| Alarm watch | Setting daily alarms to prompt taking medications, routine breaks or pauses, or time-specific actions |

Data sources: 1) Killam C, Cautin RL, Santucci AC. Assessing the enduring residual neuropsychological effects of head trauma in college athletes who participate in contact sports. *Arch Clin Neuropsychol.* Jul 2005;20(5):599–611. 2) Parenté R, Herrmann D. *Retraining Cognition: Techniques and Applications.* 2nd ed. Austin, TX: Pro-ed; 2002. 3) Duff MC, Proctor A, Haley K. Mild traumatic brain injury (MTBI): assessment and treatment procedures used by speech-language pathologists (SLPs). *Brain Inj.* Sep 2002;16(9):773–787. 4) Moffat N. Strategies of memory therapy. In: Wilson BA, Moffat N, eds. *Clinical Management of Memory Problems.* Rockville, MD: Aspen; 1984. 5) Oberg L, Turkstra LS. Use of elaborative encoding to facilitate verbal learning after adolescent traumatic brain injury. *J Head Trauma Rehabil.* Jun 1998;13(3):44–62. 6) O'Neil-Pirozzi TM, Strangman GE, Goldstein R, et al. A controlled treatment study of internal memory strategies (I-MEMS) following traumatic brain injury. *J Head Trauma Rehabil.* Jan–Feb 2010;25(1):43–51. 7) Stringer AY. *Ecologically Oriented Neurorehabilitation of Memory.* Los Angeles, CA: Western Psychological Services; 2007. 8) Turkstra LS, Bourgeois M. Intervention for a modern day HM: errorless learning of practical goals. *J Med Speech-Lang Path.* 2005;13:205–212.

PATIENT HANDOUT: DAILY AND WEEKLY PLANNING

Background

You will be most effective with your memory aid if you establish consistent daily and weekly procedures for adding information to your system and reviewing information you have already inputted.

- A **daily planning routine** will ensure that you see notes and information in a timely fashion.
- A **weekly planning routine** will help you anticipate upcoming events (and coordinate with others) and put prompts into the system for the week ahead.

- Decide on a consistent time of day (morning or evening) for daily planning and stick to it.
- Decide on a consistent day of the week for weekly planning.
- During the planning process, follow each step as listed on your checklist.
- Check off each step after it is completed.
- Remember, you will establish a habit if you consistently repeat the steps involved in planning.

Your clinician will guide you through developing a daily and weekly planning procedure that addresses your needs and preferences.

Here are examples:

EVENING PLANNING ROUTINE

STEPS:	M	T	W	Th	F	Sa	Su
1. Review "to do" list							
2. Check off all completed tasks and forward undone tasks to tomorrow							
3. Review tomorrow's appointments							
4. Set cell phone to alarm 1 hour before the appointment							
5. Make a note on tomorrow's planner page to remind you to do this procedure again							

WEEKLY PLANNING ROUTINE

STEPS: WEEK OF:							
1. Review your appointments for the week ahead; make sure all are recorded on calendar							
2. Make notes to yourself to do your exercise program on M, W, & F							
3. Check the family calendar and transfer relevant information to the planner							
4. Ask Sarah if she needs you to help in some way next week; if so write notes on appropriate days							
5. Make a note on next Saturday's planner page as a reminder to do this procedure again							

DAILY PLANNING ROUTINE

STEPS:	M	T	W	Th	F	Sa	Su

WEEKLY PLANNING ROUTINE

STEPS: Week of:							

PATIENT HANDOUT: MEMORY STRATEGY–INTENTIONAL READING

What Is Intentional Reading?

- An approach to reading that requires the reader to intentionally go through stages of memory, actively focusing attention and encoding new information.
- This strategy can be helpful if you have trouble paying attention when reading or if you have difficulty remembering what you read.

How You Do It

1. Have a pen and paper available when you start reading.
2. Divide your paper vertically into halves.
3. On the <u>**left side**</u> of the paper, write down **important facts or key points.**
   - This ensures that you sustain attention long enough to process the information.
   - It ensures that you slow down your reading pace to allow for note taking.
   - It ensures that you encode information.
   - It requires you to isolate the most important components of the text.
   - It ensures that you understand the main point of the information.
4. On the <u>**right side**</u> of the paper, write down your **thoughts, questions, and opinions**.
   - What questions come to mind related to the content?
   - What does this material remind you of?
   - Are there any diagrams or pictures that can capture the content better than words?
5. Look back at the reading material to see if you can answer your own questions. Keep your paper to remind you of what you read in case you need it later.

Example

Intentional Reading Form	
Important facts/information	• **Questions** • **Reminds me of . . .** • **Diagrams/charts** • **Things I need to look up**

PATIENT HANDOUT: TEN WAYS TO IMPROVE YOUR MEMORY

Defense and Veterans Brain Injury Center

This tool is to be used as a patient education resource during a visit with your provider. Developed by subject matter experts from the Department of Defense and Veterans Administration (Version 2: 4 May 2009) Defense and Veterans Brain Injury Center, 11300 Rockville Pike, Suite 707 Rockville, MD 20852. Telephone: (301) 589-1175. Fax: (301) 230-1976. Website: www.dvbic.org

1. **Get seven to eight hours of sleep.** Keep a quiet, cool environment. Go to sleep at the same time nightly. Don't nap. Avoid high-energy video games/movies/television prior to bedtime. Avoid exercise before bedtime.
2. **Write it down.** Keep a notebook and pen with you and write things down, it will keep you on track and help remind you of important things, like taking your medication. Day planners or small calendars also help.
3. **Avoid alcohol, tobacco, excessive caffeine, and energy drinks.** These increase sleep problems, anxiety, blood pressure levels, and overall stress.
4. **Prioritize.** Make a list of things that need to be taken care of, place them in order of importance, and check them off when completed.
5. **Get a routine.** Put your keys in the same spot every day. Park in the same areas. Being consistent helps memory and lowers anxiety.
6. **Keep mentally active.** Work crossword puzzles. Read a book. Play a board or card game, like solitaire or concentration. Learn something new every day.
7. **Decrease your stress level.** Don't take on too much at one time. Keep stress to a minimum. Stress hormones can damage your brain and add to depression and anxiety. Learn to say "no" when you're feeling overwhelmed. Ask for help when you need it. Make time for you.
8. **Stay physically active.** Take the dog for a walk. Take the stairs instead of the elevator. Small spurts of exercise add up. The higher blood flow to your brain helps promote cell growth. Exercising is also a mood booster and helps with mental clarity.
9. **Feed your brain.** Eat high-quality foods at regular intervals. Fish, colorful fruits and vegetables, milk, eggs, whole grain breads, nuts, and beans all help keep the brain and body healthy.
10. **Avoid further brain injury.** Consider swimming, walking, or running instead of playing football or boxing. Wear a helmet when riding your bike or motorcycle. Drive safely. Stay sober.

PATIENT HANDOUT: UNDERSTANDING EXECUTIVE FUNCTIONS

People make thousands of decisions every day. Most of these decisions are automatic and habitual (eg, reaching for a stick shift to change gears). However, when faced with unfamiliar or highly complex situations, decision making becomes conscious and deliberate (eg, finding a new route when blocked by road construction).

Most everyday activities fall into one of two categories:

1. Automatic tasks (skilled performance, habits, and routines)
2. Unfamiliar, changing, or complex tasks

People rely on the frontal lobe of their brains to organize their approach to unfamiliar, changing, and complex tasks. The frontal lobe of the brain is responsible for high-level thinking skills called "executive functions."

Executive functions describe two main categories of thinking skills: self-regulation and problem solving.

Self-Regulation

Self-regulation involves:
- Initiation
- Self-awareness
- Inhibition (regulating emotional responses)
- Resisting distractions/paying attention
- Appreciating obstacles and problems
- Mental flexibility (knowing when and how to change course)

Problem Solving

Problem solving involves:
- Understanding the problem
- Generating possible ideas and solutions
- Appreciating limits and restrictions of various solutions
- Prioritizing
- Anticipating consequences
- Making decisions

You may be less effective with executive functions when you are stressed or depressed, or if you have experienced a concussion. Inefficiencies in self-regulation and problem solving will be become more pronounced when you are fatigued, in pain, stressed, experiencing negative thoughts, or when there are distracters in the environment.

The first step in addressing this issue is to try to understand in which areas your performance might break down. For example, do you know what you need to do but you can't get started? Do you get started, but can't change course even when you know what you're doing is not moving you toward the intended goal?

Review the list of skills associated with self-regulation and problem solving on **Patient Handout: Rating Your Executive Function Skills.** Mark an "X" in each area where you see a personal strength and in each area you perceive as a weakness.

The second step in addressing this issue is to identify and then practice strategies that can help you maintain efficient and effective performance of your tasks and life roles. Work with your clinician to determine the strategies that are best for you.

PATIENT HANDOUT: RATING YOUR EXECUTIVE FUNCTION SKILLS

Executive Functions	Strength	Weakness
Self-Regulation		
Initiation: Can I get myself started?		
Focus: Can I resist distractions and stick to task?		
Self-monitor: Do I know when I've made a mistake?		
Mental flexibility: Can I change a plan when needed to reach my goal?		
Problem Solving		
Identification: Do I recognize when there is a problem?		
Flexibility: Can I think of more than one way to approach a problem?		
Evaluation: Do I know which plan is the best one to reach my goal?		
Prioritization: When faced with multiple problems, do I know which one to work on first, second, etc?		
Recognizing consequences: Am I able to predict how a plan will work, or am I surprised by the outcome?		
Decision making: Can I make decisions or do I get lost in the process and never really decide on what to do?		
Emotional Regulation		
Emotional regulation: Can I keep a clear head when solving problems, or does irritability, anger, or other emotion lead to poor decision making?		
Self-awareness of emotions and decision making: Can I recognize the situations that trigger irritability and anger and use strategies to keep my thinking clear?		

PATIENT HANDOUT: STRATEGIES FOR PROBLEM IDENTIFICATION

Problem Identification

The sooner a problem is recognized, the sooner you will be able to begin the process of problem solving, and the better the outcome is likely to be. Paying attention to cues within a situation, including your own emotions and the reactions of others around you, can signal that things may not be going as well as you would like and indicate that a problem exists.

Emotion Cues

Feelings of frustration, anxiety, irritation, and anger may be signs of problems that need to be addressed. Many of these emotions are uncomfortable and often a first response is to avoid thinking about these emotions. Instead try to:

- step back and observe the emotion and how it feels.
- avoid actively doing anything about the emotion; simply observe it, neither blocking it nor holding on to it.
- identify the emotion.
- focus on the underlying problem by asking yourself where the emotion is coming from.

Social Cues

Problems may be signaled by the reactions of others around us. As you interact with others:

- pay attention to how they respond to you. Look for expressions of irritation, frustration, or lack of engagement.
- if the situation permits and you are comfortable bringing this up, ask the person you are talking with if there is anything wrong. If not, you may ask others present in the group, at a later time, if they noticed any problems in the situation.
- begin the problem-solving process if problems are identified.

Outcome Cues

When problem-solving approaches fail, it is often because of one of two reasons: the problem has not been fully understood or the current approach to the problem is flawed.

- Review the entire problem sequence using Patient Handout: Problem-Solving Process to identify any weakness in problem identification or planning.
- Problems in self-monitoring may result in undetected errors that can undermine the success of the plan. Use the "pausing" strategy (see Patient Handout: Strategies to Improve Self-Regulation–Pausing) at intervals through the problem-solving process to help you identify mistakes that can be corrected.

PATIENT HANDOUT: EMOTIONAL SELF-MANAGEMENT WORKSHEET

Problems with emotional regulation can present as a significant barrier to problem solving. When people become frustrated, irritated, or angry, their thinking becomes less clear and they may say and do things that work against them and undermine their goal accomplishment. Many times people feel that irritability and anger "come out of nowhere" to cause difficulties. However, there are often recognizable early warning signs that, when identified, can signal the beginnings of irritability or anger that can turn into loss of emotional control.

The Emotional Self-Management Worksheet helps you:

- analyze situations where you have experienced difficulties with emotional regulation, and
- develop strategies to maintain the emotional control that supports good decision making and problem solving.

In the first column, you are asked to recall the physical characteristics, specific behaviors, cognitive signs, and emotions that led up to the problem situation. This allows you to identify patterns that can indicate that you may have difficulty controlling emotions. For example, you may notice that headaches, fatigue, a strained-sounding voice, and difficulty concentrating are frequent indicators of subsequent loss of emotional control. In the second column, you identify the context where a loss of emotional control occurred (eg, where you were, who was there, and what was occurring) to describe patterns that may give you insights into what situations serve to trigger a loss of emotional control. For example, you may notice frequent difficulty when you come home from work and are discussing your day with your spouse while your children are running around and yelling to get your attention. In the third column, you describe your reaction (eg, what you thought, what you felt, and what you did).

Typically, what we think strongly influences how we feel, and in turn what we do. Changing patterns of thinking in stressful situations can have a significant impact on how you feel and how you respond. Identifying early warning signs and triggers of emotional dyscontrol allows you to develop strategies that will help you keep your cool in challenging situations. Strategies to keep calm under stress include:

- **Relaxation breathing**. Using relaxation breathing takes practice but can be a powerful strategy for maintaining a sense of calm in stressful conditions.
  - Inhale slowly, counting to 3 or 4 as you inhale.
  - Exhale slowly and double the count of the exhalation. For example, if you inhale to a count of 3, exhale to a count of 6.
  - As you exhale, think of an image that is compatible with being calm and relaxed.
- **Positive self-talk.** We all have a little voice in our head that tells us what to do. This is normal. When things seem to go wrong, sometimes that voice becomes negative (eg, "I'm too slow," "I can't do this like I used to," "They are always working against me"). This pattern of thinking can impact subsequent feelings and behavior and result in emotional control difficulties that undermine problem solving. Develop a list of positive self-talk statements that you can use in difficult situations (eg, "I don't have to rush, I can take my time," "I'll relax and do my best work," "People are doing their best to support me"). Positive thinking tends to create positive feelings that translate into greater emotional stability and control. This ultimately results in better problem solving.

Before the Reaction	Context (situation)	My Reaction
Physical indicators (eg, headache, fatigue, pain, jaw tension)	Earlier events (eg, late for work and feeling rushed, argument with spouse)	What did I think?
Behavioral indicators (eg, loud voice, tapping foot)	Where did the difficulty occur?	What did I feel?
Cognitive indicators (eg, confusion, trouble following conversation, feeling rushed)	Who was present?	What did I do?
Emotional indicators (eg, feelings of, irritability, anger, embarrassment)	What was the situation?	What was the outcome?

PATIENT HANDOUT: STRATEGIES TO IMPROVE SELF-REGULATION--PAUSING

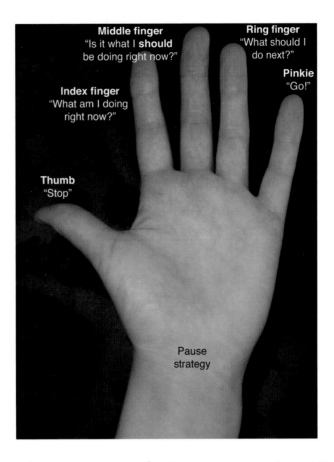

Figure 7-6. Pausing, a strategy that can improve your thinking in many ways, refers to taking a moment to align your brain and your body and to think calmly about what you are doing at the present time. It is helpful when you feel overwhelmed, distracted, or absentminded. Pausing can be used throughout the day and in almost every situation. Use your hand as a cue to think about the five steps involved in pausing.

PATIENT HANDOUT: STRATEGIES TO IMPROVE INITIATION

Sometimes people find that they just do not have the "get-up-and-go" that they had before a brain injury. These are some strategies to help you improve initiation.

Step 1

The first step to improving your initiation is to figure out what the barrier is. Difficulty with initiation can be caused by a variety of factors:

- decreased awareness of what needs to be done
- lack of energy needed to start or see things through
- inability to break tasks down into achievable steps
- difficulty with prioritization
- difficulty knowing when to do what
- fear of being interrupted
- lack of desire
- inability to generate ideas of things to do
- difficulty tracking time
- difficulty staying on task/attending
- perfectionism
- procrastination
- different priorities
- inability to function under pressure
- pain

Step 2

Next, identify the life management skills or strategies that can help you move beyond that barrier. The strategies need to match the barriers. Strategies for the common issues are suggested below.

Fatigue/Pain

- Pacing; taking a break
- Balanced lifestyle (good nutrition, sleep, exercise)

Executive Issues (difficulty with organization, planning, and attention)

- Checklists; external prompts (alarms)
- Stop notes
- Environmental adaptations
- Development of routines or habits

Overwhelmed

- Divide and conquer
- Problem-solving approaches
- Pausing; prioritization

Emotional Contributors

- Work with a psychologist

PATIENT HANDOUT: BUILDING HABITS AND ROUTINES

The Benefits of Structure

After illness or injury (or even another life change, such as retirement), individuals find themselves without structure or automatic habits and routines. This can lead to decreased time-management skills, disorganization, decreased productivity, and increased everyday memory errors. Inefficiencies like these make a person feel a sense of loss and decreased self-confidence. However, one of the best ways to get back on track is to set up new patterns of activity and repeat them consistently until they become new habits and routines.

Here are some suggestions for adding structure to your daily life:

- Get up at the same time every day.
- Reestablish personal care routines.
- Use a calendar and a daily planning checklist.
- Be responsible for creating and maintaining your own schedule.
- Carve out time in your day for a balanced life: scheduled appointments, regular contribution to home management tasks, and time for hobbies and social engagements.
- If work is not yet a reasonable goal, consider volunteering. Set up regular times and expectations.
- Create reasonable expectations; set goals for yourself and ask someone you trust to help hold you accountable.
- Set up a recurring task schedule for tasks of priority (see example below). Schedule tasks of importance for certain days of the week and make an effort to adhere to the new regimen.

Example Worksheet

Tasks	M	T	W	Th	F	Sa	Su
Morning aerobic exercise							
Sort mail inbox							
Check bank balance							

PATIENT HANDOUT: GENERATIVE THINKING STRATEGIES

What is Generative Thinking?

Generative thinking refers to the ability to come up with a variety of options or alternate solutions to problems or task approaches. It is a frontal lobe function and very susceptible to fatigue, stress, pain, and negative thoughts.

Generative thinking enables people to come up with a number of possible solutions to a given problem. By generating a number of possible solutions, the individual can evaluate them and ultimately select the best one. Generative thinking prevents people from getting locked in to only one approach.

Strategies That Help People Generate a Variety of Options and Solutions

Consider these options if you feel like you just can't come up with alternate solutions (and especially when the one you're using is ineffective).

- Leave the task or situation, do something else for a while, and come back later. Often a break will free your thinking and other circumstances may prompt new ideas.
- Brainstorm with another person.
- Gather more background information.
- Think about similar problems in the hope that it will enable you to think differently about your problem or task at hand.

If you experience difficulty with generative thinking as you perform tasks that are easy and familiar, you may simply need to use the pausing strategy to self-reflect.

- Are your personal factors under control?
- Are the situational factors making this more difficult?

PATIENT HANDOUT: PROJECT PLANNING STRATEGY–DIVIDE AND CONQUER

Instructions

This worksheet guides you through the process of developing a project plan before you begin work. Use this worksheet to organize your approach to unfamiliar, complex, or overwhelming tasks and for projects that will span multiple days.

1. List the major task components in the shaded rows, but don't worry about putting them in order.
2. List specific action items under each major task component. Again, list them as they come to mind; don't worry about putting them in order.
3. Put all the action items in order once you have listed them on the worksheet.
4. Assign yourself deadlines for key steps, if desired. Add "to-dos" to your planner.

Project:		
Order	**Task List**	**Deadlines**

Example

Project:	Clean out the garage	
Order	**Task List**	**Deadlines**
	Get rid of all trash and recycling	9/4
1	Get some large trash bags from Menards	
3	Remove/sort recycling	
2	Set up/label bags–metal, glass, newspaper	
4	Take to recycling center	
5	Clear out/bag all trash	
	Figure out and install new storage options	9/8
9	Talk to Sarah about what we want to add to the garage	
11	Go to Home Depot–buy supplies	
10	Ask Keith to help me install stuff and block out time for this	
12	Install storage items	
13	Put stuff away	
	Give away kid stuff that we no longer need	9/4
6	Talk to kids about which of their bikes, wagons etc they no longer use or want	
8	Pack up stuff in truck and bring to Goodwill	
7	Decide if there are any other non-kid things that we want to give to Goodwill	
	Clean the floor and put items away	9/18
14	Buy sweeping compound at Menards	
15	Move the vehicles out of the garage	
16	Sweep and then hose garage down	
17	Put everything back	

PATIENT HANDOUT: PROBLEM-SOLVING PROCESS

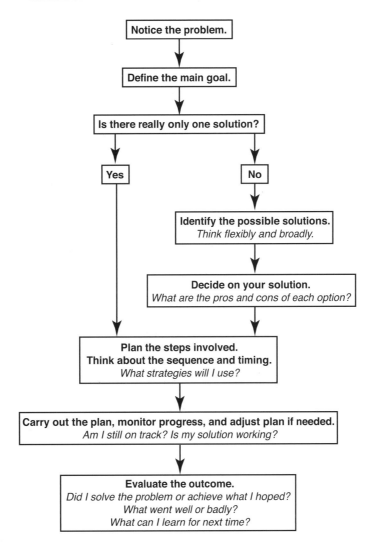

Figure 7-7. Steps in the problem-solving process.

Date:		
Problem Noticed:		
1. Main Goal:		
2. If there is really only one obvious solution, go to section 5 and plan the steps. If there is more than one possible solution, go to section 3.		

3. Alternative solutions	Pros	Cons

4. Decision:		
5. Plan:		

Steps	Strategies	Done: ✓
1.		
2.		
3.		
4.		
5.		
6.		
7.		
8.		
9.		
10.		

Remember to monitor and evaluate! Are things going well? If not, do you need to change your plan?

PATIENT HANDOUT: STRATEGY–PRIORITIZATION

Taking the time to figure out what is most important can help you manage time and accomplish what matters most, despite fatigue and pain.

Make Sure Your Actions are Aligned with Your Priorities Each Day

Step 1

Write out your to-do list. This allows you to clear space in your mind for more important things.

Step 2

Rate each task on the list using urgent/important categories.[1]

- High urgency/high importance: These are tasks that have time deadlines and serious consequences if they are not achieved promptly. These need to be fit into your current day plans as able. **[JUST DO IT]**
- Low urgency/high importance: These are tasks that are important to you, but there is no immediate deadline pending. It is important to schedule time to address these tasks. By planning for them, you may avoid always having urgent/important tasks dominating your time. **[PLAN FOR IT]**
- High urgency/low importance: These are tasks that have deadlines but the consequences are not as high. If it is important to other people in your life, delegate the task to them. If a task must be completed by you, it is often less tiring to "just do it" than continue to carry it over from day to day. Consider deleting the task from your list if it is truly not important. **[JUST DO IT, DELEGATE IT, OR DELETE IT]**
- Low urgency/low importance: These tasks are not important to you and do not have immediate deadlines. It is worth asking yourself if it needs to be done at all, does it matter to someone else, or do you want to ignore it until it becomes urgent or you have more time. **[DELEGATE, DELETE, OR IGNORE IT]**

Step 3

Make sure that tasks rated as high urgency/high importance and low urgency/high importance are added to your cell phone, planner, or calendar.

1. Covey SR. *The 7 Habits of Highly Effective People*. New York, NY: Simon and Schuster, Inc; 1989.

REFERENCES

1. Terrio H, Brenner LA, Ivins BJ, et al. Traumatic brain injury screening: preliminary findings in a U.S. Army Brigade Combat Team. *J Head Trauma Rehabil.* 2009;24(1):14–23.

2. Radomski MV, Weightman MM, Davidson L, Rodgers M, Bolgla R. Clinical Practice Guidance: Occupational Therapy and Physical Therapy for Mild Traumatic Brain Injury. Falls Church, VA: Army Office of the Surgeon General, Rehabilitation and Reintegration Division; 2010. Internal document.

3. Cornis-Pop M, Mashima PA, Roth CR, et al. Guest editorial: cognitive-communication rehabilitation for combat-related mild traumatic brain injury. *J Rehabil Res Dev.* Oct 2012;49(7):xi–xxxii.

4. Helmick K. Cognitive rehabilitation for military personnel with mild traumatic brain injury and chronic post-concussional disorder: Results of April 2009 consensus conference. *NeuroRehabilitation.* 2010;26(3):239–255.

5. McCrory P, Meeuwisse W, Johnston K, et al. Consensus statement on Concussion in Sport–the 3rd International Conference on Concussion in Sport held in Zurich, November 2008. *J Sci Med Sport.* May 2009;12(3):340–351.

6. Mittenberg W, Tremont G, Zielinski RE, Fichera S, Rayls KR. Cognitive-behavioral prevention of postconcussion syndrome. *Arch Clin Neuropsychol.* 1996;11(2):139–145.

7. Levin HS, Goldstein FC, MacKenzie EJ. Depression as a secondary condition following mild and moderate traumatic brain injury. *Semin Clin Neuropsychiatry.* Jul 1997;2(3):207–215.

8. Baum CM, Katz N. Occupational therapy approach to assessing the relationship between cognition and function. In: Marcotte TD, Grant I, eds. *Neuropsychology of Everyday Functioning.* New York, NY: Guildord Press; 2010: 62–90.

9. Radomski MV. Assessing abilities and capacities: cognition. In: Radomski MV, Trombly Latham CA, eds. *Occupational Therapy for Physical Dysfunction.* Philadelphia, PA: Lippincott Williams & Wilkins; 2008: 260–283.

10. Turkstra LS, Coelho C, Ylvisaker M. The use of standardized tests for individuals with cognitive-communication disorders. *Semin Speech Lang.* Nov 2005;26(4):215–222.

11. World Health Organization. *International Classification of Functioning, Disability and Health.* Geneva, Switzerland: World Health Organization; 2001.

12. Doninger NA, Bode RK, Ehde DM, Knight K, Bombardier CH, Heinemann AW. Measurement properties of the Neurobehavioral Cognitive Status Examination (Cognistat) in traumatic brain injury rehabilitation. *Rehabil Psychol.* 2006;51:281–288.

13. Engelhart C, Eisenstein N, Meininger J. Psychometric properties of the Neurobehavioral Cognitive Status Exam. *Clin Neuropsychol.* 1994;8:405–415.

14. Kiernan R, Mueller J, Langston JW. *Cognistat 2013 Manual.* Fairfax, CA: Cognistat, Inc; 2013.

15. Katz N, Elazar B, Itzkovich M. Validity of the Neurobehavioral Cognitive Status Examination (Cognistat) in assessing patients post CVA and healthy elderly in Israel. *Israel J Occup Ther.* 1996;5:E185–E198.

16. Blostein PA, Jones SJ, Buechler CM, Vandongen S. Cognitive screening in mild traumatic brain injuries: analysis of the neurobehavioral cognitive status examination when utilized during initial trauma hospitalization. *J Neurotrauma.* Mar 1997;14(3):171–177.

17. Engelhart C, Eisenstein N, Johnson V, et al. Factor structure of the Neurobehavioral Cognitive Status Exam (COGNISTAT) in healthy, and psychiatrically and neurologically impaired, elderly adults. *Clin Neuropsychol.* Feb 1999;13(1):109–111.

18. Ruchinskas RA, Singer HK, Repetz NK. Cognitive status and ambulation in geriatric rehabilitation: walking without thinking? *Arch Phys Med Rehabil.* Sep 2000;81(9):1224–1228.

19. Kiernan RJ, Mueller J, Langston JW, Van Dyke C. The Neurobehavioral Cognitive Status Examination: a brief but quantitative approach to cognitive assessment. *Ann Intern Med.* Oct 1987;107(4):481–485.

20. Chan CC, Lee TM, Fong KN, Lee C, Wong V. Cognitive profile for Chinese patients with stroke. *Brain Inj.* Oct 2002;16(10):873–884.

21. Nabors NA, Millis SR, Rosenthal M. Use of the Neurobehavioral Cognitive Status Examination (Cognistat) in traumatic brain injury. *J Head Trauma Rehabil.* 1997;12:79–84.

22. Randolph C. *Repeatable Battery for the Assessment of Neuropsychological Status: Manual.* San Antonio, TX: Psychological Corporation; 1998.

23. Strauss E, Sherman EM, Spreen O. *A Compendium of Neuropsychological Tests: Administration, Norms, and Commentary.* 3rd ed. New York, NY: Oxford University Press; 2006.

24. Randolph C. *Repeatable Battery for the Assessment of Neuropsychological Status (RBANS) Supplement 1.* Upper Saddle River, NJ: Pearson Education, Inc; 2008.

25. Killam C, Cautin RL, Santucci AC. Assessing the enduring residual neuropsychological effects of head trauma in college athletes who participate in contact sports. *Arch Clin Neuropsychol.* Jul 2005;20(5):599–611.

26. Moser RS, Schatz P. Enduring effects of concussion in youth athletes. *Arch Clin Neuropsychol.* Jan 2002;17(1):91–100.

27. Randolph C, Tierney MC, Mohr E, Chase TN. The Repeatable Battery for the Assessment of Neuropsychological Status (RBANS): preliminary clinical validity. *J Clin Exp Neuropsychol.* Jun 1998;20(3):310–319.

28. McKay C, Casey JE, Wertheimer J, Fichtenberg NL. Reliability and validity of the RBANS in a traumatic brain injured sample. *Arch Clin Neuropsychol.* Jan 2007;22(1):91–98.

29. Wilk CM, Gold JM, Bartko JJ, et al. Test-retest stability of the Repeatable Battery for the Assessment of Neuropsychological Status in Schizophrenia. *Am J Psychiatry.* May 2002;159(5):838–844.

30. McKay C, Wertheimer JC, Fichtenberg NL, Casey JE. The repeatable battery for the assessment of neuropsychological status (RBANS): clinical utility in a traumatic brain injury sample. *Clin Neuropsychol.* Mar 2008;22(2):228–241.

31. Helm-Estabrooks N. *Cognitive Linguistic Quick Test (CLQT).* San Antonio, TX: The Psychological Corporation; 2001.

32. Blyth T, Scott A, Bond A, Paul E. A comparison of two assessments of high level cognitive communication disorders in mild traumatic brain injury. *Brain Inj.* 2012;26(3):234–240.

33. Parashos SA, Johnson ML, Erickson-Davis C, Wielinski CL. Assessing cognition in Parkinson disease: use of the cognitive linguistic quick test. *J Geriatr Psychiatry Neurol.* Dec 2009;22(4):228–234.

34. Woodcock RW, McGrew KS, Mather N. *Woodcock-Johnson III Tests of Cognitive Abilities.* Itasca, Il: Riverside Publishing; 2001.

35. Parrish C, Roth C, Roberts B, Davie G. Assessment of cognitive-communication disorders of mild traumatic brain injury sustained in combat. *Perspectives on Neurophysiology and Neuroginic Speech and Language Disorder.* 2009;19(47-57).

36. Jones WP, Loe SA, Krach SK, Rager RY, Jones HM. Automated neuropsychological assessment metrics (ANAM) and Woodcock-Johnson III Tests of Cognitive Ability: a concurrent validity study. *Clin Neuropsychol.* Mar 2008;22(2):305–320.

37. Dean RS, Woodcock RW. *The WJ-R and Bateria-R Neuropsychological Assessment: Research Report Number 3*. Itasca, IL: Riverside Publishing; 1999.

38. Robertson IH, Ward T, Ridgeway V, Nimmo-Smith I. The structure of normal human attention: the Test of Everyday Attention. *J Int Neuropsychol Soc.* 1996;2(6):525–534.

39. Chan RC, Lai MK. Latent structure of the Test of Everyday Attention: convergent evidence from patients with traumatic brain injury. *Brain Inj.* Jun 2006;20(6):653–659.

40. Chan RC. Attentional deficits in patients with closed head injury: a further study to the discriminative validity of the test of everyday attention. *Brain Inj.* Mar 2000;14(3):227–236.

41. Baddeley AD, Emslie H, Nimmo-Smith I. *The Speed and Capacity of Language Processing (SCOLP) Test.* Bury St Edmunds, UK: Thames Valley Test Company; 1992.

42. Parle J, Roberts L, Wilson S, et al. A randomized controlled trial of the effect of thyroxine replacement on cognitive function in community-living elderly subjects with subclinical hypothyroidism: the Birmingham Elderly Thyroid Study. *J Clin Endocrinol Metab.* Aug 2010;95(8):3623–3632.

43. Saxton JA, Ratcliff G, Dodge H, Pandav R, Baddeley AD, Ganguli M. Speed and capacity of language processing test: normative data from an older American community-dwelling sample. *Appl Neuropsychol.* 2001;8(4):193–203.

44. Hinton-Bayre AD, Geffen G, McFarland K. Mild head injury and speed of information processing: a prospective study of professional rugby league players. *J Clin Exp Neuropsychol.* Apr 1997;19(2):275–289.

45. Ponsford J, Willmott C, Rothwell A, et al. Impact of early intervention on outcome following head injury in adults. *J Neurology, Neurosurg Psychiatry.* 2002;73(3):330–332.

46. Oram J, Geffen GM, Geffen LB, Kavanagh DJ, McGrath JJ. Executive control of working memory in schizophrenia. *Psychiatry Res.* Jun 15 2005;135(2):81–90.

47. Snow P, Powell M. *The Language Processing and Production Skills of Young Offenders: Implications for Enhancing Prevention and Intervention Strategies.* Canberra, AU: Australian Institute of Criminology; 2002. Report to Criminology Research Council on Grant 23/00-01. http://www.criminologyresearchcouncil.gov.au/reports/200001-23.html. Accessed August 13, 2013.

48. Papagno C, Baddeley AD. Confabulation in a dysexecutive patient: implication for models of retrieval. *Cortex.* Dec 1997;33(4):743–752.

49. Ponsford J, Willmott C, Rothwell A, et al. Factors influencing outcome following mild traumatic brain injury in adults. *J Int Neuropsychol Soc.* 2000;6(5):568–579.

50. Wilson BA, Watson PC, Baddeley AD, Emslie H, Evans JJ. Improvement of simply practice? The effects of twenty repeated assessments of people with and without brain injury. *J Int Neuropsychol Soc*, 2000; 6: 469-479.

51. Baddeley AD, Emslie H, Nimmo-Smith I. The Spot-the-Word test: a robust estimate of verbal intelligence based on lexical decision. *Br J Clin Psychol.* Feb 1993;32(Pt 1):55–65.

52. Comerford VE, Geffen GM, May C, Medland SE, Geffen LB. A rapid screen of the severity of mild traumatic brain injury. *J Clin Exp Neuropsychol.* Jun 2002;24(4):409–419.

53. Lucas SK, Carstairs JR, Shores EA. A comparison of methods to estimate premorbid intelligence in an Australian sample: data from the Macquarie University Neuropsychological Normative Study (MUNNS). *Aust Psychol.* 2003;38:227–237.

54. Roth R, Isquith P, Gioia G. *Behavior Rating Inventory of Executive Function-Adult Version (BRIEF-A).* Lutz, FL: Psychological Assessment Resources, Inc; 2005.

55. Brown TE, Holdnack J, Saylor K, et al. Effect of atomoxetine on executive function impairments in adults with ADHD. *J Atten Disord.* Feb 2011;15(2):130–138.

56. Wilson BA, Evans JJ, Alderman N, Burgess P. The development of an ecologically valid test for assessing patients with a dysexecutive syndrome. *Neuropsychol Rehabil.* 1998;8:213–228.

57. Chamberlain E. Test review: Behavioural assessment of the dysexecutive syndrome. *J Occup Psychol, Employ Disabil.* 2003;5:33–37.

58. Erez AB, Rothschild E, Katz N, Tuchner M, Hartman-Maeir A. Executive functioning, awareness, and participation in daily life after mild traumatic brain injury: a preliminary study. *Am J Occup Ther.* Sep–Oct 2009;63(5):634–640.

59. MacDonald S. *Functional Assessment of Verbal Reasoning and Executive Strategies.* London, UK: CCD Publishing; 2005.

60. Isaki E, Turkstra L. Communication abilities and work re-entry following traumatic brain injury. *Brain Inj.* May 2000;14(5):441–453.

61. Hagen C, Malkmus D, Durham P. Levels of cognitive functioning, rehabilitation of the brain-injured adult: Comprehensive physical management. Downey, CA: Professional Staff Association of Rancho Los Amigos Hospital; 1979.

62. Adamovich B, Henderson J. *Scales of Cognitive Ability for Traumatic Brain Injury: Normed Edition.* Austin, TX: Texas Pro-ed; 1992.

63. Wills P, Clare L, Shiel A, Wilson BA. Assessing subtle memory impairments in the everyday memory performance of brain injured people: exploring the potential of the extended Rivermead Behavioural Memory Test. *Brain Inj.* Aug 2000;14(8):693–704.

64. Wilson BA, Cockburn J, Baddeley AD. *The Rivermead Behavioural Memory Test.* London, UK: Pearson Assessment; 1985.

65. Wilson BA, Cockburn J, Baddeley AD, Hiorns R. The development and validation of a test battery for detecting and monitoring everyday memory problems. *J Clin Exp Neuropsychol.* Dec 1989;11(6):855–870.

66. Chung JC, Man DW. Self-appraised, informant-reported, and objective memory and cognitive function in mild cognitive impairment. *Dement Geriatr Cogn Disord.* 2009;27(2):187–193.

67. Koso M, Hansen S. Executive function and memory in posttraumatic stress disorder: a study of Bosnian war veterans. *Eur Psychiatry.* Apr 2006;21(3):167–173.

68. Schat A, van den Broek WW, Mulder PG, Birkenhager TK, van Tuijl R, Murre JM. Changes in everyday and semantic memory function after electroconvulsive therapy for unipolar depression. *J ECT.* 2007;23:153–157.

69. Makatura TJ, Lam CS, Leahy BJ, Castillo MT, Kalpakjian CZ. Standardized memory tests and the appraisal of everyday memory. *Brain Inj.* 1999;5:355–367.

70. Lezak MD, Howieson DB, Loring DW. *Neuropsychological Assessment.* 4th ed. New York, NY: Oxford University Press; 2004.

71. Toglia JP. *The Contextual Memory Test.* San Antonio, TX: Harcourt Assessments; 1993.

72. Gillen G. *Cognitive and Perceptual Rehabilitation: Optimizing Function.* St Louis, MO: Mosby, Inc; 2009.

73. Asher IE, ed. *Occupational Therapy Assessment Tools: An Annotated Index.* 3rd ed. Bethesda, MD: American Occupational Therapy Association, Inc; 2007.

74. Kaplan EF, Goodglass H, Weintraub S. *The Boston Naming Test*. 2nd ed. Philadelphia, PA: Lippincott Williams and Wilkins; 2001.

75. Pontón MO, Satz P, Herrera L, et al. Normative data stratified by age and education for the Neuropsychological Screening Battery for Hispanics (NeSBHIS): initial report. *J Int Neuropsychol Soc.* Mar 1996;2(2):96–104.

76. Brooks J, Fos LA, Greve KW, Hammond JS. Assessment of executive function in patients with mild traumatic brain injury. *J Trauma.* Jan 1999;46(1):159–163.

77. Heaton RK, Miller SW, Taylor MJ, Grant I. *Revised Comprehensive Norms for an Expanded Halstead-Reitan Battery: Demagraphically Adjusted Neuropsychological Norms for African American and Caucasian Adults*. Lutz, FL: Psychological Assessment Resources; 2004.

78. Ivnik RJ, Malec JF, Smith GE, Tangalos EG, Peterson RC. Neuropsychological test norms above age 55: COWAT, BNT, MAE Token, WRAT-R Reading, AMNART, Stroop, TMT, and JLO. *Clin Neuropsychol.* 1996;10:262–278.

79. Lucas JA, Ivnik RJ, Smith GE, et al. Mayo's Older African Americans Normative Studies: Norms for Boston Naming Test, Controlled Oral Word Association, Category Fluency, Animal Naming, Token Test, WRAT-3 Reading, Trail Making Test, Stroop Test, and Judgment of Line Orientation. *Clin Neuropsychol.* Jun 2005;19(2):243–269.

80. Mitrushina MM, Boone KB, Razani J, D'Elia LF. *Handbook of Normative Data for Neuropsychological Assessment*. 2nd ed. New York, NY: Oxford University Press; 2005.

81. Van Gorp WG, Satz P, Kiersch ME, Henry R. Normative data on the Boston Naming Test for a group of normal older adults. *J Clin Exp Neuropsychol.* Dec 1986;8(6):702–705.

82. Nicholas LE, Brookshire RH, MacLennan DL, Schumacher JG, Porrazzo S. The Boston Naming Test: Revised administration and scoring procedures and normative information for non-brain-damaged adults. *Clin Aphasiology.* 1988;18:103–115.

83. Killgore WD, Adams RL. Prediction of Boston Naming Test performance from vocabulary scores: Preliminary guidelines for interpretation. *Percept Mot Skills.* Aug 1999;89(1):327–337.

84. Henderson LW, Frank EW, Pigatt T, Abramson RK, Houston M. Race, gender and educational level effects on Boston Naming Test scores. *Aphasiology.* 1998;12:901–911.

85. Riva D, Nichelli F, Devoti M. Developmental aspects of verbal fluency and confrontation naming in children. *Brain Lang.* Feb 1 2000;71(2):267–284.

86. Zec RF, Markwell SJ, Burkett NR, Larsen DL. A longitudinal study of confrontation naming in the "normal" elderly. *J Int Neuropsychol Soc.* Oct 2005;11(6):716–726.

87. Fastenau PS, Denburg NL, Mauer BA. Parallel short forms for the Boston Naming Test: psychometric properties and norms for older adults. *J Clin Exp Neuropsychol.* Dec 1998;20(6):828–834.

88. Franzen MD, Haut MW, Rankin E, Keefover R. Empirical Comparison of Alternate Forms of the Boston Naming Test. *Clin Neuropsychol.* 1995;9:225–229.

89. Graves RE, Bezeau SC, Fogarty J, Blair R. Boston naming test short forms: a comparison of previous forms with new item response theory based forms. *J Clin Exp Neuropsychol.* Oct 2004;26(7):891–902.

90. Saxton JA, Ratcliff G, Munro CA, et al. Normative data on the Boston Naming Test and two equivalent 30-item short forms. *Clin Neuropsychol.* Nov 2000;14(4):526–534.

91. Mitrushina MM, Satz P. Repeated testing of normal elderly with the Boston Naming Test. *Aging (Milano).* Apr 1995;7(2):123–127.

92. Dikmen SS, Heaton RK, Grant I, Temkin NR. Test-retest reliability and practice effects of expanded Halstead-Reitan Neuropsychological Test Battery. *J Int Neuropsychol Soc.* May 1999;5(4):346–356.

93. Axelrod BN, Ricker JH, Cherry SA. Concurrent validity of the MAE visual naming test. *Arch Clin Neuropsychol.* Jul 1994;9(4):317–321.

94. Schefft BK, Marc Testa S, Dulay MF, Privitera MD, Yeh HS. Preoperative assessment of confrontation naming ability and interictal paraphasia production in unilateral temporal lobe epilepsy. *Epilepsy Behav.* Apr 2003;4(2):161–168.

95. Kohn SE, Goodglass H. Picture-naming in aphasia. *Brain Lang.* Mar 1985;24(2):266–283.

96. Tweedy JR, Schulman PD. Toward a functional classification of naming impairments. *Brain Lang.* Mar 1982;15(2):193–206.

97. Beatty WW, Monson N. Lexical processing in Parkinson's disease and multiple sclerosis. *J Geriatr Psychiatry Neurol.* Jul-Sep 1989;2(3):145–152.

98. Henry JD, Crawford JR. Verbal fluency deficits in Parkinson's disease: a meta-analysis. *J Int Neuropsychol Soc.* Jul 2004;10(4):608–622.

99. Lezak MD, Whitham R, Bourdette D. Emotional impact of cognitive insufficiencies in multiple sclerosis (MS) [Abstract]. *J Clin Exp Neuropsychol.* 1990;12:50.

100. Testa JA, Ivnik RJ, Boeve B, et al. Confrontation naming does not add incremental diagnostic utility in MCI and Alzheimer's disease. *J Int Neuropsychol Soc.* Jul 2004;10(4):504–512.

101. Ashman TA, Cantor JB, Gordon WA, et al. A comparison of cognitive functioning in older adults with and without traumatic brain injury. *J Head Trauma Rehabil.* May–Jun 2008;23(3):139–148.

102. Kerr C. Dysnomia following traumatic brain injury: an information-processing approach to assessment. *Brain Inj.* Nov–Dec 1995;9(8):777–796.

103. McDonald S, Flanagan S, Rollins J. *The Awareness of Social Inference Test.* Bury St Edmonds, UK: Thames Valley Test Company; 2002.

104. McDonald S, Bornhofen C, Shum D, Long E, Saunders C, Neulinger K. Reliability and validity of The Awareness of Social Inference Test (TASIT): a clinical test of social perception. *Disabil Rehabil.* Dec 30 2006;28(24):1529–1542.

105. McDonald S, Flanagan S. Social perception deficits after traumatic brain injury: interaction between emotion recognition, mentalizing ability, and social communication. *Neuropsychology.* Jul 2004;18(3):572–579.

106. McDonald S, Flanagan S, Rollins J, Kinch J. TASIT: a new clinical tool for assessing social perception after traumatic brain injury. *J Head Trauma Rehabil.* May–Jun 2003;18(3):219–238.

107. McDonald S, Tate R, Togher L, et al. Social skills treatment for people with severe, chronic acquired brain injuries: a multicenter trial. *Arch Phys Med Rehabil.* 2007;89(9):1648–1659.

108. Chung YS, Mathews JR, Barch DM. The effect of context processing on different aspects of social cognition in schizophrenia. *Schizophr Bull.* Feb 25 2010:1–9.

109. Sparks A, McDonald S, Lino B, O'Donnell M, Green MJ. Social cognition, empathy and functional outcome in schizophrenia. *Schizophr Res.* Sep 2010;122(1–3):172–178.

110. Rankin KP, Salazar A, Gorno-Tempini ML, et al. Detecting sarcasm from paralinguistic cues: anatomic and cognitive correlates in neurodegenerative disease. *Neuroimage.* Oct 1 2009;47(4):2005–2015.

111. Douglas JM, O'Flaherty CA, Snow P. Measuring perception of communicative ability: the development and evaluation of the La Trobe communication questionnaire. *Aphasiology.* 2000;14:251–268.

112. Grice P. Logic in conversation. In: Cole P, Morgan P, eds. *Studies in Syntax and Semantics.* Vol 3. New York, NY: Academic Press; 1975:44–58.

113. Douglas JM, Bracy CA, Snow PC. Measuring perceived communicative ability after traumatic brain injury: reliability and validity of the La Trobe Communication Questionnaire. *J Head Trauma Rehabil.* Jan–Feb 2007;22(1):31–38.

114. Kertesz A. *The Western Aphasia Battery.* New York, NY: Grune and Stratton; 1982.

115. Nicholas LE, Brookshire RH. Comprehension of spoken narrative discourse by adults with aphasia, right-hemisphere-brain damage, or traumatic brain injury. *Am J Speech Lang Pathol.* 1995;4:69–81.

116. Duff MC, Proctor A, Haley K. Mild traumatic brain injury (MTBI): assessment and treatment procedures used by speech-language pathologists (SLPs). *Brain Inj.* Sep 2002;16(9):773–787.

117. Brookshire RH, Nicholas LR. *Discourse Comprehension Test.* Minneapolis, MN: BRK Publishers; 1997.

118. Goodglass H, Kaplan E. *The Boston Diagnostic Aphasia Examination.* Boston, MA: Lea and Febiger; 1983.

119. Disimoni FG, Keith RL, Darley FL. Prediction of PICA overall score by short versions of the test. *J Speech Hear Res.* Sep 1980;23(3):511–516.

120. Nicholas LE, Brookshire RH. Consistency of the effects of rate of speech on brain-damaged adults' comprehension of narrative discourse. *J Speech Hear Res.* Dec 1986;29(4):462–470.

121. Mortera MH. Instrument development in brain injury rehabilitation: Part I. *Phys Disabilities Special Interest Section Q.* 2006a;29(3):1–4.

122. Mortera MH. Instrument development in brain injury rehabilitation: Part II. *Phys Disabilities Special Interest Section Q.* 2006b;29(4):1–2.

123. Mortera MH. The Mortera-Cognitive Screening Measure. New York, NY: Columbia University; 2004.

124. Frattali CM, Thompson CK, Holland AL, Wohl CB, Ferketic MM. *The American Speech-Language-Hearing Association Functional Assessment of Communication Skills for Adults (ASHA FACS).* Rockville, MD: ASHA; 1995.

125. Granger CV, Hamilton BB. The Uniform Data System for medical rehabilitation report of first admissions for 1990. Am J Phys Med Rehabil. 1992; 71: 108-113.

126. Cicerone KD, Dahlberg C, Kalmer K, et al. Evidence-based cognitive rehabilitation: recommendations for clinical practice. *Arch Phys Med Rehabil.* 2000;81:1596–1615.

127. Cicerone KD, Mott T, Azulay J, et al. A randomized controlled trial of holistic neuropsychologic rehabilitation after traumatic brain injury. *Arch Phys Med Rehabil.* Dec 2008;89(12):2239–2249.

128. Consensus conference. Rehabilitation of persons with traumatic brain injury. NIH Consensus Development Panel on Rehabilitation of Persons With Traumatic Brain Injury. *JAMA.* 1999;282(10):974–983.

129. Tsaousides T, Gordon WA. Cognitive rehabilitation following traumatic brain injury: assessment to treatment. *Mt Sinai J Med.* Apr 2009;76(2):173–181.

130. Cicerone KD, Langenbahn DM, Braden C, et al. Evidence-based cognitive rehabilitation: updated review of the literature from 2003 through 2008. *Arch Phys Med Rehabil.* Apr 2011;92(4):519–530.

131. Canter GJ. Observations on neurogenic stuttering: a contribution to differential diagnosis. *Br J Disord Commun.* Oct 1971;6(2):139–143.

132. Ruff RM, Jamora CW. Myths and mild traumatic brain injury. *Psychol Inj Law.* 2009;2:34–42.

133. Trudel TM, Nidiffer FD, Barth JT. Community-integrated brain injury rehabilitation: treatment models and challenges for civilian, military, and veteran populations. *J Rehabil Res Dev.* 2007;44(7):1007–1016.

134. Dikmen SS, Machamer J, Temkin N. Mild head injury: facts and artifacts. *J Clin Exp Neuropsychol.* 2001;23(6):729–738.

135. Ruff RM. Two decades of advances in understanding of mild traumatic brain injury. *J Head Trauma Rehabil.* Jan–Feb 2005;20(1):5–18.

136. Vanderploeg RD, Curtiss G, Luis CA, Salazar AM. Long-term morbidities following self-reported mild traumatic brain injury. *J Clin Exp Neuropsychol.* 2007;29(6):585–598.

137. Hoge CW, McGurk D, Thomas JL, Cox AL, Engel CC, Castro CA. Mild traumatic brain injury in U.S. Soldiers returning from Iraq. *New Eng J Med.* 2008;358(5):453–463.

138. Vanderploeg RD, Belanger HG, Curtiss G. Mild traumatic brain injury and posttraumatic stress disorder and their associations with health symptoms. *Arch Phys Med Rehabil.* Jul 2009;90(7):1084–1093.

139. American Speech-Language-Hearing Association. *Rehabilitation of Children and Adults With Cognitive-Communication Disorders After Brain Injury.* Rockville, MD: ASHA; 2003. Technical Report. http://www.asha.org/policy/TR2003-00146/. Accessed August 13, 2003.

140. Coelho CA, DeRuyter F, Stein M. Treatment efficacy: cognitive-communicative disorders resulting from traumatic brain injury in adults. *J Speech Hear Res.* Oct 1996;39(5):S5–17.

141. Kennedy MR, Coelho C, Turkstra L, et al. Intervention for executive functions after traumatic brain injury: a systematic review, meta-analysis and clinical recommendations. *Neuropsychol Rehabil.* Jun 2008;18(3):257–299.

142. Kleim JA, Jones TA. Principles of experience-dependent neural plasticity: implications for rehabilitation after brain damage. *J Speech Lang Hear Res.* Feb 2008;51(1):S225–239.

143. Sohlberg MM, Turkstra LS. *Optimizing Cognitive Rehabilitation: Effective Instructional Methods.* New York, NY: Guilford Press; 2011.

144. Cifu D, Hurley R, Peterson M, et al. VA/DoD Clinical Practice Guideline for Management of Concussion/Mild Traumatic Brain Injury. *J Rehabil Res Dev.* 2009;46(6):CP1–CP68.

145. Hartley LL. *Cognitive-Communicative Abilities Following Brain Injury: a Functional Approach.* New York, NY: Thomson Delmar Learning; 1995.

146. Ehlhardt LA, Sohlberg MM, Kennedy MR, et al. Evidence-based practice guidelines for instructing individuals with neurogenic memory impairments: what have we learned in the past 20 years? *Neuropsychol Rehabil.* Jun 2008;18(3):300–342.

147. Miller WR, Rollnick S. *Motivational Interviewing: Preparing People for Change.* New York, NY: Guilford Press; 2002.

148. Crosson B, Barco PP, Velozo CA, et al. Awareness and compensation in postacute head injury rehabilitation. *J Head Trauma Rehabil.* 1989;4:46–54.

149. Tennyson RD, Rasch M. Linking cognitive learning theory to instructional prescriptions. *Instr Sci.* 1988;17:369–385.

150. Comper P, Bisschop SM, Carnide N, Tricco A. A systematic review of treatments for mild traumatic brain injury. *Brain Inj.* 2005;19(11):863–880.

151. Ponsford J. Rehabilitation interventions after mild head injury. *Curr Opin Neurol.* 2005;18(6):692–697.

152. Montgomery GK. A multi-factor account of disability after brain injury: implications for neuropsychological counseling. *Brain Inj.* 1995;9(5):453–469.

153. Roth CR, Bibeau R. Post-deployment stuttering resulting from brain injury or stress? Paper presented at: Combat and Operational Stress Control Conference; April 27, 2011; San Diego, CA.

154. Borg J, Holm L, Peloso PM, et al. Non-surgical intervention and cost for mild traumatic brain injury: results of the WHO Collaborating Centre Task Force on Mild Traumatic Brain Injury. *J Rehabil Med.* Feb 2004(43 Suppl):76–83.

155. Atkinson RC, Shiffrin RM. The control of short-term memory. *Sci Am.* 1971;225(2):82–90.

156. Miller GA. The magical number seven, plus or minus two: some limits on our capacity for processing information. *Psychol Rev.* 1956;63:81–97.

157. Cicerone KD. Remediation of "working attention" in mild traumatic brain injury. *Brain Inj.* Mar 2002;16(3):185–195.

158. Stuss DT, Stethem LL, Hugenholtz H, Picton T, Pivik J, Richard MT. Reaction time after head injury: fatigue, divided and focused attention, and consistency of performance. *J Neurol Neurosurg Psychiatry.* Jun 1989;52(6):742–748.

159. Sohlberg MM, Mateer CA. The assessment of cognitive communicative functions in head injury. *Topic Lang Disord.* 1989;9(2):15–33.

160. Felmingham KL, Baguley IJ, Green AM. Effects of diffuse axonal injury on speed of information processing following severe traumatic brain injury. *Neuropsychology.* Jul 2004;18(3):564–571.

161. Defense Centers of Excellence for Psychological Health & Traumatic Brain Injury. *Co-occurring Conditions Toolkit: Mild Traumatic Brain Injury and Psychological Health.* 2nd ed. Arlington, VA: DCOE; 2011. http://www.dcoe.health.mil/Content/Navigation/Documents/Co-occurring%20Conditions%20Toolkit%20-%20Mild%20Traumatic%20Brain%20Injury%20and%20Psychological%20Health.pdf. Accessed August 14, 2013.

162. Sohlberg MM, Mateer CA. *Cognitive Rehabilitation: An Integrative Neuropsychological Approach.* New York, NY: Guilford; 2001.

163. Kurland J. The role that attention plays in language processing. *Perspect Neurophysiol Neurogenic Speech Lang Disord.* 2011;21:47–54.

164. Dahlberg CA, Cusick CP, Hawley LA, et al. Treatment efficacy of social communication skills training after traumatic brain injury: a randomized treatment and deferred treatment controlled trial. *Arch Phys Med Rehabil.* Dec 2007;88(12):1561–1573.

165. Mittenberg W, Strauman S. Diagnosis of mild head injury and the postconcussion syndrome. *J Head Trauma Rehabil.* Apr 2000;15(2):783–791.

166. Guskiewicz KM, McCrea M, Marshall SW, et al. Cumulative effects associated with recurrent concussion in collegiate football players: the NCAA Concussion Study. *JAMA.* Nov 19 2003;290(19):2549–2555.

167. Wilson BA. *Memory Rehabilitation: Integrating Theory and Practice.* New York, NY: Oxford; 2009.

168. Schacter DL, Tulving E. *Memory System 1994.* Cambridge, MA: Massachusetts Institute of Technology Press; 1994.

169. Cicerone KD, Dahlberg C, Malec JF, et al. Evidence-based cognitive rehabilitation: updated review of the literature from 1998 through 2002. *Arch Phys Med Rehabil.* Aug 2005;86(8):1681–1692.

170. Gillette Y, dePompei R, Goetz E; University of Akron. PDA intervention plan: implementing electronic memory and organization aids. BrainLine.Org website. http://www.brainline.org/content/2008/11/pda-intervention-plan-implementing-electronic-memory-and-organization-aids.html. Accessed August 14, 2013.

171. Gosnell J, Costello JM, Shane H. Using a clinical approach to answer "What communication apps should we use?." *Perspect Augment Altern Commun.* 2011;20(3):87–96.

172. Gordon WA, Cantor J, Ashman T, Brown M. Treatment of post-TBI executive dysfunction: application of theory to clinical practice. *J Head Trauma Rehabil.* Mar–Apr 2006;21(2):156–167.

173. Amberg J. Becoming a civilian. *Duty, Honor, Country…& Credit.* Chicago, IL: The Council for Adult and Experiential Learning (CAEL) Forum and News; 2010. http://www.cael.org/pdfs/128_2010dutyhonorcountryandcreditforumandnews. Accessed November 27, 2013.

174. Cicerone KD. Evidence-based practice and the limits of rational rehabilitation. *Arch Phys Med Rehabil.* Jun 2005;86(6):1073–1074.

175. Walter Reed Army Institute of Research Land Combat Study Team. *Battlemind Training I: Transitioning From Combat to Home.* Washington, DC: WRAIR; 2006. http://www.ptsd.ne.gov/pdfs/WRAIR-battlemind-training-Brochure.pdf. 2006; Accessed August 14, 2013.

176. Gordon WA, Zafonte R, Cicerone K, et al. Traumatic brain injury rehabilitation: state of the science. *Am J Phys Mede Rehabil.* 2006;85(4):343–382.

177. Kennedy MRT, Coehlo C. Self-regulation after traumatic brain injury: a framework for intervention of memory and problem solving. *Semin Speech Lang.* 2005;24(4):242–255.

178. Rath JF, Simon D, Langenbahn DM, Sherr LR, Diller L. Group treatment of problem-solving deficits in outpatients with traumatic brain injury: a randomized outcome study. *Neuropsychol Rehabil.* 2003;13:461–488.

179. Covey SR. *The 7 Habits of Highly Effective People.* New York, NY: Simon and Schuster, Inc; 1989.

180. Ylvisaker M, Turkstra LS, Coelho C. Behavioral and social interventions for individuals with traumatic brain injury: a summary of the research with clinical implications. *Semin Speech Lang.* Nov 2005;26(4):256–267.

181. Department of Defense; Department of Veterans Affairs. VA/DoD Clinical Practice Guideline for Management of Concussion/Mild Traumatic Brain Injury. Washington, DC: VA/DoD. http://www.healthquality.va.gov/mtbi/concussion_mtbi_full_1_0.pdf. Accessed August 14, 2013.

182. Raskin SA, Mateer CA. *Neuropsychological Management of Mild Traumatic Brain Injury.* New York, NY: Oxford; 2000.

183. Morton MV, Wehman P. Psychosocial and emotional sequelae of individuals with traumatic brain injury: a literature review and recommendations. *Brain Inj.* Jan 1995;9(1):81–92.

184. Castro CA, Hoge CW, Cox AL. Battlemind Training: Building Soldier Resiliency. Paper presented at: Human Dimensions in Military Operations–Military Leaders' Strategies for Addressing Stress and Psychological Support; Neuilly-sur-Seine, France; 2006. http://ftp.rta.nato.int/public//PubFullText/RTO/MP/RTO-MP-HFM-134///MP-HFM-134-42.pdf. Accessed August 14, 2013.

185. MacLennan DL, Cornis-Pop M, Picon-Nieto M, Sigford B. The prevalence of pragmatic communication impairments in traumatic brain injury. *Premier Outlook.* 2002;3(4):38–45.

186. Dahlberg CA, Hawley L, Morey C, Newman J, Cusick CP, Harrison-Felix C. Social communication skills in persons with post-acute traumatic brain injury: three perspectives. *Brain Inj.* Apr 2006;20(4):425–435.

187. Struchen MA, Pappadis MR, Sander AM, Burrows CS, Myszka KA. Examining the contribution of social communication abilities and affective/behavioral functioning to social integration outcomes for adults with traumatic brain injury. *J Head Trauma Rehabil.* Jan–Feb 2011;26(1):30–42.

188. Struchen MA, ed Social communication interventions. In: High WM, Sander MA, Struchen MA, Hart KA, eds. *Rehabilitation for Traumatic Brain Injury*. New York, NY: Oxford; 2005.

189. DeNil L, Jokel R, Rochon E. Etiology, symptomology, and treatment of neurogenic stuttering. In: Conture EG, Curlee RF, eds. *Stuttering and Related Disorders of Fluency*. 3rd ed. New York, NY: Thieme; 2007: 326–343.

190. Helm-Estabrooks N. Stuttering associated with acquired neurologic disorders. In: Curlee RF, ed. *Stuttering and Related Disorders of Fluency*. New York, NY: Thieme; 1999: 255–268.

191. Andy OJ, Bhatnagar SC. Stuttering acquired from subcortical pathologies and its alleviation from thalamic perturbation. *Brain Lang*. May 1992;42(4):385–401.

192. Heuer RJ, Sataloff RT, Mandel S, Travers N. Neurogenic stuttering: further corroboration of site of lesion. *Ear Nose Throat J*. Mar 1996;75(3):161–168.

193. Baumgartner J, Duffy JR. Psychogenic stuttering in adults with and without neurologic disease. *J Med Speech Lang Path*. 1997;5:75–95.

194. Roth CR, Aronson AE, Davis LJ, Jr. Clinical studies in psychogenic stuttering of adult onset. *J Speech Hear Disord*. Nov 1989;54(4):634–646.

195. Roth CR, Manning K. Post-deployment stuttering resulting from brain injury or stress? Paper presented at: Annual Convention of the American Speech-Language-Hearing Association. New Orleans, LA; 2009.

196. Craig AR, Franklin JA, Andrews G. A scale to measure locus of control of behaviour. *Br J Med Psychol*. Jun 1984;57(Pt 2):173–180.

197. Duffy JR. *Motor Speech Disorders Substrates, Differential Diagnosis, and Management*. 2nd ed. St Louis, MO: Elsevier Mosby; 2005.

198. Maguire GA, Riley GD, Franklin DL, Gottschalk LA. Risperidone for the treatment of stuttering. *J Clin Psychopharmacol*. Aug 2000;20(4):479–482.

199. Baumgartner JM. Acquired psychogenic stuttering. In: Curlee RF, ed. *Stuttering and Related Disorders of Fluency*. New York, NY: Thieme; 1999: 269–299.

Chapter 8

DUAL-TASK ASSESSMENT AND INTERVENTION

MARGARET M. WEIGHTMAN, PhD, PT[*] AND KAREN McCULLOCH, PhD, PT[†]

[*] Clinical Scientist/Physical Therapist, Courage Kenny Research Center, 800 East 28th Street, Mail Stop 12212, Minneapolis, Minnesota 55407-3799
[†] Professor, Division of Physical Therapy, Department of Allied Health Sciences, School of Medicine, University of North Carolina at Chapel Hill, 321 South Columbia Street, CB 7135 Bondurant Hall, Suite 3024, Chapel Hill, North Carolina 27599-7135

DUAL-TASK ASSESSMENT AND INTERVENTION

Introduction

Persons with traumatic brain injury (TBI), and specifically with concussion/mild traumatic brain injury (c/mTBI), have been shown to have statistically significant slower gait speed and reduced stability under dual-task conditions compared to healthy controls.[1-3] These differences may be subtle and difficult to detect with simple clinical measures, but could be devastating for a deployed service member in a war zone and may affect reintegration into work and community environments. Issues related to assessment and intervention for postural control and attention issues, specifically in dual-task conditions following brain injury, have been reviewed.[4] Similarly, Al-Yahya[5] has published a systematic review of the use of dual-task methodology to assess cognitive motor interference that occurs while walking, and suggests the overall effect of cognitive tasks was most prominently detected in measures of gait speed.

There is a clear need to develop valid and reliable assessment tools to evaluate recovery and the effects of intervention on dual-task deficits after c/mTBI to establish definitive therapy assessment and treatment standards for both service members and the civilian patient population. Although a specific and appropriate dual-task test clearly relevant for service members with c/mTBI cannot be recommended at this time, some options are available. Dual-task "cost," or decrement in skill level (error) or time to complete a task when two or more tasks are done simultaneously could be monitored to assess recovery and the effect of intervention. The Functional Gait Assessment[6] is a clinical test of walking containing items that require patients to perform more than one task, such as walking while turning one's head or walking around objects. The Walking and Remembering Test (WART) has been shown to be reliable and feasible in persons with acquired brain injury.[7] A dual-task questionnaire[8] has only been used in one study, but may provide information on the average difficulty of everyday tasks that require dual tasking and may grossly identify persons who report dual-task difficulty.

Research on specific interventions for issues such as postural control, attention, and dual or multiple tasks in persons with c/mTBI is in its infancy, although small studies show using dual-task training methods in older adults may be useful to improve balance.[4,8,9] Early findings indicate the importance of training specificity. Therapists are encouraged to design individualized intervention strategies with military overtones (ie, obstacle courses, map reading, carrying a load, speed, visual scanning, time constraints) for service members who have attention deficits in dual-task situations. It is important to begin with simple interventions and move to more complex tasks as appropriate. When it is appropriate to progress, real-life tasks are encouraged and should involve functional skills for balance, gait, visual-spatial, and cognitive tasks trained in progressively more challenging dual-task conditions.

This section of the Toolkit provides assessments and interventions that are considered **practice options** based on the level of evidence available at this time. Therapists are encouraged to consider this area of assessment and intervention for those service members who obtain maximum scores on standard motor and cognitive assessment tools, yet still report deficits.

DUAL-TASK ASSESSMENT

Introduction

In a clinical setting, measures of dual-task performance typically involve using observation and readily available equipment, such as simple walkways, obstacle courses, stopwatches, objects to carry, and lists of rote cognitive tasks (alphabet, serial subtractions, simple questions to answer). Some physical therapy departments have dynamic posturography equipment (such as the Neurocom [Natus Medical Incorporated, Clackamas, OR] or Proprio [Perry Dynamics Proprio Reactive Balance Systems, Decatur, IL] systems) and can assess more sensitive measures of postural control (eg, postural sway) during different sensory conditions or while combining a cognitive task overlay. No dual-task test combinations have been validated in service members with c/mTBI, but several studies of individuals with sports concussion have described methods to detect dual-task performance problems. This dual-task assessment section provides some options for evaluating an individual service member. Testing in an evaluative way, by comparing baseline information to follow-up testing for an individual, is a reasonable approach. Guidelines to interpret individual results in comparison to group findings are not available at this time.

DUAL-TASK PERFORMANCE ASSESSMENTS

Purpose/Description

A number of measures have been suggested for measuring dual-task performance to assess how impairments in attention may affect performance in balance and walking in persons with brain injury, including the WART,[10] the Timed Up and Go (TUG; Cognitive) test,[11] and a walking and spoken sentence verification task.[8] In general, dual-task assessment involves measuring baseline performance on a single motor task (eg, time to complete fast walking for a specified distance) and measuring single-task performance on a cognitive task (eg, repeating the months of the year backwards from the current month, or serially subtracting 7 from 100). In the dual-task condition, both tasks are performed at the same time. This dual-task testing is used as an experimental approach in cognitive psychology to understand the processes of skilled performance,[12] but also has implications for real-life situations that require doing more than one thing at a time.

Recommended Instrument Use

The scenarios provided are examples of the concept. Alternate motor and cognitive tasks can be substituted as appropriate, but must be consistently applied for an individual subject. There is insufficient information on norms or retest reliability for young adults of military age to provide information on sensitivity, specificity, or minimal detectable change (MDC) of these types of scenarios.

It is important to remember that neurologically intact persons will show reductions in performance in dual-task versus single-task conditions if the task combination is sufficiently challenging. Individuals who have mTBI may also be able to successfully do two tasks at the same time without performance decrement if the two tasks are very simple (eg, standing still while listening to instructions). If, while under clinical observation, the clinician feels a service member shows evidence of attention impairments that may affect task performance, a dual-task assessment for the individual service member may be appropriate. This information could be used for follow-up testing and comparison for that individual. Group comparisons are not appropriate at this time.

Administration Protocol/Equipment/Time

Example protocols are shown below and require a stopwatch. Other requirements depend on task protocol. To quantify reductions in performance,

dual-task costs can be calculated as a percentage (eg, 10% dual-task cost for walking speed). This calculation requires a baseline measurement of single-task performance so dual-task performance can be interpreted. Relative dual-task cost[4] can be figured by adjusting for single-task performance (control for slower or faster usual walking speed; Exhibit 8-1).

Ideally, dual-task costs are figured for both the motor and the cognitive task. Cognitive task performance may be computed by looking at accuracy of responses (eg, to serial subtraction or number of correct responses). If only motor dual-task costs are measured, it is possible that costs are occurring with the cognitive task and are undetected. Dual-task costs can occur in either or both of the two tasks.

Groups Tested With This Measure

Dual-task costs for walking and cognitive tasks have been measured in community-dwelling older adults.[5,10] A randomized controlled trial evaluated the effectiveness of a cognitive-motor dual-task training program in persons with acquired brain injury and used walking distance completed in 2 minutes or clicking a handheld mechanical counter while verifying the correctness of simple sentences (eg, "Dogs have wings." "Dogs have four legs.").[8] The TUG test was used under single-task versus dual-task conditions for identifying elderly individuals who are prone to falling. While the TUG test was found to be a sensitive and specific measure for identifying community-dwelling adults who are at risk for falls, the ability to predict falls was not enhanced by adding a secondary task to the TUG test.[11]

Interpretability

- Norms: not available for the specific tasks used in these examples. Young adults demonstrated relative dual-task costs for walking time at an average of 2% to 3% in a test of the WART,[10] whereas older adults had a reduction in walking speed of 4%. Digit span dual-task costs were on average 8% to 9% for younger adults and 15% for older adults in the WART.[10]

  In measures of anterior displacement (velocity in m/sec) of the center of mass during level walking comparing 15 college-aged volunteers who had sustained a concussion to 15 uninjured controls (all

323

EXHIBIT 8-1

EQUATION FOR FIGURING RELATIVE DUAL-TASK COST

$$DTCwalk = \frac{(DTwalk - STwalk)}{STwalk} \times 100$$

DT: dual task
DTC: dual-task cost
ST: single task

---

participants were involved in athletics and concussed participants had sustained a grade 2 concussion [symptoms lasting longer than 15 minutes without loss of consciousness]), the normal controls showed a dual-task cost of 5.7% while the concussed participants showed a 10.1% cost on day 2 following concussion. Single-task conditions involved walking with undivided attention, while dual-task conditions involved walking while simultaneously completing simple mental tasks, such as spelling five-letter words in reverse, subtraction by sevens, and reciting the months of the year in reverse order.[13] Dual-task deficits were retested at days 5, 14, and 28, and some deficits lingered.

- MDC: not available for this specific example. If the patient's score is less than the MDC value, it is considered indistinguishable from measurement error.
- Reliability estimates: not available for the example tasks used in this Toolkit
- Internal consistency: not available
- Interrater: Reliability for walking time in the WART (intraclass correlation coefficient [ICC] [2,1]) was .98 for younger adults and .99 for older adults.[10]
- Intrarater: not available
- Test-Retest: ICC (2,1) for young adults for single-task trials of walking a narrowed path were .83 to .92; for a dual-task trial of walking time, ICC was .76.[10]

Validity Estimates: not available for the example tasks used in this population

- Content/Face: not available
- Criterion: not available
- Construct: Older adults were slower and remembered shorter digit spans with greater dual-task costs than younger adults.[10]

Selected References

Abernethy B. Dual-task methodology and motor skills research: some applications and methodological constraints. *J Hum Mov Stud.* 1988;14:101–132.

Evans JJ, Greenfield E, Wilson BA, Bateman A. Walking and talking therapy: improving cognitive-motor dual-tasking in neurological illness. *J Int Neuropsychol Soc.* Jan 2009;15(1):112–120.

McCulloch K. Attention and dual-task conditions: physical therapy implications for individuals with acquired brain injury. *J Neurol Phys Ther.* 2007;31(3):104–118.

McCulloch KL, Mercer V, Giuliani C, Marshall S. Development of a clinical measure of dual-task performance in walking: reliability and preliminary validity of the Walking and Remembering Test. *J Geriatr Phys Ther.* 2009;32(1):2–9.

Parker TM, Osternig LR, Lee HJ, Donkelaar P, Chou LS. The effect of divided attention on gait stability following concussion. *Clin Biomech (Bristol, Avon).* May 2005;20(4):389–395

Shumway-Cook A, Brauer S, Woollacott M. Predicting the probability for falls in community-dwelling older adults using the Timed Up & Go Test. *Phys Ther.* Sep 2000;80(9):896–903.

DUAL-TASK COST EXAMPLE 1: WALKING AND REMEMBERING TEST[10]

Equipment/Set-Up

A walkway, stopwatch, and a list of single-digit random numbers (see below) are required. On a marked, narrowed, 7.5-inch-wide (19 cm), 20-foot-long (6.1 m) walkway, mark an additional 5 feet (.91 m) from the start and end of the walkway (total 30 ft) for acceleration and deceleration.

Step 1: Single-Task Walking (Fast Pace)

To determine the time it takes to walk a 7.5-inch-wide, 20-foot-long walkway at a fast pace, start the subject at the beginning of the acceleration zone and begin timing when the subject's first foot crosses the start line marker onto the walking path. Finish timing when the subject's front foot crosses the finish line. Ask the subject to walk as fast as he or she can between the tape lines and to keep his or her feet between the lines until reaching the cone (or other object) at the end of the deceleration zone. Remind the subject to:

- keep feet between the tape lines (the trial does not count if the subject's foot touches the tape line more than twice during the trial), and
- avoid running; this is a test of fast walking.

Record the time to the tenths of a second. Record the average of two trials:

Trial 1 (sec)_____ Trial 2 (sec)_____ Average _____

Step 2: Digit Span Testing

The purpose of this step is to determine the longest digit span the subject can recall after a delay equivalent to the average time to walk in the single-task condition (Step 1, above). The longest digit span correct for at least one trial is used in the dual-task condition and is considered to be 100% correct for assessing cognitive errors. Discontinue testing after the patient scores 0 correct on both trials (Table 8-1). Administer both trials of each item even if the patient passes trial 1. Score 0 to 1 point for each response.

Give the patient the following instructions: "I'm going to say some numbers that I want you to remember after a brief delay. Listen carefully to the numbers, and use any method except writing or talking to help you remember them. When I give

you the cue 'now,' repeat the numbers to me."

Take longest digit span correct after the time delay (in seconds, determined in Step 1) for at least one trial to use in Step 3.

dual-task condition: _____ (number of digits)

Step 3: Dual-Task Walking (Fast Pace)

Use the longest digit string (from Step 2) the subject was able to recall at least once with the time delay (from Step 1) for the dual-task testing, then combine the two tasks. Give the patient the following instructions:

"Now we are going to combine walking with remembering numbers. We will do this task twice. I am going to say some numbers that I want you to remember until we get to the end of the walking path. You may use any method you choose to remember the numbers, except saying them out loud. Walk as quickly as you can but take care not to step off the path. I will walk beside you and time you from when you first step onto the path. Continue walking until I say 'now,' then repeat the numbers you have been concentrating on while you were walking."

TABLE 8-1

DIGIT SPAN TESTING

Item/Trial		Response: Record subject's response after time delay (to nearest second)[*] _____ seconds	Score
1. Trial 1	6-4-3-9		
Trial 2	7-2-8-6		
2. Trial 1	4-2-7-3-1		
Trial 2	7-5-8-3-6		
3. Trial 1	6-1-9-4-7-3		
Trial 2	3-9-2-4-8-7		
4. Trial 1	5-9-1-7-4-2-8		
Trial 2	4-1-7-9-3-8-6		
5. Trial 1	5-8-1-9-2-6-4-7		
Trial 2	3-8-2-9-5-1-7-4		
6. Trial 1	2-7-5-8-6-2-5-8-4		
Trial 2	7-1-3-9-4-2-5-6-8		
Total score			

*Determined from average of two trials in single-task walking (fast pace).

Present the number of digits from the list below that the subject can recall from digit span testing above (eg, you would say "5 1 9 6 3" if the patient can recall five digits above.)

Trial 1   Digits presented: 5 1 9 6 3 8 4 1 9 3
Digits recalled: _____
Steps off path: _____
Seconds to complete trial (to tenths of
  second): _____

Trial 2   Digits presented: 8 7 1 9 2 4 3 6 9 5
Digits recalled: _____
Steps off path: _____
Seconds to complete trial (to tenths of
  second): _____

Note: If space considerations warrant, any standard distance can be used, with markers at the start and finish line, and 3 to 5 feet before

for acceleration and deceleration. A standard distance must be used consistently with each patient to make comparisons over time. Also, if the subject can only recall two or three digits correctly, use that number in the dual-task trial and consider it 100%.

Example Calculations

Single-task (from Step 2) walking speed 20 ft (6.1 m):
Trial 1: <u>9.5 sec</u>   Trial 2: <u>9.1 sec</u>
Average (STwalk;): <u>9.3 sec</u>

Dual-task (from Step 3) walking speed 20 ft (6.1 m):
Trial 1: <u>10.5 sec</u>   Trial 2: <u>10.3 sec</u>
Average (DTwalk;): <u>10.4 sec</u>

$$\text{DTCwalk} = \frac{(10.4 - 9.3)}{9.3} \times 100; \text{DTCwalk} = 11.8\%$$

DUAL-TASK EXAMPLE 2: COGNITIVE ERROR DURING WALKING AND REMEMBERING TEST

Using the number of digits that the subject repeated correctly in Step 2 above as 100%, determine the number of digits that the subject repeated correctly after the combined fast-walking and digit-span recall from Step 3 above.

Note: Subjects sometimes get partial spans correct. Partial credit can be given if:

- first or last digit is correct,
- any digits adjacent to first or last digit are correct, or
- there is a correct sequence of three anywhere in span.

Example Calculations

Subject A was able to recall seven digits from Step 2; therefore, that number becomes 100%. If, during Step 3, the subject is able to recall only six of the seven presented numbers (missing any number in

the span), his or her dual-task cost is calculated by the following:

6/7 × 100 = 85.7% correct in the dual-task condition

Therefore, the dual-task cost is 100% − 85.7%; or 14.3%.

Subject B was able to recall nine digits from Step 2; therefore that number becomes 100%. During Step 3, the subject recalls the nine-digit span as follows:

Correct: 3-7-4-8-1-6-2-9-3
Patient recall: 3-7-8-4-1-6-2-3

The first two are correct (3, 7), the second two transposed (both incorrect), the next three correct (1, 6, 2), one digit is omitted (9), and the last is correct (3). Therefore, the total number of correct digits is 6/9, or 67% correct.

DUAL-TASK ASSESSMENT EXAMPLE 3: TANDEM WALK WITH COGNITIVE TASK

Ask the subject to walk heel to toe as fast as possible down a 20-foot (6.1 m) tape line, instructing the subject to make sure to touch heel to toe and stay on the tape. Ask the subject to turn at the end of the line and walk heel to toe as fast as possible back to the starting point. Begin timing when the subject's first foot touches the tape line and finish timing when the subject's first foot steps off the tape line at the

beginning. Record the time to the tenths of a second and take the average of two trials. Ask the subject to repeat the phonetic alphabet (Table 8-2) to ensure the service member can complete the cognitive task in a single-task condition. Then combine the two tasks and record the average of two trials. For the trial to count, the service member may make no more than two steps that are not heel to toe.

Standardized Start Line Instructions

Step 1: Single Task Tandem Walking

Give the subject the following instructions:

"Walk heel to toe as fast as you can safely walk to the end of the tape, turn, and return to walk off the end of the tape on this end of the line. Try to keep your feet on the tape line and make sure the heel of one foot touches the toe of the other foot all the way down the line. Go as fast as you can. Ready . . . Begin."

Trial 1 (sec)_____ Trial 2 (sec)_____ Average_____

Step 2: Cognitive Task

Give the patient the following instructions: "Recite the phonetic alphabet." If the service member cannot correctly recite the phonetic alphabet, another cognitive task should be substituted to ensure the cognitive task can be accomplished in a single-task condition. Repeating the phonetic alphabet backwards could also be substituted.

Step 3: Dual-Task Tandem Walking

Give the patient the following instructions:

"Now I would like you to combine these two tasks. Remember, please walk heel to toe down the tape line as fast as you can safely walk to the end of the line, turn, and return to this end of the tape. Keep your feet on the line, go as fast as you can, *and* recite the phonetic alphabet. Remember to speak loud enough so I can hear you, and start over reciting the alphabet if you finish before you are done walking. Ready . . . Begin."

Trial 1 (sec)_____ Trial 2 (sec)_____ Average_____

Note: If space considerations warrant, any standard distance can be used, but the standard distance must be used consistently with each patient to make comparisons over time.

TABLE 8-2

PHONETIC ALPHABET

Letter	Phonetic letter
A	Alpha
B	Bravo
C	Charlie
D	Delta
E	Echo
F	Foxtrot
G	Golf
H	Hotel
I	India
J	Juliet
K	Kilo
L	Lima
M	Mike
N	November
O	Oscar
P	Papa
Q	Quebec
R	Romeo
S	Sierra
T	Tango
U	Uniform
V	Victor
W	Whiskey
X	X-ray
Y	Yankee
Z	Zulu

Example Calculations

Single-task tandem walking speed 40 ft (12.2 m):
Trial 1: <u>16.7sec</u>   Trial 2: <u>16.5 sec</u>
Average (STwalk;): <u>16.6 sec</u>

Dual-task tandem walking speed 40 ft (12.2 m):
Trial 1: <u>17.6 sec</u>   Trial 2: <u>17.0 sec</u>
Average (DTwalk;): <u>17.3 sec</u>

$$DTCwalk = \frac{(17.3-16.6)}{16.6} \times 100 \; ; DTCwalk = 4.2\%$$

This example would indicate a 4.2% slower tandem walking speed under dual-task conditions.

DUAL-TASK QUESTIONNAIRE

Purpose/Description

The dual-task questionnaire is used to obtain information relating to everyday difficulties with dual tasking.

Recommended Instrument Use

This questionnaire has only been used in one study. It does appear to give information on the average difficulty of everyday tasks that require dual tasking and may grossly identify persons who report dual-task difficulty. It should not be used to follow change over time until further evaluated psychometrically.

Administration Protocol/Equipment/Time

This is a brief, 10-question, pencil-and-paper survey that should take less than 2 to 3 minutes (Form 8-1).

Groups Tested With This Measure

This measure has been used in people with dual-tasking difficulties arising from acquired brain injury (stroke and TBI) between 6 and 280 months following injury with a range of premorbid intellectual abilities.[8]

Interpretability

The average questionnaire response in persons with acquired brain injury who underwent a 5-week, cognitive-motor dual-tasking training program improved from 2.09 (standard deviation 0.68) to 1.71 (standard deviation 0.56) using a 5-point, 0-to-4 scale, with a "4" indicating very often and a "0" indicating never.[8]

- Norms: not available
- MDC: not available. If the patient's score is less than the MDC value, it is considered indistinguishable from measurement error.

Reliability Estimates

- Internal consistency: not applicable
- Interrater: not available
- Intrarater: not available
- Test-Retest: a control group of persons with acquired brain injury (stroke and TBI) between 6 and 280 months after injury with a range of premorbid intellectual abilities (r = 0.69)[8]

Validity Estimates

- Content/Face: Questions include tasks with which everyone experiences difficulty from time to time.[8]
- Criterion: not available
- Construct: control group of persons with acquired brain injury (stroke and TBI) between 6 and 280 months after injury with a range of premorbid intellectual abilities showed no evidence of a difference between test occasions (P = 0.752). Subjects who underwent a 5-week, cognitive-motor dual-tasking training program showed a significant improvement in average questionnaire response (P < 0.10),[8] although the difference was not significant after intention to treat analysis.

Selected Reference

Evans JJ, Greenfield E, Wilson BA, Bateman A. Walking and talking therapy: improving cognitive-motor dual-tasking in neurological illness. *J Int Neuropsychol Soc.* Jan 2009;15(1):112–120.

SECTION 2: DUAL-TASK INTERVENTION

Purpose/Background

Although impairments in motor/postural and cognitive components of dual-task performance are recognized in individuals with c/mTBI, research on specific interventions for the issues of attention and dual or multiple tasks in these individuals is in its infancy.[4,8,9] Early findings seem to indicate the importance of training specificity; that is, the ability to generalize from one type of dual-task training (eg, a cognitive-motor task versus two motor tasks) has not been found consistently.[8] Training in the combination of cognitive and motor tasks together

does seem to offer benefits over single-task balance training and may transfer to a cognitive-motor test that has not been practiced.[14,15]

Experts suggest that training scenarios be tasks relevant to the real-life home and occupational situations for each individual. Suggested interventions include tasks carried out in progressively more complex environments and under increasingly more difficult multitask conditions. Interventions should involve motor, manual, visual-spatial, and cognitive tasks, with a goal of assisting the service member in improving his or her ability to perform everyday tasks in complex environments. Summary

FORM 8-1

DUAL-TASKING QUESTIONNAIRE

The following questions are about problems that everyone experiences from time to time, but some of which happen more often than others. We want to know how often these things have happened to you **in the past few weeks**. There are five options, ranging from *very often* to *never*, or *not applicable (N/A)*. Please circle the appropriate response.

Do you have any of these difficulties?

1. Paying attention to more than one thing at a time.

very often (4)   often (3)   occasionally (2)   rarely (1)   never (0)   N/A

2. Needing to stop an activity to talk.

very often (4)   often (3)   occasionally (2)   rarely (1)   never (0)   N/A

3. Being unaware of others speaking to you when doing another activity.

very often (4)   often (3)   occasionally (2)   rarely (1)   never (0)   N/A

4. Following or taking part in a conversation where several people are speaking at once.

very often (4)   often (3)   occasionally (2)   rarely (1)   never (0)   N/A

5. Walking deteriorating when you are talking or listening to someone.

very often (4)   often (3)   occasionally (2)   rarely (1)   never (0)   N/A

6. Busy thinking your own thoughts, so not noticing what is going on around you.

very often (4)   often (3)   occasionally (2)   rarely (1)   never (0)   N/A

7. Spilling a drink when carrying it.

very often (4)   often (3)   occasionally (2)   rarely (1)   never (0)   N/A

8. Spilling a drink when carrying it and talking at the same time.

very often (4)   often (3)   occasionally (2)   rarely (1)   never (0)   N/A

9. Bumping into people or dropping things if doing something else as well.

very often (4)   often (3)   occasionally (2)   rarely (1)   never (0)   N/A

10. Difficulty eating and watching television or listening to the radio at the same time.

very often (4)   often (3)   occasionally (2)   rarely (1)   never (0)   N/A

Total Score = _____.
Sum of 1–10/10
Total is average rating per question

feedback given to patients on their performance with regard to number of errors (ie, number targets not identified or number of balance losses) and information on their performance (ie, distractions seen as the reason for their loss of balance) may be helpful in providing insight on safety issues and areas for improvement.

Strength of Recommendation: Practice Option

Preliminary evidence has shown training-specific improvement in cognitive-motor and balance tasks in community-dwelling adults at risk for falls[9] and those with acquired brain injury.[8] The use of sports or activities such as t'ai chi ch'uan to improve dual-task abilities have been suggested,[4] although efficacy findings are mixed.[16]

EXHIBIT 8-2

SECONDARY TASKS IN TRAINING PROGRAMS

---

1. **Auditory discrimination tasks:** Patients were asked to identify the noises or voices from a compact disc such as:
   1) Identifying voices (man, woman, child)
   2) Identifying noises (hand clap, door close, dog bark, cat meow)
2. **Name things/words:** Patients were asked to name things such as types of flower, states, and men's names.
3. **Visual discrimination tasks:** Patients were shown the pictures before and after performing the balance tasks. They were asked to memorize the pictures and to respond if the pictures were the same. They were required to say "yes" if the pictures were the same and "no" if they were different.
4. **Random digit generation:** Patients were asked to randomly name the numbers between 0 and 300.
5. **Counting backward:** (eg, by twos, threes).
6. **Visual spatial task:** Patients were asked to place numbers, objects, or letters in the imagined matrixes. Then they were required to name the numbers, objects, or letters in the specific matrix cell.
7. **Visual imaginary spatial tasks:** Patients were asked to imagine and tell the road direction (eg, the road direction from their home to the post office).
8. **N-Back task:** Patients were asked to recite numbers, days, or months backward (eg, December, November, . . . January).
9. **Subtract or add number to letter:** Patients were asked to give the letter as a result of the equation (eg, k–1=j).
10. **Remembering things:** Patients were asked to memorize telephone numbers, prices, objects, or words.
11. **Tell story:** Patients were asked to tell any story such as what they did in the morning, what they did on their vacation, and so on.
12. **Tell opposite direction of action:** Patients were asked to name the opposite direction of their actions. For example, they were required to name "left" when they move their right leg.
13. **Spell the word backward:** Patients were asked to spell a word backward such as "apple," "bird," and "television."
14. **Say any complete sentence:** Patients were asked to say any complete sentence.
15. **Stroop task:** Patients were asked to name the color of the ink while ignoring the meaning of the word.

Reproduced with permission from: Silsupadol P, Siu KC, Shumway-Cook A, Woollacott MH. Training of balance under single- and dual-task conditions in older adults with balance impairment. *Phys Ther.* 2006;86(2):269–281, Appendix 2, p 281. Copyright 2006, American Physical Therapy Association. This material is copyrighted, and any further reproduction or distribution is prohibited.

TABLE 8-3

EXAMPLE OF DUAL-TASK TRAINING WHILE VARYING INSTRUCTIONAL SET

	Secondary Activities	Focus B/S[*]	Balance (no. of missteps) Left	Right	Verbal Responses No. of Responses	No. of Errors
Balance Activities						
Stance Activities						
1. Semi-tandem, eyes open, alternation	Spell words forward	80/20				
2. Semi-tandem, eyes closed arm alternation	Spell words backward	20/80				
3. Draw letter with right foot	Name any words that start with letter A–K	20/80				
4. Draw letters with left foot	Name any words that start with letter L–X	80/20				
5. Perturbed standing holding a ball	Remember prices (eg, bill payment)	20/80				
6. Perturbed standing holding a ball	Remember prices (eg, groceries)	80/20				
Transitional Activities						
Gait Activities						
7. Walk, narrow base of support	Count backward by 3	80/20	0	6	25	0
8. Walk, narrow base of support	Count backward by 3	20/80	7	27	28	0
9. Walk, narrow base of support, step sideways, backward avoiding the obstacles (holding a basket)	Remember words	80/20				
10. Walk, narrow base of support, step sideways, backward avoiding the obstacles (holding a basket)	Remember words	20/80				
11. Walk and kick a ball to hit the cans	Tell the opposite direction of the ball	20/80				
12. Walk and kick a ball to hit the cans	Tell the opposite direction of the ball	80/20				
13. Walk and reach and trunk twisting	Visual imaginary task (tell the road direction from home to the lab)	80/20				

[*]Focus B/S: focus on balance activities/secondary tasks (80/20: focus on balance activities; 20/80: focus on secondary tasks).

Intervention Methods

Several intervention methods can be used to improve dual tasking, including the following:

1. Provide practice opportunities and training in motivating interventions that involve dual-task activities. Include tasks that begin with simple combinations of postural control (balance and gait with cognitive tasks; see Exhibit 8-2 and Table 8-3) and cognitive and visual-spatial tasks and advance to progressively more complex environments and progressively more difficult multitasking conditions.

2. If using dual-task activities in training, vary the priority the service member puts on the tasks that are combined, a concept referred to as "instructional set" because it is generated by the therapist's instructions. Requiring a shift in attention from one task to another as directed by the therapist may improve overall "dual-task" abilities based on early intervention studies with older adults.[14] Guide this shift in attention by cues such as "this time really focus on the balance task," then "this time really concentrate on getting the cognitive task correct."

3. Progress practice opportunities to tasks that are related to the individual's specific occupational environment and to the roles that an individual is expected to resume.

4. Encourage participation in and provide education about the types of recreational sport and leisure activities that involve multiple task performance while maintaining a service member's attention and motivation.

5. See the "Points to Remember" sheet, which is included for therapists designing dual-task intervention programs.

DUAL-TASK INTERVENTIONS: THERAPIST POINTS TO REMEMBER

- Dual-task learning is likely task specific. Although there may be some generalization to similar tasks, it is important to focus on the specific types of dual tasks that need to be improved. For example, if visual-spatial tasks (scanning the environment) while under challenging postural conditions (uneven terrain) is a relevant task, the intervention strategies should be designed for those conditions.

- According to McCulloch, "The ability to generalize novel dual-task conditions to real life has not been demonstrated for patients with neurological involvement, so choosing therapy activities that are closer to real life is a reasonable approach; walking while dialing (and talking) on a cell phone, map reading, . . . way finding."[4(p116)]

- Training in single-task conditions (ie, balance) has not been shown to improve dual-task skills (ie, balance and cognitive tasks combined).

- Progress the cognitive load from simple cognitive tasks to more complex tasks and from stable postural or gait tasks to more challenging situations once the simpler tasks have been mastered.

- The "instructional set" is important; that is, it is important to set up the directions or instruction for the patient as to the focus of their attention (ie, does the patient focus on the balance or postural control task, on the cognitive task, or on both tasks equally?). Vary the "instructional set" during training.

- Providing external (extrinsic) feedback on errors and successes may improve service member learning.

- Consider the person's long-term goals, targeting environments and roles that a patient is expected to resume.

- Possible interventions strategies:
  ○ Tasks with military overtones, obstacle courses, map reading, carrying a load, speed changes, visual scanning, altered terrain.
  ○ Recreational (non-contact) sports, such as ping-pong, tennis, basketball, bicycling, or tai chi. Consider water-based therapy programs.
  ○ Simulators or virtual-reality based games (eg, Nintendo Wii) that involve postural control with visual scanning and upper extremity motor tasks.

REFERENCES

1. Fait P, McFadyen BJ, Swaine B, Cantin JF. Alterations to locomotor navigation in a complex environment at 7 and 30 days following a concussion in an elite athlete. *Brain Inj.* Apr 2009;23(4):362–369.

2. Parker TM, Osternig LR, van Donkelaar P, Chou LS. Gait stability following concussion. *Med Sci Sports Exerc.* Jun 2006;38(6):1032–1040.

3. Vallée M, McFadyen BJ, Swaine B, Doyon J, Cantin JF, Dumas D. Effects of environmental demands on locomotion after traumatic brain injury. *Arch Phys Med Rehabil.* 2006;87(6):806–813.

4. McCulloch K. Attention and dual-task conditions: physical therapy implications for individuals with acquired brain injury. *J Neurol Phys Ther.* 2007;31(3):104–118.

5. Al-Yahya E, Dawes H, Smith L, Dennis A, Howells K, Cockburn J. Cognitive motor interference while walking: a systematic review and meta-analysis. *Neurosci Biobehav Rev.* Jan 2011;35(3):715–728.

6. Wrisley DM, Marchetti GF, Kuharsky DK, Whitney SL. Reliability, internal consistency, and validity of data obtained with the functional gait assessment. *Phys Ther.* 2004;84(10):906–918.

7. McCulloch K, Blakeley K, Freeman L. Clinical tests of walking dual-task performance after acquired brain injury: feasibility and dual-task cost compared to a young adult group. *J Neurol Phys Ther.* 2005(29):213.

8. Evans JJ, Greenfield E, Wilson BA, Bateman A. Walking and talking therapy: improving cognitive-motor dual-tasking in neurological illness. *J Int Neuropsychol Soc.* Jan 2009;15(1):112–120.

9. Silsupadol P, Siu KC, Shumway-Cook A, Woollacott MH. Training of balance under single- and dual-task conditions in older adults with balance impairment. *Phys Ther.* Feb 2006;86(2):269–281.

10. McCulloch KL, Mercer V, Giuliani C, Marshall S. Development of a clinical measure of dual-task performance in walking: reliability and preliminary validity of the Walking and Remembering Test. *J Geriatr Phys Ther.* 2009;32(1):2–9.

11. Shumway-Cook A, Brauer S, Woollacott M. Predicting the probability for falls in community-dwelling older adults using the Timed Up & Go Test. *Phys Ther.* Sep 2000;80(9):896–903.

12. Abernethy B. Dual-task methodology and motor skills research: some applications and methodological constraints *J Hum Mov Stud.* 1988;14:101–132.

13. Parker TM, Osternig LR, Lee HJ, Donkelaar P, Chou LS. The effect of divided attention on gait stability following concussion. *Clin Biomech (Bristol, Avon).* May 2005;20(4):389–395.

14. Silsupadol P, Shumway-Cook A, Lugade V, et al. Effects of single-task versus dual-task training on balance performance in older adults: a double-blind, randomized controlled trial. *Arch Phys Med Rehabil.* 2009;90(3):381–387.

15. Silsupadol P, Lugade V, Shumway-Cook A, et al. Training-related changes in dual-task walking performance of elderly persons with balance impairment: a double-blind, randomized controlled trial. *Gait Posture.* 2009;29(4):634–639.

16. Hall CD, Miszko T, Wolf SL. Effects of Tai Chi intervention on dual-task ability in older adults: a pilot study. *Arch Phys Med Rehabil.* Mar 2009;90(3):525–529.

Chapter 9

PERFORMANCE AND SELF-MANAGEMENT, WORK, SOCIAL, AND SCHOOL ROLES

LESLIE DAVIDSON, PhD*; CAROL SMITH HAMMOND, PhD, CCC/SLP†; PAULINE MASHIMA, PhD, CCC/SLP‡; LESLIE NITTA, CCC/SLP§; JENNY OWENS, OTD¥; MARY RADOMSKI, PhD¶; MAILE T. SINGSON, CCC-SLP**; MARSEY WALLER DEVOTO, OTD††; ALINE WIMBERLY, OTR/L, CBIS‡‡; AND JOETTE ZOLLA, OT§§

INTRODUCTION

SECTION 1: SELF-MANAGEMENT ROLES
  CANADIAN OCCUPATIONAL PERFORMANCE MEASURE
  OCCUPATIONAL SELF-ASSESSMENT
  FATIGUE AND SLEEP ISSUES AFTER CONCUSSION/MILD TRAUMATIC BRAIN INJURY
  MEDICATION MANAGEMENT
  INTERVENTION: FATIGUE AND SLEEP ISSUES AFTER CONCUSSION/MILD TRAUMATIC BRAIN INJURY
  INTERVENTION: MEDICATION MANAGEMENT
  INTERVENTION: BILL PAYING AND MONEY MANAGEMENT
  CLINICIAN TIP SHEETS

SECTION 2: SOCIAL ROLES
  REENGAGING WITH SPOUSES, CHILDREN, AND FRIENDS
  ASSESSMENT OF COMMUNICATION AND INTERACTION SKILLS
  ACTIVITY CO-ENGAGEMENT SELF-ASSESSMENT
  DYADIC ADJUSTMENT SCALE
  INTERVENTION: REENGAGING WITH SPOUSES, CHILDREN, AND FRIENDS
  CLINICIAN TIP SHEETS

SECTION 3: RETURN TO SCHOOL
  RETURNING TO SCHOOL
  CLINICIAN TIP SHEETS

SECTION 4: RETURN TO DUTY
  INTERVENTION: PERFORMING WORK ROLES
  RETURN TO DUTY VALIDATION PROGRAM
  CLINICIAN TIP SHEETS

REFERENCES

SECTION 5: PATIENT HANDOUTS

*Director, Occupational Therapy, Shenandoah University, 1460 University Drive, Winchester, Virginia 22601

†Research Speech Pathologist, Audiology/Speech Pathology, Durham Veterans Affairs Medical Center, #126, 508 Fulton Street, Durham, North Carolina 27705

‡Chief, Speech Pathology Section, Department of Surgery, Otolaryngology Service, Tripler Army Medical Center, 1 Jarrett White Road, Tripler Army Medical Center, Honolulu, Hawaii 96859

§Speech-Language Pathologist, Greater Los Angeles Veterans Affairs Healthcare System, Sepulveda Ambulatory Care Center, 16111 Plumber Street, Building 200, Room 2409/Gold Team, Sepulveda, California 91343

¥Occupational Therapist, Warrior Resiliency and Recovery Center, Blanchfield Army Community Hospital, Building 2543, Room 118, 650 Joel Drive, Fort Campbell, Kentucky 42223

¶Clinical Scientist, Courage Kenny Research Center, 800 East 28th Street, Mail Stop 12212, Minneapolis, Minnesota 55407

**Speech Language Pathologist, Traumatic Brain Injury Program, Veterans Affairs Pacific Island Health Care System, Traumatic Brain Injury Clinic, Specialty Clinic Module 8, 459 Patterson Road, Honolulu, Hawaii 96819

††Occupational Therapist, Military Share Brain Injury Program, Shepherd Center, 2020 Peachtree Road Northwest, Atlanta, Georgia 30309

‡‡Formerly, Occupational Therapist, Warrior Resiliency and Recovery Center, Traumatic Brain Injury Clinic, Fort Campbell, Kentucky

§§Occupational Therapist, Brain Injury Clinic, Courage Kenny Rehabilitation Institute, Allina Health, 800 East 28th Street, Mail Stop 12210, Minneapolis, Minnesota 55407*

INTRODUCTION

Although most people recover from concussion/mild traumatic brain injury (c/mTBI) within 3 months of injury,[1] some experience symptoms that interfere with the performance of life roles and tasks related to activities of daily living (ADLs), instrumental activities of daily living (IADLs), work, and maintaining social relationships. For example, one of the most common complaints after concussion is ongoing issues with fatigue.[2] Patients report both physical and mental fatigue that affects their ability to efficiently perform daily and weekly ADLs, IADLs, and work responsibilities. Pain and cognitive inefficiencies may also make self-management tasks more effortful or error laden.

The overarching goal of occupational therapy assessment and intervention is to enable patients to return to valued roles and activities.[3] Doing so involves understanding the patient's priorities, identifying impairments and inefficiencies that interfere with performance, and intervening to enable the patient to reengage in valued roles and activities in everyday life.

SECTION 1: SELF-MANAGEMENT ROLES

CANADIAN OCCUPATIONAL PERFORMANCE MEASURE

Purpose/Description

The Canadian Occupational Performance Measure (COPM) is an individualized standardized measure that is administered during initial assessment to specify the patient's priorities for therapy and baseline status in areas of functioning; it is repeated to objectify progress toward goals and outcomes of therapy (Exhibit 9-1). The COPM is a semistructured interview that uses an ordinal scale to quantify changes in client-reported performance and satisfaction in areas of self-care, productivity, and leisure.

Recommended Instrument Use: Practice Standard

- This test is an essential inclusion in an initial occupational therapy assessment to identify patients' priorities and to inform the development of the occupational therapy intervention plan.
- It should also be readministered as an outcome measure, quantifying the extent to which the patient has experienced appreciable improvements in occupational performance.

Note: The COPM may not be appropriate for individuals who lack self-awareness of deficits.[4] In these situations, family members may be invited to participate in the COPM interview, presuming their treatment priorities are endorsed by the patient.[4,5]

Administration Protocol/Equipment/Time

The COPM is comprised of the administration manual, scoring cards, and test worksheet. It takes 20 to 40 minutes to administer as follows:

1. The therapist asks the client to identify issues of concern in areas of self-care, productivity, and leisure.
2. The client rates the importance of these issues using a 1-to-10 scale (10 signifying most importance).
3. The client chooses up to five areas to be the focus of occupational therapy intervention.

EXHIBIT 9-1

CANADIAN OCCUPATIONAL PERFORMANCE MEASURE

The Canadian Occupational Performance Measure can be found in the following: Law M, Baptise S, McColl MA, Carswell A, Polatajko H, Pollock N. *Canadian Occupational Performance Measure.* 2nd ed. Toronto, Canada: Canadian Association of Occupational Therapists–Association Canadienne d'Éducation Publications; 1994. Available through Canadian Associations of Occupational Therapists: www.caot.ca.

4. The client rates his or her current level of performance and satisfaction for each area of concern again using a 1-to-10 scale (10 representing the highest level of performance and satisfaction).

5. After a negotiated period of occupational therapy intervention, the client again rates his or her performance and satisfaction for the (up to) five areas addressed in occupational therapy.

Groups Tested With This Measure

The COPM has been tested on and used to measure outcomes of occupational therapy services with a variety of diagnostic groups, such as those with traumatic brain injury (TBI),[6,7] including c/mTBI.[4,5] The COPM has been used with other diagnostic groups[8] (see the list of important references at www.caot.ca/copm/description.html for more information).

Interpretability

The COPM was designed to measure outcomes of therapy based on the individual client's priorities and perceptions of status and improvement. Although COPM scores have been evaluated in aggregate to evaluation program outcomes,[4,5] the COPM is not a norm-referenced measure.[9] Rather, it was designed to measure occupational performance as individually defined.[9]

Scoring

The occupational therapist calculates the total performance score by adding the performance scores of up to five areas, then dividing by the number of problem areas (obtaining an average from 1 to 10). The total satisfaction score is calculated in the same manner. The difference between initial evaluation and subsequent scores (change score) can be used to measure treatment outcome.[8]

Minimal Detectable Change

The minimal detectable change (MDC) at 95% (MDC_{95}) was calculated based on data from the COPM test-retest evaluation involving 26 community-dwelling individuals with stroke and yielded the following[10]:

*   COPM performance $MDC_{95} = 1.65$
*   COPM satisfaction $MDC_{95} = 1.82$

This means that a patient's before and after scores (pre-post score) would need to change by 1.65 for the COPM performance score and by 1.82 for the COPM satisfaction score to be 95% confident that true change occurred (rather than measurement error).

Minimal Clinically Importance Differences

As cited by Trombly and colleagues,[4] Law et al reported that COPM performance and COPM satisfaction change scores exceeding 2 represent clinically significant change.[11]

Responsiveness Estimates

The COPM appears to be sensitive to the before-after effects of treatment and to treatment versus nontreatment for individuals with brain injury. Numerous studies have reported statistically significant differences in pre-post COPM performance and satisfaction scores of clients with acquired brain injury (including mTBI) associated with occupational therapy intervention.[4,5,7] Jenkinson and colleagues[6] reported statistically significant COPM performance changes based on 10 clients with brain injury (P = 0.018), and relative ratings (P = 0.008) for those who received community-based outpatient intervention; change scores for the same period for a similar group (n = 15) who did not receive intervention and that of their relatives did not reach statistical significance.

Reliability and Validity Estimates

Interrater Reliability

Interrater reliability (as determined by comparing client's performance self-ratings and that of relatives) is acceptable. Jenkinson and colleagues[6] found that COPM performance ratings for participants and that of their relatives were not significantly different. In an outpatient occupational therapy outcomes study, clients with TBI and their family members did independent ratings of COPM performance at admission, discharge, and follow-up.[4] Similar to the Jenkinson's[6] findings, there were no significant differences in patient-relative ratings at any of these intervals.

Interrater Agreement

Interrater agreement (as determined by comparing problem prioritization when the COPM was administered by two occupational therapists) is moderate. The COPM was administered twice (average of 7 days between) to 95 patients with various diagnoses who were newly referred to outpatient occupational therapy.[12] Sixty-six percent of the activities prioritized at the first administration were prioritized at the second.

Test-Retest

Test-retest reliability for client COPM performance and satisfaction ratings is good. Cup and colleagues[10] administered the COPM twice to patients with stroke (mean interval of 8 days) and found high levels of correlation between the first and second sets of COPM scores. The Spearman's rho correlation coefficient for test-retest performance scores was 0.89 (P < 0.001) and 0.88 (P < 0.001) for test-retest satisfaction scores.

Test-retest reliability for problem identification is moderate. In the same study, of the 115 problems identified during the first administration of the COPM, 64 (56%) were also identified at the second administration.[10]

Concurrent (Criterion) Validity

Treatment-related changes in the COPM score for persons with TBI are consistent with other measures of self-reported goal achievement. Sixteen outpatients with TBI (some mild) who received outpatient occupational therapy realized statistically significant improvements in self-identified goals as measured by admission-discharge comparisons on goal attainment scaling (P < .001), COPM performance (P < .001), and satisfaction measures (P < .001).[4]

Discriminant Validity

Unique problems may be evaluated with the COPM. Cup and colleagues[10] found that the COPM measures a different construct than other stroke-related activity-participation standardized measures, including the Barthel Index, Frenchay Activities Index, and Stroke Adapted Sickness Impact Profile-30. None of the scores on the standardized measures of function significantly correlated with the COPM but they all significantly correlated with one another.

OCCUPATIONAL SELF-ASSESSMENT

Purpose/Description

The Occupational Self-Assessment (OSA; Exhibit 9-2)[13] is a paper-and-pencil self-report designed to help occupational therapists understand patients' self-perceptions of occupational competence, valued areas of functioning, priorities, and the perceived impact of the environment on performance. This information may be used in treatment planning, as a means to develop patient-therapist rapport and partnership,[14] and to document outcomes of care.[15]

The OSA is composed of two parts. Part I includes a series of statements about everyday activities (eg, "concentrating on my tasks"). These statements were derived from the Model of Human Occupation[16] and relate to skills and occupational performance, habituation, and volition.[14] The patient uses a four-point scale to rate his or her competence specific to each statement, then uses a four-point scale to indicate the extent to which the area is important to him or her (Exhibit 9-3). Finally, the patient reviews the list to select the four areas he or she aspires to change. Part II involves a series of statements that measure environmental supports.

Recommended Instrument Use: Practice Option

The OSA may be used to establish treatment priorities during the occupational therapy evaluation process. For some patients who have difficulty generating ideas or conversation about problem areas, the OSA may be preferable to the less-structured COPM.

Administration Protocol/Equipment/Time

Clinicians should refer to the administration manual for detailed instructions specific to

---

EXHIBIT 9-2

OCCUPATIONAL SELF-ASSESSMENT

The Occupational Self-Assessment is available from:

> Model of Human Occupation Clearinghouse
> Department of Occupational Therapy
> University of Illinois at Chicago
> 1919 West Taylor Street
> Chicago, IL 60612
> www.moho.uic.edu

EXHIBIT 9-3

OCCUPATIONAL SELF-ASSESSMENT—MYSELF

Step 1: Below are statements about things you do in everyday life. For each statement, circle how well you do it. If an item does not apply to you, cross it out and move on to the next item.

Step 2: Next, for each statement, circle how important this is to you.

Step 3: Choose up to 4 things about yourself that you would like to change. You can also write comments in this space.

Name: _____ **Date:** _____

	I have a problem doing this.	I have some difficulty doing this.	I do this well.	I do this extremely well.	This is not so important to me.	This is important to me.	This is more important to me.	This is most important to me.	I would like to change.
Concentrating on my tasks.	Lots of problems	Some difficulty	Well	Extremely well	Not so important	Important	More important	Most important	
Physically doing what I need to do.	Lots of problems	Some difficulty	Well	Extremely well	Not so important	Important	More important	Most important	
Taking care of the place where I live.	Lots of problems	Some difficulty	Well	Extremely well	Not so important	Important	More important	Most important	

Reproduced with permission from Baron K, Kielhofner G, Iyenger A, Goldhammer V, Wolenski J. *A User's Manual for the Occupational Self Assessment (OSA)*. Version 2.2. Chicago, IL: University of Illinois at Chicago; 2006: 48.

administration and scoring. It takes approximately 30 minutes to administer and discuss the OSA; the manual, score sheet, and a pencil are required.

Groups Tested With This Measure

The OSA has been tested on persons with physical disabilities as well as those with psychiatric disabilities[15]; it has been translated into multiple languages.

Interpretability

Norms

No norms are reported.

Scoring

OSA responses are used in a collaborative process. Therapists should particularly take note of activities that are both rated as problematic *and* of great value to the patient and use this information to guide treatment planning.

Mean Detectable Change

No information reported.

Reliability and Validity Estimates

Rasch analysis was used in three iterative studies involving over 500 subjects.[17] Findings suggest good internal validity and that it is adequately sensitive and reliable in distinguishing between levels of perceived occupational competence.

FATIGUE AND SLEEP ISSUES AFTER CONCUSSION/MILD TRAUMATIC BRAIN INJURY

Patients often report ongoing fatigue issues after sustaining concussion.[2] Patients may report both physical and mental fatigue that affects their ability to efficiently perform their daily and weekly ADLs, IADLs, and work responsibilities. Problems with fatigue and sleep typically require medical management, which includes comprehensive assessment. Occupational therapists may contribute to that effort and inform their intervention plan by formal and informal patient interviews and by administering standardized assessment tools (eg, Epworth Sleepiness Scale[19] [ESS], Fatigue Severity Scale[20] [FSS]).

Strength of Recommendation

The US Department of Veterans Affairs (VA) and Department of Defense (DoD) Clinical Practice Guideline for Management of Concussion/Mild Traumatic Brain Injury[18] does not recommend any specific fatigue or sleep assessments over others. The assessments described in this section are considered options.

Assessments

Epworth Sleepiness Scale

The ESS (available at www.epworthsleepinessscale.com/about-epworth-sleepiness/) is a self-administered, eight-item questionnaire used to measure daytime sleepiness in adults.[19] The ESS involves rating how likely people are to fall asleep in eight different situations or activities (scale of 0 to 3). It does not ask how often people actually fall asleep in these situations; just the chance of doing so. The total ESS score provides an estimate of a person's level of sleepiness in daily life but does not specify what factors contribute to sleepiness or diagnose specific conditions. It measures one aspect of a person's sleep-wake health status.

Recommended Instrument Use: Practice Option. If patients describe daytime sleepiness as a barrier to their performance of everyday tasks, the ESS may be used as a baseline measure of sleep-wake health status.

Administration Protocol/Equipment/Time. Most people can answer the ESS independently in 2 or 3 minutes. Only the questionnaire and a pencil or pen are needed.

Groups Tested With This Measure. The ESS was normed on healthy adults and has been used with various clinical populations, including adults with TBI.[21] However, its use with persons who have sustained c/mTBI is unknown.

Interpretability

Scoring. The total ESS score is the sum of the eight items; scores range from 0 to 24 (the higher the score, the higher the person's daytime sleepiness).

Norms. A study of healthy Australian adults (N = 72) reported an average ESS score of 4.6 (95% confidence interval 3.9 to 5.3). The normal range was defined as 0 to 10, although approximately 10% to 20% of the general population has ESS scores greater than 10.[22]

Responsiveness estimates. The ESS may not be suitable for retest over periods of days or weeks (given the instructions to rate likelihood of sleepiness in "recent times").

Reliability Estimates

Internal consistency. There is a high level of internal consistency as assessed by Cronbach's alpha (0.88 to 0.74 in four different groups of patients).[22]

Test-retest. Total ESS scores are reliable over a period of months (rho = 0.82).[22]

Validity Estimates

Construct. The ESS measures average sleep propensity in eight situations. The ESS scores differ between normal subjects and individuals with obstructive sleep apnea, which is known to increase sleepiness.[22]

Fatigue Severity Scale

The FSS (available at www.mainedo.com/pdfs/FSS.pdf) is designed to evaluate the impact fatigue has on a patient. A recent systematic review of fatigue measures suggested that the FSS demonstrated good psychometric properties and has the ability to detect change over time.[23]

Recommended Instrument Use: Practice Option. Occupational therapists may administer the FSS when patients indicate that fatigue is a barrier to their performance of everyday tasks. The FSS total score can help the therapist determine when referral to a physician for further evaluation is in order.

Administration Protocol/Equipment/Time. The FSS contains nine statements. The patient rates the severity of his or her fatigue symptoms by reading each statement and then circling a number from 1 to 7, based on how accurately it reflects his or her condition during the past week and the extent to which he or she agrees or disagrees that the statement applies. The higher the value, the stronger the agreement with the statement.

Groups Tested With This Measure. The FSS has been used to assess fatigue in many clinical populations, including individuals with multiple sclerosis, stroke, Parkinson's disease,[23] and mild to moderate TBI.[24]

Interpretability

Scoring. Two scoring methods have been described: summing a total score and calculating an average score. A total score (obtained by summing ratings of the nine statements) of 35 or less suggests that the individual may not be suffering from fatigue. Patients who score 36 or more should be referred to a physician for further evaluation.[25]

The average score is calculated by dividing the total score by nine.[21] People with depression alone score approximately 4.5.[24]

Mean Detectable Change. The MDC_{95} was calculated based on data from an FSS test-retest evaluation involving 11 individuals with systemic lupus erythematosus or multiple sclerosis.[21]

FSS MDC_{95} = 1.44. This means that a patient's pre-post score would need to change by 1.44 for the FSS score to be 95% confident that true change occurred (rather than measurement error).

Reliability Estimates

Internal Consistency. Good internal consistency (Cronbach's alpha = 0.88–0.95)[21]

Test-Retest. Eleven subjects (five with systemic lupus erythematosus, six with multiple sclerosis) were retested after an average of 10 weeks, in which no change in fatigue was clinically anticipated. Paired *t* test differences were not significant; correlation coefficient was 0.84.[21]

Validity Estimates

Convergent. FSS scores are correlated with other measures of fatigue, including the Multidimensional Assessment of Fatigue and Rhoten Fatigue Scale.[23]

MEDICATION MANAGEMENT

Many individuals with c/mTBI report forgetfulness and organization problems. As a result and for a variety of reasons, patients with c/mTBI may have difficulty keeping track of their medications and remembering to take them as prescribed. For example, patients may be taking medications prescribed by more than one physician or have received instructions about medication at a time

FORM 9-1

MEDICATION MANAGEMENT PERFORMANCE OBSERVATION

Instructions

The following observation checklist may be used to help the therapist determine what aspect of medication management is problematic for a given patient. Ideally, this observation may occur in the patient's room (as an inpatient setting), during a home visit, or if the patient brings his or her medications to an outpatient session.

Identifying Medications

- Can the patient locate all of his or her medication bottles? Are they stored together in the same place? Does the patient keep medications in a specific place in the house or on his or her person?
- Can the patient identify the names of the pills, what they look like, and their purpose?

Organizing Medications

- Does the patient have a written schedule of his or her medications?
- How are the medications organized (eg, day, time of day, both)?
- Does the patient use a pill box?

Opening Medication Containers

- Can the patient open bottles with childproof caps?
- Can the patient open bottles with regular caps?

Using Vision to Read Labels and Recognize Medications

- Can the patient identify what the medication looks like and distinguish the differences between medications?
- Can the patient read the prescriptions on the bottles?
- Does the patient understand what the prescriptions mean?

Memory Strategies and Medication Schedules

- Does the patient use a pill box?
- Can the patient fill his or her pill box accurately?
- Does the patient have a written schedule for taking medications?
- Does the patient use a checklist?
- Does the patient remember when to take the medications?
- Does the patient have a system for remembering to take the medications? If so, what (eg, alarms, reminders from someone else, etc)? Does the patient take his or her medications around meals and or bedtime?

Refilling Medications

- Does the patient know the name of his or her prescribing physician? Does the patient know the doctor's telephone number?
- Can the patient recognize when medications need to be refilled?
- Does the patient know how to refill the medication?
- Can the patient report or find the name and number of the pharmacy?
- Does the patient remember to pick up refills after ordering them?
- If the patient took too much medication, would he or she know what to do?
- If the patient took too little medication, would he or she know what to do?

Adapted with permission from Marsey Waller Devoto, MSOT, OTD; Assistant Professor and Fieldwork Coordinator, Brenau University, School of Occupational Therapy College of Health Sciences, 500 Washington St Southeast, Gainesville, GA 30501; 2013.

when they have been less able to attend to or remember the information. Because medication management is an extremely important component of any patient's recovery, especially for those with brain injury, it is important to assess the extent to which patients with c/mTBI are adhering to their medication regimen.

If clients are not managing their medications well, they may present with drowsiness, decreased attention skills, and overall inability to efficiently manage pain and stress. If a client is taking medications regularly and as prescribed, the treatment team is better able to understand the client's baseline and potential. It is also helpful to collaborate with nursing staff and doctors to determine whether a client's medications should be changed.

Assessment will be optimally effective in this realm if an interdisciplinary approach, involving but not limited to nursing, physical therapy, and speech language pathology, is used to understand this and other problems associated with c/mTBI.

Strength of Recommendation: Practice Option

There are no standardized or validated methods described in the literature for assessing the extent to which individuals with c/mTBI understand and are able to manage their medications. However, assessment in this area is consistent with standard occupational therapy practices and reported as valuable by occupational therapists working with individuals with c/mTBI.

Assessment

Screen all patients with c/mTBI for any issues that they may have with medication management. The first screen may be done during the client's initial interview, during which it is important to determine the following:

- whether the client understands the medications he or she takes,
- what the doses and schedules are,
- whether or not the client remembers to take his or her medications,
- who prescribed the medication,
- the purpose of the medications, and
- the extent to which the client follows his or her medication regimen as prescribed.

If the interview indicates that the patient has difficulties with some aspect (or several aspects) of medication management, use more formal methods for determining where the performance breakdown lies. Use a self-report questionnaire with additional follow-up questions and observe functional performance (see Patient Handout: Medication Management Self-Report Questionnaire and Form 9-1).

Determine how the client manages his or her medication and whether or not the management system is effective. Define the organization systems he or she uses (pill organizer, medication list, spouse), memory aids (checklist reminders, alarms, etc), and strategies for identifying medications and dosages (medication list). Once the areas of breakdown are identified, you can address each area individually.

INTERVENTION: FATIGUE AND SLEEP ISSUES AFTER CONCUSSION/MILD TRAUMATIC BRAIN INJURY

Patients report both physical and mental fatigue that affects their ability to efficiently perform daily and weekly ADLs, IADLs, and work responsibilities. Fatigue can be minimized or restored with rest and fatigue management strategies. It is important that individuals understand the best methods of managing fatigue while simultaneously working on increasing their activity tolerance. Therefore, occupational therapists provide education about fatigue and sleep hygiene and help patients employ strategies that maximize energy and productivity as they regain their activity tolerance.

Many of the strategies described in this section

of the toolkit require the service member to "work smarter, not harder." This means making decisions about how to manage one's workload and tasks and when to take breaks, strategies that may appear to be at odds with some aspects of military culture. Therapists should prepare for service member rebuttals such as, "I can't take breaks whenever I want to." Therapists help patients appreciate that their command is supportive of their recovery process and that even if some strategies are not feasible on the job, they may be helpful for aspects of life that are under service members' control.

Intervention Methods

1. Provide patient education regarding fatigue and contributing factors (see Patient Handout and Clinician Tip Sheet: Fatigue Management and Factor Awareness; also www.nhlbi.nih.gov/health/public/sleep/healthy_sleep.pdf).
2. Help the patient identify and implement individualized fatigue management and sleep hygiene strategies (see Patient Handout and Clinician Tip Sheet: Taking Breaks, Pacing; also www.helpguide.org/mental/stress_relief_meditation_yoga_relaxation.htm).
3. Remind patients and therapists of executive and attention strategies that apply to fatigue management, such as pausing and compensatory cognitive strategies (see Chapter 7: Cognition Assessment and Intervention).

Strength of Recommendation: Practice Standard

Recommendations for fatigue management and sleep hygiene are supported by the VA/DoD Clinical Practice Guideline for Management of Concussion/Mild Traumatic Brain Injury.[19]

INTERVENTION: MEDICATION MANAGEMENT

It is important for clients to take their medication regularly and as prescribed to increase independence and maximize rehabilitation potential. It is also important for patients to establish accountability and competency in managing their own medication.

Strength of Recommendation: Practice Option

There is no empirical evidence to guide practice in this area; however, intervention is consistent with standard occupational therapy practices and reported as valuable by occupational therapists working with individuals with c/mTBI.

Intervention Methods

- Address barriers to medication management (as identified during assessment) in a systematic fashion (see Clinician Tip Sheet: Intervention Planning for Medication Management).
- Develop a comprehensive list of medications, coordinating with nursing staff if possible (see Exhibits 9-4 and 9-5).
- Determine which strategies will best facilitate consistent adherence to the medication regimen (see Strategies to Improve Medication Management Clinician Tip Sheets: Pill Organizers, Checklists and Routines, and Alarms and Reminders).

EXHIBIT 9-4

EXAMPLE MEDICATION SUMMARY

Medicine	Dose	Time (s)	Reason	Prescribing Doctor
Zoloft	40 mg 3x/day	0800 & 1800	Depression	Dr. Smith
Nexium	40 mg	0800	Stomach pain	Dr. Jones
Zanaflex	4 mg	0800	Headache	Dr. Hope

EXHIBIT 9-5

EXAMPLE MEDICATION SCHEDULE

Morning

Medicine	Dose/Route	Time	Reason
Nexium	40 mg by mouth	0800	Stomach pain
Zanaflex	4 mg by mouth	0800	Headache

After Lunch/Midday

Medicine	Dose/Route	Time	Reason
Zanaflex	4 mg by mouth	1400	Muscle pain

Bedtime

Medicine	Dose/Route	Time	Reason
Prazosin	1 mg /1–2 tabs by mouth	At bedtime	Sleep/PTSD/BP
Zanaflex	4 mg by mouth	At bedtime	Muscle pain
Seroquel	400 mg by mouth	2200	Sleep

As Needed

Medicine	Dose/Route	Time	Reason
Midrin	2 tabs by mouth	At onset of headache & 2 tabs every 6 hours as needed	Headaches
Motrin	200 mg (6 tabs)	Once a day as needed	Pain

BP: blood pressure
PTSD: posttraumatic stress disorder

INTERVENTION: BILL PAYING AND MONEY MANAGEMENT

Purpose/Background

Brain injury, including c/mTBI, may affect how a person feels, processes information, and executes functional tasks, including those related to bill paying and money management. Injury-related symptoms (decreased attention, memory, or executive functions), changes in routine, fatigue, and accompanying mood disorders sometimes make it difficult for patients to pay bills on time, organize personal paperwork, and effectively manage their money. Occupational therapists help patients employ strategies and techniques to reestablish competence in this important area of self-management.

Intervention will be optimally effective in this realm if:

- the patient understands that performance problems in this area do not reflect personal incompetence. Rather, the temporary after-effects of c/mTBI combined with personal (eg, pain, headache) and situational (eg, distracting environment) factors make the task more challenging at present.
- the patient has implemented some form of memory back-up system (such as a day planner) that can be used to address personal financial tasks.

Strength of Recommendation: Practice Option

There is no empirical evidence to guide practice in this area. Intervention is consistent with standard occupational therapy practice and reported as valuable by occupational therapists working with individuals with c/mTBI.

Intervention Methods

- Talk with the patient to figure out the specific symptoms or factors that contribute to problems with money management. Also, ask the patient to describe in detail his or her current processes for task performance as well as those used in the past when, presumably, he or she had fewer problems. For example, find out answers to questions of this nature:

○ What happens to the bills when they arrive in the mail?

○ When do you tend to pay bills? At a routine time during the week or month? On weekends or after work?

○ Where in the home is the activity performed?

○ How and where are financial records stored?

• Use this information to identify processes or strategies that may improve task performance. Effective processes or strategies may involve modifying daily routines (ie, sorting mail to avoid disorder, confusion, and worry associated with losing bills amid junk mail) or using checklists or worksheets to organize bill-paying procedures to ensure accuracy (see the following Patient Handouts and Clinician Tip Sheets: Organizing the Mail, Establishing a Budget, Bill Paying, Using a Smartphone or Planner to Manage Money, and AAA Worksheet; and Patient Handouts: Budget Planning Worksheet, Budget Tracking Worksheet, and Money Management [packet]).

CLINICIAN TIP SHEET: FATIGUE MANAGEMENT—FACTOR AND STRATEGY AWARENESS

Purpose/Background

Occupational therapists help patients address problems with fatigue by:

• providing education on healthy living, including information related to managing fatigue;

• helping the patient identify strategies to improve sleep and address fatigue; and

• supporting and reinforcing the process of implementing new strategies and habits through structure and reinforcement.

Patient Handout: Fatigue Management–Factor and Strategy Awareness summarizes four key avenues for addressing fatigue by establishing and maintaining 1) good sleep hygiene practices, 2) good nutrition and hydration, 3) regular exercise or activity, and 4) stress-reduction practices.

Instructions

The handout incorporates information and opportunities for a patient's self-reflection. The patient and therapist discuss these reflections and together identify new strategies that might help (the therapist may also refer the patient to other professionals). For example:

• If a patient reports difficulty falling asleep due to ongoing issues with pain, a referral to his or her primary doctor may be indicated to investigate the source of the pain

or the medications the individual is taking.

• If the patient reports difficulty falling asleep and also reports excessive caffeine use or napping behaviors, these areas may need to be changed.

• If the patient reports falling asleep readily but waking up often with nightmares, the recommendation may be a referral to a psychologist or physician.

Occupational therapists support implementation of fatigue management and sleep strategies by incorporating them into homework assignments and reinforcing behaviors that optimize the patient's energy level and rest. Occupational therapists also support fatigue management and improved sleep patterns by helping patients learn and then implement appropriate stress-relief skills. This might include learning relaxation techniques such as deep breathing, progressive muscle relaxation, mindfulness meditation, and guided imagery (see www.helpguide.org/mental/stress_relief_meditation_yoga_relaxation.htm). During clinic sessions, therapists help patients select and learn techniques then provide homework assignments that support implementation on a routine basis.

Remember, occupational therapists use in-depth conversation with the patient about his or her fatigue, activity, and sleep patterns to inform referrals to other providers. Occupational therapy intervention that emphasizes education and implementation of sleep and fatigue management strategies contributes to interdisciplinary efforts to address this important aspect of functioning.

CLINICIAN TIP SHEET: HELPING PATIENTS LEARN AND IMPLEMENT FATIGUE MANAGEMENT STRATEGIES

Purpose/Background

Many individuals view fatigue management strategies (such as taking breaks or pacing) as forms of laziness or weakness. It is important that therapists help patients see these techniques as means by which they perform at their optimum level.

The patient handouts on these topics are designed to facilitate discussions that help patients reflect on their physical and mental responses to fatigue. Once they identify their symptoms and current patterns, patients need assistance exploring and implementing alternative strategies, including taking preemptive breaks that can give them greater staying power, pacing, and managing personal and situational factors (see Chapter 7, Cognitive Assessment and Intervention).

In general, implementing fatigue management strategies in daily life involves effective use of compensatory cognitive strategies, self-reflection, and self-awareness.

Effective Use of Compensatory Cognitive Strategies

As is the case whenever people are engaged in changing patterns of behavior, it is easy to forget one's best intentions amid the challenges and distractions of everyday life. Therefore, occupational therapists help patients build on their skills with compensatory cognitive strategies to optimize the likelihood that they will remember to use fatigue management strategies in the course of their everyday activities. This includes the following:

- Using stop notes. Taking a moment to leave yourself a written note as to where you left off and what to do next (after a break or when the task is resumed the next day) can be a useful compensatory strategy. Many patients report reluctance to take breaks because they will forget where they were; stop notes help eliminate that concern.
- Preplanning fatigue management strategies. Generative thinking can be taxing and very difficult, especially when an individual is fatigued. That is why it is very important that patients plan for fatigue in advance, when they are not tired. This may involve generating a possible "break" list in therapy and having numerous options for breaks when at home or work, or spreading essential or desired tasks throughout the week.
- Using alarm prompts for starting and stopping breaks or initiating scheduled tasks. Sometimes patients get so engaged in the task at hand that they simply forget to monitor symptoms that might otherwise indicate the need for a break. As a result, they do not stop until it is simply too late. Setting an hourly alarm for a fatigue status check might encourage a brief preemptive break and increase staying power for the work session. Similarly, setting an alarm for 10 minutes could signal a return to the task after a brief break or initiate a scheduled task.

Self-Reflection and Self-Awareness

Self-reflection and self-awareness are essential to the successful use of fatigue management strategies. Patients need to be mindful of their daily to-do lists, priorities, and activity tolerance.

They need to know:

- when to take a break,
- how long the break needs to be, and
- what to do during a break or if stopping for the day and trying again another time is a better option. For example, simply stopping for the day may be the best option if headache pain is out of control and continued effort is likely to both exacerbate pain and result in error-laden output.

Remember, therapists can contribute to improved patient self-awareness in this realm by providing simulated work tasks at therapy sessions in which the patient practices implementing these strategies and analyzes his or her performance afterwards (see AAA Worksheet in Chapter 7, Cognitive Assessment and Intervention).

CLINICIAN TIP SHEET: INTERVENTION PLANNING FOR MEDICATION MANAGEMENT

General Guidelines

Identify one area to work on at a time. Start with a compiled, comprehensive list of medications. If the patient is taking several medications, use a pill organizer. Establish daily and weekly routines as they relate to medication. Link assessment findings with intervention plans (Table 9-1).

TABLE 9-1

INTERVENTION PLANNING

Assessment Issue	Yes	No
Can patient open the medication bottle?	Nothing needs to be addressed	Request easy-open bottles from the pharmacy. Use adaptive equipment like a rubber bottle opener.
Can patient read the prescription?	Nothing needs to be addressed	Type prescription in large print and tape to outside of the bottle. Use adaptive equipment, such as a magnifier. If the above suggestions are ineffective, color code the medication and link the coding to a comprehensive medication list.
Can patient identify medications, dosages, and purpose of medication?	Even if the client has a good handle on his/her medication, it is recommended that he/she develop a wallet list of medications (and laminate it, if possible).	Develop a list of medications for the wallet (and laminate if possible). Review the medications list with the patient to make sure he/she understands.
Does the patient understand how to follow the directions of the prescribed medications?	Even if the client has a good handle on his/her medication, it is recommended that he/she develop a medication schedule. This can be posted at home (on the refrigerator).	Develop a medication schedule that can be posted at home. It is important to review the schedule with the client and have the client use it to fill his/her pill box. Emphasize to the patient and family the importance of keeping the medication schedule updated and double check to make sure the schedule matches the prescription guidelines on the bottles.
Can patient develop a schedule to follow to take all of his/her medications?	Use a medication schedule comprised of all medications from all doctors.	Use medication schedule comprised of all medications from all doctors. In addition, it may be helpful to consider using a pill box divided into different times of the day and days of the week.
Can patient organize his/her medications (ie, does he/she have a pill box, etc)?	This is usually the case if someone takes fewer than three medications. Nothing needs to be addressed.	Use some form of medication box or organizer. When determining which pill box is the best fit for your patient, it is important to remember the simplest option that meets all of your client's needs is usually the best option. If you cannot find the ideal pill box, adapt a similar one. When deciding on the right pill box, consider the following: • How often does patient take medications (once a day, twice a day, etc)? • How many pills does the patient take? • Does patient have PRN meds? If so, how often can he/she take them, and is there a maximum amount? • Will he/she need to take some of the medications when away from home?

(Table 9-1 *continues*)

Table 9-1 *continued*

Can patient follow a schedule and take medications on time?	Post a medication schedule as a back-up.	Help the patient develop a medication schedule and routine. It is helpful to anchor these routines to routines that are already in place in a client's daily schedule (such as eating meals). In addition, it is important to determine what types of cues would be effective for the client. Just as there are many types of pill boxes, there are also many different strategies and devices. When determining the best cuing system for your client, it is important to determine what systems your client already uses and what has been successful. For example, some clients like to use alarms on their cell phones, whereas other people use CATs or watch reminders. Again, try the simplest options first. Types of cuing systems may include: cell phone alarms, CAT alarms/schedules, day planner schedule checklists, and watch alarms. Your client should practice these strategies at home as well as in the clinic. Initially, the client may need additional cuing from family members. However, as the client develops a medication routine, less cuing may be needed.
Does patient know when and how to refill his/her medication?	Nothing needs to be addressed	Have the client fill the pill box at the same scheduled time every week (eg, Sunday evenings). At this time, have patient check to see if any refills are needed. When the client determines what medications need to be refilled, make a list with the name of the medication, prescription number, prescribing doctor, name of pharmacy, and telephone number of the pharmacy. Then, with the clinician or family member, the client can practice calling in a prescription or taking the prescription to the pharmacy to be refilled.

CAT: cognitive assistive technology
PRN: pro re nata (as needed)

CLINICIAN TIP SHEET: STRATEGIES TO IMPROVE MEDICATION MANAGEMENT—MEDICATION LIST

Start intervention by helping the patient compile a comprehensive list of medications (see Exhibit 9-4). It is important that patients know what medications they are taking for several reasons. Patients often see several doctors, all of whom may prescribe medications. It is help- ful for these doctors to know what medications a patient is taking to provide the best care. It is also important for patients to take ownership of their care, knowing what medications they take and why.

CLINICIAN TIP SHEET: STRATEGIES TO IMPROVE MEDICATION MANAGEMENT—MEDICATION SCHEDULE

Develop a medication schedule to help clients fill their pill organizers (see Exhibit 9-5). Divide the schedule into the different times the medications should be taken.

CLINICIAN TIP SHEET: STRATEGIES TO IMPROVE
MEDICATION MANAGEMENT—EMERGENCY CARD

An emergency card is another helpful resource to develop for your client (Figure 9-1; a free card template is available at: www.medids.com/free-id.php).

Emergency Medical Card *(see also reverse)*

Name: _____ DOB: __/__/____

Address: _____

_____

Phone: _____ Blood Type: _____

Primary Care Physician

name: _____ phone: _____

Emergency Contact

name: _____ phone: _____

Medical Conditions:

Medications:

Allergies:

Figure 9-1. Emergency wallet medical card.

CLINICIAN TIP SHEET: STRATEGIES TO IMPROVE
MEDICATION MANAGEMENT—DAILY CHECKLIST

It is important to anchor medication times to a patient's current routines (ie, morning medications taken at breakfast, midday medications taken with lunch, evening medications taken at dinner). It is recommended that clients schedule times to refill their medications pillbox, preferably at the same time every week using a medication sheet. To help develop these medication routines, it may be important to develop checklists as reminders (Exhibit 9-6). These checklists should be posted in a visible area, such as the bathroom mirror.

CLINICIAN TIP SHEET: STRATEGIES TO IMPROVE
MEDICATION MANAGEMENT—MEMORY AIDS

Patients may be able to identify medications and organize them in a pill organizer, but if they cannot remember to take them as scheduled, the organization system is useless. Therefore, memory aids are important components to the success of medication management.

Occupational therapy intervention incorporates selecting a memory aid based on the patient's needs

---

EXHIBIT 9-6

SAMPLE CHECKLIST

Morning Checklist	Afternoon Checklist	Evening Checklist
1. Brush teeth	1.	1.
2. Take shower	2.	2.
3. Get dressed	3.	3.
4. Eat breakfast	4.	4.
5. Take meds	5.	5.
6. Get keys, wallet, planner	6.	6.

---

and abilities and training the patient to use it (see also Chapter 7, Cognitive Assessment and Intervention). Because there are a multitude of memory aids, from checklists to cell phones to watches, it is necessary to match the client's needs and abilities to the appropriate memory aids (eg, smart watch, cell phone, watch with alarms, checklist, day planner, spouse or loved one calling or reminding client to take medications during scheduled time). Try the simplest option that meets your client's needs first and progress from there. Many electronic devices and other aids can be explored through a simple Internet search.

Discuss or observe the following:

- What systems does the client already have in place and use? Does the client often use a cell phone for reminders? Does the client use a day planner?
- Does the client already have a structured schedule and home environment?
- What is the client's current cognitive level? Can he or she follow one-step, two-step, or multistep directions? Does the client get confused handling multiple applications? Can the client tolerate multiple alarms, or will that just be confusing? Can the client follow and understand the alarms if he or she cannot set them?
- Is the client able to solve basic functional problems?
- Does the client understand written, pictorial, and verbal directions?
- Does the client initiate participating in ADLs?
- Does the client prefer high technology or low technology?
- Does the client respond to external cues?

Does the client hear the alarm, not notice it, or just turn it off and forget what it is for?
- Did the client wear a watch before experiencing cognitive difficulties?
- How simple is the equipment to use? Which equipment functions are important and which would lead to greater confusion? Is one type or brand of watch better than another for the specific client? Therapists should test the equipment and be able to operate it before asking the patient to do so.
- Does the client have vision impairments? Can he or she read, including complex materials?
- Does the client need multiple alarms?
- Is cost a factor?

In addition to anchoring medication times to patients' current routines, it is also important to educate clients and their families on storing the pill organizer (as well as the pill boxes) in the same place; that way clients do not get confused or frustrated every time they fill their pill box.

Adequately train patients to operate the memory aids and provide opportunities to practice on a regular basis. Several high-tech memory aids may be complex to operate; however, with good instruction, repetition, and practice, it is possible for someone to learn to operate the equipment effectively. Provide simple, written out, step-by-step directions to set the device (these instructions can be given to all clients who use the same device), then have the client follow the directions step by step with you. You may need to use chaining techniques to help the patient learn this new information. **Remember,** memory devices may get lost or break, so patients with problems managing medication may need back-up from a spouse or another source.

CLINICIAN TIP SHEET: ORGANIZING THE MAIL

Purpose/Background

Establish a strategy with the patient on how to organize mail to stay on top of paying bills on time; provide simulated activity so the patient gains experience with the process (Table 9-2).

Directions

1. Talk with the patient to figure out what specific symptoms and factors contribute to problems with organizing the mail.
2. Review Patient Handout: Organizing the Mail, adapting recommended procedures for the individual patient's circumstances.
3. If the patient indicates a willingness to try this strategy at home, have him or her complete the simulated work task described below.
4. After providing instructions, ask the patient to complete the AAA worksheet before, during, and after task performance (see also Techniques to Promote Engagement and Learning in Chapter 7, Cognitive Assessment and Intervention).
5. Based on simulation performance, modify strategy recommendations as needed.

6. Assign homework to implement some or all aspects of the recommended strategy.

Task: Organizing the Mail

1. Provide the patient with the following: an "Incoming Mail" box filled with junk mail and important mail items; sticky notes.
2. Ask the patient to perform steps 2, 4, 5, and 6 as specified on the corresponding patient handout.
3. Observe performance as described below.

Performance Measures (Evaluate the Following)

1. Ability to prioritize and organize mail
2. Length of time to complete the task before becoming frustrated and fatigued
3. Effect of task modifications on performance
4. Extent to which patient can employ other strategies for managing personal and situational factors during task performance
5. Amount of assistance needed to complete task (eg, independent, requires supervision [specify why], needs cues [specify the nature and frequency of cues], or needs hands-on assistance [specify the nature of the assistance and amount])

TABLE 9-2

TASK ANALYSIS FOR THE SIMULATED WORK TASK: ORGANIZING MAIL

Skills Targeted	Task Analysis
Attention	Ability to complete task without interruptions due to distractions
Memory	Ability to follow instructions
Problem solving	Ability to plan and then modify the plan as needed
Organization/self-structuring	Appropriate and effective use of office supplies and materials

CLINICIAN TIP SHEET: ESTABLISHING A BUDGET

Purpose/Background

The purpose of this task is to establish a budget, allow clients to make appropriate payments on time, and become better organized (Table 9-3).

Directions

Develop a spreadsheet with the client to break down his or her budget (involve the client's spouse, if applicable) based on income, bills that need to be

TABLE 9-3

TASK ANALYSIS FOR SIMULATED WORK TASK: BUDGETING

Skills Targeted	Task Analysis
Attention	Ability to complete task without interruptions
Memory	Ability to follow recall information about income and other details provided
Problem solving	Ability to plan and then modify the plan as needed
Organization/self-structuring	Appropriate and effective ways to use budget sheet

paid, and other expenses. Structure the task according to the client's needs.

Task Description

1. Assist the patient in identifying monthly income and expenses. If the patient is unable to organize a budget, ask a family member for assistance (see Patient Handout: Budget Planning Worksheet).
2. Ask the patient to fill out the budget tracking worksheet (see Patient Handout: Budget Tracking Worksheet and completed example).
3. Observe performance as described below.

Performance Measures (Evaluate the Following)

1. Ability to identify income and expenses
2. Length of time to complete the task before becoming frustrated and fatigued
3. Effect of task modifications on performance
4. Extent to which the patient can employ other strategies for managing personal and situational factors during task performance
5. Amount of assistance needed to complete the task (eg, independent, requires supervision [specify why], needs cues [specify the nature and frequency of cues], or needs hands-on assistance [specify the nature of the assistance and amount])

CLINICIAN TIP SHEET: BILL-PAYING ACTIVITY

Purpose

The purpose of this task is to assess and improve the client's sustained attention during money management and promote correct task completion (Table 9-4).

Directions

1. Talk with the patient to figure out the specific symptoms or other factors that contribute to problems with bill paying.
2. Review Patient Handout: Bill Paying, adapting recommended procedures for the individual patient's circumstances.
3. If the patient indicates a willingness to try this strategy at home, have him or her complete the simulated work task (described below).
4. After providing instructions, ask the patient to complete the AAA Worksheet before, during, and after task performance (see also "Techniques to Promote Engage-

ment and Learning" in Chapter 7, Cognitive Assessment and Intervention).
5. Based on simulation performance, modify strategy recommendations as needed.
6. Assign homework to implement some or all aspects of the recommended strategy.

Task Description

1. Provide the money management packet to the client and ask him or her to complete the task by reading the instructions (see procedure on patient handout). Explain to the client that you are trying to assess his or her ability to follow instructions and complete a basic money management task.

Performance Measure (Evaluate the Following)

1. Ability to write a check properly
2. Ability to calculate the account
3. Ability to use prompts or cues from the therapist to adjust task performance

TABLE 9-4

SIMULATED WORK TASK: BILL PAYING

Skills Targeted	Task Analysis
Attention	Ability to complete task without interruptions due to distractions
	Ability to write a check and balance the account by alternating attention between the two tasks
Working memory	Ability to do math without using a calculator
Problem solving	Ability to identify errors with task, fix the problem when it arises

4. Ability to manage personal and situational factors during task performance
5. Amount of assistance needed to complete the task (eg, independent, requires supervision [specify why], needs cues [specify the nature and frequency of cues], or needs hands-on assistance [specify the nature of the assistance and amount])

CLINICIAN TIP SHEET: USING A SMARTPHONE OR PLANNER TO HELP MANAGE MONEY

Purpose

The purpose of this task is to improve the efficiency and accuracy of the client's ability to perform financial management tasks by using memory back-ups (Table 9-5).

Directions

Talk with the client about his or her ability to recall and retain information during complex everyday tasks associated with money management. Talk about devices that can help the client complete tasks without relying on others for help (eg, a daily organizer or cognitive assistive technology [CAT]).

Task Description

Provide the patient with a CAT or memory aid tool, such as a daily organizer with a calendar, and identify strategies for inputting prompts into the tools or devices; have the patient demonstrate back the proper techniques.

Performance Measure (Evaluate the Following)

1. Ability to attend to the task
2. Ability to follow two- to four-step instructions
3. Ability to use prompts or cues from therapist to adjust task performance
4. Ability to manage personal and situational factors during task performance
5. Amount of assistance needed to complete the task (eg, independent, requires supervision [specify why], needs cues [specify the nature and frequency of cues] or needs hands-on assistance [specify the nature of the assistance and amount])

TABLE 9-5

TASK ANALYSIS REGARDING MEMORY AID TO MANAGE MONEY

Skills Targeted	Task Analysis
Sustained and alternating attention	Ability to complete task without interruptions due to distractions
	Ability to put information into a CAT and go between two different programs to complete task
Memory	Ability to remember the steps to use a CAT appropriately

CAT: cognitive assistive technology

SECTION 2: SOCIAL ROLES

REENGAGING WITH SPOUSES, CHILDREN, AND FRIENDS

Activity engagement associated with the roles of friend, spouse, and parent changes as service members go on lengthy and often serial deployments. Once commonplace, everyday interactions turn into long-distance communications through letters, telephone and video calls, and emails. Role strains are common throughout and following deployment. The challenges of reintegration with family and friends may be exacerbated by symptoms related to c/mTBI and the associated psychosocial strain.[27] Awareness and insight into specific interpersonal stressors, role shifts, and the needs of others may provide a foundation for healthy reengagement with family and friends. Stressors with family and friends may influence overall perceptions of well-being and affect performance in areas such as work, school, and social settings. Occupational therapists explore service members' social and family roles to help them successfully reenter their home communities.

While this section of the toolkit summarizes occupational therapy evaluation tools and methods that may enable the therapist to better understand patients' challenges with role resumption and social interaction, it is important for occupational therapists to be mindful of their scope of practice and confine services to their areas of expertise associated with activities, occupations, and roles. Evaluations by and referrals to other professionals, such as social workers, psychologists, chaplains, and counselors may also be needed. All professionals involved in helping a service member reestablish family and social roles should be committed to team communication and to reinforcing interdisciplinary strategies that advance carry-over and minimize frustration and confusion for all involved.

Recommended Instrument Use

The following assessments may be used in service members who have returned home with c/mTBI and present challenges of reengagement with spouses, children, or friends (Table 9-6). These may have been identified by the service members themselves or by another interested party.

Note: The COPM is described in the self-management section of the toolkit. The COPM may be used to assess childcare concerns and to inform the intervention plan. However, even if service members with children do not identify parenting issues among their top five priorities, the occupational therapist should explore this area of functioning with the patient.

TABLE 9-6

EVALUATION OPTIONS BASED ON KEY SOCIAL RELATIONSHIPS

Evaluation	Spouse	Children	Friends
Canadian Occupational Performance Measure[1]	X	X	X
Assessment of Communication and Interaction Skills[2]	X	X	X
Activity Co-engagement Self-assessment[3]	X	X	X
The Dyadic Adjustment[4]	X		

1) Law M, Baptise S, McColl MA, Carswell A, Polatajko H, Pollock N. *Canadian Occupational Performance Measure.* 2nd ed. Toronto, ON: Canadian Association of Occupational Therapists–Association Canadienne d'Éducation Publications; 1994. 2) Kielhofner G. *A Model of Human Occupation: Theory and Application.* 3rd ed. Philadelphia, PA: Lippincott Williams & Wilkins; 2002. 3) Davidson LF. *Activity Co-engagement Self-assessment.* Winchester, VA: Shenandoah University; 2009. 4) Spanier GB. Measuring dyadic adjustment: new scales for assessing the equality of marriage and similar dyads. *J Marriage Fam.* 1976;38:15–28.

ASSESSMENT OF COMMUNICATION AND INTERACTION SKILLS

The Assessment of Communication and Interaction Skills (ACIS)[28] is a structured observation rating scale that explores the interaction of an individual during occupational engagement or in a group setting (Exhibit 9-7). This tool addresses the domains of physicality, information exchange, and relations; observations of competencies and deficiencies inform treatment planning (Exhibit 9-8).

EXHIBIT 9-7

ASSESSMENT OF COMMUNICATION AND INTERACTION SKILLS

The Assessment of Communication and Interaction Skills is available from:

Model of Human Occupation Clearinghouse
Department of Occupational Therapy
University of Illinois at Chicago
1919 West Taylor Street
Chicago, IL 60612
www.moho.uic.edu

Recommended Instrument Use: Practice Option

This test may be a helpful inclusion in an occupational therapy evaluation when the patient or others indicate that communication and social functioning interfere with task performance.

This assessment must be conducted in an environment and with a task that has been specifically chosen for and by the client and concerned loved one (spouse, child, etc). The task must have structured and unstructured elements, a moderate to high risk of unpredictability or challenges, and require the dyad to engage in activities both in a parallel (eg, both cutting their own vegetables) and cooperative format (they are serving dinner from one central dish and must negotiate how to share resources). Spouse-patient activities could include cooking and eating dinner, paying bills and reviewing finances, playing with the children, or planning a trip. Parent-child activities might include structured play (eg, a board game), unstructured play (eg, playing make believe), storytelling, or assisting with homework.

Administration Protocol/Equipment/Time

Clinicians should refer to the administration manual for detailed instructions specific to administration and scoring. It takes 20 to 60 minutes to administer the ACIS, depending on the task. The manual, score sheet, and a pencil are all the equipment that is required.

As the patient engages in an individual or group activity, the therapist observes three aspects of so-cial functioning (physicality, information exchange, and relations). Skills related to each domain (20 verbs) are rated using a four-point scale (competent, questionable, ineffective, deficit). In the case of a dyad activity, the therapist may rate the performance of both individuals simultaneously.

Groups Tested With This Measure

The test was developed for adults with psychiatric illness, but version 4.0 can be used to assess communication and interaction issues associated with any condition or illness.[29]

Interpretability

Norms

No norms are reported.

Scoring

As the patient engages in an individual or group activity, the therapist observes three aspects of social functioning: 1) physicality, 2) information exchange, and 3) relations. Skills related to each domain (20 verbs) are rated using a four-point scale (competent, questionable, ineffective, or deficit).

Mean Detectable Change

No information reported.

Reliability Estimates

Internal Consistency/Interrater and Intrarater Reliability

Rasch analysis was used to evaluate internal consistency and rater reliability. Authors described good internal consistency and evidence of intrarater and interrater reliability.[28]

Validity Estimate

Construct

Using Rasch analysis, the ACIS discriminated between varying levels of communication and interaction skill as reported by Asher.[29]

ACTIVITY CO-ENGAGEMENT SELF-ASSESSMENT

The Activity Co-Engagement Self-Assessment (ACeS) is designed to help the occupational therapist better understand the patient's engagement in activities with loved ones, including types of activities performed together, potential barriers to activity engagement, and perceived self characteristics

357

EXHIBIT 9-8

ACIS SUMMARY SHEET

Client:				Examiner:		
Observation situation:						
Age:	Sex:		Diagnosis:			
Adaptations:			Inpatient:		Outpatient:	
Ethnicity:	White		Black	Hispanic	Asian	Native American

Competent (4): Competent performance that supports communication/interaction and yields good interpersonal/group outcomes. Examiner observes no evidence of a deficit.

Questionable (3): Questionable performance that places at risk communication/interaction and yields uncertain/interpersonal group outcomes. Examiner questions the presence of a deficit.

Ineffective (2): Ineffective performance that interferes with communication/interaction and yields undesirable interpersonal/group outcomes. Examiner observes a mild to moderate deficit.

Deficit (1): Deficit performance that impedes communication/interaction and yields unacceptable group outcomes. Examiner observes a severe deficit (risk of damage, danger, provocation, or breakdown of interpersonal group relations).

Physicality					Comments:
Contacts	4	3	2	1	
Gazes	4	3	2	1	
Gestures	4	3	2	1	
Maneuvers	4	3	2	1	
Orients	4	3	2	1	
Postures	4	3	2	1	
Information Exchange					Comments:
Articulates	4	3	2	1	
Asserts	4	3	2	1	
Asks	4	3	2	1	
Engages	4	3	2	1	
Expresses	4	3	2	1	
Modulates	4	3	2	1	
Stares	4	3	2	1	
Speaks	4	3	2	1	
Relations					Comments:
Collaborates	4	3	2	1	
Conforms	4	3	2	1	
Focuses	4	3	2	1	
Relates	4	3	2	1	
Respects	4	3	2	1	
Comments:					

as they relate to engaging in activities with others (Form 9-2). In addition, the patient is asked to identify areas of strength and areas for improvement. This tool can be used for self-evaluation and reflection (when used in conjunction with a video observation and analysis). Goal setting and strategy implementation may also be incorporated after ACeS administration.[27]

Recommended Instrument Use: Practice Option

The ACeS may be used when concerns about communication or interaction between the patient and his or her children, spouse (or significant other), siblings, or close friends have been identified. If patients have not had opportunities to engage in activities with their loved ones, this assessment will not be useful. The therapist may administer all sections or individual sections, based on the patient's circumstances. Findings from the assessment and self-reflections may be used for goal writing, family activity treatment sessions, and to help guide education and strategy adoption. **Note**: The patient identifies a particular loved one (eg, daughter, son, or spouse) and fills out the questionnaire with that *single individual* in mind.

Groups Tested with this Measure

These methods have not been formally tested on any groups.

Interpretability

Supplemented by findings from standardized assessments, the results from the ACeS will provide the occupational therapist with information that can be used throughout the occupational therapy process. For the purpose of goal setting, the ACeS will provide a subjective comparison of preinjury/postinjury coactivity engagement, self-perceived relationship traits, and patient priorities regarding traits and resumption of activities with loved ones. This information allows for a client-centered focus when developing treatment goals and interventions. In addition, subjectively reporting participation barriers may provide the therapist with insights into deficits not identified through standardized measures or observation. Patient responses can be used as a source for making treatment decisions, including environmental modification recommendations and strategy adoption. Additionally, the relationship trait questionnaire can be used for goal setting, self-reflection through video self-observation, and self-monitoring across the continuum of treatment.

Norms

There are no established norms for this self-report tool.

Mean Detectable Change

MDC is not established.

Responsiveness, Reliability, and Validity Estimates

Responsiveness, reliability, and validity estimates are not established.

DYADIC ADJUSTMENT SCALE

The Dyadic Adjustment Scale (DAS)[30] is a 32-question self-report questionnaire exploring adjustments in partner relationships. The DAS measures four areas associated with marital or relationship adjustment: (1) consensus on issues important to marital functioning, (2) dyadic satisfaction, (3) dyadic cohesion, and (4) expression of affection.

Partners are asked to rate the extent of agreement or disagreement in fifteen areas (eg, religion, leisure interests and activities, family finances, household tasks). Respondents are asked to indicate how often they engage in behaviors relating to marriage (eg, confiding in mate, quarreling with mate), how often they engage in activities together and how they feel about where the relationship is going.

Recommended Instrument Use: Practice Option

The DAS can be used with any couple, married or unmarried.[30] For the purpose of service members with c/mTBI, it may be used when resumption of spousal roles and associated activities has been identified as a concern. This evaluation should be done in conjunction with other assessment tools designed to gain an understanding of activity engagement, self-perception of parenting, and goals.

Administration Protocol/Equipment/Time

The DAS is given to married or partnered couples and can be administered as a paper-and-pencil task or in the course of an interview. Although the

FORM 9-2

ACTIVITY CO-ENGAGEMENT SELF-ASSESSMENT

Background

Spending time engaged in enjoyable activities with loved ones is one way of reestablishing relationships as you return home. The following questions have been designed to help your occupational therapist understand more about the activities you do with your loved ones (children, spouse, significant other [SO], etc) as well as the challenges you may face when spending time together. Please make an effort to answer questions as honestly as you are able. This information will help us set goals and plan treatment for your occupational therapy.

I am answering the questions that follow based on spending time and sharing activities with my (select **one**):

____ child/children

____ spouse or significant other

____ close friend(s) or sibling(s)

____ other (specify):

Here is more information about my loved ones (as identified above).

Child/children	Spouse/SO	Friend(s) or siblings(s)	Other
Name(s):	Name:	Name:	Name:
Age(s):	Age:	Age:	
	# of years together:	Nature of relationship:	Nature of relationship:

PART I: SPENDING TIME TOGETHER

This assessment describes my relationship with my (choose one):____ child/children ____ spouse ____ friend

1) List the activities you and your loved one(s) <u>routinely</u> did together prior to your last deployment and injury and how often you did them (ie, going to the movies twice a month; going to the park every Saturday).
2) List the activities you and your loved one are currently doing together.
3) List the activities you would like to engage in with your loved one on a routine or more frequent basis.
4) What activities have you and your loved done together within the past week?
5) Which of the following issues are barriers that make it difficult for you to enjoy activities with your loved one? **Circle the response that best applies to you.**

	Yes	No	Sometimes
I have pain during activities.	Y	N	S
I have headaches during activities.	Y	N	S
I get dizzy during activities.	Y	N	S
I get angry during activities.	Y	N	S
I can't tolerate bright lights.	Y	N	S
I experience feelings of nausea.	Y	N	S
I become frustrated.	Y	N	S
I don't like to be touched.	Y	N	S

(**Form 9-2** *continues*)

Form 9-2 *continued*

I can't pay attention to the game or activity.	Y	N	S
I feel like a bad person.	Y	N	S
I don't have enough time.	Y	N	S
No one listens to me.	Y	N	S
I get tired during activities.	Y	N	S
I have no transportation.	Y	N	S
The noise level bothers me.	Y	N	S
I don't know what to do with my loved one(s).	Y	N	S
I don't share the same interests with my loved one(s).	Y	N	S

PART II: HOW I CURRENTLY SEE MYSELF

Circle the appropriate response to how you see yourself as a (**circle one**) parent/spouse/friend.

My loved one would describe me as:	**Never**	**Occasionally**	**Usually**
Kind	N	O	U
Strict	N	O	U
Patient	N	O	U
Lazy	N	O	U
Selfish	N	O	U
Loving	N	O	U
Fair	N	O	U
Mean	N	O	U
Supportive	N	O	U
Unreliable	N	O	U
Caring	N	O	U
Encouraging	N	O	U
Nervous	N	O	U
Absent	N	O	U
Moody	N	O	U
Easygoing	N	O	U
Tolerant	N	O	U
Generous	N	O	U
Funny	N	O	U
Flexible	N	O	U
Forgiving	N	O	U
Committed	N	O	U
Respectful	N	O	U
Trustworthy	N	O	U
Bossy	N	O	U
Cooperative	N	O	U

(**Form 9-2** *continues*)

Form 9-2 *continued*

1) The things I do best as a parent/spouse/friend are:

2) The things I would like to be better at as a parent/spouse/friend are:

---

amount of time it takes to complete the assessment is not indicated, the author suggests that it takes only a few minutes. The evaluation may be given to both partners independently or individual partners at any given time.[30]

Groups Tested With This Measure

The scale has been used to evaluate partner adjustment across the demographic continuum since its development in 1976. It has not been used with couples where one has sustained TBI.

Interpretability

Scoring

Responses to the 32 items each carry a number value that can be summed to determine subscale scores and a total score. The scale ranges from 0 to 151.[30] Occupational therapists will likely gain more insight regarding patient-spouse relationships by reviewing subscale scores and patients' responses to individual items rather than trying to interpret a total score.

Mean Detectable Change

MDC is not available.

Responsiveness Estimates

Responsiveness estimates are not available.

Reliability Estimates

Internal consistency. Internal consistency reliability was determined for the DAS as well as the component subscales. This included 0.96 for the DAS; 0.90 for the dyadic consensus subscale; 0.94 for the dyadic satisfaction subscale; 0.86 for the dyadic cohesion subscale; and 0.73 for the affectional expression subscale.[30]

Validity Estimates

Content validity. The 32 items were selected from an initial pool of approximately 300 items based on consensus among three judges that the item was indicative of marital adjustment.[30]

Criterion validity. The scale was administered to 218 married people and a sample of 94 individuals who were divorced. Each of the 32 items in the scale correlated significantly with the external criterion of marital status.[30]

Construct validity. The DAS is significantly correlated with other published marital adjustment scales (0.86 among married respondents; 0.88 among divorced respondents).[30]

INTERVENTION: REENGAGING WITH SPOUSES, CHILDREN, FRIENDS

Professionals involved in helping service members reestablish family and social roles should be committed to team communication and reinforcing interdisciplinary strategies that advance carry-over and minimize frustration and confusion for all involved.

The following evaluation and interventions strategies are based on the behavioral/cognitive-behavioral conceptual frame of reference. This frame of reference is based on the premise that cognitive processes are responsible for behaviors. In addition, adaptive responses are behavior based; feedback from adaptive responses change our cognitive processes as well as our behavior (Figure 9-2). For example, say your patient is a mechanic and has recently had a difficult time attending to his work tasks at the end of the day. This is typically when he cleans up his workstation, puts all of his tools away, and completes his paperwork for all the activities done throughout his shift. His problems with attention at the end of the shift have led to numerous errors in paperwork and organization of his workspace. His poor attention (cognitive processes) has led to behavior issues (poor organization and errors), which have led to "maladaptive responses," including increased anxiety in the workplace, avoiding work activities, and general performance issues.

To turn this around, the therapist can provide assistance in structuring paperwork and returning tools and items to their storage places throughout the day. That way, his final tasks of the day (sweeping, general cleaning) require less attention and are better matches for his abilities at that time of day. Changing the structure and organization of the workday (cognitive processes) leads to better performance, which leads to habit formation, increased performance, and reinforcement of the new way of doing things.

If therapists suggest strategies that provide pa-

tients with adaptive responses, they must provide therapy, reinforcement, and feedback that shapes behavior.[31] In addition to the environment and context, it is assumed a number of inherent capacities will influence the feedback loop. These may include attention, memory, orientation, processing skills, perception, and interpretation. According to the behavioral/cognitive-behavioral conceptual model of practice, a therapist can affect change in three ways:

1. by working with the client to adopt adaptive behaviors in the context of relationships and abandon maladaptive ones,
2. by facilitating adaptive skill development, and
3. by working to change unsubstantiated perceptions of performance that may impair productive activity role resumption.

The strategies and interventions suggested for reengagement with friends, spouses, and children are based on these principles.

Recommended Use

The following may be used with service members who have returned home with c/mTBI and present challenges of reengagement with spouses, children, or friends. These challenges may have been identified by the service members themselves or by another interested party. Family members or friends must be available and committed to implement the following recommendations.

Strength of Recommendation: Practice Option

There is little empirical evidence to guide practice in this area; however, intervention is consistent with standard occupational therapy practices and reported as valuable by occupational therapists working with individuals with c/mTBI.

Intervention Methods

Reengaging as a Parent

Therapists will choose appropriate interventions based on their experience and knowledge of an individual patient's needs. It is strongly recommended the therapist work with the patient and child during sessions to provide feedback and modeling.

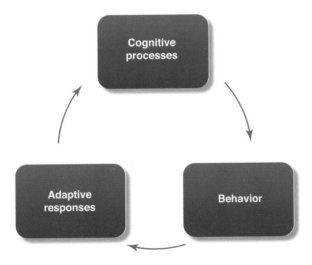

Figure 9-2. Behavioral/cognitive behavioral conceptual frame of reference.

1. Provide education regarding parenting skills (see Patient Handout: Understanding Your Child's World—Toddler).

2. Help the patient understand and assess the demands of various child play activities and cognitive demands (see Patient Handout and Clinician Tip Sheet: Understanding the Structure of Play and Parent-Child Activities, and Patient Handout: Understanding the Environment of Play and the Role of Cooperation in Child-Related Activities).

3. Help the patient identify and use multiple resources for post-deployment family support (see Clinician Tip Sheet: Utilizing Resources for Family Reengagement).

4. Help the patient understand how and why c/mTBI may impact parenting (see Chapter 7, Cognitive Assessment and Impairment, "Multifactor Model Explaining Performance Declines after mTBI" and "Understanding Human Information Processing").

Reengaging With a Spouse

1. Provide education regarding common issues for spouses after deployment (see Patient Handout: Reconnecting with Your Spouse or Significant Other).

2. Help the patient understand and assess the demands of various roles his or her spouse has adopted during deployment and assist in role reengagement (see Patient Handout and Clinician Tip Sheet: Reengaging in Household Roles and Activities, and Patient Handout: Dividing Roles With Your Spouse).

3. Help the patient understand how and why c/mTBI may impact his or her relationship with his or her spouse (see Chapter 7, Cognitive Assessment and Impairment, "Multifactor Model Explaining Performance Declines After mTBI" and "Understanding Human Information Processing").

CLINICIAN TIP SHEET: UNDERSTANDING THE STRUCTURE OF PLAY, ROLES OF ENVIRONMENT, AND COOPERATION IN PARENT-CHILD ACTIVITIES

Background

Service members who return from lengthy and serial deployments will often find that returning to family roles presents a challenge. Symptoms associated with c/mTBI may only exacerbate these challenges. Potential issues associated with parenting should be discussed before patients return home or after they have returned and issues have been identified.

The role of the occupational therapist is to gain an understanding of the patient's parental role performance anxieties and concerns, and provide education and strategies to facilitate role resumption. To do this effectively, the therapist must be aware of the cognitive and social-emotional issues that may place barriers between the patient and effective role performance, as well as with task elements, such as levels of structure and the cooperative continuum in parent-child play. It is also important that the therapist have a grasp on child developmental play so as to suggest and present appropriate activities.

Therapy Approaches to Improving Resumption of Parent Roles

1. Goals associated with parent-child interaction should be developed in collaboration with the patient (and spouse if appropriate).

2. Evaluation tools, such as the COPM and ACeS, and observation should be used to discuss strengths and areas of concern.

3. If possible, evaluation and interventions should include a large observation component; the therapy clinic should have a number of developmentally appropriate toys as well as a "safe and private" play space.

4. When choosing play activities for the clinic, use those that span the continuum of structure to provide opportunities to rehearse and adopt strategies and skills.

5. Provide education about play and structure (Table 9-7).

6. Parent-child clinic work should be planned in advance, with the patient generating activity ideas. Facilitate identification of activities that are unstructured, semistructured, and structured, and plan on at least one activity in each area.

7. Have the patient predict his or her performance. Use predications based on previously generated goals.

8. The parent-child session will include a brief overview of the session and, if appropriate,

TABLE 9-7

GUIDE FOR PROVISION OF STRUCTURE

Level of Structure	Examples of Activities	Cognitive Demands Associated With Level of Structure
Structured (typically this level of structure is not tolerated by infants and toddlers. At the age of 5, children begin to successfully engage in more structured play)	Model building, some cooking activities (eg, baking, construction tasks, board games, video game, many sports)	Organization and planning, sequencing, error detection and correction, attention to detail, memory, time management, ability to shift focus, ability to understand and follow rules and directions
Semi-structured (toddlers to adult-aged kids)	Puzzles, arts and crafts, pretend play, some sports, some video games	Task initiation, organization and planning, error detection and correction, flexibility, time management, attention
Unstructured (all ages)	Some arts and crafts, such as free drawing and play dough, sand play, water play, dancing	Task initiation, creative thinking, planning and organization, flexibility, time management

the child's predication of how the session may go based on the activities chosen.

9. The therapist will provide added or decreased structure, grade task materials for increased or decreased collaboration, and cue for strategy implementation.

10. A reflection will be done immediately after the session. If the activity was videotaped, the therapist and the patient should review the tape.

11. If indicated, the therapist will provide modeling behaviors for parent-child interaction.

12. Help the patient identify how much structure is needed in play activities to op-

timally interact with his or her children at home (see Table 9-7). Therapists can have some control over the level of structure by changing game rules, adding directions, or modifying activity-based play goals.

13. Help the patient determine what types of cognitive strategies might improve his or her ability to satisfactorily engage with his or her children during play. Provide opportunities (via homework or in-clinic activities with children) for the patient to practice these strategies.

14. The patient will keep a parent-child activity log to review with the therapist in person or by email.

CLINICIAN TIP SHEET: REENGAGING IN HOUSEHOLD ROLES AND ACTIVITIES

Background

Role conflict is a source of marital stress following deployment even in healthy service members[32]; the addition of potential inefficiencies associated with c/mTBI can increase the conflict surrounding role reengagement and negotiation. Role participation, performance, and satisfaction can be evaluated through interview, the COPM, and the ACeS (spouse version). In addition, the associated patient handout can be used as an evaluative and therapeutic tool in the clinic.

Therapists may also help patients resume home roles and responsibilities in the following ways.

- Help partners realistically prioritize. When working with patients and their partners on role negotiation, it is important to evaluate the skills necessary to perform identified roles and the context in which they are going to be done. For example, if a patient wants to resume the role of money management (banking, bill paying, and budgeting), the therapist must explore the subtasks the patient must do successfully to fully complete those tasks. In addition, performance evaluation must be consistent with the context. Are money management activities done online only, offline only, or a combination of the two? Using the strategies introduced in Chapter 7 (Cognitive Assessment and Intervention) can help when dividing role tasks and activities needed to fully participate in areas that are a priority.

- Work with both partners during treatment sessions. Address role resumption in a partnership between the patient and the spouse. Provide strategies and skills to facilitate negotiation and successful collaboration.
- Include information about cognitive task demands. Incorporate an education dimension to therapy; provide information about cognitive task demands as related to role activities and assist in determining appropriate levels of performance.
- Engage in real-life activities as they relate to roles. Create budgets based on the couple's income and expenses, make sandwiches, do laundry, plan vacations. Observe communication styles and points of conflict during these tasks and provide feedback and suggestions to improve performance.
- Become a partner in scheduling role activities (see calendar example located in associated patient handout). This can be done face to face or through email. The journal entries completed individually by the patient and spouse will help you better understand barriers to optimal performance.
- Reflect with the couple. Consider videotaping observations of co-occupational engagement. You may want to employ the ASIS to structure activity negotiation and engagement. The ASIS can also be used by the couple to evaluate performance during video reflections.

Remember, as a rehabilitation specialist, your job is to work with the couple to help them successfully divide and conquer.

Selected References

Defense Centers of Excellence for Psychological Health and Traumatic Brain Injury. *Reintegrating Into Family Life After Deployment.* http://www.realwarriors.net/active/afterdeployment/familylife.php. Accessed September 12, 2013.

Minnesota National Guard. Beyond The Yellow Ribbon: Bringing Soldiers and Their Families All The Way Home. http://www.minnesotanationalguard.org/btyr/. Accessed September 12, 2013.

SECTION 3: RETURN TO SCHOOL

RETURNING TO SCHOOL

Service members who have sustained c/mTBI are typically younger adults acquiring vocational skills or training to qualify for promotion, or veterans returning to school to pursue new careers. Persisting cognitive and psychosocial difficulties present as significant barriers to successful classroom participation and learning.[33,34] Students with a history of TBI report studying longer and with more effort, and require greater use of study strategies than they did prior to sustaining their injuries.[35] Moreover, they have greater difficulties with memory, executive functions, socialization, and academic skills than students without TBI.[36,37] While the majority of research investigating return to school has focused on students with moderate to severe TBI, subtle challenges in physical, cognitive, behavioral, and social areas have been reported by students with c/mTBI. Cognitive symptoms (eg, memory, attention) and psychosocial problems (eg, aggression, depression, reduced frustration tolerance) impact their transition to college.[38]

Because psychosocial factors appear to impact academic performance for students with c/mTBI,[36] the clinician should consider comorbidities that may be associated with postdeployment, such as hypervigilance, irritability, low frustration tolerance, depressed mood, fatigue, sleep dysfunction, headache, dizziness, balance, vision and hearing problems, and pain (see Clinician Tip Sheet: Postdeployment Factors and Academic Performance). Facilitating return to school involves assessing skills specific to academic performance (see Clinician Tip Sheet: Needs Assessment–Return to School), and teaching compensatory strategies (see clinician tip sheets and patient handouts in this section, and in Chapter 7, Cognitive Assessment and Intervention). The initial assessment identifies the service member's current academic status or plan, performance level, and goals to guide the intervention plan. In addition to instruction on strategies to enhance academic performance, service members may benefit from guidance applying for admission, facilitating success by matching their performance level with academic program demands, and advocating for accommodation services (see Clinician Tip Sheet: College Accommodations for Students With Cognitive Disabilities).

Strength of Recommendation: Practice Option

Although empirical guidelines for return to school after TBI do not exist, the literature indicates that cognitive and psychosocial challenges associated with TBI are strongly correlated with the difficulties people experience as they return to school. There are numerous practice guidelines for treating cognitive and psychosocial sequelae of TBI.[36,39–43] This knowledge can be used to develop rehabilitation models that go beyond standard academic accommodations and provide effective cognitive and behavioral strategies that support successful return to school after c/TBI.

Intervention Methods

1. Complete a needs assessment (see Clinician Tip Sheet: Return to School Needs Assessment, and Patient Handout: Return to School Needs Assessment/Essential Skills for College Success).
2. Provide patient education (see Clinician Tip Sheet: Postdeployment Factors and Academic Performance and Clinician Tip Sheet: College Accommodations for Students With Cognitive Disabilities).
3. Teach strategies to improve reading comprehension (see Patient Handout: Study Reading Systems and Clinician Tip Sheet: Reading Strategies).
4. Teach strategies to improve note taking (see Clinician Tip Sheet and Patient Handout: Note-Taking Strategies).
5. Teach test-taking strategies (see Clinician Tip Sheet and Patient Handout: Test-Taking Strategies).

Selected References

Cicerone KD, Langenbahn DM, Braden C, et al. Evidence-based cognitive rehabilitation: updated review of the literature from 2003 through 2008. *Arch Phys Med Rehabil.* Apr 2011;92(4):519–530.

Cook J. Higher education: an attainable goal for students who have sustained head injuries. *J Head Trauma Rehabil.* 1991;6:64–72.

Ip RY, Dornan J, Schentag C. Traumatic brain injury: factors predicting return to work or school. *Brain Inj.* Jul 1995;9(5):517–532.

Kennedy MRT, Coelho C, Turkstra LS, Ylvisaker M, Sohlberg MM, Yorkston K, Chiou HH, Kan PF. Intervention for executive functions after traumatic brain injury: a systematic review, meta-analysis and clinical recommendations. *Neuropsychol Rehabil.* 2008;18:257–299.

Kennedy MRT, Krause MO. Academic experiences of adults with and without traumatic brain injury using the College Survey for Students with Brain Injury (CSS-BI). *Eighth World Conference on Brain Injury.* Washington, DC, March 13, 2010.

Kennedy MR, Krause MO, Turkstra LS. An electronic survey about college experiences after traumatic brain injury. *Neurol Rehabil.* 2008;23(6):511–520.

Laforce R Jr, Martin-MacLeod L. Symptom cluster associated with mild traumatic brain injury in university students. *Percept Mot Skills.* Aug 2001;93(1):281–288.

Sohlberg MM, Avery J, Kennedy M, et al. Practice guidelines for direct attention training. *J Med Speech-Lang Path.* 2003;11(3):xix–xxxix.

Sohlberg MM, Kennedy MRT, Avery J, et al. Evidenced-based practice for the use of external memory aids as a memory compensation technique. *J Med Speech-Lang Path.* 2007;15(xv–li).

Sohlberg MM, Turkstra LS. *Optimizing Cognitive Rehabilitation: Effective Instructional Methods.* New York, NY: Guilford Press; 2011.

Stewart-Scott AM, Douglas JM. Educational outcome for secondary and postsecondary students following traumatic brain injury. *Brain Inj.* 1998;12:317–331.

Ylvisaker M, Turkstra L, Coehlo C, et al. Behavioural interventions for children and adults with behaviour disorders after TBI: a systematic review of the evidence. *Brain Inj.* Jul 2007;21(8):769–805.

CLINICIAN TIP SHEET: RETURN-TO-SCHOOL NEEDS ASSESSMENT

Background

Assessing changes in cognitive function and self-awareness and identifying strengths and weaknesses and barriers to learning is critical when designing an intervention plan to facilitate a service member's return to school. The Essential Skills for College Success[44] survey helps identify potential challenges in returning to school that can be used in conjunction with other assessment tools to evaluate cognitive deficits. It is a self-assessment scale for students who have been deployed to rate their level of difficulty in academic skills and predict their success in college. Survey areas include listening, note taking, reading, remembering, organizing, writing papers, working in groups, and making presentations. Periodic reassessment using this tool provides a way to quantify outcome measures (see Patient Handout: Return to School Needs Assessment/Essential Skills for College Success Handout).

Ongoing assessment of the service member's school performance enables interdisciplinary team members (eg, vocational rehabilitation counselors, mental health providers, social workers) to identify and address needs, as they arise, to facilitate school success. Assessment results also provide support for the clinician to advocate for appropriate adaptations, modifications, and accommodations for the service members (see College Accommodations for Students With Cognitive Disabilities; also see Clinician Tip Sheet: Electronic Memory and Organization Aids–Smartphone and Mobile Applications in Chapter 7, Cognition Assessment and Intervention).

Selected Reference

Zarzecki MA, Crawford E, Smith Hammond C. Essential Skills for College Success, VHA Evolving Paradigms II. *Polytrauma Conference.* Las Vegas, NV; September 22, 2009.

CLINICIAN TIP SHEET: POSTDEPLOYMENT SYMPTOMS THAT CAN INFLUENCE ACADEMIC PERFORMANCE

Background

The return-to-school transition for service members with c/mTBI can be complicated by psychosocial comorbidities.[36] Postdeployment symptoms may include hypervigilance,[45] irritability and low frustration tolerance, anxiety, sleep dysfunction and fatigue, physical symptoms (eg, pain, headache, dizziness, balance, and vision and hearing problems), medication side effects, depressed mood, memory deficits, and attention and concentration difficulties.[46]

Clinicians should consider the influence of these deployment-related symptoms on the student's ability to attend to and comprehend lectures, take notes, recall information, write papers, comprehend and retain reading material, and study for and take tests. The following postdeployment symptoms and suggestions are intended to help clinicians understand the potential influence of symptoms and provide strategies to decrease their impact on academic performance.

- **Hypervigilance** is a symptom associated with the constant need to monitor the environment for potential danger.[45] In the school setting, this may divide the student's attention and interfere with the ability to process information presented in the classroom and while studying or taking tests. Service members often manage hypervigilance by acclimating to the campus environment and classroom prior to the start of the classes, and by sitting in a location within a classroom that allows them to monitor all individuals in the room, with their back against a wall or facing the door, ready for rapid evacuation.
- **Irritability and low frustration tolerance** may be triggered by disrespectful behaviors

of classmates that do not align with military standards of conduct. This may include classmates talking during a lecture, not completing work in a timely manner, or challenging authority figures. Additionally, service members may become frustrated by the increased time and effort involved in learning new information. Self-regulation and behavioral management strategies can facilitate successful reintegration into the academic setting. Promote understanding that learning requires time and effort, and that effective behavior- and time-management strategies can help reduce the frustration and anxiety associated with returning to school.

- **Fatigue and sleep dysfunction** are common postdeployment symptoms[47,48] that may interfere with attention and concentration and impact reading efficiency and lecture understanding. For management strategies, refer to Patient Handout: Fatigue Management–Factor and Strategy Awareness.
- **Medications** for pain, sleep, and mental health conditions may have side effects that impact alertness and interfere with attention, concentration, and the ability to retain information. Providing feedback to prescribing physicians regarding negative side effects will assist in efficient medication management.
- **Physical symptoms** associated with postdeployment, such as pain, headache, dizziness, balance, vision, and hearing problems[49,50] can interfere with receiving and interpreting written and spoken information. Pain tends to command attention and may compromise the ability to dedicate full attention to lectures and course work, as well as influence class attendance. Physician consultation to manage physical symptoms that interfere with school performance is important.
- **Anxiety, worry, and stress** may result in thoughts that interfere with the ability to attend to, concentrate on, process, and retrieve information. Anxiety may divert concentration during class and increase vulnerability to thought intrusions. Anxiety may also interfere with test taking and make it difficult to initiate assignments when feeling overwhelmed, which contributes to procrastination. Behavioral, organizational, and time-management strategies can assist with initiating and accomplishing assignments, managing anxiety, stress, and feeling overwhelmed.
- **Unrealistic expectations** can interfere with return to school after deployment. Military training provides service members with skills to successfully execute their education plan, including the ability to focus and perform under pressure. Encourage service members to approach college as their next mission, realizing that success is possible with the use of compensatory strategies. Patience, perseverance, and realistic expectations are important to their school success.

Selected References

Cifu DX, Blake C. *Overcoming Post-Deployment Syndrome. A Six-Step Mission to Health*. New York, NY: Demos Medical Publishing; 2011.

Goodrich GL, Kirby J, Cockerham G, Ingalla SP, Lew HL. Visual function in patients of a polytrauma rehabilitation center: a descriptive study. *J Rehabil Res Dev*. 2007;44(7):929–936.

Helfer TM, Jordan NN, Lee RB. Postdeployment hearing loss in U.S. Army soldiers seen at audiology clinics from April 1, 2003, through March 31, 2004. *Am J Audiol*. 2005;14(2):161–168.

Hoge CW, McGurk D, Thomas JL, Cox AL, Engel CC, Castro CA. Mild traumatic brain injury in U.S. Soldiers returning from Iraq. *N Engl J Med*. 2008;358(5):453–463.

Iverson GL, Langlois JA, McCrea MA, Kelly JP. Challenges Associated with Post-Deployment Screening for Mild Traumatic Brain Injury in Military Personnel. *Clin Neuropsychol*. 2009;23(8):1299–1314.

Lew HL, Poole JH, Vanderploeg RD, et al. Program development and defining characteristics of returning military in a VA Polytrauma Network Site. *J Rehabil Res Dev*. 2007;44(7):1027–1034.

Vasterling JJ, Brewin CR. *Neuropsychology of PTSD. Biological, Cognitive, and Clinical Perspectives.* New York, NY: Guilford Press; 2005.

CLINICIAN TIP SHEET: READING STRATEGIES

Background

Reading strategies can be passive or active. Active strategies are more effective because they require purposeful effort to increase meaning by developing relationships between information presented and previous knowledge and experiences, making judgments and predictions about the information, and creating connections between different ideas. College-level reading requires active participation on the part of the reader to facilitate recall of information.[52]

Three Components of Reading Strategies

To optimize the use of reading strategies, preparation involves controlling internal conditions (eg, pain, stress, fatigue) and the external study environment (eg, noise, distractions), and employing strategies that can assist with redirecting attention focus. For information on strategies to manage personal and environmental factors that may distract or prevent optimal studying, refer to Clinician Tip Sheet: Understanding the Multifactor Model of Functioning After Concussion in Chapter 7, Cognitive Assessment and Intervention). Effective reading strategies have components that address organization, isolation, and elaboration.[53]

Organization Strategies

Organization strategies activate the readers' attention before they begin to read by cueing their awareness regarding their knowledge on the topic and connections to new information. Strategies include:

- **Previewing**. Previewing or scanning material prior to reading for comprehension activates previous knowledge about the topic, aids in organization, and establishes the purpose for reading the text. This step is similar to looking at the picture on a jigsaw puzzle box prior to putting the pieces together or knowing the scope of a mission before planning (see Patient Handout: Study Reading Systems).
- **Graphic or concept mapping.** This may be used as a pre- or postreading strategy to process and organize information in a visual format. This is done while reading by creating timelines, tree diagrams, or web-shaped diagrams that connect main ideas with supporting details and requires the ability to identify relationships between and among ideas. Concept mapping software is available that can help with this tactic (eg, Inspiration 9, which can be downloaded from www.inspiration.com/).

Isolation Strategies

Isolation strategies include underlining, highlighting, and note taking. Selecting key points from a text reduces the amount of information to retain.

- **Underlining and highlighting** are passive methods that can help focus attention on the text being read and require the reader to identify the main idea of passages or paragraphs and discriminate between important and unimportant information.
- **Note taking** while reading is an active strategy that involves transforming written text into information that is meaningful to the reader. By organizing information into main points and supporting details, readers are able to self-monitor how well they understand the information, relate new information to previous knowledge, and make judgments and predictions. Note taking is effective only when notes are in the reader's own words and are reviewed after they are written.[52]

Elaboration Strategies

Elaboration strategies include self-questioning and rehearsing information aloud. These strategies facilitate an awareness of relationships between new information with prior knowledge and information that is inferred.

- **Self-questioning strategy** requires the reader to ask *who, what, when, where, how,* and, more importantly, *why* questions while reading. Self-questioning focuses attention, prompts retrieval of information, helps readers self-monitor their comprehension, encourages prediction of test questions, and fosters a deeper processing of information.

- **Rehearsing information aloud** is a strategy in which readers "teach" themselves new information by restating it in their own words. Rewording new information requires readers to associate new concepts

with prior knowledge, summarize key ideas, and reflect on personal reactions.

These strategies are effective with regular information review. Rereading information is a passive review technique that does not result in the same degree of retention that can be achieved through actively retrieving information multiple times.[54]

Selected References

Holschuh JP, Aultman LP. Comprehension Development. In: Flippo RF, Caverly DC, eds. *Handbook of College Reading and Study Strategy Research*. 2nd ed. New York, NY: Routledge; 2009: 121–144.

Hooper CH. *Practicing College Learning Strategies*. 5th ed. Belmont, CA: Wadsworth, Cengage Learning; 2010.

Mulcahy-Ernt PI, Caverly DC. Strategic Study-Reading. In: Flippo RF, Caverly DC, eds. *Handbook of College Reading and Study Strategy Research*. 2nd ed. New York, NY: Routledge; 2009: 177–198.

CLINICIAN TIP SHEET: NOTE TAKING

Background

Note taking is a critical aspect of achieving academic success and is required in multiple contexts and formats, including when listening to lectures, briefings, or instructions, and while reading textbooks, articles, or onscreen text. Although college students spend approximately 80% of class time listening to lectures,[55] they typically record incomplete notes, including only 20% to 40% of the important lecture ideas.[56,57]

Note taking is a complex and demanding cognitive activity involving attending to oral instructions or written text, selecting important facts and concepts, manipulating information in working memory, interpreting information, deciding what to record, and writing or typing the information. These almost simultaneous demands are made on multiple cognitive processes.

- During lectures, the time urgency of selecting and recording key points while comprehending new information places significant demands on executive functioning and memory. Although the typical speaking speed is approximately two to three words per second, the average writing speed is approximately 0.2 to 0.3 words per second.[58]
- Postdeployment factors that may impede the complex task of note taking include difficulty with attention, reduced speed of processing, decreased working memory,

and problems with executive functioning (see Clinician Tip Sheet: Deployment Related Factors That Can Influence Academic Performance).

Methods to Improve Note Taking

Methods to improve note taking and facilitate learning from lectures based on generative theories of learning include improving the completeness of notes, making relationships among lecture ideas, and making relationships between lecture ideas and prior knowledge. Self-questioning and summarizing are more effective strategies than taking and reviewing notes because they require a student to construct their own meaning of the lecture. This underscores the importance of summarizing and revising notes after classes.[59]

Instructors can improve note taking in lectures by providing students with a list of main ideas or topics and subtopics to improve selective attention and guide note taking on the most important information.[60]

Methods to Organize Notes

Methods to organize notes include the Cornell method, two-column method, margin notes, outlining, mapping, charting, topic and concept cards (flashcards), side notes for onscreen text, and intentional reading for written text (see Patient Handout: Memory Strategy–Intentional Reading).

Additional resources on note-taking methods include the following:

- Academic Skills Center, Dartmouth College. www.dartmouth.edu/~acskills/ success/notes.html.
- California Polytechnic State University Student Academic Services, Academic Skills Center. www.sas.calpoly.edu/asc/ ssl/notetakingsystems.html.
- Penn State University Center for Academic Achievement. www.sl.psu.edu/Documents/Note_Taking_Strategies.pdf.
- Stanford University Office of Accessible Education, Strategies for Academic Success, Suggestions for Note Taking. www. stanford.edu/dept/undergrad/cgi-bin/ drupal_ual/sites/default/files/common/ docs/ctl_notetaking.pdf.
- Princeton University, The McGraw Center for Teaching & Learning. www.princeton. edu/mcgraw/library/for-students/.

Assistive Technology Aids

Assistive technology aids may improve note taking, provided they do not serve as a distraction. The following are common aids for note taking:

- digital audio/voice recorders that record spoken information for future reference to reconcile with written notes.
- smart pens that provide simultaneous audio recording of lecture and visual recording of notes that can be downloaded onto a computer.
- laptop computers and tablets for taking notes in lectures.
- text-to-speech software that converts text to audio.
- applications for note taking on computers and tablets.
- software applications for taking notes on electronic text that allow side-by-side on-screen note taking and editable portable document format (PDF) files.

Selected References

Armbruster BB. Taking notes from lectures. In: Flippo RF, Caverly DC, eds. *Handbook of College Reading and Study Strategy Research*. 2nd ed. New York, NY: Routledge; 2009:220–248.

Cohn E, Cohn S, Bradley J. Notetaking, working memory, and learning principles of economics. *J Econ Educ.* 1995;26:291–307.

Kiewra KA. A review of note taking: the encoding-storage paradigm and beyond. *Educ Psychol Rev.* 1989;1:147–172.

Kiewra KA. Students' note-taking behaviors and the efficacy of providing the instructor's notes for review. *Contemp Educ Psychol.* 1985;10:378–386.

O'Donnell A, Dansereau DF. Learning from lectures: effects of cooperative review. *J Exp Educ.* 1993;61:116–125.

Piolat A, Olive T, Kellogg RT. Cognitive effort during notetaking. *Appl Cogn Psychol.* 2005;19:291–312.

CLINICIAN TIP SHEET: TEST-TAKING STRATEGIES

Meeting assignment deadlines and having adequate time to study for tests is dependent upon efficient organization and prioritization. The key to managing time is developing a study schedule based on accurate judgments of the time required to learn and retain new information, complete reading and writing assignments, and review and study for tests. Although schedules are modified according to pain, fatigue, and mood levels, a study schedule will provide the structure that supports motivation, enhances efficiency, and helps avoid procrastination.

A realistic study schedule will also help reduce anxiety by providing a visual timeline for completing course assignments and preparing for tests. This is critical for service members whose educational benefits depend on them passing college courses. In military service, service members are required to develop clearly defined goals, adhere to stringent deadlines, and fulfill duty responsibilities. Course syllabi offer this same structure. The following are suggestions that will promote success in time management and preparing for tests.

- Based on the patient's strengths and preferences, select a planner system (eg, paper planner or calendar, smartphone, tablet computer, dry-erase board) to consolidate school, study, and personal commitments, including exam dates from course syllabi. This will provide a visual overview and engage the patient in planning and prioritizing tasks.
- Assist the patient in establishing realistic timelines by estimating time needed to complete tasks (eg, reading and creating a study guide for each chapter). Have the patient predict, then compare the actual time required to complete tasks to increase self-awareness and time management.
- Guide the patient to use the planner to track daily task progress and review, reorganize, and reprioritize to-do lists as needed to allow adequate time to prepare and study for tests.
- Inform the patient of accommodation services for test taking available through the school.
- Reinforce strategies that enhance retention, such as making associations with prior knowledge and experiences, generating questions about the information, and creating visual tools, such as concept maps, timelines, notes, or webs. These strategies increase the meaningfulness of information and enhance recall.
- Help the patient identify and minimize or eliminate distracters that interfere with concentration and learning. Distracters may be internal or personal (eg, hunger, fatigue, pain, medication effects, depression, anxiety, anger, irritability) or external or environmental (eg, poor lighting, noise, uncomfortable chair, cluttered desk, incoming phone calls, text or email messages).
- Develop redirection strategies to lengthen the time of effective studying (eg, positive self-talk, standing and stretching, getting a drink of water to get back on track).
- Teach strategies to improve recall and retention of information (eg, distributed across multiple sessions rather than "cramming" in a mass practice session).[61]

Selected References

Baddeley AD, Eysenck M, Anderson M. *Memory*. New York, NY: Psychological Press; 2009.

University Seminar at Middle Tennessee State University, Study Skills Help Page, Learning Strategies for Success, http://frank.mtsu.edu/~studskl/.

CLINICIAN TIP SHEET: COLLEGE ACCOMMODATIONS FOR STUDENTS WITH COGNITIVE DISABILITIES

Americans With Disabilities Act Amendments Act of 2008

In accordance with the Americans with Disabilities Act Amendments Act of 2008, students with TBI or PTSD are entitled to receive services and accommodations for symptoms that may affect their academic performance.[62] Colleges and universities have adopted nondiscrimination policies and procedures to support the full participation of students requesting accommodation services, programs, and activities (Exhibit 9-9).

All colleges and universities have some kind of office for students with disabilities that provides reasonable accommodations and support for students with documented disabilities at no charge. Confidential information is shared with classroom instructors only with the student's permission.

To initiate services and accommodations, documentation from a qualified professional is needed to verify the presence of a disability and potential impact within an academic setting. To ensure timely service, a request for services should be submitted several weeks prior to the start of the semester. Check with each college for its specific requirements. Guidelines for disability documentation are available through the Association on Higher Education and Disabilities (www.ahead.org/resources/best-practices-resources/elements).

Although resources vary among colleges, types of accommodations may include:

- early class registration and registration assistance
- academic counseling
- extended time to take exams
- extended time to complete projects, papers,

EXHIBIT 9-9

AMERICANS WITH DISABILITIES ACT AMENDMENTS ACT OF 2008

The Americans With Disabilities Act Amendments Act (ADAAA) of 2008 defines a disability as "a physical or mental impairment that substantially limits one or more major life activities." It states that "an individual would be substantially limited in a major life activity if the individual's major life activity or activities are materially restricted as to the condition, manner or duration under which he or she performs the activity as compared to most people."

According to the ADAAA, major life activities include: "seeing, hearing, sleeping, walking, standing, lifting, bending, speaking, breathing, learning, reading, concentrating, thinking, communicating and working." An impairment may be substantially limiting even if its impact is only episodic. Prescribed medications may further impair academic performance.

The invisible nature of postdeployment symptoms makes it necessary for the student to self-identify. In the college setting, nondisclosure of limitations is a significant issue, in part because individuals do not want to be considered as disabled by either themselves or others.[1] Additionally, career fields (eg, security, criminal justice, law enforcement) may require background checks in which certain disability history may not be favorable.[2]

---

1) Church TE. Helping student-veterans poses unique challenges. *Disability Compliance in Higher Education*. 2008;13(4). 2) Burnett SE, Segoria J. Collaboration for military transition students from combat to college: it takes a community. *J Postsecondary Educ Disabil*. 2009;22(1):233–238.

---

and assignments

- exams in a distraction-reduced area
- note-taking assistance
- tutoring (also available through campus learning centers)
- lecture notes prior to class, if available
- being allowed to stand during class to relieve body pain
- use of recording devices during class (digital recorders)
- assistive technology to convert speech to text, digital text to speech, or documents to alternative formats or sizes
- alternate format exams

Additional accommodation resources may be available through the following sources:

- **Tutorial Assistance Program:** Tutorial assistance is available through the Veterans Affairs Post 9-11 GI Bill for students "receiving VA educational assistance at the half time or more rate and who have a deficiency in a subject making tutoring necessary." Toll free number: 1-888-442-4551.
- **Computer/Electronic Accommodations Program:** The Computer/Electronic Accommodations Program (www.tricare.mil/cap) serves active duty service members and federal employees with disabilities to ensure they receive appropriate accommodations (eg, assistive technology) and services to support their recovery, rehabilitation, and reintegration.

Selected References

Burnett SE, Segoria J. Collaboration for military transition students from combat to college: it takes a community. *J Postsecondary Educ Disabil*. 2009;22(1):233–238.

Church TE. Helping student-veterans poses unique challenges. *Disability Compliance Higher Educ*. 2008;13.

Additional Resources

Montgomery College, Maryland. http://cms.montgomerycollege.edu/EDU/Plain.aspx?id=10283. Accessed September 13, 2013.

US Department of Veteran's Affairs. http://www.GIBILL.va.gov/resources/education%5Fresources/programs/tutorial_assistance_program.html. Accessed September 13, 2013.

US Equal Employment Opportunity Commission. http://www.eeoc.gov/laws/statutes/adaaa.cfm. Accessed September 13, 2013.

SECTION 4: RETURN TO DUTY

INTERVENTION: PERFORMING WORK ROLES AND RETURN TO DUTY

In addition to impacting performance in self-care, home management, and family- and community-based activities, c/mTBI can significantly disrupt an individual's ability to function in job roles. Perceived inadequacy in one's occupation can undercut personal competency and self-efficacy, which may, in turn, have a detrimental effect on productivity and work quality.

Recent research on return to work following head injury has attempted to answer questions such as the following:

- What are the rates of return to work?
- What factors are indicators of successful return to work?
- What interventions are effective in enhancing return to work?

Answers to these questions can be complicated by variables including injury severity, variations in the definition of return to work, and availability of vocational rehabilitation services.

A review by Shames, Treger, Ring, and Giaquintoon suggests that injury severity and lack of self-awareness may be the most significant indicators of failure to return to work.[63] Specifically, a strong correlation was found between self-awareness and favorable employment outcome.[64] Associations have also been made between failure to return to work and psychiatric history, violent mechanism of injury, and prior alcohol or drug use.[65] Impaired cognition, including inattention, impaired memory, slower processing speed, and decreased verbal skills seem to interfere with return to work as well.[66]

Civilian literature focusing on c/mTBI reveals that only 12% of patients with c/mTBI following motor vehicle accidents were able to return to full premorbid level of employment, with 30% able to return to modified work.[67]

Occupational therapy intervention in this realm embodies two complementary approaches: 1) instruction in compensatory cognitive strategies that is functionally compatible with the service member's job requirements (see Cognitive Assessment and Intervention for more information about compensatory cognitive strategies); and 2) completion of simulated work tasks of increasing realism to evoke an adaptive response to challenges. Simulated work tasks may incorporate implementation, rehearsal, and refinement of compensatory strategies.

When addressing issues related to return to work, it is important to consider the following:

- When instructing service members in the use of cognitive compensatory strategies, be sure to discuss their implementation in the work environment. Brainstorm with the service member about what types of adaptive equipment and strategies will be feasible in training and combat.
- Consider the impact of stress on job performance. Rehabilitation clinicians often instruct patients to learn to control their environments and approaches to limit stress when possible. However, it is unrealistic to think that stress will be controllable in combat. It is important to allow real-world time constraints, environmental distractions, activity complexities, multitasking demands, and anxiety-provoking stimuli to be present during some therapeutic activities when preparing service members to return to work.
- Ensure therapy moves from static to dynamic, structured to unstructured, controlled to uncontrolled, and predictable to unpredictable. By placing service members in realistic situations, occupational therapists can facilitate adaptive responses, both neuroplastic and compensatory. The desired outcome is that when the conditions of performance are stressed, the functional impact of identified deficits will be diminished or remediated.
- Note that traditional cognitive testing may not fully reveal deficits, which may only be evident under real-world demands. When setting goals, combine testing results with observations during functional vocational simulations to pinpoint specific areas of deficiency.

Strength of Recommendation: Practice Option

There is little empirical evidence to guide practice in this area; however, intervention is consistent with standard rehabilitation practices and reported as valuable by clinicians working with individuals with c/mTBI.

Intervention Methods

Intervention methods include the following tasks.

- Remedial activities based on Soldier's Manual of Common Tasks[68] (see related patient handouts and clinician tip sheets), including the following:
  ○ locating topographical symbols on a military map,
  ○ determining the grid coordinates of a point on a military map, and
  ○ performing first aid for bleeding of an extremity.
- Vocational simulations of moderate complexity (see related patient handout and therapist tool), such as:
  ○ administrative tasks, and
  ○ job-specific tactical simulations.
- Return-to-duty performance validation (see related patient handout and clinician tip sheet).

Note: The remedial and simulated return-to-duty tasks described in this toolkit are designed for service members who have demonstrated at least basic competency using compensatory motor, visual, or cognitive strategies.

RETURN-TO-DUTY PERFORMANCE VALIDATION PROGRAM

The following is a **practice option** that has been adopted at Fort Campbell, Kentucky. It is continually being developed and refined, and it is understood that this program may be difficult to replicate at other locations due to the variable availability of and cooperation among the many parties involved. However, the concept of "performance validation" is central to occupational therapy intervention related to determining a service member's readiness to return to duty.

The Return-to-Duty Performance Validation Program is a multidisciplinary, functional assessment that takes place over 10 treatment sessions. It is the last step in the TBI treatment process and incorporates a "top down" evaluative approach.

During the program, service members participate in both didactic and real-life, application-based training activities. Many of the training activities are those that are supported by the installation and regularly used by units for training. During the activities, service members are evaluated based on overall performance and independence. Team members from several therapeutic disciplines are involved, including occupational therapy, physical therapy, and mental health. Each provider assesses behavior according to his or her scope of practice. Specifically, occupational therapists comment on visual, cognitive, and fine motor skills; physical therapists comment on balance and vestibular reactions; and mental health providers comment on managing psychological stress and anxiety (Form 9-3).[69]

The performance validation sessions are arranged to present service members with gradually increasing task complexity and psychological demand. In doing so, occupational therapists can assess the service member's ability to generalize strategies learned and implemented in the clinic to approximations of real-world situations. Service members are monitored closely by mental health providers and participate in weekly biofeedback sessions to learn to actively control adverse reactions to stress. If service members display balance deficits that impact task performance, they then participate in physical therapy sessions targeting compensatory strategies.

The "critical tasks" involved in Fort Campbell's Return-to-Duty Performance Validation Program are outlined below. This progression may not be possible to replicate everywhere based on the availability of the required training and equipment; however, this task list may be modified to incorporate other common tasks that are deemed appropriate and for which resources are more readily available.

Task 1: Didactic Review of Eagle First Responder Skills, Followed by Practice Exercise

Review the principles of tactical combat casualty care via slideshow presentation and discussion. Practical exercises consist of basic casualty simulations to rehearse applying tourniquets, pressure dressings, and occlusive dressings for an open chest wound. Environmental distractions and stressors should be minimized to facilitate learning. The service member should:

- Verbalize understanding the difference among the three levels of care (care under fire, tactical field care, and casualty evacuation).
- Demonstrate manual carries for casualty evacuation.
- Be able to call up a 9-line medical evacuation (MEDEVAC) request based on a given scenario (radio use).
- Evaluate a casualty using "CBA" (check circulation, breathing, and airway).
- Demonstrate appropriate hemorrhage control (apply a tourniquet and a pressure dressing).
- Check for an exit wound.
- Seal an open chest wound.
- Open and maintain an airway (head tilt, chin lift [when appropriate], jaw thrust, insert a nasopharyngeal tube).
- Address tension pneumothorax (be able to identify tension pneumothorax and accurately simulate needle decompression).[68,70]

Task 2: Rollover Training Using High-Mobility Multipurpose Wheeled Vehicle Egress Assistance Trainer

High-Mobility Multipurpose Wheeled Vehicle (HMMWV) Egress Assistance Trainer (HEAT) instructors present a 20- to 30-minute class on HMMWV rollover safety. Service members then complete three rollover simulations (basic egress, egress with limited visibility [blindfolded], and egress out the turret). On the final simulation, service members must extract a simulated casualty, perform Eagle First Responder (EFR) treatment, and call up a 9-line MEDEVAC request. The service member must:

- Yell "rollover" at critical rollover angle (30 degrees).
- Demonstrate appropriate HMMWV egress techniques (speed of egress; egress under variable conditions, such as reduced vision or in water; egress out the turret).
- Demonstrate appropriate response for various roles (tank commander, driver, back seat, gunner).
- Demonstrate appropriate extraction of a casualty (may use mannequin).
- Perform EFR skills to treat casualty.

- Call up a 9-line MEDEVAC request.[68,70–72]

Task 3: Required Physical Tasks and Drill and Ceremony Review

These are physical tasks completed at various stations and supervised by participating clinicians. They may require the service member to:

- Don gas mask per Army standard (under 9 seconds).
- Don mission-oriented protective posture (MOPP) suit per Army standard.
- Describe the five levels of MOPP (0 through 4).
- Simulate casualty evacuation using combat litter.
- Complete physically demanding activities to bring heart rate to 85% of maximum heart rate without requiring intervention due to increased headache, dizziness, imbalance, or nausea. Activities may include 3- to 5-second rushes, combat rolls, push-ups, sit-ups, and the like.
- Demonstrate ability to lead and follow drill and ceremony commands according to rank or experience. The following commands are required: facing movements, forward march, column left/right, and rear march.[68]

Task 4: Zero and Qualify Weapon Using Engagement Skills Trainer

For this task, the service member must:

- Demonstrate understanding of basic marksmanship skills (steady position, aiming, breath control, and trigger squeeze).
- Zero and qualify with the assigned weapon (primarily M-4).
- Identify all parts of the weapon.
- Perform function check on weapon.
- Clear weapon.
- Demonstrate adequate visual skills, including visual recognition, accommodative facility/flexibility, visual processing speed, fixation, and hand-eye coordination.[68]

Task 5: Combat Scenarios Using Virtual Combat Convoy Trainer

In this task, service members complete two or three predetermined combat scenarios embedded with selected entities (improvised explosive devices

FORM 9-3

OCCUPATIONAL THERAPY GRADING SHEET

Return to Duty Activity: _____   Date: _____

Name	Pass/Fail*	Go/No Go	IL	Pain	Comments (judgment/safety, memory, visual skills, problem solving, planning, organization, attention, motor planning, sequencing, processing speed)

*An IL score of 1, 2, or 3 indicates a pass; an IL score of 4 or 5 indicates a fail.
IL: independence level

Independence Levels

1. Independent, no adaptations. Service member (SM) is able to complete all the tasks in the activity safely, without modification or compensations, within reasonable time. No cues are required.
2. Independent with adaptations or modifications. SM requires increased time to complete tasks, use of compensatory strategies and techniques, indirect verbal guidance or gestural guidance.
3. Acceptable level of assistance. SM requires no more help than direct verbal assistance or physical assistance. SM performs at a level that is acceptable based on rank or experience. SM will benefit from additional training.
4. Unacceptable level of assistance. SM requires that a part of the task (< 25%) be completed for them by the clinician or SM performs at a level that is unacceptable based on his or her rank or experience.
5. Dependent. SM requires that 25% or more of activity be done for them by the clinician. SM requires psychological intervention. SM unable to complete task due to physical restrictions or limitations.

Cueing Descriptions

Cueing descriptions are based on those found in the Executive Function Performing Test.[1]

No Cues Required

The SM does not require help or reassurance. Self-cueing (speaking to oneself) is acceptable.

Indirect Verbal Guidance

The SM requires verbal prompting, such as an open-ended question or an affirmation that will help him or her move on. Indirect verbal guidance should come in the form of a question, not direct instruction (eg, "What should you do now?" "What is the next step?" "What else do you need?").

Gestural Guidance

The SM requires gestural prompting. At this level, you are not physically involved with any portion of the task. Instead, you should make a gesticulation that mimics the action necessary to complete the task, or make a movement that guides the SM. You may not physically participate (eg, by handing the SM an item).

Direct Verbal Assistance

You are required to deliver a one-step command, so that you are cueing the SM to take an action.

(**Form 9-3** *continues*)

Form 9-3 *continued*

Physical Assistance

You are physically assisting the SM with the step, but you are not doing it for him or her. You may hold/steady/prepare an item, but the SM is still attending to and participating in the task.

Do for the Service Member

You are required to do a portion of the task for the participant.

Cueing Guidelines

- If the SM has difficulty with any aspect of any of the tasks, you must wait at least 10 seconds (to observe processing) before giving a cue.
- Give two cues of each kind before progressing to the next cueing level.
- Give cues progressively in the order listed above.
- Do not initiate conversation during the task, and do not "cheerlead" (ie, do not give positive or negative feedback).

1) Baum CM, Connor LT, Morrison T, Hahn M, Dromerick AW, Edwards DF. Reliability, validity, and clinical utility of the Executive Function Performance Test: a measure of executive function in a sample of people with stroke. *Am J Occup Ther.* Jul–Aug 2008;62(4):446–455.

[IEDs], rocket-propelled grenades, noncombatants, friendly forces, etc). The service member must:

- Demonstrate appropriate radio use.
- Demonstrate adequate visual scanning and attention to visible threats, such as IEDs, rocket-propelled grenades, and snipers.
- Demonstrate adequate safety and judgment.
- Navigate through a virtual scenario (laterally and directionally) using a map and given route.
- Demonstrate adequate communication within the team.
- Perform respective role (driver, tank commander, gunner, etc) without assistance.[68]

Task 6: Care Under Fire Scenario at Medical Skills Training Center Using Simulation Mannequins

Service members complete three medical training scenarios of escalating psychological demand and cognitive complexity. The first iteration involves caring for a mannequin on a litter with the lights on and loud music playing. The second iteration involves caring for a mannequin on the floor with the lights on, combat sounds (low), strobe flashing (low), and simulated smoke. The third iteration involves caring for a mannequin on the floor with debris (simulating explosion), lights out, combat sounds (high), strobe flashing (high), and simulated smoke. Service members must:

- Demonstrate understanding of the difference between the three levels of care (care under fire, tactical field care, and casualty evacuation).
- Demonstrate appropriate radio use by calling up a 9-line MEDEVAC request based on the given scenario.
- Evaluate the casualty using "CBA" (check circulation, breathing, and airway).
- Control hemorrhage by applying a tourniquet or pressure dressing.
- Check for an exit wound.
- Seal an open chest wound.
- Open and maintain an airway (head tilt, chin lift [when appropriate], jaw thrust, insert a nasopharyngeal tube).
- Address tension pneumothorax (identify tension pneumothorax and accurately simulate needle decompression).
- Demonstrate acceptable level of independence when under stressful conditions (combat sounds, reduced vision, strobe light, fog, visually distressing images).[68]

Task 7: Didactic Review of Land Navigation Followed by Practical Exercise

This activity involves a classroom-style presentation of basic land navigation skills, followed by a practical exercise in which 8-digit grid coordinates are used to locate three specific features on a map and determine the distance and azimuth between the three points. The service member must:

- Demonstrate appropriate protractor use and be able to determine 8-digit grid coordinates.
- Correctly identify topographical symbols on a military map.
- Correctly identify colors on a military map.
- Correctly identify marginal information on a military map.
- Correctly identify terrain features.
- Calculate distance between two points.
- Correctly determine azimuth between two points.
- Verbalize understanding the use of a pace count.
- Demonstrate appropriate use of compass to shoot azimuth.[68]

Task 8: Completion of Judgmental Shooting Scenarios Using Engagement Skills Trainer

Service members work as a team to complete five to seven preselected "collective" shooting scenarios, followed by 5 to 10 "shoot/no-shoot" scenarios. Scenarios are selected based on increasing realism and the complexity of the skills required. Service members must:

- Demonstrate adequate visual and perceptual skills, including visual recognition, accommodation, visual fields, contrast sensitivity, visual attention and scanning of sector of fire, visual processing speed, fixation, and hand-eye coordination.
- Demonstrate adequate communication within the team.
- Respond accurately and efficiently to weapon malfunction.
- Demonstrate good judgment and follow the rules of engagement.
- Lack impulsivity.
- Demonstrate weapon safety at all times.[68]

Task 9: Three- To Five-Point Land Navigation Course

In this activity, the service member completes land navigation tasks individually under supervision of participating providers (maximum distance between points of 350 m). The service member must:

- Demonstrate appropriate protractor use and determine 8-digit grid coordinates.
- Correctly identify topographical symbols on a military map.
- Correctly identify colors on a military map.
- Correctly identify marginal information on a military map.
- Correctly identify terrain features.
- Calculate distance between two points.
- Correctly determine azimuth between two points.
- Demonstrate appropriate use of pace count (able to track pace count while navigating).
- Demonstrate appropriate compass use.
- Use terrain association when possible.
- Demonstrate adequate visual scanning and awareness of surroundings.
- Demonstrate problem-solving capabilities if point cannot be located.
- Demonstrate cognitive flexibility.[68]

Task 10: Combat Simulation/Improvised Explosive Device Lane in a Squad-Sized Element

The mission during this activity is to keep from being "mortally" wounded while evaluating, treating, and evacuating a casualty following a simulated IED attack. The team is provided with paintball guns and is opposed by two or three training personnel acting as the opposing force. The service member must:

- Independently perform assigned role (eg, squad leader, medical provider, additional personnel assigned to establish security).
- Demonstrate appropriate "reaction to contact."
- Establish a perimeter.
- Move casualty to a covered position if necessary.
- Perform EFR skills (care under fire) to evaluate and treat casualty.
- Demonstrate appropriate radio use to call up situation reports (SITREPS) and 9-line MEDEVAC request.
- Demonstrate appropriate "break from contact."
- Use combat litter to evacuate casualty to collection point.
- Perform tactical field care once casualty is out of enemy fire.
- Demonstrate good judgment and overall safety.
- Demonstrate adequate awareness of surroundings.

- Demonstrate appropriate communication within team.[68]

Activity Preparation

Setup

Recommended equipment for the above-mentioned tasks includes clipboards, stopwatches, compasses, protractors, military maps, training aids, mannequins, moulage, a small-arms generator and simulated IEDs from the training support center, water cooler, sunscreen, bug spray, smoke machine, night vision goggles, flashlights, two-way radios, paintball guns, modular integrated communications helmets, body armor, face shields, gas masks, and Joint Service Lightweight Integrated Suit Technology suits ("J-List" suits that provide protection against chemical attack). Access to the following training entities is also recommended: HEAT, Engagement Skills Trainer, Virtual Combat Convoy Simulator, and Medical Skills Training Center.

Brief Soldier

Tell the service member the following:

You have been selected to participate in a therapeutic program designed to assess your readiness to return to duty. This program will serve as the capstone of your therapy and will incorporate all elements of your rehabilitation thus far. The multidisciplinary assessment team includes professionals from occupational therapy, physical therapy, and mental health. The physicians involved in your care will use input from participating therapists to customize your treatment and discharge plans, which may include returning you to duty or initiating a military occupational specialty medical retention board or medical evaluation board.

Performance Measures

An occupational therapy grading sheet was developed specifically for the Return-to-Duty Performance Validation Program at Fort Campbell (see Form 9-3). It is not yet validated and is merely a proposed option for performance assessment. Physical therapy and mental health providers may wish to design a similar grading sheet for use during return-to-duty program sessions. Overall "go/no go" status for each session is based on collaboration among providers. At the conclusion of the program, all involved providers meet to discuss patient performance and discharge recommendations. Each participant is then invited to meet with the team to go over the recommendations.

Selected References

Baum C, Connor LT, Morrison T, Hahn M, Dromerick AW, Edwards DF. Reliability, validity, and clinical utility of the Executive Function Performance Test: a measure of executive function in a sample of people with stroke. *Am J Occup Ther*. 2008;62:446–455.

Baum C, Morrison T, Hahn M, Edwards DF. *Executive Function Performance Test*. http://ot.wustl.edu/about/resources/executive-function-performnce-test-efpt-308. Accessed October 16, 2013.

Ruff RM, Marshall LF, Crouch J, et al. Predictors of outcome following severe head trauma: follow-up data from the Traumatic Coma Data Bank. *Brain Inj*. 1993;7(2):101–111.

Ruffolo CF, Friedland DF, Dawson DR, Colantonio A, Lindsay PH. Mild traumatic brain injury from motor vehicle accidents: factors associated with return to work. *Arch Phys Med Rehabil*. 1999;80(4):392–398.

Shames J, Treger I, Ring H, Giaquinto S. Return to work following traumatic brain injury: trends and challenges. *Disabil Rehabil*. 2007;29(7):1387–1395.

Sherer M, Bergloff P, Levin E, High WM Jr, Oden KE, Nick TG. Impaired awareness and employment outcome after traumatic brain injury. *J Head Trauma Rehabil*. 1998;13(5):52–61.

Wagner A, Hammond F, Sasser H, Wiercisiewski D. Return to productive activity after TBI: relationship with measures of disability, handicap and community reintegration. *Arch Phys Med Rehabil*. 2002;83:107–114.

CLINICIAN TIP SHEET: TOPOGRAPHICAL SYMBOLS ON A MILITARY MAP

Purpose/Background

This activity requires obtaining a 1:50,000-scale military map (these may be available through a military post's training and support center, or the service member may be able to bring one to treatment). Use the associated patient handout to go over the topographical symbols with the service member. If you do not have a military background, take this opportunity to allow the patient to instruct you; this will give you an idea of the service member's level of functional performance in this area. Challenging the patient's teaching skills is also beneficial from an occupational standpoint, as nearly all service members will be faced with the responsibility to train others in their jobs at some time during their career.

Activity Preparation

Setup

- On a 1:50,000-scale military map, circle each item of marginal information (Table 9-8) found on the map.

- Randomly letter the circled items A through J.
- Circle 10 items or features on the map itself, which are indicated by color. Choose two of each color (red, blue, green, red-brown, etc).
- Randomly number each colored item 1 through 10. The potential items are listed below.
- Have a sheet of paper and a pencil available for the service member.

Brief Soldier

Tell the service member to letter the paper A through J and 1 through 10. Tell the service member to write down the name of the item contained in each lettered and numbered circle on the map.

Success or failure for each item is rated as "Go" or "No Go," respectively.

Skills Addressed

Static visual attention, visual identification, working memory, and figure ground are all addressed with this activity.

TABLE 9-8

PERFORMANCE MEASURES FOR TOPOGRAPHICAL SYMBOLS ON A MILITARY MAP

Measure	Go	No Go
Identified the sheet name		
Identified the sheet number		
Identified the contour interval		
Identified the grid-magnetic angle (mils or degrees)		
Identified the legend		
Identified the bar scales		
Identified the declination diagram		
Identified the grid reference box		
Identified the adjoining map sheets diagram		
Identified the elevation guide		
Identified 2 of 2 specific human-made features (shown in black on the map)		
Identified 2 of 2 water features (blue on the map)		
Identified 2 of 2 vegetation features (green on the map)		
Identified 2 of 2 human-made features (eg, main roads or build-up areas; shown in brown or red-brown on the map)		
Identified 2 of 2 contour lines (shown in brown or red-brown on the map)		

CLINICIAN TIP SHEET: DETERMINE GRID COORDINATES OF A POINT ON A MILITARY MAP

Purpose/Instructions

This activity requires a 1:50,000-scale military map and a protractor (these may be available through a military post's training and support center, or the service member may be able to bring one to treatment). You will also need a copy of *The Soldier's Manual of Common Tasks*.[68] Use the associated patient handout to review how to determine grid coordinates with the service member. If you do not have a military background, take this opportunity to allow the patient to instruct you; this will give you an idea of the service member's level of functional performance in this area. Challenging the patient's teaching skills is also beneficial from an occupational standpoint, as nearly all service members will be faced with responsibility to train others in their jobs at some time during their career.

Note, the patient handout instructs service members how to determine 6-digit grid coordinates.[68] You may find that service members are more familiar with using 8-digit grid coordinates, as this method is preferable for use during actual land navigation. Therefore, the following activity has been designed to use 8-digit grid coordinates.

Activity Preparation

Setup

Provide the service member with a 1:50,000-scale military map, protractor, paper, and pen or pencil.

Brief the Soldier

Instruct the service member to find the 8-digit grid for a specific human-made object or terrain feature of the therapist's choice. Pick an object using the legend at bottom of map, such as a church, windmill, mine, building, or route marker. Alternatively, provide the exact coordinates and ask the service member to find what object is at that location.

Performance Measures

Observe for the following abilities and use your observations to measure performance. See how the patient:

- uses the correct protractor according to map's scale (1/50,000 m).
- looks for the correct symbol or coordinates.
- uses the protractor appropriately (moving it along the map from left to right and from bottom to top).
- places protractor correctly (horizontal line of protractor is lined up with the horizontal line of the map and vertical line of the protractor is lined up with the vertical lines of the map, going straight over top of the object).
- places the zone identifiers in front of coordinates.
- identifies correct object or grid coordinates.
- uses appropriate strategies to remember objects or coordinates while working.
- completes task in a functional time limit.
- completes task with no verbal cues.

Skills Addressed

This activity assesses static visual attention, figure ground, procedural memory, sequencing, precision, and hand-eye coordination.

To Make the Activity Harder

- List several objects or coordinates at a time for the service member to locate.
- Pick objects that are more difficult to locate or are in busy locations.
- Give the service member a time limit.
- Have the service member complete another task simultaneously (scanning) or add background noise for additional stimulation.

To Make the Activity Easier

- Have the service member locate just one object or coordinate at a time.
- Pick objects that are more easily seen.

CLINICIAN TIP SHEET: PERFORM FIRST AID FOR BLEEDING OF AN EXTREMITY

Instructions

This activity could be performed in a small-group setting. Review techniques then divide patients into groups of two for practical rehearsal. Observe speed, problem-solving, fine-motor coordination, response to stress, and procedural memory. Activity can be graded up or down for complexity, stress, required speed, and the like.

Activity Preparation

Setup

Use the same field dressing repeatedly. Have materials available for a pressure dressing (wadding and cravat or a strip of cloth). Have one service member play the part of the casualty and another apply the field and pressure dressing. Use moulage or mark a place on the casualty's arm or leg to simulate a wound. For applying a tourniquet, use a mannequin or simulated arm or leg (padded length of 2-by-4-inch wood with a glove or boot on one end) with a field dressing appropriately placed on the arm or leg. **Under no circumstances will a live simulated casualty be used to evaluate the application of a tourniquet.** Place the tourniquet materials (a stick and one or two pieces of cloth) nearby.

Brief Soldier

Tell the service member to take the first aid steps

TABLE 9-9

PERFORMANCE MEASURES FOR ACTIVITY: PERFORM FIRST AID FOR EXTREMITY BLEEDING

Step	Go	No Go
1. Uncovered the wound		
2. Applied a field dressing		
3. Applied manual pressure and elevated the arm or leg, if necessary		
4. Applied a pressure dressing, if necessary		
5. Applied a tourniquet, if necessary		
6. Performed steps 1–5, as necessary, in sequence		

required to put on a field dressing and, if necessary, apply a pressure dressing on the casualty's wound (Table 9-9). When testing the first step (uncovering the wound), you can vary the test by telling the service member that clothing is stuck to the wound or that a chemical environment exists. After steps two and three (applying a field dressing and applying manual pressure to the extremity), tell the service member that the bleeding has not stopped. After step four, tell the service member the bleeding is continuing and ask him or her to describe the wound and perform first aid.

CLINICIAN TIP SHEET: JOB-SPECIFIC TACTICAL SIMULATION 1– DYNAMIC VISUAL SCANNING ACTIVITY

Purpose/Instructions

These types of activities will vary based on the service member's military occupational specialty. Simulations can be modified to target specific skill areas.

- A forward observer can complete a visual scavenger hunt using a spotting scope and scanning for specific landmarks at a distance of 100 to 300 meters.
- A medic can complete tactical casualty combat care simulations.
- A combat engineer may calculate breaching charges based on given scenarios.
- An upper-enlisted member may prepare and execute briefings.

Keep in mind that creativity is the key when creating these activities. Also, feel free to rely on the individual service member to guide your approach. The knowledge and experience of your patients can be a valuable resource in developing occupational therapy return-to-work programming.

Activity Preparation

Setup

There are many variations to this activity. The goal, however, is always the same: challenge the patient to adequately attend to specific visual stimuli in a dynamic, real-world environment. The activity can take place in the hospital, post exchange, commissary, or outside. Desired stimuli can range from large items, such as car makes and models, to small items, such as wedding bands. Provide yourself and the patient with a pen or pencil and a small notepad.

Brief Soldier

Instruct the patient that he or she will be required to scan for desired stimuli while walking through a busy environment. Reiterate the importance of staying alert and focused while using effective search patterns.

Performance Measures

To determine accuracy, divide the patient's scanning totals by your own. For example, if the patient spotted 15 soldiers wearing Army combat uniforms and you spotted 21, his or her accuracy would be 71%.

Skills Addressed

This activity addresses selective, divided, and alternating visual attention, dynamic visual acuity, and working memory.

To Make the Activity Harder

The activity can be made more difficult by adding additional dual-task elements, such as having the patient keep track of one or both of the totals internally, or having the patient complete a secondary task while performing visual scanning (ie, locate items on a grocery list).

To Make the Activity Easier

The task can be simplified by reducing the number of required stimuli, completing the task in a less distracting environment, and removing dual-task elements.

CLINICIAN TIP SHEET: JOB-SPECIFIC TACTICAL SIMULATION 2– TARGET DETECTION VISUAL SCANNING ACTIVITY

Activity Preparation

Setup

This activity mimics a tactical training task performed by many service members. The activity requires advanced set-up and a large, relatively flat outdoor space. Select 10 small (3 to 5 inch) military items (eg, a pin, badge, compass, and protractor). Scatter the items on the ground in a lane that is approximately 20 to 30 meters wide. Have the patient use binoculars or a spotting scope to locate and identify the items from approximately 25 to 75 meters away. Materials include a scope or binoculars, 10 military items, pen or pencil, and a small notepad.

Brief Soldier

Instruct the service member that he or she will be required to scan for desired stimuli scattered within a designated lane. Upon locating each target, the patient attempts to identify it and write a detailed description of the item on the notepad.

Performance Measures

To determine accuracy, divide the patient's scanning totals by 10. If the patient spotted 7 out of the 10 items, accuracy would be 70%.

Skills Addressed

Visual discrimination, visual closure, figure ground, selective attention, and accommodation are addressed in this activity.

To Make the Activity Harder

To make the activity harder, increase difficulty by partially obscuring some of the items from view, choosing smaller items, and enforcing a time constraint.

To Make the Activity Easier

To make the activity easier, simplify the task by using larger items and reducing distance.

CLINICIAN TIP SHEET: DUTY ROSTER ACTIVITY

Activity Preparation

Setup

Provide the service member with the handout, a blank Duty Roster Activity form (Department of the Army 6 [DA-6]), calendar, and a pencil.

Brief Soldier

Instruct the service member to use given information and the previous month's DA-6 form to complete the following month's schedule. If the patient requires cues, follow these 10 general rules:

1. Write out all the days of the month across the top.
2. Highlight vertically the weekends and holidays (these are the "weekend" duty cycle).
3. Place a lower case "a" in the upper right hand corner of the days that certain service members will be absent.
4. Based on the last weekday and weekend from the previous month (given), begin filling in the numbers from left to right, keeping in mind that there are two simultaneous duty cycles: weekday and weekend. For example, an individual could be in the fourth duty slot for weekdays, but the nineteenth duty slot for weekends.
5. When you get to number 20 in either duty cycle, fill in the lower right hand corner of the square to signify "duty" for a service member on that particular day.
6. When a duty day falls on a day a service member will be on leave, duty goes to the next highest-ranking service member (#19).
7. The service member who misses duty because of leave performs duty the next day that he or she is back for that particular duty cycle. The following day after that, he or she becomes number 1.

8. The person who does duty in the stead of someone who is on leave cycles back to number 1 the day after completing substitute duty (staying in the same duty cycle).
9. A service member will never pull duty two days in a row. If the two duty cycles (weekend and weekday) coincide so that a person will have two duty days in a row, follow the same process described in numbers 7 and 8.

Performance Measures

Assess service members based on the level of cueing required, organization of approach, attention to details, cognitive flexibility, and problem solving. To determine the accuracy of the service member's response, you must correct by hand because there are multiple correct responses for the duty roster.

Skills Addressed

Organizational skills, planning, sequencing, executive functions, following written instructions, working memory, and attention to detail are all addressed with this activity.

To Make the Activity Harder

To make the activity harder, increase the number of fictional sergeants on the duty roster, increase the number of accommodations required, provide a time limit, increase distractions, or introduce a second task to complete simultaneously.

To Make the Activity Easier

Decrease the number of sergeants on the duty roster, decrease the number of accommodations required, allot more time for completion, and set up the activity in a controlled environment with few distractions to make the activity easier.

CLINICIAN TIP SHEET: TRAINING SCHEDULE

Activity Preparation

Setup

Provide the service member with the handout, a blank weekly calendar, and a pencil.

Brief the Soldier

Instruct the service member to complete the training schedule following the guidelines on the handout.

Skills Addressed

This activity addresses organizational skills, planning, sequencing, following written instructions, attention to detail, working memory, and executive functions.

To Make the Activity Harder

To make the activity harder, increase the number of activities to schedule, decrease flexibility by requiring training activities to take place at certain times, provide a time limit, increase environmental distractions, or introduce a second task to complete simultaneously.

To Make the Activity Easier

To make the activity easier, decrease the number of scheduled activities, increase flexibility by removing assigned times, or limit environmental distractions.

Definition of Terms From Patient Handout

- NCOER: Noncommissioned Officer Evaluation Report
- EO class: Equal Opportunity class
- NCODP: Noncommissioned Officer Development Program

CLINICIAN TIP SHEET: DRESS UNIFORM ERROR DETECTION

Instructions

Incorrectly place 5 to 10 badges on the Army Service Uniform jacket. Score the number of inappropriately placed badges the service member is able to identify and correct. The total score will be factored out of the number of badges initially put on the jacket. For correct placements, refer to Army Regulation 670-1 or the US Army Uniform Guide.[69,70]

Activity Preparation

Setup

Provide service members with the handout, the dress uniform jacket, a ruler, and a US Army Uniform Guide.[70]

Brief Soldier

Explain to the service member that some or all of the badges on the dress jacket are not correctly placed and it is his or her job to pin them in the correct locations.

Skills Addressed

This activity addresses skills such as visual scanning, memory, fine motor skills, attention to detail, and following directions.

To Make the Activity Harder

To make this activity harder, increase the number of badges on the jacket and make initial (incorrect) placement of badges similar to the correct placement, simulate interruptions (set a timer to go off, set up a phone to ring, add an additional task to complete), give the service member a time limit for completion, or have the service member complete the activity in a distracting environment.

To Make the Activity Easier

Decrease the number of badges on the jacket and make initial (incorrect) placement of badges obvious, complete activity in a controlled environment with little noise or distraction, or allot more time for completion to make the task easier.

REFERENCES

1. Ruff RM. Two decades of advances in understanding of mild traumatic brain injury. *J Head Trauma Rehabil.* Jan–Feb 2005;20(1):5–18.

2. de Leon MB, Kirsch NL, Maio RF, et al. Baseline predictors of fatigue 1 year after mild head injury. *Arch Phys Med Rehabil.* 2009;90:956–965.

3. American Occupational Therapy Association. Occupational therapy practice framework: domain and process. *Am J Occup Ther.* 2008;62:625–683.

4. Trombly CA, Radomski MV, Davis ES. Achievement of self-identified goals by adults with traumatic brain injury: phase I. *Am J Occup Ther.* 1998;52:810–818.

5. Trombly CA, Radomski MV, Trexel C, Burnet-Smith SE. Occupational therapy and achievement of self-identified goals by adults with acquired brain injury: phase II. *Am J Occup Ther.* Sep–Oct 2002;56(5):489–498.

6. Jenkinson N, Ownsworth T, Shum D. Utility of the Canadian Occupational Performance Measure in community-based brain injury rehabilitation. *Brain Inj.* Nov 2007;21(12):1283–1294.

7. Phipps S, Richardson P. Occupational therapy outcomes for clients with traumatic brain injury and stroke using the Canadian Occupational Performance Measure. *Am J Occup Ther.* 2007;61:328–334.

8. Carswell A, McColl MA, Baptise S, Law M, Polatajko H, Pollock N. The Canadian Occupational Performance Measure: a research and clinical literature review. *Can J Occup Ther.* 2004;71:210–222.

9. Law M, Baptise S, McColl MA, Carswell A, Polatajko H, Pollock N. *Canadian Occupational Performance Measure.* 2nd ed. Toronto, ON: Canadian Association of Occupational Therapists–Association Canadienne d'Éducation Publications; 1994.

10. Cup EHC, Scholte op Reimer WJM, Thijssen MCE, van Kuyk-Minis MAH. Reliability and validity of the Canadian Occupational Performance Measure in stroke patients. *Clin Rehabil.* 2003;17:402–409.

11. Law M, Polatajko H, Pollock N, McColl MA, Carswell A, Baptise S. Pilot testing of the Canadian Occupational Performance Measure: Clinical and measurement issues. *Can J Occup Ther.* 1994;61:191–197.

12. Eyssen IC, Beelen A, Dedding C, Cardol M, Dekker J. The reproducibility of the Canadian Occupational Performance Measure. *Clin Rehabil.* Dec 2005;19(8):888–894.

13. Baron KB, Kielhofner G, Goldhammer V, Wolenski J. *A User's Manual for the Occupational Self-Assessment.* Chicago, IL: University of Illinois at Chicago; 1998.

14. Baron KB, Kielhofner G, Iyenger A, Goldhammer V, Wolenski J. *A User's Manual for the Occupational Self Assessment (OSA).* Chicago, IL: University of Illinois at Chicago; 2006.

15. Kielhofner G, Forsyth K. Measurement properties of a client self-report for treatment planning and documenting therapy outcomes. *Scand J Occup Ther.* 2001;8:131–139.

16. Kielhofner G. *A Model of Human Occupation: Theory and Application.* 2nd ed. Baltimore, MD: Lippincott Williams & Wilkins; 1995.

17. Kielhofner G, Forsyth K, Kramer J, Iyenger A. Developing the Occupational Self-Assessment: the use of Rasch analysis to assure internal validity, sensitivity and reliability. *Br J Occup Ther.* 2009;72:94–104.

18. Management of Concussion/mTBI Working Group. VA/DoD Clinical Practice Guideline for Management of Concussion/mTBI. *J Rehabil Res Dev.* 2009;46(6):CP1–CP68.

19. Johns MW. Reliability and factor analysis of the Epworth Sleepiness Scale. *Sleep.* Aug 1992;15(4):376–381.

20. Krupp LB, LaRocca NG, Muir-Nash J, Steinberg AD. The fatigue severity scale. Application to patients with multiple sclerosis and systemic lupus erythematosus. *Arch Neurol.* Oct 1989;46(10):1121–1123.

21. Masel BE, Scheibel RS, Kimbark T, Kuna ST. Excessive daytime sleepiness in adults with brain injuries. *Arch Phys Med Rehabil.* Nov 2001;82(11):1526–1532.

22. Johns M. The Official website of the Epworth Sleepiness Scale. http://epworthsleepinessscale.com/about-epworth-sleepiness/. Accessed September 19, 2013.

23. Whitehead L. The measurement of fatigue in chronic illness: a systematic review of unidimensional and multidimensional fatigue measures. *J Pain Symptom Manage.* Jan 2009;37(1):107–128.

24. Merritta C, Cherian B, Macaden AS, John JA. Measurement of physical performance and objective fatigability in people with mild-to-moderate traumatic brain injury. *Int J Rehabil Res.* Jul 9 2009.

25. National Women's Health Resource Center, Inc. Healthy Living Web page. The Fatigue Severity Scale. http://www.healthywomen.org/content/article/fatigue-severity-scale-fss. Accessed September 19, 2013.

27. Davidson LF. *Activity Co-engagement Self-assessment.* Winchester, VA: Shenandoah University; 2009.

28. Forsyth K, Lai J, Kielhofner G. The assessment of communication and interaction skills (ACIS): measurement properties. *Br J Occup Ther.* 1999;62:69-74.

29. Asher IE, ed. *Occupational Therapy Assessment Tools: An Annotated Index.* 3rd ed. Bethesda, MD: American Occupational Therapy Association; 2007.

30. Spanier GB. Measuring dyadic adjustment: new scales for assessing the equality of marriage and similar dyads. *J Marriage Fam.* 1976;38:15–28.

31. Ikiugu MN. *Psychosocial Conceptual Practice Models in Occupational Therapy: Building Adaptive Capability.* St Louis, MO: Mosby Elsevier; 2007.

32. Gambardella LC. Role-exit theory and marital discord following extended military deployment. *Perspect Psychiatr Care.* Jul 2008;44(3):169–174.

33. Cook J. Higher education: an attainable goal for students who have sustained head injuries. *J Head Trauma Rehabil.* 1991;6:64–72.

34. Ip RY, Dornan J, Schentag C. Traumatic brain injury: factors predicting return to work or school. *Brain Inj.* Jul 1995;9(5):517–532.

35. Stewart-Scott AM, Douglas JM. Educational outcome for secondary and postsecondary students following traumatic brain injury. *Brain Inj.* Apr 1998;12(4):317–331.

36. Kennedy MR, Krause MO, Turkstra LS. An electronic survey about college experiences after traumatic brain injury. *NeuroRehabilitation.* 2008;23(6):511–520.

37. Kennedy MRT, Krause MO. Academic experiences of adults with and without traumatic brain injury using the College Survey for Students with Brain Injury (CSS-BI). *Eighth World Conference on Brain Injury.* Washington, DC, March 13, 2010.

38. Laforce R Jr, Martin-MacLeod L. Symptom cluster associated with mild traumatic brain injury in university students. *Percept Mot Skills.* Aug 2001;93(1):281–288.

39. Cicerone KD, Langenbahn DM, Braden C, et al. Evidence-based cognitive rehabilitation: updated review of the literature from 2003 through 2008. *Arch Phys Med Rehabil.* Apr 2011;92(4):519–530.

40. Sohlberg MM, Avery J, Kennedy M, et al. Practice guidelines for direct attention training. *J Med Speech Lang Pathol.* 2003;11(3):xix-xxxix.

41. Sohlberg MM, Kennedy MRT, Avery J, et al. Evidenced-based practice for the use of external memory aids as a memory compensation technique. *J Med Speech Lang Pathol.* 2007;15:xv–li.

42. Sohlberg MM, Turkstra LS. *Optimizing Cognitive Rehabilitation: Effective Instructional Methods.* New York, NY: Guilford Press; 2011.

43. Ylvisaker M, Turkstra L, Coehlo C, et al. Behavioural interventions for children and adults with behaviour disorders after TBI: a systematic review of the evidence. *Brain Inj.* Jul 2007;21(8):769–805.

44. Zarzecki MA, Crawford E, Smith Hammond C. Essential Skills for College Success, VHA Evolving Paradigms II. *Polytrauma Conference*. Las Vegas, NV. September 22, 2009.

45. Vasterling JJ, Brewin CR. *Neuropsychology of PTSD. Biological, Cognitive, and Clinical Perspectives*. New York, NY: Guilford Press; 2005.

46. Cifu DX, Blake C. *Overcoming Post-Deployment Syndrome. A Six-Step Mission to Health*. New York, NY: Demos Medical Publishing; 2011.

47. Hoge CW, McGurk D, Thomas JL, Cox AL, Engel CC, Castro CA. Mild traumatic brain injury in US. Soldiers returning from Iraq. *New Eng J Med*. 2008;358(5):453–463.

48. Iverson GL, Langlois JA, McCrea MA, Kelly JP. Challenges Associated With Post-Deployment Screening for Mild Traumatic Brain Injury in Military Personnel. *Clin Neuropsychol*. 2009;23(8):1299–1314.

49. Goodrich GL, Kirby J, Cockerham G, Ingalla SP, Lew HL. Visual function in patients of a polytrauma rehabilitation center: A descriptive study. *J Rehabil Res Dev*. 2007;44(7):929–936.

50. Helfer TM, Jordan NN, Lee RB. Postdeployment hearing loss in US Army soldiers seen at audiology clinics from April 1, 2003, through March 31, 2004. *Am J Audiol*. 2005;14(2):161–168.

51. Lew HL, Poole JH, Vanderploeg RD, et al. Program development and defining characteristics of returning military in a VA Polytrauma Network Site. *J Rehabil Res Devt*. 2007;44(7):1027–1034.

52. Mulcahy-Ernt PI, Caverly DC. Strategic study-reading. In: Flippo RF, Caverly DC, eds. *Handbook of College Reading and Study Strategy Research*. 2nd ed. New York, NY: Routledge; 2009:177–198.

53. Holschuh JP, Aultman LP. Comprehension development. In: Flippo RF, Caverly DC, eds. *Handbook of College Reading and Study Strategy Research*. 2nd ed. New York, NY: Routledge; 2009:121–144

54. Hooper CH. *Practicing College Learning Strategies*. 5th ed. Belmont, CA: Wadsworth, Cengage Learning; 2010.

55. Armbruster BB. Taking notes from lectures. In: Flippo RF, Caverly DC, eds. *Handbook of College Reading and Study Strategy Research*. 2nd ed. New York, NY: Routledge; 2009:220–248.

56. Kiewra KA. Students' note-taking behaviors and the efficacy of providing the instructor's notes for review. *Contemp Educ Psychol*. 1985;10:378–386.

57. O'Donnell A, Dansereau DF. Learning from lectures: effects of cooperative review. *J Exper Educ*. 1993;61:116–125.

58. Piolat A, Olive T, Kellogg RT. Cognitive effort during notetaking. *Appl Cogn Psychol*. 2005;19:291–312.

59. Kiewra KA. A review of note taking: the encoding-storage paradigm and beyond. *Educ Psychol Rev*. 1989;1:147–172.

60. Cohn E, Cohn S, Bradley J. Notetaking, working memory, and learning principles of economics. *J Econ Educ*. 1995;26:291–307.

61. Baddeley AD, Eysenck M, Anderson M. *Memory*. New York, NY: Psychological Press; 2009.

62. ADA Amendments Act of 2008, 42 USC § 12101 (2008).

63. Shames J, Treger I, Ring H, Giaquinto S. Return to work following traumatic brain injury: trends and challenges. *Disabil Rehabil*. 2007;29(7):1387–1395.

64. Sherer M, Bergloff P, Levin E, High WM Jr, Oden KE, Nick TG. Impaired awareness and employment outcome after traumatic brain injury. *J Head Trauma Rehabil*. Oct 1998;13(5):52–61.

65. Wagner A, Hammond F, Sasser H, Wiercisiewski D. Return to productive activity after TBI: relationship with measures of disability, handicap and community reintegration. *Arch Phys Med Rehabil.* 2002;83:107–114.

66. Ruff RM, Marshall LF, Crouch J, et al. Predictors of outcome following severe head trauma: follow-up data from the Traumatic Coma Data Bank. *Brain Inj.* Mar–Apr 1993;7(2):101–111.

67. Ruffolo CF, Friedland JF, Dawson DR, Colantonio A, Lindsay PH. Mild traumatic brain injury from motor vehicle accidents: factors associated with return to work. *Arch Phys Med Rehabil.* Apr 1999;80(4):392–398.

68. US Department of the Army. *Soldier Training Publication STP 21-1-SMCT. Soldier's Manual of Common Tasks Warrior Skills Level I.* Washington, DC: DA; 2012.

69. Ringler WG. *U.S. Army Uniform Guide (Look Sharp!).* Huntsville, TX: Ringler Enterprises, Inc; 2012.

70. US Department of the Army. *Wear and Appearance of Army Uniforms and Insignia.* Washington, DC: DA; 2005. Army Regulation 670-1.

71. Baum CM, Connor LT, Morrison T, Hahn M, Dromerick AW, Edwards DF. Reliability, validity, and clinical utility of the Executive Function Performance Test: a measure of executive function in a sample of people with stroke. *Am J Occup Ther.* Jul–Aug 2008;62(4):446–455.

72. Army Study Guide website. *9 Line MEDEVAC Request.* Foster City, CA: QuinStreet, Inc. http://www.armystudyguide.com/content/army_board_study_guide_topics/First_Aid/9-line-medevac-request.shtml. Accessed September 19, 2013.

SECTION 5: PATIENT HANDOUTS

PATIENT HANDOUT: MEDICATION MANAGEMENT SELF-REPORT QUESTIONNAIRE

Instructions

Your answers to these questions will help us ensure you take the medications prescribed by your doctor. Please select or provide the answer to each question that best fits your situation or circumstances.

1. Do you know the names of your medications and what they look like? If yes, please list them.
   ___ Yes, all of them.
   ___ Yes, some of them.
   ___ No, none of them.

   _____
   _____
   _____

2. Do you know the purpose and dosages of your medications? If so, please list below.
   ___ Yes, all of them.
   ___ Yes, some of them.
   ___ No, none of them.

   _____
   _____
   _____
   _____

3. Do you keep a current list of your medications?
   _____ Yes   _____ No
4. Do you have a schedule for taking your medications (ie, morning, lunch, evening)?
   ___ Yes, I do for all medications I take.
   ___ Yes, I do, but only for some medications I take.
   ___ No, I do not have a schedule.
5. Do you know when to take your medication(s)?
   _____ Yes   _____ No
6. Can you open the containers?
   _____ Yes   _____ No
7. Can you read the prescription on the bottle?
   _____ Yes   _____ No
8. Do you understand how to follow the prescription?
   _____ Yes   _____ No
9. How do you organize your medications? Do you use a pill box or do you take the pills directly out of the bottles?

   _____
   _____

10. How do you remember to take your medications?

    _____
    _____

11. Do you know how to refill your medications? Do you know who to call? Do you know who and when to call and how to pick up your refills?
    _____ Yes   _____ No

Example: _____
_____
_____

12. Do you carry your doctor's name and telephone number with you?
    _____ Yes   _____ No

PATIENT HANDOUT: FATIGUE MANAGEMENT–FACTOR AND STRATEGY AWARENESS

Background

After concussion, you may find that you tire more readily during both physical and mental tasks. It is important to actively work on managing your fatigue to avoid unnecessary errors and frustrations and to put your effort into regaining your previous level of activity tolerance.

You can manage fatigue by maintaining:

1. good sleep hygiene practices,
2. good nutrition and hydration,
3. regular exercise/activity, and
4. stress reduction practices.

Maximizing Your Energy as You Recover

This handout is designed to help you explore each of the four factors that comprise fatigue management so you and your therapist can identify strategies that might help you improve your energy and activity tolerance. Read each section and answer questions about your current habits, then discuss your answers with your occupational therapist and together identify possible strategies that you can evaluate in your daily life.

Sleep Hygiene

- Sleep hygiene pertains to all behavioral and environmental factors that precede **sleep** and may interfere with **sleep.**
- The following practices help people establish restful and satisfying sleep patterns.
    - Wake up and go to bed at consistent times.
    - Avoid stimulants, such as caffeinated beverages and nicotine, after 2:00 pm.
    - Avoid alcoholic drinks before bed.
    - Minimize distractions in your bedroom (this includes television).
    - Relax before bed so you can unwind before sleep.
    - Limit naps to no longer than 30 minutes; avoid napping after 3:00 pm.
    - Exercise and stay active during the day. Try to exercise every day, but not within 5 hours of bedtime.

Components of Your Sleep Routine	Your Current Habits	Strategy (N/A if no problems are reported)
What time do you awake/get up?		
What time do you go to bed?		
What do you typically do right before going to bed at night (read, watch TV, etc)?		
Do you nap during the day?		
If yes, how often and how long?		

Sleep Characteristics	Your Current Habits	Strategy (N/A if no problems are reported)
Do you fall asleep readily?		
Do you stay asleep?		
Do you wake up feeling rested?		
Other:		

Nutrition and Hydration

Your body needs well-balanced meals and consistent hydration to heal optimally. If you do not know what good nutrition entails, it may benefit you to meet with a nutritionist to review guidelines and options.

Nutrition Characteristics (how would you describe your nutrition at the following meals)	Your Current Habits	Strategy (N/A if no problems are reported)
Breakfast		
Snack		
Lunch		
Snack		
Dinner		
Other:		

Regular Exercise

If cleared by your medical doctor, it is important to resume physical activities. Exercise helps brain function and builds activity tolerance. Consult with your therapist to assure an effective exercise regimen.

Exercise Characteristics	Current Habits	Strategy (N/A if no problems are reported)
What is your current routine in terms of endurance or aerobic exercise (frequency, time of day, and nature of the exercise)?		
What is your current routine in terms of strengthening exercise (frequency, time of day, and nature of the exercise)?		

Stress Reduction

It is important to resume or develop stress-reduction skills. These skills vary from individual to individual, and include regularly engaging in activities that help you reduce your stress level.

Stress-Reduction Activities	Current Habits	Strategy (N/A if no problems are reported)
What kinds of everyday activities help you reduce stress?		
How often do you engage in these activities? Daily, weekly, monthly?		

FURTHER RESOURCES

- Additional information on sleep hygiene can be found at: http://www.nhlbi.nih.gov/health/public/sleep/healthy_sleep.pdf.
- Detailed stress-relief techniques can be found at: http://helpguide.org/mental/stress_relief_meditation_yoga_relaxation.htm.

PATIENT HANDOUT: TAKING BREAKS

Overview

As you recover from concussion/mild traumatic brain injury (c/mTBI), you can manage fatigue and optimize performance by knowing how to pace yourself. Sometimes this means stepping away from your work for a few moments to regroup so you can continue to perform at your best.

Managing fatigue involves knowing:

1) when to take a brief break, and
2) what to do during a brief break that will rejuvenate you.

Steps you can take:

1) Pre-plan what to do during a brief break that will refresh you.
2) Come up with some additional things to do when you need a brief break (see example below).

WHAT TO DO WHEN YOU NEED A BREAK

1. Take a brief walk.	6.
2. Do stretching exercises.	7.
3. Get a drink of water.	8.
4.	9.
5.	10.

Recognizing When You Need to Take a Break

Be aware of any **physical symptoms** that indicate you may need a break, including:

- headache or tension
- irritability
- eye strain
- increased fatigue
- increased frustration
- decreased ability to concentrate
- other:

Be aware of cognitive inefficiencies that impede task performance, such as:

- increasing number of errors
- increasing need to start over or not remembering what you did last
- inability to see the big picture, understand the whole of the task
- task feels harder than it should be
- other:

An increase in physical symptoms or cognitive inefficiencies signals you to stop and reflect on what to do next.
Options:

- Determine if you need a break, should shift to another task, or if you are done for the day.
- Leave yourself a "stop note," which allows you to resume where you left off when you come back.
- Determine approximately how long a break you need to resume the task refreshed. Set an alarm if needed.

- Return to the task. Read your stop note and seamlessly resume the task.

REMEMBER: Sometimes the goal is to work smarter rather than harder!

PATIENT HANDOUT: PACING

Activity tolerance refers to your capacity for physical output and stamina on a given day. After concussion or other injuries, people work to regain their activity tolerance by doing as much as they are able without under- or over-doing.

In the early stages of recovery (or any time you feel busy or overwhelmed), it can be helpful to view your activity tolerance as a limited resource that needs to be budgeted. Much like a checking account, if your activity tolerance is not well managed, there can be penalties and it can take a long time to recover.

Pacing is a strategy that enables you to maximize your activity tolerance and thereby manage fatigue.

How Pacing Works

Consider the activities that you need to perform throughout a week:

- personal tasks,
- home-management tasks,
- care of others / social tasks,
- medical appointments, and
- work and community tasks.

Pacing yourself involves scheduling these tasks throughout the course of the week (with rest breaks scheduled as well) so your activity tolerance can be used wisely and restored to functional levels with rest. If an event or project requires you to use all of your activity tolerance in one fell swoop, you will need to plan to rest before and after to help restore that budget.

Begin by tracking the areas that you are primarily responsible for on the grid below. Choose days of the week on which you will try to perform these tasks; make sure you are spreading them out throughout the week and not over-taxing yourself on any particular day. Here's an example of part of a completed grid; fill out your own on the next page.

EXAMPLE RESPONSIBILITIES GRID

Task	Sun	Mon	Tues	Wed	Thurs	Fri	Sat
Personal							
Physical therapy appointments			X		X		
Physical therapy home exercises		X		X		X	
Household							
Grocery shopping							X
Home repair tasks							X
Work							
Duty assignment		X	X	X	X	X	

RESPONSIBILITIES GRID

Task	Sun	Mon	Tues	Wed	Thurs	Fri	Sat
Personal							
Household							
Care of others							
Medical							
Social							
Work/Community							

REMEMBER: Meeting your task responsibilities as you recover does not involve an all-or-none phenomenon. Pacing allows you to continue to perform essential or desired tasks as you thoughtfully schedule them over the course of the week.

PATIENT HANDOUT: MEDICATION SUMMARY

Medicine	Dose	Time(s)	Reason	Prescribing Doctor
	mg/day			Dr.
	mg/day			Dr.
	mg/day			Dr.
	mg/day			Dr.
	mg/day			Dr.
	mg/day			Dr.
	mg/day			Dr.
	mg/day			Dr.

PATIENT HANDOUT: MEDICATION SCHEDULE

Morning

Medicine	Dose/Route	Time	Reason

After Lunch/Mid Day

Medicine	Dose/Route	Time	Reason

Bedtime

Medicine	Dose/Route	Time	Reason

As Needed

Medicine	Dose/Route	Time	Reason

PATIENT HANDOUT: ORGANIZING THE MAIL

Receiving mail on a daily basis can be overwhelming at times, especially because getting junk mail is inevitable. Having a systemized method of mail management can reduce irritation and allow better awareness of necessities when it comes to paying bills.

Here are some ideas for how you can get organized:

1. Set up a system and game plan.
    *   Obtain the supplies needed to get organized: a box for incoming mail, a shredder, a filing cabinet or file box, file folders, marker, and a calendar, cognitive assistive technology (CAT), or day planner.
    *   Talk with your significant other and establish a specific place in which to put all incoming mail as it arrives. For example, use the kitchen, bedroom, or home office.
    *   Purchase a 13-by-10-inch box, label it "Incoming Mail," and put it in the designated place (as above). Consider purchasing a clear plastic bin for this purpose.
2. Sort the contents of the Incoming Mail box once per week.
    *   Once a week, with your significant other, go through the mail and sort it into two piles: junk mail and important mail.
        *   Junk mail: any mail that is not important to you (such as credit offers, advertisements, newsletters)
        *   Important mail: any mail that you need (such as utility bills, credit card bills, mortgage bill / statement, car payment, tax information, receipts)
3. To prevent identity theft, shred all junk mail. If you do not want to shred all junk mail, at least shred your name and address before recycling the rest.
4. Further sort your important mail pile.
    *   Create a temporary sorting space. Clear off a table top surface or floor space.
    *   Use sticky notes to help you sort. Create a sticky note for each category of important mail that you observed when you separated out the junk mail, such as utility bills, credit card bills, mortgage bill/statement, car payment, tax information, receipts.
    *   Place the sticky notes around the table and sort important mail accordingly. After sorting, return the sticky notes to the Incoming Mail box for reuse.
5. File your important mail by categories.
    *   Label file folders based on the categories above.
    *   Make sure one folder is labeled "Unpaid Bills."
6. Put papers into their respective file folders and store in the file or file box.
7. Examine each bill in the Unpaid Bills folder; write the due date on the outside of each envelope.
8. Make reminders for yourself in your CAT, day planner, or calendar on the days on which you actually intend to write checks or pay the bill or bills.

REMEMBER: If you set up and maintain a mail-sorting procedure on a weekly basis, you will reduce the stress of going through mail and be more organized when it comes to paying your bills.

PATIENT HANDOUT: ESTABLISHING A BUDGET

Keeping a budget is difficult for most people, even those without concussion. Having consistent and simple methods for keeping track of your money (to avoid over- or underpayment of bills) can be particularly helpful as people recover from the aftereffects of concussion.

Staying on top of your finances involves three key steps:

1. Estimating your monthly expenses
2. Tracking your actual monthly income and expenses
3. Maintaining bank account balances

Improving Your Budgeting and Financial Management

1. Determine why your financial management process breaks down.
2. Do you have a good handle on what your actual expenses are each month?
3. Are you spending more each month than you estimate?
4. Are you keeping records of what you actually spend each month?
5. Do you have an effective accounting system in place?
6. Set up your own record-keeping systems (see Patient Handout: Budget Planning Worksheet).
7. Use a calculator to make sure your records are accurate.
8. Work with your spouse (or other family members) to set joint financial management goals and work as a team to achieve them. Decide on who is responsible for what based on each person's strengths. Set aside a time each week to log expenses and bank transactions and to problem solve together.

REMEMBER: Learning good financial management habits takes time and practice; be patient with yourself if your first (second or third) efforts are not perfect.

FURTHER RESOURCES

There are several Internet sources that can help you with budget planning, such as:

- http://www.womens-finance.com/monthlybudget.shtml
- http://www.docstoc.com/docs/7923811/Budget-Planner-Worksheets
- http://www.free-financial-advice.net/create-budget.html

PATIENT HANDOUT: BUDGET PLANNING WORKSHEET

Step 1: Estimate your typical income and expenses for each month. Fill in the "Estimated Amounts" column below.

Income and Expense Categories		Estimated amounts
Estimated monthly income	Your monthly take-home pay	
	Your spouse's monthly take-home pay	
	Other work income	
	Financial gifts	
	Investment income	

Estimated Income Total

Estimated monthly expenses	Rent or mortgage	
	Utility: electricity or gas	
	Utility: water	
	Telephone/cell phone/Internet	
	Garbage	
	Groceries	
	Car payment	
	Clothing	
	Gasoline	
	Leisure/eating out	
	Childcare	
	Other:	
	Other:	

Income and Expense Categories

	Other:	

Estimated Expense Total

Step 2: Compare your estimated expense total to your income total.

- If your estimated expenses are greater than your estimated income, determine what expenses you might pare down.
- If your estimated expenses are greater than your estimated income, determine how you might generate more income or if you can afford to dip into your savings.

Step 3: Examine the actual amounts of money available in your bank account(s).

Actual Amount in Checking Account	Actual Amount in Savings Account

PATIENT HANDOUT: BUDGET TRACKING WORKSHEET

Step 1: Transfer your income and expense estimates from the Budget Planning Worksheet.
Step 2: Record your starting bank balances at the beginning of the month.
Step 3: Work with your family members to keep track of what you actually spend this month.
Step 4: At the end of the month, record bank balances and compare estimated to actual monthly expenses.
Step 5: Adjust budget as needed.

Example

Income and Expense Categories		Estimated amounts	Actual amounts for the month of:
Monthly income	Your monthly take-home pay	$2,322.32	$2,322.32
	Your spouse's monthly take-home pay	$1,543.65	$1,543.65
	Other work income		
	Financial gifts		
	Investment income		
Income Total			
Monthly expenses	Rent or mortgage	$950.56	$950.56
	Utility: electricity or gas	$130	$120.76
	Utility: gas/water	$60–70	$57.90
	Telephone/cell phone/internet	$136.10	$136.10
	Garbage/trash	$40.34	$40.34
	Groceries	$110–130	$122.42
	Car payment	$428	$428
	Clothing		$0
	Gasoline	$110–$140	$129.90
	Leisure/eating out	$100–$140	$132
	Childcare		
	Other:		
	Other:		
	Other:		
Expense Total		**$2,065.44–$2,165.44**	**$2,117.98**

Checking account balance at beginning of month	Savings account balance at beginning of month
$2,342.40	$3,245.89

Analysis

- Did I meet my financial goals this month?
  Yes
- What, if anything, do I want to change to better manage my budget next month?
  Eat out less.

PATIENT HANDOUT: BUDGET TRACKING WORKSHEET

Income and Expense Categories		Estimated amounts	Actual amounts for the month of:
Monthly income	Your monthly take-home pay		
	Your spouse's monthly take-home pay		
	Other work income		
	Financial gifts		
	Investment income		
Income Total			
Monthly expenses	Rent or mortgage		
	Utility: electricity or gas		
	Utility: water		
	Telephone/cell phone/Internet		
	Garbage/trash		
	Groceries		
	Car payment		
	Clothing		
	Gasoline		
	Leisure/eating out		
	Childcare		
	Other:		
	Other:		
	Other:		
	Expense Total		

Account	Balance at beginning of month	Balance at end of month
Checking		
Savings		

Analysis

- Did I meet my financial goals this month?

- What, if anything, do I want to change to better manage my budget next month?

PATIENT HANDOUT: BILL PAYING

People can minimize the stress and effort involved in bill paying by setting up monthly routines and procedures for this activity. This is particularly helpful as people recover after concussion.

The following are two examples of bill-paying procedures that you may consider when optimizing your own efficiency in this area.

1. Set up automatic withdrawal/bill-paying with your bank, vendors, and utilities.
   - Several banks and service companies try to make it more convenient for clients to pay their monthly bills by offering to take owed money directly out of a client's bank account.
   - As a consumer, you can call vendors and set up a day for the merchant to take the money out of your account. You will need an email account to receive confirmations and notices from your bank.
   - You can schedule payments to go out of your account in the beginning or towards the end of the month, which reduces the stress of paying a bill every week or so.
   - Use a spreadsheet to keep track of your payments and how much money is due monthly.
   - Balance your account to make sure you have enough money to be withdrawn. Your bank should also send you a new electronic statement to review after any change occurs to your account.
2. Pay your bill by writing a check, mailing the bill, and maintaining the balance of your account.
   - Set up your work space, removing as many distractions as possible.
   - Collect the supplies and materials you need for the task (eg, checkbook, pen, calculator, stamps, checkbook register, deposit slips, notepaper).
   - Make a list of the bills that need to be paid.
   - Write the check for the first bill on your list.
     - Record the check number (top right corner) on the checkbook register.
     - Fill in the appropriate details (eg, date, payee, amount).
     - Write the amount paid in your checkbook register and subtract from your bank balance.
     - Put the check and bill stub in the envelope and seal the envelope. Stamp and add your return address.
   - Cross the bill off your list.
   - Move on to the next bill.
   - Repeat the above steps until all bills are crossed off your list.
   - Put all the bills in the mail.

BALANCING YOUR ACCOUNT (EXAMPLE)

Date	Check No.	Payment type and details (check, credit, deposit; payee)	Amount paid	Deposit	Balance
Example 1/10/14		Credit card payment: Groceries at Kroger's	$156.43	00	Before trans: $1,342.30 After: $1,185.87 Before trans: $1,185.87 After: Before trans: After: Before trans:

PATIENT HANDOUT PACKET: MONEY MANAGEMENT

The goal of this task is to perform financial transactions in which you come up with the correct account balance at the end.

1. Start with a balance of **$1,233.45** in your account.
2. Use the sample blank checks (Figure 9-3) provided to pay the following bills in this order:
   - Wayne's Lawn Care (Figure 9-4)
   - Gas and water bill (Figure 9-5)
   - Charter Cable bill (Figure 9-6)
3. Deposit the following using the sample deposit slip (Figure 9-7):
   - Refund form Wal-Mart: $53.24
   - Check from Kalvin Smith: $476.57
4. Calculate your new account balance.

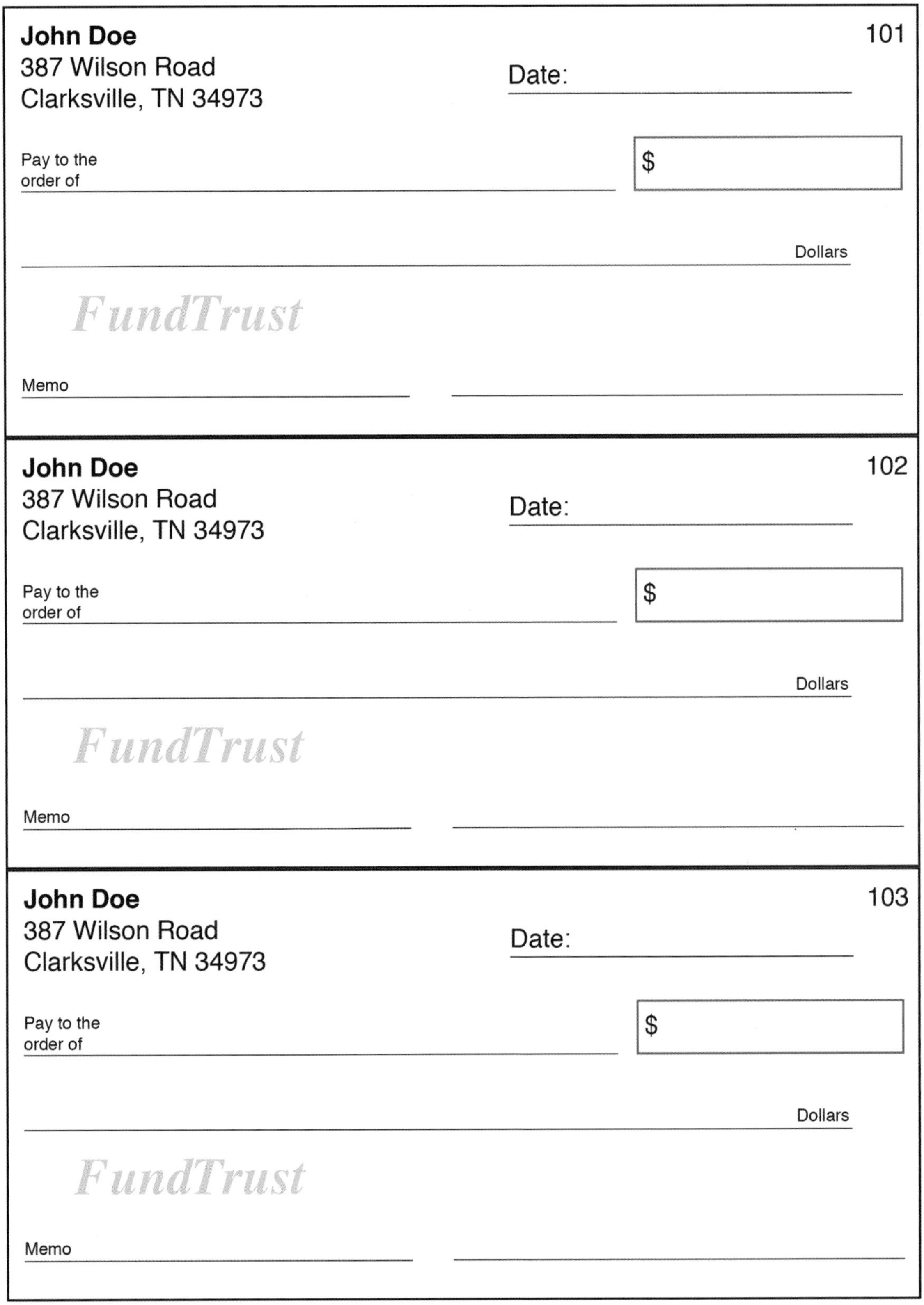

John Doe
387 Wilson Road
Clarksville, TN 34973

101

Date: _____

Pay to the
order of _____ $ [   ]

_____ Dollars

FundTrust

Memo _____   _____

John Doe
387 Wilson Road
Clarksville, TN 34973

102

Date: _____

Pay to the
order of _____ $ [   ]

_____ Dollars

FundTrust

Memo _____   _____

John Doe
387 Wilson Road
Clarksville, TN 34973

103

Date: _____

Pay to the
order of _____ $ [   ]

_____ Dollars

FundTrust

Memo _____   _____

Figure 9-3. Sample blank checks.

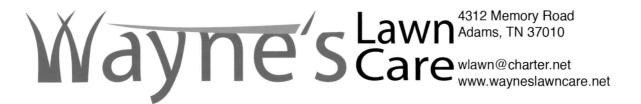

4312 Memory Road
Adams, TN 37010
wlawn@charter.net
www.wayneslawncare.net

Customer:
  John Doe
  387 Wilson Road
  Clarksville, TN 34973

Account #	984928
Invoice #	3865
Invoice Date	14 September 2013

Terms:

Item		
Aerate Lawn	Invoice subtotal	$80.00
	Tax	$0.00
	Invoice total	$80.00
	Total payments for this invoice	$0.00
	Balance due for this invoice	$80.00
	Balance dues from previous invoices	$0
	Total amount owed	$80.00

Figure 9-4. Sample lawn care bill.

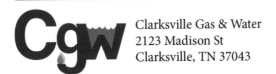
Clarksville Gas & Water
2123 Madison St
Clarksville, TN 37043

Account # 358762987
Billing cycle 4 Dec 2012 – 3 Jan 2013
Payment due by 4 Feb 2013

Customer Information: John Doe
387 Wilson Rd
Clarksville, TN 37043

Meter Location: 387 Wilson Rd
Clarksville, TN 37043

Billing Statement

Payments Received

2 Jan 2013 - $90.14

Outstanding Balance

$0.00

Charges this period		
Gas	$11.65	Reading 2000–2011
Water	$30.61	Reading 73383–73777
Sewer	$43.65	
Tax	$2.91	
Total	**$88.82**	

Usage History	**Previous**	**Type**	**Usage**	**Charge**
Account # 358762987	Nov	Water	2100 Gallons	0
Water meter #	Nov	Gas	900 Cubic Feet	0
Gas meter #	Oct	Water	1200 Gallons	0
	Oct	Gas	2700 Cubic feet	0

Important message

Effective July 13th customer acct number will be changing. Please notify bank or payment services you used to pay your bill.
Look for new numbers on bill after July 13th. Go to CGW website or call 931-098-9786.

- - - - - - - - - - - *Make checks payable to: Clarksville Gas and Water* -

Figure 9-5. Sample gas and water bill.

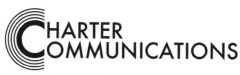

CHARTER COMMUNICATIONS

P.O. Box 31269
Clarksville, TN 34243

Security code
14th of Next Month

John Doe
387 Wilson Road
Clarksville, TN 34973

Account #   20497992875
Phone #   (931)386-9873
Contact us: for billing or questions
visit us @ www.charter.com, or call 1-888-Get Charter

Account Information:
Thank you for choosing Charter Communications. We appreciate your prompt payment and value you as a customer. Charter brings your home to life.

Summary:	
Previous Balance	$80.19
Payment Received	$80.19
Balance Forward	$0
Charter Cable Services	$44.99
Charter Internet Services	$29.99
Adjustments, Taxes and Fees	$5.21
Total Due	**$80.19**

Charter Communications • P.O. Box 31269 • Clarksville, TN 34243

Figure 9-6. Sample cable bill.

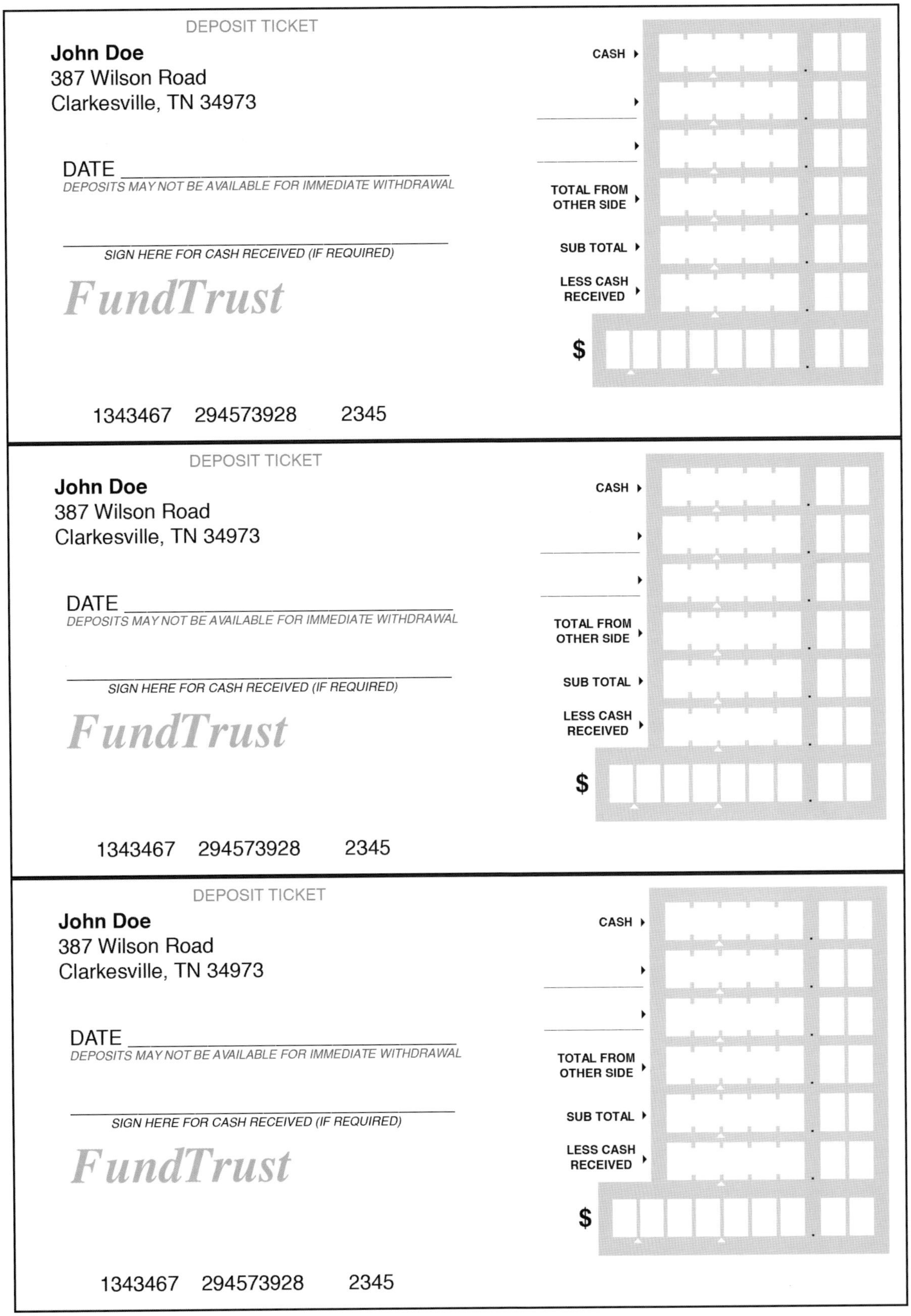

DEPOSIT TICKET

John Doe
387 Wilson Road
Clarkesville, TN 34973

DATE ______________________
DEPOSITS MAY NOT BE AVAILABLE FOR IMMEDIATE WITHDRAWAL

____
SIGN HERE FOR CASH RECEIVED (IF REQUIRED)

FundTrust

CASH ▸
▸
▸
TOTAL FROM OTHER SIDE ▸
SUB TOTAL ▸
LESS CASH RECEIVED ▸
$

1343467 294573928 2345

DEPOSIT TICKET

John Doe
387 Wilson Road
Clarkesville, TN 34973

DATE ______________________
DEPOSITS MAY NOT BE AVAILABLE FOR IMMEDIATE WITHDRAWAL

____
SIGN HERE FOR CASH RECEIVED (IF REQUIRED)

FundTrust

CASH ▸
▸
▸
TOTAL FROM OTHER SIDE ▸
SUB TOTAL ▸
LESS CASH RECEIVED ▸
$

1343467 294573928 2345

DEPOSIT TICKET

John Doe
387 Wilson Road
Clarkesville, TN 34973

DATE ______________________
DEPOSITS MAY NOT BE AVAILABLE FOR IMMEDIATE WITHDRAWAL

____
SIGN HERE FOR CASH RECEIVED (IF REQUIRED)

FundTrust

CASH ▸
▸
▸
TOTAL FROM OTHER SIDE ▸
SUB TOTAL ▸
LESS CASH RECEIVED ▸
$

1343467 294573928 2345

Figure 9-7. Sample deposit slips.

CHECKBOOK REGISTER ACTIVITY

Date	Check #	Payment Type (Check, Credit, Deposit)	Amount Paid	Deposit	Balance: $1,233.45
					Before trans:
					After:
					Before trans:
					After:
					Before trans:
					After:
					Before trans:
					After:
					Before trans:
					After:
					Before trans:
					After:
					Before trans:
					After:
					Before trans:
					After:

PATIENT HANDOUT: USING A SMARTPHONE OR PLANNER TO MANAGE MONEY

The calendar on your cell phone, organizer, or day planner comes in handy for keeping track of your money and making sure you pay your bills on time. By using the calendar feature, you can input specific times and dates to remind you of when you intend to pay certain bills.

Using a Cell Phone to Create Reminders

- Go to the calendar setting and select a date.
- Type "pay bills" in the subject line.
- Set a reminder alarm for 3 days prior to due date.
- When the phone reminder goes off, make sure you write a check, post the envelope, and mail the payment.
- Consider adding a reminder note to your planner just in case your alarm doesn't go off as planned.

Using a Planner or Organizer to Manage Money

- When you receive a bill, open it and write the due date on the outside of the envelope.
- Decide by what date you must pay and mail the bill so it will be paid on time.
- Make a note on the calendar prompting you to pay a given bill on the date specified. If your budget allows, try to specify one or two days each month to pay all your bills.
- Establish a daily routine for reviewing your planner; that way you will see bill-paying prompts on the days you specified.

PATIENT HANDOUT: UNDERSTANDING YOUR CHILD'S WORLD—INFANT (0–1 YEAR OLD)

Age-Appropriate Behaviors

Infants' understanding of the world around them is based on their age and their life experiences. We would not expect a 3-year-old to be able to sit for a 30-minute conversation, but we would not think twice about asking a 17-year-old to do the same. Successful engagement with your child is somewhat dependent on your ability to understand the world in which they live. This handout is designed to help you identify age-appropriate play activities that the two of you can do successfully.

How Does My Child Play?

Infants learn through play. During the first year of life, infants' play is exploratory and we are often unable to identify their activity as play. They do this through contact with others, playing with their hands and feet, and engaging in the world around them; remember, their world is only what they see in front of them at any given moment. Babies are interested in others who talk, sing, and explore their world. Infants will seek out parents or siblings as their first choice for play "toys."

What Games Does My Infant Play?

Games such as peek-a-boo, dancing with the child in your arms, floor play, and singing games are all effective ways to engage infants and help them learn about the world around them. Looking at picture books and listening to music are wonderful ways to share time with your infant. As your baby grows and begins to roll and crawl, toys that move, such as trucks and trains, will provide turn-taking activities.

Activities for Infants 0 to 6 Months Old

- Talk and sing when you are doing activities like changing, bathing, or feeding the child.
- Play with your child's toes and fingers, and say the names of body parts.
- Place high contrast and colorful objects where the baby can see and begin to reach for them.
- Walk with the infant and rock, sing songs, and bounce.
- Engage in floor time as well as other positions during play.
- Play with toys that make sounds (soothing) and play music.[1]

Activities for Infants 6 to 12 Months Old

- Play peek-a-boo and other hiding games.
- Promote crawling and pulling up in safe places.
- Promote playing with toys that react when they are touched or squeezed.
- Provide teething toys.
- When your child is upset, console by rocking and holding.
- Let your child fill containers and dump them out.
- Provide your child with pots, pans, and a wooden spoon.
- Change toys often when babies get bored with them.[1]

What are Typical Infant Behaviors?

Don't be surprised if your infant seems to be enjoying your time together one minute and is screaming the next. Infants are not able to understand subtle changes in their bodies, so they may be content and happy while the two of you play, only to realize they are hungry, wet, and unhappy about it. This quick turn of events will require you to quickly change your behavior as well. The "turn on a dime" behaviors seen in infants, although frustrating, are a normal part of the developmental process.

Parenting an Infant After Sustaining Concussion

- Infants are exhausting not only because of their sleep patterns but because they require constant attention. This becomes more evident once they are mobile. Be aware of your level of fatigue as this can influence your thinking skills and overall performance.
- You will have to be attentive to your child or be aware of what he or she is doing almost all of the time. Dual tasking, like watching television, playing video games, or talking with/texting friends while watching your infant may be unsafe.
- If you have issues with memory, double check the safety of your surroundings; close doors, latch safety gates, and keep hot or sharp items out of reach.
- Ask for help when you need it. If you need a brief break, place your infant in a safe place (such as a crib) and leave the room. Your child will be fine for a few minutes while you reset.
- Never leave your child alone in the home without supervision by an adult or child older than 14.
- Incorporate cognitive strategies you have used for other activities, such as work and school, to the home and your role as a parent.
- Most of all, have fun!

Takeaways

Use this space to list three activities you will do with your infant.

1.

2.

3.

1. National Network for Child Care. Helping infants learn. In: Lopes M, ed. *CareGiver News*. 1993:4. Amherst, MA: University of Massachusetts Cooperative Extension.

**PATIENT HANDOUT: UNDERSTANDING YOUR CHILD'S WORLD—
TODDLER (1–3 YEARS OLD)**

Age-Appropriate Behaviors

A child's understanding of the world around them is based on his or her age and his or her life experiences. We wouldn't expect a 3-year-old to be able to sit for a 30-minute conversation but we wouldn't think twice about asking a 17-year-old to do the same. Successful engagement with your child is somewhat dependent on your ability to understand the world in which they live. This handout is designed to help you identify age-appropriate play activities that the two of you can do successfully.

How Does My Child Play?

Toddlers are active learners who are continuing to develop the fine and gross motor skills they will need as they get older. At this age, they are becoming more interested in other children and will begin to play alongside them. Younger toddlers will have difficulty sharing and cooperating, so it is a good idea to have enough materials for you and your child to complete an activity. That being said, encourage turn-taking while speaking and playing. Language development is on the rise during these years. In addition, your toddler may look to you to model play behavior and copy what you have done.

What Does My Toddler Play?

Children this age will spend hours putting things in containers and dumping them out. They will begin building with sand, play dough, and clay. They become increasingly interested in music and dance. These gross motor activities also include outdoor playgrounds, walks, and throwing and chasing balls. Toddlers will put things in their mouth as a means of exploration, so be sure to watch these children carefully.

Toddlers love to play with a variety of household objects and will often toss a fancy doll for a 99-cent kitchen spoon. Activities and toys encourage the child's imagination, and as you play with your toddler, promote imaginative and dramatic play. Some toys the two of you can enjoy together include blocks, riding toys, dolls, pots and pans, stuffed animals, dress-up clothes, cars/trucks/trains, books, some arts and crafts, and music.

Activities for Toddlers

- Fill and dump containers.
- Make play dough.
- Sink or water table play (be sure the child is supervised at all times).
- Pretend play and building. Ask your local appliance shop for a cardboard box from a refrigerator or other large appliance. Cut doors and windows in the box to make a playhouse.
- Draw with different-sized crayons. Different sizes help with toddlers' fine motor skills and hand muscle development.
- Messy play. Finger paint with shaving cream mixed with food coloring.
- Jumping. Place pillows, cushions, or a mattress on the floor and let your toddler bounce and jump.
- Playground play. Some swings, climbing equipment, and low slides are appropriate for this age group.
- Go for lots of walks. Encourage your toddler to practice walking and running.
- Help your toddler practice climbing stairs.
- Play house with dolls and housekeeping props, such as plastic dishes and spoons.[1]

What are Typical Toddler Behaviors?

Because their language skills are just beginning to emerge, toddlers have a difficult time expressing their needs and feelings. This is often the source of the toddler "meltdown." Be aware of the pre-meltdown signs during play. These may include physically changing their space, decreased eye contact, increased laughter, or sudden fatigue.

Toddlers are movers who constantly run from one activity to another. Although they need structure to predict what comes next, highly structured activities like board games and play with numerous rules are difficult and can become a source of frustration for the child and the caregiver.

Interacting With a Toddler

- Provide choices; if the parent or caregiver provides two choices for an activity, the child feels in control of their environment and activities. Instead of saying, "It's time to read a book," say, "Would you like to read a book and then brush your teeth or would you like to brush your teeth first and then read a book?"
- Acknowledge the toddler's feelings. Instead of saying, "There's no reason to be upset that you spilled the bubbles," say "I can see you're sad about spilling that container of bubbles. Would you like to make more?"
- Avoid environments that require the child to stay still and quiet for long periods of time.
- Be flexible in your activities and the time you spend with each one.
- Set limits to help the child understand what is expected.
- Provide positive reinforcements during games and activities.
- Let the child know how much you enjoy playing with him/her.
- Position yourself at eye level with the child during games and activities, when possible.
- Most of all, have fun!

Takeaways

In the space below, list three activities you will do with your toddler.

1.

2.

3.

1. National Network for Child Care; Miller L. Play activities for children birth to nine years. *Family Day Care Facts*. Amherst, MA: University of Massachusetts. 1991.

PATIENT HANDOUT: UNDERSTANDING THE STRUCTURE OF PLAY
AND PARENT-CHILD ACTIVITIES

Background

The elements of play may seem routine on the surface. Games such as patty-cake, building with Legos (Lego Systems, Inc, Enfield, CT), imaginary pirates, or a backyard game of basketball, despite their familiarity, are complex and fall within a continuum of structure and cooperation.

Throughout the therapy process, an emphasis has been placed on your ability to identify skills that are strengths and some that present a challenge. Self-reflections on task demands and the strategies you have adopted can easily be translated into the activities you do with your children. If needed, effective planning and strategy implementation can make the wonderful and challenging job of parenting a positive experience for you and your children. This handout provides some suggestions that may help you understand which, if any, strategies you may use when spending time with your child (**Figure 9-8**).

What are the Structures of Play?

All activities and play have some type of structure. They typically fall into three categories: structured, semi-structured, and unstructured.

"Structure" refers to the level of variability that an activity allows in order to successfully complete it. For example, in the areas of play, a **structured** activity may be building a model. To complete an airplane model correctly, you must perform the steps in a specific order (eg, you would not put the wings on without first having a stable body). Successful completion of one step is based on successful completion of previous ones.

A **semi-structured** task is an activity that presents with a logical sequence, but there are a number of different ways to reach the end (eg, constructing a puzzle). You are given the materials to complete the task and you know exactly what the final product will look like, but there is an infinite number of ways you can go from the first step (eg, opening the box and pouring out the puzzle pieces) to the final step (eg, fitting the last piece).

An **unstructured** activity is one in which the directions and rules are minimal. An unstructured play activity you may engage in with your child is sand play; you have the materials (sand) but there are few rules or outcome expectations identified. As the two of you play together, unstructured play may quickly become semi-structured as you negotiate what you may build, how to go about it, and what it may look like in the end.

The Importance of Understanding Activity and Play Structure After Concussion

The various levels of structure in play activities will require you to use different cognitive skill sets. These skill sets become even more critical when engaging in an activity with another person, especially a child. Because various levels of structure, as related to play, will tax different cognitive skills, you may use various cognitive strategies to make the activities easier for you.

Level of Structure	Examples of Activities	Cognitive Demands Associated with Level of Structure
Structured (typically this level of structure is not tolerated by infants and toddlers. At the age of 5, children begin to engage in more structured play successfully).	Model building, some cooking activities (eg, baking), construction tasks, board games, video games, many sports	Organization and planning, sequencing, error detection and correction, attention to detail, memory, time management, ability to shift focus, ability to understand and follow rules and directions
Semi-structured (toddlers to adult-age children)	Puzzles, arts and crafts, pretend play, some sports, some video-games	Task initiation, organization and planning, error detection and correction, flexibility, time management, attention
Unstructured (all ages)	Some arts and crafts, such as free drawing and play dough, sand play, water play, dancing	Task initiation, creative thinking, planning and organization, flexibility, time management

> **REMEMBER: When choosing play activities to do with your children, be sure to consider the level of structure in the activity and how the structure may present cognitive demands; being aware of potential challenges can greatly increase the success and enjoyment of the activities you choose to do with your child.**

Takeaways

Consider the following questions as you plan activity time with your children.

- Currently, what level of structure works best for you as you play with your children?
- What cognitive strategies might make fun time with your children more satisfying and enjoyable for you and them?

PATIENT HANDOUT: UNDERSTANDING THE ENVIRONMENT OF PLAY AND THE ROLE OF COOPERATION IN CHILD-RELATED ACTIVITIES

Environment of Play

We spend time with our families in every environment imaginable: home, grocery store, places of worship, parks, friends' homes, schools, libraries, and others. Each of these settings presents different environmental conditions that may influence your ability to engage with your child.

Take a moment to review the following list of environmental characteristics. For each environmental characteristic, rate the extent to which it helps or detracts from "fun time" with your child by placing a checkmark in the appropriate column.

Environmental Characteristic	Helps me enjoy my time with my child	Detracts from my time with my child	Neither – No effect on my time with my child
Crowds			
Light and glare			
Noise (volume)			
Noise (in the background)			
Temperature (hot or cold)			
Time of day			
Colors in a room			
How the environment is organized			
Physical space (too large or too small)			
Knowledge of exits			
Other:			
Other:			

When planning activities with the family, be aware of how these environmental factors may influence your ability to make this a successful experience for you and your children. Here are some suggestions.

- Go to the playground early in the day or later in the evening when it will be less crowded and you will be less distracted. If you have light sensitivity, the early morning and evening hours will make it a more pleasant experience for you.
- During shopping activities, avoid big stores if possible. Go to a smaller local store where there are fewer distractions for you and your child.
- Plan family activities around the time of day you feel most able to participate. This may be early in the morning or later in the afternoon.
- If you have concerns about public places, be sure to spend some time exploring the space to alleviate those concerns. This will help you better engage with your family members.
- Be aware of the environmental demands and use the strategies you have learned with your therapist to successfully engage with your family members.

Takeaways

In the space below, list two things that, based on this information, you will do next time you take your children out for a fun activity in the community.

1.

2.

Activities and Collaboration

Similar to a continuum of structure, when engaging in activities with your child, the activity you choose has an element of collaboration and cooperation. Often the amount of cooperation can be modified by providing more materials or taking away materials. In general, activities that require cooperation tend to involve greater levels of communication and satisfaction. Consider how you can orchestrate the cooperation and interaction characteristics of an activity by how you set up a simple family meal.

If you are having a family dinner and each person is given a plate of food that comes from the kitchen, there is little need to ask for things on the table. All the family members have what they need at every given time during the meal, but there are fewer requirements for communication. This situation places low demand on family cooperation. Conversely, if you sit down at the table with the food in the middle and family members are expected to serve themselves (family style), the situation is conducive to more collaboration and discussion. This situation places high demand on family cooperation, but provides the opportunity to practice healthy cooperation and negotiation.

The nature of participating in activities with your child, be it a family dinner or a play task, is basically the same. Think about the activity ahead of time and consider how you are feeling as you begin the activity with your child. Make choices about just how much cooperation you want to build into the activity. For example, if one or both of you are tired, you may decide to work in parallel on your model airplane. Minimize the conversation or sharing by working on separate task components. If you are interested in increasing the likelihood of working cooperatively together, work together on one component of the model airplane or limit the availability of tools and materials so that you need to share.

Insight into how various activities influence collaboration between you and your child is important when choosing activities that will promote a healthy reengagement after your injury. Remember that children younger than 3 will have a hard time sharing and collaborating on a project, so have materials for both of you to use.

> **REMEMBER: Sharing supplies and materials during an activity generally leads to greater levels of communication and cooperation.**

Takeaways

Think of one activity that you enjoy with your child or children. List three things you can change about how you organize or perform this activity to increase the cooperation and communication involved.

1.

2.

3.

PATIENT HANDOUT: RECONNECTING WITH YOUR SPOUSE OR SIGNIFICANT OTHER

Background

Returning to a loved one after deployment can fill you with anticipation and excitement as well as apprehension. The emotions are even more complex if you are coming home with injuries. This handout provides some basic information to prepare you for the process of reconnecting with your spouse or significant other; we encourage you to seek out other resources that are available to you as well.

Points to Keep in Mind

After your return home, the "new normal" may take weeks to months to establish. It is normal for things to be awkward between you and your spouse at first. Be open to communication, be flexible, share your experiences, and listen to your loved one's concerns.

Remember that you may continue to experience issues associated with your concussion after returning home. Sometimes people experience symptoms as they encounter new challenges or try to function in the less-structured environments of home. Despite the possibility of physical and cognitive consequences of your injuries, returning to the role of "present spouse" after a long absence is both exciting and anxiety provoking for you and your loved one. Be patient with yourself and your spouse during the first 6 months to year; the process of reengaging takes time.

Share

Share your feelings with your spouse about what is going on and what has happened to you. Encourage your loved one to share his or her feelings as well. Listen to what your loved one shares and validate his or her feelings; both of you have gone through a number of changes and have experienced quite a bit on your own. The best way for the two of you to reengage is to communicate and spend time talking and sharing.

Educate

Educate your spouse about mTBI, what it is, and behaviors often associated with this diagnosis. Your partner may not understand why you are sleeping so much, avoiding bright lights, having constant headaches, or failing to pay attention. Let your loved one know how the injury has impacted you and what you have done during the rehabilitation process to decrease the associated symptoms. Help him or her become part of your recovery process.

Ask

Ask questions about how the household was managed while you were gone. Your loved one had to adopt a new routine, which may have included taking care of kids, assisting other military spouses and providing support, paying bills, dealing with family-related health issues, and doing yard work and home maintenance, to name a few. Do not be critical of those tasks that may have fallen to the bottom of the priority list and be sure to acknowledge the significant amount of work your loved one did during your absence. Your partner may love to return many of these duties to you. Discuss this with your loved one and work on slowly resuming "normal" household and partner duties.

Communicate

Communicate your needs and let your partner know why you ask for things. Your spouse may have planned a full schedule with friends and family upon your return home. If you feel as though you are unable to tolerate a busy schedule, ask to begin slowly and work with your spouse on scheduling events and activities.

Use Resources

Use the resources available to members of the military who are returning home with or without an injury. Reconnecting can be difficult for both you and your partner, and support may be needed. Bring your spouse to your rehabilitation sessions so treatments and goal setting can include his or her concerns as well as your own.

Teach

Teach your partner many of the strategies you have adopted to ensure success in different areas; he or she can act as a reinforcer or reminder for strategy use. If needed, incorporate these into home and family routines.

FURTHER RESOURCES

The following are additional places where you can find help returning to family life after deployment.

- Beyond The Yellow Ribbon: Bringing Soldiers and Their Families All the Way Home. http://www.beyondtheyellowribbon.org/home. A website of the Minnesota National Guard. Accessed October 25, 2013.
- Reintegrating into Family Life After Deployment. A website provided by the Defense Centers of Excellence. http://www.realwarriors.net/active/afterdeployment/familylife.php. Accessed October 25, 2013.

PATIENT HANDOUT: REENGAGING IN HOUSEHOLD ROLES AND ACTIVITIES

Background

During your absence, your loved one became responsible for running the home and all the responsibilities related to the household. At times, the additional responsibility was welcome. Success may have generated a sense of accomplishment and contribution not felt before. At the same time, the additional responsibilities may have become burdensome and presented unwelcome challenges.

Resuming the traditional roles each of you had prior to your deployment and injury may be difficult; however, assuming your partner will continue with all he or she had taken on is unrealistic. This handout and the worksheet that follows are designed to help you and your partner identify ways in which you can work together at home. Use the worksheet as a way to negotiate role resumption and develop new routines together.

Considerations for Discussion Between You and Your Partner as You Reestablish Household Roles

- Am I limited by any deficits or problems (physical, cognitive, visual, social, emotional) that will prevent me from successfully resuming a role?
- Do I currently have any activity restrictions that may prevent me from successfully resuming a role (ie, driving)?
- Are there any other barriers that prevent me from resuming a role (ie, motivation, interest, time, lack of competence)?
- What roles are most important for me to resume and what roles are most important for my partner to maintain?
- What roles do I not wish to resume or take on, and what roles does my partner hope to relinquish?
- Do my partner and I argue over any of the identified roles and associated activities? If so, what is the source of the argument (we both want to do it, neither of us wants to do it, being critical of the other's performance or style)?

Once you and your spouse have determined how to reassign home and family responsibilities, it is important to develop a plan and reflect on role negotiation and performance as a team. Set aside a time each week to coordinate your household family activities for the upcoming week. Use daily planners and calendars to help organize and develop these together.

Example

Week of 12/20	Laundry	Yard Work	Cooking	Take Kids to School	Pick up Kids	Pay Bills
Monday			Joe	Joe	Jane	Jane
Tuesday			Jane	Jane	Joe	
Wednesday	Jane		Joe	Joe	Jane	
Thursday			Jane	Jane	Joe	
Friday			Joe	Joe	Jane	
Saturday	Jane		Eat out			
Sunday		Joe	Together			

Keep a journal and identify when role conflict occurred between you and your spouse and what was done to resolve the conflict. Talk together about the conflict to gain the other's perspective. Bring the journal entries and calendars to therapy and use these as a source of discussion and reflection on performance.

REMEMBER: Communication with your partner is key to successful role negotiation.

PATIENT HANDOUT: DIVIDING UP ROLES WITH YOUR SPOUSE

This handout is to be completed by the patient's spouse. An alternative version may be developed to explore predeployment roles and desire to resume.

PART A:

The purpose of this worksheet is to explore roles you participated in before, during, and after your partner's deployment. Roles in the areas of home management, finances, parenting, future planning, and work distribution are considered.

Role	Before Deployment	During Deployment	After Deployment	Desire to Continue (Yes or No)
Home Management				
Shopping				
Cleaning				
Home repair				
Yard work				
Laundry				
Pet care				
Cooking				
Finances				
Budgeting				
Bill paying				
Banking				
Insurance				
Wills				
Credit cards				
Mortgage				
Parenting				
Discipline				
Transportation				
Scheduling				
Medical issues				

Help with school				
Volunteering for kid activity				
Morning routine				
Bedtime routine				
Gift buying				

Other

Auto repair				
Vacation plans				
Moving-related activity				
Visitors				
Retirement planning				
Other				

PART B:

- List those roles you want to relinquish:

- List those roles you want to maintain:

- Which roles are areas of conflict with your partner?

- Which roles are you willing to negotiate on?

Data source: Gambardella LC. Role-exit theory and marital discord following extended military deployment. *Perspect Psychiatr Care.* Jul 2008;44(3):169–174.

**PATIENT HANDOUT: RETURN TO SCHOOL NEEDS ASSESSMENT—
ESSENTIAL SKILLS FOR COLLEGE SUCCESS**

Name: _____ Date _____

Check all that apply:

_____ I am enrolled in school this semester.

_____ I am planning on enrolling in school within the year.

_____ I am a part-time student.

_____ I am a full-time student.

Directions: Using the scale below each item, please rate how difficult is it (or if you are not in school at present, how concerned you are regarding the items below) for you to:

1. Listen to instructor and take notes at the same time

   0 = not at all   1= a little bit   2 = moderately   3 = quite a bit   4 = extremely

2. Pay attention to the instructor because you are distracted by people or situations that seem threatening

   0 = not at all   1= a little bit   2 = moderately   3 = quite a bit   4 = extremely

3. Stay awake in class

   0 = not at all   1= a little bit   2 = moderately   3 = quite a bit   4 = extremely

4. Pay attention to the instructor because your mind wanders

   0 = not at all   1= a little bit   2 = moderately   3 = quite a bit   4 = extremely

5. Ask the instructor a question or for clarification and additional explanation

   0 = not at all   1= a little bit   2 = moderately   3 = quite a bit   4 = extremely

6. Focus while reading at home

   0 = not at all   1= a little bit   2 = moderately   3 = quite a bit   4 = extremely

7. Focus while reading at work or school

   0 = not at all   1= a little bit   2 = moderately   3 = quite a bit   4 = extremely

8. Remember what you have learned when taking a test

   0 = not at all   1= a little bit   2 = moderately   3 = quite a bit   4 = extremely

9. Organize notes from lectures

   0 = not at all   1= a little bit   2 = moderately   3 = quite a bit   4 = extremely

10. Decide what to write about in a paper

    0 = not at all   1= a little bit   2 = moderately   3 = quite a bit   4 = extremely

11. Write a paper (including locating, collecting, and organizing the information needed to write the paper)

    0 = not at all   1= a little bit   2 = moderately   3 = quite a bit   4 = extremely

12. Finish homework projects, assignments, and papers on time

    0 = not at all   1= a little bit   2 = moderately   3 = quite a bit   4 = extremely

13. Remember to bring completed assignments to class

    0 = not at all   1= a little bit   2 = moderately   3 = quite a bit   4 = extremely

14. Start working on a project or assignment (paper) so you have plenty of time to complete (not starting at the last minute)

    0 = not at all   1= a little bit   2 = moderately   3 = quite a bit   4 = extremely

15. Remember verbal instructions for complex projects

    0 = not at all   1= a little bit   2 = moderately   3 = quite a bit   4 = extremely

16. Complete assigned reading material

    0 = not at all   1= a little bit   2 = moderately   3 = quite a bit   4 = extremely

17. Work with others on group assignments

    0 = not at all   1= a little bit   2 = moderately   3 = quite a bit   4 = extremely

18. Write so others can read and understand what you have written

    0 = not at all   1= a little bit   2 = moderately   3 = quite a bit   4 = extremely

19. Make oral presentations in class

    0 = not at all   1= a little bit   2 = moderately   3 = quite a bit   4 = extremely

20. Stay motivated to put your best effort into school for the entire semester

    0 = not at all   1= a little bit   2 = moderately   3 = quite a bit   4 = extremely

21. Keep a balance between school and other things going on in your life (eg, family, job, health, etc)

    0 = not at all   1= a little bit   2 = moderately   3 = quite a bit   4 = extremely

22. Keep your emotions (anger, frustration) toward instructors and fellow classmates under control

    0 = not at all   1= a little bit   2 = moderately   3 = quite a bit   4 = extremely

23. How hopeful are you that you will succeed in school?

    0 = not at all   1= a little bit   2 = moderately   3 = quite a bit   4 = extremely

---

PATIENT HANDOUT: STUDY-READING SYSTEMS

[S]URVEY, [Q]UESTION, [R]EAD, [R]ECORD, [R]ECITE, [R]EVIEW

This handout outlines "SQ4R," a system designed to assist your comprehension and retention of material while reading.

SURVEY*

Preview the entire book

- ❑ Survey the introduction or preface
- ❑ Survey the table of contents
- ❑ Survey appendices, glossaries, and references
- ❑ Flip through the pages to see how the information is organized

Preview the chapter

- ❑ Read the introductory section and make predictions about the content
- ❑ Read the headings and subheadings
- ❑ Look for pictures, graphs, charts, and tables
- ❑ Read the summary at the end of the chapter

QUESTION†

- ❑ Read the questions at the end of the chapter for main concepts and important details
- ❑ Develop your own who, what, how, when, where, which, and why questions about the information
- ❑ Compare the information with your opinions and previous knowledge
- ❑ Understand the main ideas of pictures, graphs, charts, and tables
- ❑ Look up unfamiliar words

READ/RECORD‡

- ❑ Read the text in a systematic manner from start to end
- ❑ Take notes either in the book or on notepaper
- ❑ Summarize the information in your own words; if you are having difficulty, implement a strategy to overcome barriers (eg, reduce the demands, shorten your study time, eliminate distractions, or take a break)

RECITE§

- ❑ Recite answers to questions aloud in your own words, check your notes or the text for accuracy, ask for clarification if you don't understand the information
- ❑ Provide examples cited in the text or from your own knowledge or experiences

REVIEW¥

- ❑ Review your notes and test yourself frequently to retain information for the test
- ❑ Define new vocabulary
- ❑ Write a summary of the chapter using your own words

---

*Similar to briefing or overview of mission.
†Similar to operational guidelines.
‡Similar to perform duties, carry out mission, record.
§Similar to debriefing.
¥Similar to after-action report.

FURTHER RESOURCES

- Holschuh JP, Aultman LP. Comprehension development. In: Flippo RF, Caverly DC, eds. *Handbook of College Reading and Study Strategy Research*. 2nd ed. New York, NY: Routledge; 2009:121–144.
- Robinson FP. *Effective Study*. New York, NY: Harper & Brothers; 1946.

PATIENT HANDOUT: NOTE-TAKING STRATEGIES

Note taking plays a critical role in academic success and is required in multiple contexts and formats, including listening to lectures or instructions and taking notes while reading textbooks, articles, or on-screen electronic text. Note taking during lectures requires you to attend to and process information, select key details, and write or type notes while simultaneously processing incoming information. A second major aspect of note taking comes after the lecture, when you revise your notes to summarize, fill in, or clarify information.

Invest the time to implement the following suggestions before, during, and after the lecture.

Before the Lecture

Prepare yourself to learn by[1,2]:

- Arriving early to class to select a seat where you will not be distracted.
- Checking the course syllabus or purpose of the briefing to anticipate what the instructor is likely to present.
- Reading assignments before class to understand main ideas, formulate questions, and become familiar with terminology.
- Doing a quick review of previous lecture notes.

During the Lecture

Listen actively by[1]:

- Developing the intention to learn in the lecture and getting involved in the ideas being presented.
- Developing notes that will allow quick review of key concepts that are likely to be on the test.
- Asking or answering questions and seeking clarification while the information is fresh in your mind.
- Generating questions and formulating answers of information that might be on the test.

If you lose concentration[1]:

- Use "self-talk" to manage attention lapses (eg, "I will relax, breathe, and refocus on what I am doing").
- Leave space between points and paragraphs if you miss information so you can fill in blanks later.
- Keep a notecard in view to remind you to focus.
- Write down cues to help remind you of the topic.
- Use a smartpen or audio recorder to retrieve missed information.

How to take notes and what to write down[1–3]:

- Take notes consistently, but do not try to write down every word; focus on facts, definitions, or formulas
- Translate ideas into your own words.
- If the instructor is using slides, write down the main idea from each slide.
- Write main ideas with a few supporting details. Organize as you write:
  - Leave space to elaborate (eg, information from your textbook that complements the lecture).
  - Use indentation to distinguish major from minor supporting points.
  - Develop a system of abbreviations and symbols.
  - Draw pictures or diagrams to help visualize information (mapping).
- Be aware of the following cues that may signal the importance of topics or details and highlight them in your notes:
  - Information reviewed from past classes.

- Information repeated or restated during class, recapped at the end of class, or written on the board.
- Amount of time spent on a point and number of examples provided.
- Word hints, such as, "This is key information," "Make sure you understand this," "These are the key points," "Got it?"
- Nonverbal cues from the lecturer, such as pauses, change in intonation, and gestures.

After the Lecture[1,3]

- Take 5 minutes to review your notes after class to change, organize, add, delete, summarize, or clarify information.
- Review and revise your notes to fill in missing information, highlight key information, or link new information to your existing knowledge base.
- Write down key words to cue your recall of important information.
- Formulate questions that may be asked on a quiz.
- If you do not understand information presented during the lecture, check your textbook, or request clarification from the instructor after class or during office hours.
- Review your notes at regular intervals to keep the information in your memory.

REMINDER: Test preparation starts the first day of class with note taking and developing a study schedule.

FURTHER RESOURCES

- Penn State University, Center for Academic Achievement. http://www.sl.psu.edu/Documents/Note_Taking_Strategies.pdf. Accessed October 28, 2013.
- James Madison University. Learning Toolbox. http://coe.jmu.edu/LearningToolbox/index.html. Accessed October 28, 2013.
- California Polytechnic State University, Student Academic Services, Academic Skills Center. Lecture Notes. http://www.sas.calpoly.edu/asc/ssl/lecturenotes.html. Accessed October 28, 2013.

PATIENT HANDOUT: TEST-TAKING STRATEGIES

Before the Test

- Develop a schedule to review notes and study guides, and self-test.
- Make sure that you attend the class meeting before the exam. The teacher often provides information about the material that will be on the test or other information that may be helpful.
- Request accommodations through the Office for Students With Disabilities (or similar) on campus if needed (eg, taking the test in a nondistracting environment).
- Arrive early to allow yourself time to prepare your mind and body to perform optimally and secure a preferred seat in the classroom.

During the Test

- Survey the test to quickly develop a "plan of attack."
  - Allocate your time accordingly (eg, you may need more time to answer essay questions).
  - Consider answering the easy questions first.
- Read instructions and questions. Underline key points to consider when responding. Ask for clarification if you don't understand.
- For multiple-choice questions:
  - Think of the answer before you read the choices.
  - Eliminate obvious wrong answers.
  - Consider that technically worded choices are not always the correct answer.
- For true-or-false questions, attend to qualifiers and keywords (eg, usually, sometimes, generally, always, or never).
- For essay questions:
  - Make an outline before writing the essay to organize your thoughts.
  - Answer the questions completely. Some may have multiple components.
  - Avoid long introductions or conclusions.
  - If the question asks for facts, don't provide opinions.
- Mark difficult questions. Revisit these later if you have time.
- Answer all questions if there is not a penalty for guessing.
- Proofread your work to correct errors (eg, spelling, grammar, and punctuation) that may lower your grade.

FURTHER REFERENCES

- Hooper CH. *Practicing College Learning Strategies*. 5th ed. Belmont, CA: Wadsworth Publishing; 2009: 192–227.
- California Polytechnic State University Student Academic Services, Academic Skills Center. http://sas.calpoly.edu/asc/ssl/objectivetesttaking.html. Accessed October 28, 2013.
- Landsburgher J. Study Guides and Strategies Web site. *Ten Tips for Terrific Test Taking*. http://www.studygs.net/tsttak1.htm. Accessed October 28, 2013.
- Southwestern University Center for Academic Success. Test Taking Strategies. http://www.southwestern.edu/offices/success/assistance/skilldevelopment/testtaking.php. Accessed October 28, 2013.
- Test Taking Tips. http://www.testtakingtips.com/. Accessed October 28, 2013.

PATIENT HANDOUT: TOPOGRAPHICAL SYMBOLS ON A MILITARY MAP

Conditions

You are given a standard 1:50,000-scale military map.

Standards

Identify topographic symbols, colors, and marginal information on a military map with 100% accuracy.

Performance Steps

1. Identify the colors on a military map.
   - Ideally, every feature on the portion of the earth being mapped is shown on the map in its true shape and size. Unfortunately, that is impossible.
   - The amount of detail shown on a map increases or decreases, depending on its scale; for example, on a map with a scale of 1:250,000, 1 inch shows 4 miles.
   - Details are shown by topographic symbols. These symbols are shown using six basic colors (see Table 1 below).

TABLE 1

COLORS ON TOPOGRAPHIC MAPS

Colors	Symbols
Black	Cultural (human-made) features (other than roads)
Blue	Water
Brown	All relief features (contour lines on old maps, cultivated land on red-light readable maps)
Green	Vegetation
Red	Major roads, built-up areas, special features on old maps
Red-Brown	All relief features and main roads on red-light readable maps

2. Identify the symbols used on a military map to represent physical features, such as physical surroundings or objects, as shown in Table 2.

TABLE 2

FEATURES ON TOPOGRAPHIC MAPS

Features	Colors	Description
Drainage	Blue	These symbols include lakes, streams, rivers, marshes, swamps, and coastal waters.
Relief	Brown	These features are normally shown by contour lines, intermediate contour lines, and form lines. In addition to contour lines, there are relief symbols to show cuts, levees, sand, sand dunes, ice fields, strip mines, and glaciers.
Vegetation	Green	These symbols include woods, scrub, orchards, vineyards, tropical grass, mangrove and marshy areas or tundra.
Roads	Red, Black, or Red-brown	These symbols are hard-surface, heavy-duty roads; hard-surface medium-duty roads; improved light-duty roads; unimproved dirt roads; and trails. On foreign road maps, symbols may differ slightly. Check the map legend for proper identification of roads.
Railroads	Black	These symbols show single-track railroads in operation; single-track railroads not in operation; double- or multiple-track railroads.
Buildings	Black, Yellow, Red, or Pink	These symbols show built-up areas, schools, churches, ruins, lighthouses, windmills, and cemeteries.

- The shape of an object on the map usually tells what it is. For example, a black, solid square is a building or a house; a round or irregular blue item is a lake or pond.
- Use both logic and color coding to determine a map feature. For example, blue represents water.
- If you see a symbol that is blue and has clumps of grass, it's a swamp.
- The size of the symbol shows the approximate size of an object. Most symbols are enlarged 6 to 10 times so that you can see them under dim light.
- Use the legend; it identifies most of the symbols used on the map.
3. Identify the marginal information found on the legend.
   - Marginal information found at the top of the map sheet:
     ◦ The top left corner contains the geographic location of the map area and the scale of the map.
     ◦ The top center shows the name of the map sheet.
     ◦ The top right corner contains the map edition, map series, and the map sheet number.
   - Marginal information at the bottom of the map sheet:
     ◦ The lower left corner of the map contains the legend, the name of the agency that prepared the map, the map sheet number, and the map sheet name.
     ◦ The bottom center contains the bar scales in meters, yards, miles, and nautical miles; the contour interval of the contour lines; the grid reference box; the declination diagram; and the G-M angle (mils or degrees).
     ◦ The lower right corner contains the elevation guide, the adjoining map sheet diagram, and the boundaries box, which shows any boundaries that may be on the map.

PATIENT HANDOUT: DETERMINE GRID COORDINATES OF A POINT ON A MILITARY MAP

Conditions

Given a standard 1:50,000 scale military map, a 1:50,000 grid coordinate scale, pencil, paper, and a point on the map for which coordinates must be determined.

Standards

Determine the six-digit grid coordinates for the point on the map with a 100-meter tolerance (grid coordinates must contain the correct two-letter 100,000 meter-square identifier).

Training and Evaluation

Training information outline:

1. To keep from getting lost, a soldier must know how to determine his or her location. A combat area has no street addresses, but a military map can help you identify a location accurately. The map has vertical lines (top to bottom) and horizontal lines (left to right). These lines form small squares 1,000 meters on each side called "grid squares."
2. The lines that form grid squares are numbered along the outside edge of the map picture. No two grid squares have the same number.
3. The precision of a point location is shown by the number of digits in the coordinates: the more digits, the more precise the location.
   - 1996: a 1,000-meter grid square.
   - 192961: to the nearest 100 meters.
   - 19269614: to the nearest 10 meters.

Exercise

1. Use the figures in *The Soldier's Manual of Common Tasks* to complete this exercise. Your address is grid square 1181. How do you know this? Start from the left and read right until you come to 11, the first half of your address. Then read up to 81, the other half. Your address is somewhere in grid square 1181.
2. Grid square 1181 gives your general neighborhood, but there is a lot of ground inside that grid square. To make your address more accurate, just add another number to the first half and another number to the second half so your address has six numbers instead of four.
   - To get those extra numbers, pretend that each grid square has 10 lines inside it running north and south, and another 10 running east and west. This makes 100 smaller squares. You can estimate where these imaginary lines are.
   - Suppose you are halfway between grid line 11 and grid line 12. Then the next number is 5, and the first half of your address is 115. Now suppose you are also 3/10 of the way between grid line 81 and grid line 82. Then the second half of your address is 813. (If you were exactly on line 81, the second part would be 810). Your address is 115813.
   - The most accurate way to determine the coordinates of a point on a map is to use a coordinate scale. You do not have to use imaginary lines; you can find the exact coordinates using a coordinate scale and protractor (Graphic Training Aid 5-2-12) or a plotting scale. Each device has two coordinating scales, 1:25,000 meters and 1:50,000 meters. Make sure you use the correct scale.
3. Locate the grid square in which the point is located (the point should already be plotted on the map, for example, Point A.
   - The number of the vertical grid line on the left (west) side of the grid square is the first and second digits of the coordinates.
   - The number of the horizontal grid line on the bottom (south) side of the grid square is the fourth and fifth digits of the coordinates.

4. To determine the third and sixth digits of the coordinates, place the coordinate scale on the bottom horizontal grid line of the grid square containing Point A.
5. Check to see that the zeroes of the coordinate scale are in the lower left (southwest) corner of the map grid square.
6. Slide the scale to the right, keeping the bottom of the scale on the bottom grid line until Point A is under the vertical (right hand) scale. On the bottom scale, the 100-meter mark nearest the vertical grid line provides the third digit, 5. On the vertical scale, the 100-meter mark nearest Point A provides the sixth digit, 3. Therefore, the six-digit grid coordinate is 115813.
7. To determine the correct two-letter 100,000-meter square identifier, look at the grid reference box in the margin of the map.
8. Place the 100,000-meter square identifier in front of the coordinate, GL 11508133.

Content for this activity is reproduced from: US Department of the Army. *Soldier's Manual of Common Tasks, Warrior Skills Level 1.* Washington, DC: DA; 2009. http://www.25idl.army.mil/commontasks.pdf. Accessed April 23, 2014.

PATIENT HANDOUT: PERFORM FIRST AID FOR BLEEDING OF AN EXTREMITY

Conditions

You have a casualty who has a bleeding wound of the arm or leg. The casualty is breathing. Necessary equipment and materials include the casualty's first aid packet, materials to improvise a pressure dressing (wadding and cravat or strip of cloth), materials to elevate the extremity (blanket, shelter half, poncho, log, or any available material), rigid object (stick, tent peg, or similar object), and a strip of cloth.

Standards

Control bleeding from the wound following the correct sequence. Place a field dressing over the wound with the sides of the dressing sealed so it does not slip. Check to ensure the field and pressure dressing does not have a tourniquet-like effect. Apply a tourniquet to stop profuse bleeding not stopped by the dressings, or for missing arms and legs.

Performance Standards

1. Uncover the wound, unless clothing is stuck to the wound or if you are in a chemical environment. **Do not remove protective clothing in a chemical environment**; apply dressings over the protective clothing.

Note: *If an arm or leg has been cut off, go to step 5.*

2. Apply the casualty's field dressing.
   - Apply the dressing, white side down, directly over the wound.
   - Wrap each tail, one at a time, in opposite directions around the wound so the dressing is covered and both sides are sealed.
   - Tie the tails into a nonslip knot over the outer edge of the dressing, not over the wound.

Warning

Field and pressure dressings should not have a tourniquet-like effect. The dressing must be loosened if the skin beyond the injury becomes cool, blue, or numb.

   - Check the dressing to make sure it is tied firmly enough to prevent slipping without causing a tourniquet-like effect.
3. Apply manual pressure and elevate the arm or leg to reduce bleeding, if necessary.
   - Apply firm manual pressure over the dressing for 5 to 10 minutes.
   - Elevate the injured part above the level of the heart unless a fracture is suspected and has not been splinted.
4. Apply a pressure dressing if the bleeding continues.
   - Keep the arm or leg elevated.
   - Place a wad of padding directly over the wound.
   - Place an improvised dressing over the wad of padding and wrap it tightly around the limb.
   - Tie the ends in a nonslip knot directly over the wound.
   - Check the dressing to make sure it does not have a tourniquet-like effect.

Note: *If the bleeding stops, watch the casualty closely, and check for other injuries. If heavy bleeding continues, apply a tourniquet.*

Warning

The only time a tourniquet should be applied is when an arm or leg has been cut off, or when heavy bleeding cannot be stopped by a pressure dressing. If only part of a hand or foot has been cut off, the bleeding should be stopped using a pressure dressing.

---

5. Apply a tourniquet.
   - Make a tourniquet at least 2 inches wide.
   - Position the tourniquet.
     - Place the tourniquet over the smoothed sleeve or trouser leg if possible.
     - Place the tourniquet around the limb 2 to 4 inches above the wound, between the wound and the heart but not on a joint or directly over a wound or a fracture.
     - Place the tourniquet just above and as close as possible to the joint when wounds are just below a joint.
   - Apply the tourniquet.
     - Tie a half knot.
     - Place a stick (or similar object) on top of the half knot.
     - Tie a full knot over the stick.
     - Twist the stick until the tourniquet is tight around the limb and bright red bleeding has stopped.

Note: *In case of an amputation, dark oozing blood may continue for a short time.*

   - Secure the tourniquet. The tourniquet can be secured using the ends of the tourniquet band or with another piece of cloth as long as the stick does not unwind.

Note: *If a limb is completely amputated, the stump should be padded and bandaged (do not cover the tourniquet). If possible, severed limbs or body parts should be saved and transported with, but out of sight of, the casualty. The body parts should be wrapped in dry, sterile dressing; placed in a dry plastic bag; and placed in a cool container (do not soak in water or saline or allow to freeze). If your location in the field or during combat does not allow for the correct preserving of parts, do what you can to keep it sterile and prepare it to be transferred.*

   - Do not loosen or release a tourniquet once it has been applied.
   - Mark the casualty's forehead with a letter *T* using a pen, mud, the casualty's blood, or whatever is available.
6. Watch the casualty closely for life-threatening conditions, check for other injuries (if necessary), and treat for shock.

Content for this activity are reproduced from: US Department of the Army. *Soldier's Manual of Common Tasks, Warrior Skills Level 1.* Washington, DC: DA; 2009. http://www.25idl.army.mil/commontasks.pdf. Accessed October 28, 2013.

PATIENT HANDOUT: JOB-SPECIFIC TACTICAL SIMULATION 1— DYNAMIC VISUAL SCANNING ACTIVITY

Visual scanning and attention to detail are critical skills for any service member. In this task, you will be challenged to scan your environment for two specific visual stimuli:

1. People wearing glasses
2. People wearing hats

To keep track of your accuracy, you will be asked to keep a tally of the number of people you see that meet the descriptions above. Your totals will be compared with your therapist's.

People wearing hats   **People wearing glasses** _____

PATIENT HANDOUT: JOB-SPECIFIC TACTICAL SIMULATION 2— TARGET DETECTION ON VISUAL SCANNING ACTIVITY

Visual scanning and attention to detail are critical skills for any service member. In this task, you will be challenged to hone your visual skills to locate and identify specific static visual targets. Use the scope and/or binoculars to locate and describe as many military items as you can.

1. _____
2. _____
3. _____
4. _____
5. _____
6. _____
7. _____
8. _____
9. _____
10. _____

PATIENT HANDOUT: DA-6/DUTY ROSTER ACTIVITY

Instructions

Using January's duty roster (DA-6), fill out the February duty roster. The last weekday and last weekend have been given to you. Be sure you always have someone on duty during a week and weekend. Weekday duty and weekend duty are considered two separate duty times; weekday duty numbers carry over to the next weekday, and weekend numbers carry over to the next weekend.

- All weekends and holidays are to be highlighted; holidays are considered weekends.
- If you have a service member who wants time off (pass or leave) a lowercase "a" should be placed in the days that service member wants off.
- The numbers will continue to increase while the service member is on pass or leave.

You must accommodate for the following special circumstances:

- 15 FEB 10 is President's Day and is a federal holiday for the division.
- SGT Foxtrot wants 22, 23, 24 FEB off to take his sick mother to the hospital.
- SGT Charlie wants 3 FEB off to take care of his kids.
- SGT Kilo wants 6 FEB off for hunting because it is rabbit season.
- SGT Alpha wants 26 FEB off because he is moving into his new apartment.

EXAMPLE DUTY ROSTER

DUTY ROSTER		NATURE OF DUTY				ORGANIZATION				FROM *(Date)*		TO *(Date)*	
GRADE	NAME	Month		JAN						FEB			
		Day	29	30	31	1	2	3	4	5	6	7	8	9	10	11	12	13	14	15	16	17	18	19	20	21	22	23	24	25	26	27	28
SGT	Alpha		15	1	2																														
SGT	Bravo		16	2	3																														
SGT	Charlie		17	3	4																														
SGT	Delta		18	4	5																														
SGT	Echo		19	5	6																														
SGT	Foxtrot		◣	6	7																														
SGT	Golf		1	7	8																														
SGT	Hotel		2	8	9																														
SGT	Indigo		3	9	10																														
SGT	Juliet																																	
SGT	Kilo																																	
SGT	Lima																																	
SGT	Mike																																	
SGT	November																																	
SGT	Oscar																																	
SGT	Papa																																	
SGT	Quebec																																	
SGT	Romeo																																	
SGT	Sierra																																	
SGT	Tango																																	

DA FORM 6, JUL 1974   PREVIOUS EDITIONS OF THIS FORM ARE OBSOLETE.   For use of this form, see AR 220-45; the proponent agency is DCS, G-1.

APD LF v1.02

PATIENT HANDOUT

DUTY ROSTER		NATURE OF DUTY		ORGANIZATION		FROM *(Date)*		TO *(Date)*

GRADE	NAME	Month	JAN															FEB																								
		Day	29	30	31	1	2	3	4	5	6	7	8	9	10	11	12	13	14	15	16	17	18	19	20	21	22	23	24	25	26	27	28								
SGT	ALPHA		15	1	2																																				
SGT	BRAVO		16	2	3																																				
SGT	CHARLIE		17	3	4																																				
SGT	DELTA		18	4	5																																				
SGT	ECHO		19	5	6																																				
SGT	FOXTROT		◤	6	7																																				
SGT	GOLF		1	7	8																																				
SGT	HOTEL		2	8	9																																				
SGT	INDIGO		3	9	10																																				
SGT	JULIET		4	10	11																																				
SGT	KILO		5	11	12																																				
SGT	LIMA		6	12	13																																				
SGT	MIKE		7	13	14																																				
SGT	NOVEMBER		8	14	15																																				
SGT	OSCAR		9	15	16																																				
SGT	PAPA		10	16	17																																				
SGT	QUEBEC		11	17	18																																				
SGT	ROMEO		12	18	19																																				
SGT	SIERRA		13	19	◤																																				
SGT	TANGO		14	◤	1																																				

DA FORM 6, JUL 1974   PREVIOUS EDITIONS OF THIS FORM WILL BE USED UNTIL EXHAUSTED.   For use of this form, see AR 220-45; the proponent agency is DCSPER.

APD PE v1.00

ANSWER KEY

DUTY ROSTER		NATURE OF DUTY									ORGANIZATION												FROM *(Date)*				TO *(Date)*		

GRADE	NAME	Month	JAN											FEB																		
		Day	29	30	31	1	2	3	4	5	6	7	8	9	10	11	12	13	14	15	16	17	18	19	20	21	22	23	24	25	26	27	28
SGT	Alpha		15	1	2	16	17	18	19	◣	3	4	1	2	3	4	5	5	6	7	6	7	8	9	8	9	10	11	12	13	14	10	11
SGT	Bravo		16	2	3	17	18	◣	1	2	4	5	3	4	5	6	7	6	7	8	8	9	9	11	9	10	12	13	14	15	16	11	12
SGT	Charlie		17	3	4	18	19	20	◣	1	5	6	2	3	4	5	6	7	8	9	7	8	10	10	10	11	11	12	13	14	15	12	13
SGT	Delta		18	4	5	19	◣	1	2	3	6	7	4	5	6	7	8	8	9	10	9	10	11	12	11	12	13	14	15	16	17	13	14
SGT	Echo		19	5	6	◣	1	2	3	4	7	8	5	6	7	8	9	9	10	11	10	11	12	13	12	13	14	15	16	17	18	14	15
SGT	Foxtrot		◣	6	7	1	2	3	4	5	8	9	6	7	8	9	10	11	12	11	12	13	14	13	14	15	16	17	18	19	15	16
SGT	Golf		1	7	8	2	3	4	5	6	9	10	7	8	9	10	11	12	13	12	13	14	15	14	15	16	17	18	19	◣	16	17
SGT	Hotel		2	8	9	3	4	5	6	7	10	11	8	9	10	11	12	12	13	14	13	14	15	16	15	16	17	18	19	◣	1	17	18
SGT	Indigo		3	9	10	4	5	6	7	8	11	12	9	10	11	12	13	14	15	16	15	16	17	18	17	18	19	◣	1	2	3	19
SGT	Juliet		4	10	11	5	6	7	8	9	12	13	10	11	12	13	14	15	16	17	16	17	18	19	18	19	◣	1	2	3	4	1
SGT	Kilo		5	11	12	6	7	8	9	10	13	14	11	12	13	14	15	16	17	16	17	18	19	18	19	◣	19	1	2	3	4	1	2
SGT	Lima		6	12	13	7	8	9	10	11	14	15	12	13	14	15	16	16	17	18	17	18	19	◣	19	1	2	3	4	5	1	2
SGT	Mike		7	13	14	8	9	10	11	12	15	16	13	14	15	16	17	17	18	19	◣	1	2	3	4	5	6	2	3				
SGT	November		8	14	15	9	10	11	12	13	16	17	14	15	16	17	18	18	19	◣	19	1	2	1	2	3	4	5	6	7	3	4
SGT	Oscar		9	15	16	10	11	12	13	14	17	18	15	16	17	18	19	◣	1	2	1	2	3	3	4	4	5	6	7	8	5	6
SGT	Papa		10	16	17	11	12	13	14	15	18	19	16	17	18	19	◣	20	1	1	2	3	4	2	3	5	6	7	8	9	4	5
SGT	Quebec		11	17	18	12	13	14	15	16	19	◣	17	18	19	1	1	2	3	2	3	4	5	4	5	6	7	8	9	10	11	7	8
SGT	Romeo		12	18	19	13	14	15	16	17	◣	1	18	19	1	2	3	4	5	4	5	6	7	6	7	8	9	10	11	12	8	9
SGT	Sierra		13	19	◣	14	15	16	17	18	1	2	◣	1	2	3	4	5	4	5	6	7	6	7	8	9	10	11	12	13	9	10
SGT	Tango		14	◣	1	15	16	17	18	19	2	3	◣	1	2	3	4	5	6	5	6	7	8	7	8	9	10	11	12	13	9	10

DA FORM 6, JUL 1974   PREVIOUS EDITIONS OF THIS FORM ARE OBSOLETE.   For use of this form, see AR 220-45; the proponent agency is DCS, G-1.   APD LF v1.02

PATIENT HANDOUT: TRAINING SCHEDULE

Instructions

You are in charge of creating a weekly training schedule for your platoon. The following activities need to take place every day: physical training, first and final formations, accountability, personal hygiene, breakfast, and lunch. Lunch must be an hour and a half.

The following activities do not need to be every day, but need to be scheduled into the week's events with no gaps or overlaps:

- weapons management
- complete Department of the Army (DA) Form 2404
- warrior skill training
- counseling/noncommissioned officer evaluation reports (NCOERs)
- equal opportunity class
- noncommissioned officer development plans (NCODPs)
- preventative medicine class
- training meeting
- suicide prevention meeting

Weapons management can only take place on Tuesdays and Thursdays. Counseling/NCOERs need to be completed after 1500. Please use the attached calendar to create a weekly training schedule.

	Sunday	Monday	Tuesday	Wednesday	Thursday	Friday	Saturday
0500							
0530							
0600							
0630							
0700							
0730							
0800							
0830							
0900							
0930							
1000							
1030							
1100							
1130							
1200							
1230							
1300							
1330							
1400							
1430							
1500							
1530							
1600							
1630							
1700							
1730							
1800							

PATIENT HANDOUT: ARMY DRESS UNIFORM ERROR DETECTION

Instructions

Your job is to correct the Army dress uniform jacket in front of you. None, some, or all of the badges on the jacket are incorrectly placed. Use your knowledge and other available resources to correct the badges so the jacket is wearable.

Chapter 10

FITNESS ASSESSMENT AND INTERVENTION

MARGARET M. WEIGHTMAN, PhD, PT* AND KAREN McCULLOCH, PhD, PT†

*Clinical Scientist/Physical Therapist, Sister Kenny Research Center, 800 East 28th Street, Mailstop 12212, Minneapolis, Minnesota 55407
†Professor, Division of Physical Therapy, Department of Allied Health Sciences, School of Medicine, University of North Carolina at Chapel Hill, 321 South Columbia Street, CB 7135 Bondurant Hall, Suite 3024, Chapel Hill, North Carolina 27599

INTRODUCTION

The effects of dizziness, imbalance, pain, and overall fatigue may render it less likely that a service member will maintain his or her accustomed level of conditioning, let alone sufficient conditioning to meet the comprehensive fitness needs for military responsibilities, following concussion/mild traumatic brain injury (c/mTBI). One role of physical therapists is to encourage active lifestyles and to provide recommendations for service members whose injuries do not allow participation in previous fitness, sport, and leisure activities. Exercise may improve mood and aspects of health status in individuals with TBI.[1] Physical activity that results in increased cardiovascular fitness may improve cognitive status, including attentional control,[2] memory, and learning.[3]

RETURN TO SPORT

Guidance on a return to activity and sport following concussion is found in the sports medicine literature.[4–6] Current guidelines suggest that athletic activity should not resume until after the physical signs and symptoms of concussion are no longer present at rest or with physical exertion, and cognitive deficits are fully resolved.[5,6] The consensus statement on concussion in sport provides a six-stage return-to-play protocol.[6] Return to play is a gradual process in which the individual is monitored for symptom complaints and cognitive function at each level of increased activity. Progression through stages occurs only if the individual is asymptomatic at the current level. Typically each stage requires 24 hours, and if symptoms return at a given stage, the individual is returned to the previous stage and progressed again 24 hours later. The stages include:

1. rest/no activity: complete physical and cognitive rest.

2. aerobic exercise only, consisting of light, short duration (10–15 minutes) activity, such as swimming, walking, or stationary cycling (less than 70% maximal predicted heart rate).
3. sport-specific training (eg, running, skating).
4. noncontact drills (including cutting and other lateral movements).
5. full contact, controlled training (requires medical clearance).
6. full contact game play.

These return-to-activity guidelines for sports concussion are typically based on symptom resolution, neuropsychological tests, and balance assessments, often with preinjury tests to determine a return to baseline function prior to resuming an activity. Additional study has been called for to facilitate understanding of the pathophysiological changes and recovery of cerebral blood flow and brain metabolism following concussion.[7]

POSTCONCUSSION SYNDROME

Persistent concussive complaints have been described as postconcussion syndrome (PCS). The World Health Organization defines PCS as persistence (beyond 4 weeks) of three or more of the following symptoms at rest: headache, dizziness, fatigue, irritability, or difficulties with sleep, concentration, or memory.[8] Although concussion management guidelines developed in sport do not recommend exercise until symptoms have resolved at rest,[5,6] these guidelines do not address treatment options when symptoms do not resolve at rest or return during exertion.

Investigators at University of Buffalo are conducting studies to address alternatives for individuals with persistent symptom complaints. Progressive aerobic exercise has been used to treat individuals with PCS 3 to 6 weeks after concussion who have symptoms at rest and experience exacerbated symptoms with exercise.[9–12] This protocol begins with an incremental treadmill exercise test (standard Balke protocol) administered until the first sign of symptom exacerbation, which is then set as the athlete's maximum exercise intensity (heart rate and blood pressure). Supervised repetitive training is conducted at 80% of this predetermined symptom threshold, often resulting in improved function and reduced symptoms.[10]

The theory behind this treatment is that physiologic dysfunction affects the autoregulation of cerebral blood flow, mediated by autonomic dysfunction. This dysfunction causes exacerbated symptoms during exercise. Exercise at a level below the onset of symptom exacerbation is theorized to improve autonomic balance necessary for cerebral blood flow autoregulation, thereby reducing symptoms during exercise and at rest.

In the University of Buffalo protocol, athletes are carefully monitored during all exercise and use both personal heart rate monitors and graded symptom reports to maintain exercise intensity at subsymptom exacerbation levels.[10,12] Athletes retest at 2- to 3-week intervals to determine changes in their maximum exercise intensity level that produces onset of PCS symptoms. The athlete continues to exercise at 80% of the determined maximum intensity level. Evidence supports the safety of this subsymptom threshold aerobic exercise.[9,10,12,13]

A commonly used symptom checklist (Graded Symptom Checklist) for sports concussion is provided in the return-to-play consensus document[6] and is used during the University of Buffalo maximum exercise testing protocol. The Neurobehavioral Symptom Inventory-22[14] is an alternative to this symptom checklist that has been studied to a greater degree following military mTBI.[15]

Based on the University of Buffalo study, service members with PCS of at least 3 to 6 weeks duration may be referred for a symptom-producing exercise test to determine individual subsymptom threshold for use in an exercise program.[16] This type of program may be adapted using a bicycle ergometer (watts or other workload measure) instead of a treadmill, although the safety of this modification has not been evaluated.

Some additional considerations when evaluating a service member's fitness and developing exercise programs for use during recovery are as follows.

- It is important to assess a service member's pre- and postinjury level of participation (specifically frequency and duration) in aerobic and strengthening exercises.
- General exercise recommendations advise healthy adults aged 18 to 65 years get 30 minutes of moderate-intensity aerobic physical activity for a minimum of 5 days each week and muscular strength and endurance activities for a minimum of 2 days each week.[17]
- Therapists should determine a service member's ability to self-monitor exercise intensity through such measures as heart rate, rate of perceived exertion, and metabolic equivalents. One method to monitoring exercise intensity is to use the guideline of 50% to 85% of age-predicted maximum heart rate as the target zone for exercise, which can be found at The American Heart Association's website (www.heart.org).

- It is important to screen patients for health risk factors prior to beginning or resuming an exercise or fitness rou e.[18] Service members with risk factors should be referred for medical clearance before resuming an exercise program. Information on risk factors is also included on the American Heart Association website, including risk factor calculators for heart attack and high blood pressure (www.heart.org). Risk factors that cannot be modified include increased age (over 65), heredity (both family history of heart disease and race), and sex (males are at greater risk). Modifiable risk factors include:
  ○ high blood cholesterol and triglyceride levels
  ○ high blood pressure
  ○ diabetes and prediabetes
  ○ overweight and obesity
  ○ smoking
  ○ lack of physical activity
  ○ unhealthy diet
  ○ stress

- Service member fitness testing standards and requirements can be accessed via the Human Performance Resource Center, a Department of Defense initiative under the Force Health Protection and Readiness Program.[19]

- Guides to testing and training for the Army include the Army Physical Readiness Training Quick Reference Card (GTA 07-08-003)[20] and the *Army Physical Readiness Training Manual* (Training Circular 3-22.20).[21]

- The Comprehensive Soldier Fitness Program and requirements can be used as a fitness target as soon as appropriate in a service member's rehabilitation program to encourage military readiness (see Warfighter Fitness, below).

WARFIGHTER FITNESS

As a service member recovers from c/mTBI and resumes fitness training, the therapist should encourage activities that stress agility, flexibility, stability, speed, power, balance, coordination, and posture. These factors are promoted as essential for injury prevention and performance optimization in the Comprehensive Soldier Fitness program. This program, introduced in 2010, focuses on meeting the comprehensive needs for soldier readiness and expands beyond the prior emphasis on muscular endurance (push-ups, sit-ups) and cardiorespiratory fitness (1- to 2-mile runs) that was intended to prepare service members for annual fitness testing. All branches of the military are focused on total force fitness, noting the importance of mind, body, family, and environment for overall fitness.[22]

Newer fitness training protocols recognize the need for training specificity depending on individual military occupation specialty and mission tasks.[22] Therapists should consider the following four components of physical fitness training[23] when implementing training activities (Table 10-1). The Army Medical Department has developed detailed training regimens for service members training for duty and those who are injured (available on the Army Medical Department's intranet).[24] These resources are extensively illustrated and recommend exercises and how to progress them, as well as guide ongoing training regimens based on fitness level and stage of deployment preparation or injury recovery (Form 10-1).

TABLE 10-1

COMPONENTS OF PHYSICAL FITNESS TRAINING

Physical Fitness Components	Example Activity Types
Endurance training (repetitive activities at low workload)	Swimming Long-distance running Cycling Elliptical trainers
Mobility training (speed, balance, jumping, directional change)	Plyometrics Speed (sprint) training, including directional change
Strength training (increase ability to generate force and power)	Weight training regimes adjusting: Load Repetitions Rest time between sets Core stability programs
Flexibility training (avoid hypo- or hypermobility)	Muscle-specific static stretching programs

FORM 10-1

EXERCISE LOG

Exercise log for week of _____

Weekly Exercise Goals:			
	Goals Set	**Goals Met/Not Met**	
Number of Days of Cardiovascular Exercise			
Number of Days of Strength Training			

Date	Type of Exercise	Intensity ✓ Heart Rate ✓ RPE ✓ Repetitions/sets	**Duration** (minutes)	**Comments**
	• Aerobic • Strength Training • Other			
	• Aerobic • Strength Training • Other			
	• Aerobic • Strength Training • Other			
	• Aerobic • Strength Training			

	• Other			
	• Aerobic • Strength Training • Other			
	• Aerobic • Strength Training • Other			
	• Aerobic • Strength Training • Other			

REFERENCES

1. Gordon WA, Sliwinski M, Echo J, McLoughlin M, Sheerer MS, Meili TE. The benefits of exercise in individuals with traumatic brain injury: a retrospective study. *J Head Trauma Rehabil.* 1998;13(4):58–67.

2. Colcombe SJ, Kramer AF, Erickson KI, et al. Cardiovascular fitness, cortical plasticity, and aging. *Proc Natl Acad Sci U S A.* 2004;101(9):3316–3321.

3. Lojovich JM. The relationship between aerobic exercise and cognition: is movement medicinal? *The J Head Trauma Rehabil.* May-Jun 2010;25(3):184–192.

4. Guskiewicz KM, Broglio SP. Sport-related concussion: on-field and sideline assessment. *Phys Med Rehabil Clin N Am.* 2011;22(4):603–617, vii.

5. McCrory P, Johnston K, Meeuwisse W, et al. Summary and agreement statement of the 2nd International Conference on Concussion in Sport. *Br J Sports Med.* 2005;39:196–204.

6. McCrory P, Meeuwisse W, Johnston K, et al. Consensus statement on concussion in sport–the 3rd International Conference on Concussion in Sport held in Zurich, November 2008. *J Sci Med Sport.* 2009;12(3):340–351.

7. Len TK, Neary JP. Cerebrovascular pathophysiology following mild traumatic brain injury. *Clin Physiol Funct Imaging.* 2011;31(2):85–93.

8. World Health Organization. *International Statistical Classification of Disease and Related Health Problems.* Geneva, Switzerland: WHO; 1992.

9. Baker JG, Freitas MS, Leddy JJ, Kozlowski KF, Willer BS. Return to full functioning after graded exercise assessment and progressive exercise treatment of postconcussion syndrome. *Rehabil Res Pract.* 2012;2012:705309.

10. Leddy JJ, Kozlowski K, Donnelly JP, Pendergast DR, Epstein LH, Willer B. A preliminary study of subsymptom threshold exercise training for refractory post-concussion syndrome. *Clin J Sport Med.* 2010;20(1):21–27.

11. Leddy JJ, Kozlowski K, Fung M, Pendergast DR, Willer B. Regulatory and autoregulatory physiological dysfunction as a primary characteristic of post concussion syndrome: implications for treatment. *NeuroRehabilitation.* 2007;22(3):199–205.

12. Leddy JJ, Sandhu H, Sodhi V, Baker JG, Willer B. Rehabilitation of concussion and post-concussion syndrome. *Sports Health.* 2012;4(2):147–154.

13. Leddy JJ, Baker JG, Kozlowski K, Bisson L, Willer B. Reliability of a graded exercise test for assessing recovery from concussion. *Clin J Sport Med.* Mar 2011;21(2):89–94.

14. Cicerone KD, Kalmar K. Persistent postconcussion syndrome: the structure of subjective complaints after mTBI. *J Head Trauma Rehabil.* 1995;10:1–17.

15. Meterko M, Baker E, Stolzmann KL, Hendricks AM, Cicerone KD, Lew HL. Psychometric assessment of the Neurobehavioral Symptom Inventory-22: the structure of persistent postconcussive symptoms following deployment-related mild traumatic brain injury among veterans. *J Head Trauma Rehabil.* 2012;27(1):55-62.

16. Willer B, Leddy JJ. Management of concussion and post-concussion syndrome. *Curr Treat Options Neurol.* 2008;8(5):415–426.

17. Haskell WL, Lee IM, Pate RR, et al. Physical activity and public health: updated recommendations for adults from the American College of Sports Medicine and the American Heart Association. *Med Sci Sports Exer.* 2007;39(8):1423–1434.

18. Vitale AE, Sullivan SJ, Jankowski LW, Fleury J, Lefrancois C, Lebouthillier E. Screening of health risk factors prior to exercise or a fitness evaluation of adults with traumatic brain injury: A consensus by rehabilitation professionals. *Brain Inj.* 1996;10(5):367–375.

19. US Department of Defense. Human Performance Resource Center website. Service-Specific Resources: Army. http://hprc-online.org/physical-fitness/weight-management/service-specific-resources/army. Accessed January 7, 2014.

20. US Department of the Army. Army Physical Readiness Training Quick Reference Card. Washington, DC: DA; 2010. GTA 07-08-003. http://www.25idl.army.mil/PT/GTA_%2007-08-003.pdf. Accessed November 25, 2013.

21. US Department of the Army. *Army Physical Readiness Program.* Washington, DC: DA; 2012. Field Manual 7-22.

22. Uniformed Services University of the Health Sciences. Human Performance Research Center webpage. http://humanperformanceresourcecenter.org. Accessed November 26, 2013.

23. Roy TC, Springer BA, McNulty V, Butler NL. Physical Fitness. *Mil Med.* 2010;175(8):14–20.

24. US Department of the Army. *Soldier's Guide: Tools for the Tactical Athlete.* Washington, DC: DA; 2013. http://armymedicine.mil/Documents/Soldiers_Guide_8_7_2013.pdf. Accessed January 7, 2014.

Chapter 11

HEALTH-RELATED QUALITY OF LIFE / PARTICIPATION ASSESSMENT

MARGARET M. WEIGHTMAN, PhD, PT*; EMI ISAKI, PhD, CCC/SLP†; MARY RADOMSKI, PhD, OTR/L‡; CAROLE R. ROTH, PhD, BC-ANCDS¥

*Clinical Scientist /Physical Therapist, Courage Kenny Research Center, 800 East 28th Street, Mail Stop 12212, Minneapolis, MN 55407-3799
†Assistant Professor, Communication Sciences & Disorders, Northern Arizona University, Department of CSD, Building 66, PO Box 15045, Flagstaff, Arizona 86011-5045
‡Clinical Scientist, Courage Kenny Research Center, 800 E 28th Street, Mail Stop 12212, Minneapolis, Minnesota 55407-3799
§Division Head, Speech Pathology, Naval Medical Center San Diego, 34800 Bob Wilson Drive, Building 2/2, 2K-11R5, San Diego, California 92134-6200

INTRODUCTION

According to the World Health Organization's International Classification of Functioning, participation refers to the extent to which an individual takes part in the life areas or situations of his or her own choosing.[1] Full participation implies that the individual is capable of engaging in activities in a manner expected of a person without restrictions. Physical, occupational, and speech-language clinicians view participation as a fundamental outcome of intervention. One aspect of a participation-level measure is the assessment of health-related quality of life (HRQOL). Existing studies on HRQOL, as it relates to traumatic brain injury (TBI) of all severity levels, focus primarily on functional status and symptom measurement and do not consistently include assessments of other factors, such as depression and environmental factors.[2,3] Participation-level measures of specific problems service members with concussion/mild traumatic brain injury (c/mTBI) may exhibit are found in this toolkit under the appropriate problem area (eg, Headache Disability Index, Neck Disability Index, Patient-Specific Functional Scale, Canadian Occupational Performance Measure, and Dizziness Handicap Inventory, etc).

Many of the disease-specific measures of participation and quality of life are currently more relevant to those with moderate to severe brain injury.[4] Some examples include the following:

- **The Medical Outcomes Study 36-Item Short-Form Health Survey (SF-36)**. This is a generic tool developed for the Medical Outcomes Study[5] whose psychometric properties are extensively evaluated in multiple populations, with some work done to assess its reliability and validity in the TBI population.[6] This short form was constructed to survey health status and was designed for use in clinical practice, research, health policy evaluation, and general population surveys.[5] The standard SF-36 may be used to assess quality of life relative to active duty military personnel when a more specific version is unavailable.
- **The Mayo-Portland Adaptability Inventory–4 (MPAI-4)**.[7] This assessment can be used to evaluate individuals with acquired brain injury in the post-acute period in addition to being used for program evaluation.[8] It has been used in individuals with

mild brain injury.[8,9]
- **The Participation Objective, Participation Subjective (POPS)**. This assessment measures household and societal participation. It has typically been used in those with moderate to severe brain injury.[10]
- **The World Health Organization Quality of Life–BREF (WHOQOL-BREF)**. This is a shortened version of the World Health Organization (WHO) 100-question quality-of-life assessment that measures the impact of disease and impairment measure on four broad domains of physical health, psychological health, social relationships, and environment.[11]
- **The American Speech-Language-Hearing Association National Outcomes Measurement System (ASHA NOMS)**. This assessment includes the functional communication measures (FCMs) used by speech-language pathologists to reflect the effects of intervention on acquired cognitive-communication disorders. The FCMs include nine measures specifically relevant to mild TBI. The ASHA NOMS is recognized and accepted by the Centers for Medicare and Medicaid Services and the National Quality Forum as approved quality measures.[12]

Rehabilitation clinicians are encouraged to consider quality-of-life and participation-level measures to monitor individual service members and to evaluate programs designed to serve the active duty and veteran population. Given the absence of an appropriate military-related measure, a global measure of health status, quality of life, and/or participation would be a component of a site-specific program evaluation. Additionally, these types of assessments can provide information on an individual service member's response to intervention.

The process for determining the most appropriate HRQOL instrument is defined by the program's purpose and goals, and the instruments included here should be considered examples and not all inclusive. It is not uncommon for programs to select several instruments for measuring HRQOL in those with combat-acquired c/mTBI due to the associated complexity of patient symptoms. The purpose of this section of the toolkit is to provide the clinician with sufficient information about the instruments to assist in making an informed decision.

THE 36-ITEM HEALTH SURVEY 2.0

Purpose/Description

The SF-36 is a patient self-report questionnaire that measures health status across eight domains.[5] Four scales relate to functional status, three to well-being, and one to overall health. The overall evaluation of health is based on the general health scale. Physical functioning, role-physical, bodily pain, and general health scales contribute to the physical health summary measure. Vitality, social functioning, role-emotional, and mental health contribute to the mental health summary measure.

Recommended Instrument Use

A version of the SF-36 is available to assess health outcomes for veterans.[13,14] In the absence of a version specific to active duty personnel, the standard SF-36 may be used. Given the need to consider their health status over the prior 4 weeks, memory issues in service members with c/mTBI may make it difficult to answer the questions appropriately. There is a 1-week acute version of the SF-36 that requires recall of health status over the preceding 1 week only.

Administration Protocol/Equipment/Time

It takes approximately 15 minutes to complete the SF-36 questionnaire. Scoring is a two-step process. Initially, the patient's responses are recoded to obtain values between 0 and 100 for each item. A higher score indicates a more favorable health state. Then all the items related to each domain are averaged to obtain a domain score. Scoring instructions are available online for the SF-36, version 1, and a computerized format for scoring the SF-36, version 2, can also be found online (www.qualitymetric.com).

The SF-36 version 1, developed by RAND Health Communications (Santa Monica, CA) is available online (www.rand.org/health/surveys_tools/mos/mos_core_36item.html). In 1996, version 2 of the SF-36 was introduced by Quality Metrics (Lincoln, RI; www.qualitymetric.com). According to Quality Metrics, "The RAND-36 is an exact replica of the content of the SF-36. However, because RAND uses different scoring algorithms for two of the 8 scales (bodily pain, general health), their results for those scales are not comparable with the standard SF-36."[15] SF-36 version 2 is most often used with the scaling and wording changes and requires purchase of a user's manual.

Groups Tested With This Measure

This measure has been used on patients with mild TBI and moderate to severe brain injury. The SF-36 can also distinguish between patients with medical conditions and psychiatric disorders, and between the general population and patients with medical conditions such as kneecap replacement, rheumatoid arthritis, and dialysis.[6]

Interpretability

- Norms: not available for patients with brain injury. One study[6] has shown that patients with mild TBI have significantly lower scores on all scales than a comparison group that had no disabilities.
- Minimal detectable change (MDC): In one study of 14 brain-injured patients (Glasgow Coma Scale [GCS] score < 14) 1 year after injury, the smallest detectable difference was calculated for all SF-36 subscales and ranged from 16.24 to 41.74.[16] If the patient's score is less than the MDC value, it is considered indistinguishable from measurement error.
- Responsiveness estimates: In one study of 14 brain-injured patients (GCS < 14) 1 year after injury, standard error of the measurement values ranged from 5.86 to 25.[16] Because this represents such a large percentage of the overall scale, this tool cannot measure small changes and may be insensitive to changes in a population of brain-injured patients with mild injuries. Improvements to version 2 of the SF-36 have improved responsiveness to change and other psychometric properties.[17]

Reliability Estimates

- Internal consistency: Cronbach's alpha ranged from 0.83 to 0.91 for a group of community-dwelling patients (n = 98) that had sustained mTBI at least 1 year earlier and who had a loss of consciousness and/or confusion for less than 1 day.[6]
- Interrater: Intraclass correlation coefficient (ICC) between psychologists was studied in a sample (n = 14) of brain-injured patients at 1 year after injury. The patients were admitted to a neurosurgical service

and had GCS scores below 14. ICC ranged from 0.44 to 0.94, with the mental health subscale being the least reliable between raters.[16]

- Intrarater: not available
- Test-Retest: ICC's from 0.30 to 0.93, depending on subscale and patient population.[18] For SF-36 version 2, the reliability coefficients are typically greater than 0.70.[17]

Validity Estimates

- Content/Face: This measure appears to survey most aspects of health.
- Criterion: Strong correlations (0.50 to 0.63) were found between SF-36 scales pertaining directly to physical functioning (general health, physical functioning, physical role, bodily pain, vitality) and the physical symptoms scale of the Institute for Rehabilitation Research symptom

checklist. As expected, emotional role and mental health scores of the SF-36 were more strongly related to psychological factors than to physical factors on this checklist.[6]

Similarly strong correlations were found between the SF-36 scales and participants' Health Problems List responses (0.60 to 0.75). Robust correlations (0.52 to 0.77) were found between Beck Depression Inventory (second edition) and the SF-36 subscales. The strongest of these correlations (0.77) was between the Beck Depression Inventory and the Mental Health scale of the SF-36.[6]

- Construct: This measure has been tested for its ability to distinguish patients with multiple diagnoses, for sensitivity to change, and for correlation to numerous other disability, pain, depression, and health scales.[18]

Selected References

Findler M, Cantor J, Haddad L, Gordon W, Ashman T. The reliability and validity of the SF-36 health survey questionnaire for use with individuals with traumatic brain injury. *Brain Inj.* Aug 2001;15(8):715–723.

Ware JE, Sherbourne CD. The MOS 36-Item Short-Form Health Survey (SF-36): I. Conceptual framework and item selection. *Medical Care.* 1992;30:473–481.

MAYO-PORTLAND ADAPTABILITY INVENTORY

Purpose/Description

The MPAI-4 is a 35-item rating scale that measures problems after brain injury. It can be self-rated or rated by a clinician or significant other. It consists of 29 items in 3 subscales (Ability Index, Adjustment Index, Participation Index) intended to reflect the current status of the individual with brain injury. The additional six items not included in the MPAI-4 score are used to identify the presence of other factors that may be contributing to the individual's current status.[8] The original MPAI was designed to assist in clinical evaluation during the post-acute period following acquired brain injury (ABI), and in the evaluation of rehabilitation programs designed to serve individuals with ABI. Individuals with very severe cognitive impairment should not be given the MPAI.

Recommended Instrument Use: Practice Option

The MPAI-4 may be used by individual clinicians or rehabilitation teams for purposes of:

- **Intervention**. The MPAI-4 provides rehabilitation professionals with a brief and reliable means of assessing functioning in each of these three major domains (ability, adjustment, and participation) to help target areas for intervention and assess progress.
- **Community reintegration**. MPAI-4 items assess major obstacles to community reintegration that may result directly from brain injury, as well as problems in the social and physical environment.
- **Reevaluation**. Periodic reevaluation with MPAI-4 during post-acute rehabilitation or other intervention documents progress, efficacy, and appropriateness of the intervention.
- **Research**. Responses to the MPAI-4 by individuals with longstanding ABI and their caregivers and close acquaintances help answer questions about the future of those who are newly injured and their long-term medical, social, and economic needs.[19]

Administration Protocol/Equipment/Time

The MPAI-4 takes 5 to 10 minutes to administer. The MPAI-4 may be completed by people with ABI, their significant others, medical or rehabilitation professionals, and other designated observers who know the individual well. Scoring and interpretation of the MPAI-4 require professional training and experience. A worksheet is provided in the user manual that guides the user through scoring and rescoring items. Items are rated on a 5-point scale from 0 to 4, where 0 represents the most favorable outcome, no problem, or independence, and 4 represents severe problems.

The MPAI-4 consists of a manual and the MPAI-4 forms, which may be downloaded from The Center for Outcome Measurement in Brain Injury website, copied, and used by clinicians without fee or other charge; however, the authors retain copyright to the MPAI-4 and previous versions.

Groups Tested with this Measure

The MPAI-4 has been used in individuals with acquired TBI ranging in severity from mild to severe, as well as in individuals who have suffered neurologic trauma due to strokes and tumors. It has been used by nationally recognized rehabilitation programs for TBI, including Learning Services Corp, Rehab Without Walls, and the Mayo Clinic Acquired Brain Injury Program.[8]

Interpretability

- Norms: Data are available from two samples for comparison purposes. These data sets were both obtained for adults with ABI ranging in severity from mild to moderately severe, as well as for a small sample of individuals with stroke and other neurologic etiologies in post-acute residential, outpatient, or community-based rehabilitation. The data does not represent true "normative" data because there are no references to a non-ABI sample (for norms, see the revised edition of the Mayo-Portland Adaptability Inventory).[9]
- MDC: not available
- Responsiveness: MPAI-4 provides a broader assessment at lower levels of disability

than Disability Rating Scale.[20] Change in MPAI-4 score from pre-admission to the end of a comprehensive day-treatment program was significant (paired $t = 8.35$, $P < 0.0001$[21]).

Reliability Estimates

- Internal consistency has been determined by Rasch analysis (Person reliability = 0.88; item reliability = 0.99) and traditional psychometric indicators (Cronbach's alpha = 0.89).[8] For the three subscales, Person reliability ranged from 0.78 to 0.79, item reliability from 0.98 to 0.99, and Cronbach's alpha from 0.76 to 0.83. Subscales correlated moderately (Pearson r = 0.49–0.65) with each other and strongly with the overall scale (Pearson r = 0.82–0.86).[8]
- Interrater reliability: Person reliability for the self-MPAI was 0.84 (Person separation = 2.29 and item reliability was 0.95).[9]
- Item reliability ranged from 0.97 to 0.99.[19]

Person reliability indicates the degree to which items differentiate people. Item reliability indicates the degree to which items are related for different people. Person reliability over 0.80 and item reliability over 0.90 are desirable. Person separation is used to classify people. In Rasch analysis, a separation of at least 2 is desired.[9]

Validity Estimates

- Construct validity: 0.98[22]
- Concurrent validity: original MPAI consensus ratings correlated with Disability Rating Scale scores (r = 0.81), with Rivermead Behavioral Memory Test (r = 0.47).[9]
- Predictive validity is demonstrated in a number of studies.[21-24] Time since injury and staff-rated MPAI-4 were significant predictors of vocational independence scale scores (P < 0.01), staff-rated MPAI-4 was also predictive of time to placement (P < 0.001[22]; staff MPAI-4 ratings contributed significantly to the prediction of community-based employment at 1 year follow-up (P < 0.01[24]).

Selected References

Malec JF. The Mayo-Portland Participation Index: a brief and psychometrically sound measure of brain injury outcome. *Arch Phys Med Rehabil.* 2004;85:1989–1996.

Malec JF, Kragness M, Evans RW, Finlay KL, Kent A, Lezak MD. Further psychometric evaluation and revision of the Mayo-Portland Adaptability Inventory in a national sample. *J Head Trauma Rehabil.* Nov-Dec 2003;18(6):479–492.

Malec JF, Lezak MD. *Manual for the Mayo-Portland Adaptability Inventory (MPAI-4) for Adults, Children and Adolescents.* San Jose, CA: The Center for Outcome Measurement in Brain Injury. Revised 2008.

PARTICIPATION OBJECTIVE, PARTICIPATION SUBJECTIVE

Purpose/Description

The POPS is a 26-item instrument used to obtain the patient's as well as a societal/normative perspective for commonly occurring social activities.[10] Each of the items in the instrument is addressed with two sets of questions, which are organized into five subscales:

1) domestic life,
2) major life areas,
3) transportation,
4) interpersonal interactions and relationships, and
5) community, recreational, and civic life.

The POPS focuses on activities related to community functioning, generates the objective measure of participation and subjective measure of participation, gauges performance in terms of level of engagement, and incorporates patient preferences for individual satisfaction with his or her level of engagement and determination of importance of each activity. Creation of the subscales was based on the *International Classification of Functioning, Disability, and Health* model.[25]

Recommended Instrument Use: Practice Option

This assessment shows how a patient perceives his or her socialization. For individuals with c/mTBI, this assessment can be administered during initial evaluation. The POPS can also be readministered prior to discharge from therapy services to determine if changes have occurred in community functioning.

Administration Protocol/Equipment/Time

This assessment is administered via in-person interview. The 26-item instrument is available online. Administration time is not estimated on the website; however, the POPS can be completed in a relatively short amount of time.[10] Training and testing information is not yet available.

Groups Tested With This Measure

The POPS was developed from a multifocus research instrument, Living Life After Traumatic Brain Injury (LLATBI).[26] The LLATBI was used in multiple studies involving individuals with TBI and those without disabilities at Mount Sinai School of Medicine. The number of participation items on the LLATBI was reduced, and the POPS was developed.[10] It has been used clinically and in research to measure the outcomes of TBI interventions across the severity range, including mTBI, specifically at the level of participation at home and in the community.[10,27]

Interpretability

- Norms: LLATBI data were gathered on 454 individuals with TBI living in the community and on 121 individuals with no disability.[26]
- Scoring: Brown[10] reports that hour and frequency items are converted to base scores, which are then converted to standardized z-scores. The z-scores are weighted against mean importance ratings of the TBI sample and non-disordered sample for each item. The patient's total participation objective (PO) score is calculated as the average of the weighted z-scores for the 26 items.[10] The participation subjective (PS) score is determined by multiplying the patient's importance score by his or her satisfaction score (ranging from + 4, "most important," to − 4, "least important").[10] The patient's PS total score is the mean across the 26 activities.
- MDC: not available
- Responsiveness estimates: not available

Reliability Estimates

Adequately assessing the reliability and validity of the POPS is complex because the instrument provides both objective descriptive data as well as subjective data.[10]

- Internal consistency: not available
- Interrater: not applicable
- Intrarater: not applicable
- Test-Retest: Repeated measures of the POPS 1 to 3 weeks apart on a subsample of 65 people with TBI resulted in ICC scores ranging from 0.37 to 0.89, and the total PO score was 0.75. The ICC score of the total PS score was 0.80.[10]

Validity Estimates

- Content/Face: not available
- Criterion: not available
- Construct: This was not assessed, as Brown et al[28] determined that no measure provides a "gold standard" for comparison with the POPS at this time. Instead, Brown et al[28] developed a series of expectations of how PO and PS scores should perform if they are validly reflecting the constructs targeted by the items. The authors stated that strong support was found in the data for the expectations.

Selected References

Brown M. Participation Objective, Participation Subjective. 2006. http://www.tbims.org/combi/pops. Accessed November 19, 2013.

Brown M, Dijkers MP, Gordon WA, Ashman T, Charatz H, Cheng Z. Participation Objective, Participation Subjective: a measure of participation combining outsider and insider perspectives. *J Head Trauma Rehabil.* 2004;19(6):459–481.

Curtin M, Jones J, Tyson GA, Mitsch V, Alston M, McAllister L. Outcomes of participation objective, participation subjective (POPS) measure following traumatic brain injury. *Brain Injury.* 2011;25(3):266–273.

World Health Organization. *International Classification of Functioning, Disability and Health.* Geneva, Switzerland: World Health Organization; 2001.

WHO-QUALITY OF LIFE-BREF

Purpose/Description

The World Health Organization Quality of Life abbreviated version (WHOQOL-BREF) is a quality-of-life assessment that measures the impact of disease and impairment on daily activities and behavior, and includes measures of perceived health and disability or functional status. It assesses the individual's perceptions in the context of their culture, value systems, and personal goals, standards, and concerns. The WHOQOL-BREF includes 26 questions derived from the original WHOQOL-100 assessment[29–32] that measure the four broad domains of physical health, psychological health, social relationships, and environment. All items are rated on a 5-point scale (1 to 5).

Recommended Instrument Use: Practice Option

This WHOQOL-BREF has both clinical and research applications. It can help clinicians make judgments about the areas in which a patient is most affected by disease, treatment decisions, and to measure change in quality of life over the course of treatment. Following a review of the literature on quality-of-life assessment after TBI, an international TBI consensus group recommended the WHOQOL based on its feasibility, specificity, validity, comprehensiveness, norms psychometric quality, and international availability.[33] Research applications include clinical trials and health policy research. The WHOQOL-BREF is available in 19 languages. For further recommendations, see the WHOQOL-BREF website (www.who.int/mental_health/media/en/76.pdf).

Administration Protocol/Equipment/Time

The WHOQOL-BREF is a self-administered questionnaire; if necessary, interviewer-assisted or interview-administered forms may be used. It uses a 5-point Likert scale ranging from 1 (not at all) to 5 (completely) to answer questions based on experiences over the preceding 2 weeks. It requires 10 to 15 minutes to administer. When completed by a patient or family member, it may take 6 to 30 minutes.

Groups Tested With This Measure

The WHOQOL-BREF has been tested on adults age 18 years and older from many different populations across the world, as well as on individuals with different disorders, including spinal cord injury,[34,35] TBI across the severity range,[36,37] stroke,[38,39] dementia,[40] other neurological illnesses, human immunodeficiency virus,[41] cancer,[42] chronic pain,[43] depression,[44] and community-dwelling older adults.[45]

Interpretability

- Norms: Norms are available for different cross-cultural groups of people with various diseases. See the Rehabmeasures. org website for further reading (www.rehabmeasures.org/Lists/RehabMeasures/ PrintView.aspx?ID=937)
- MDC: not established
- Responsiveness estimates: not available

Reliability and Validity Estimates

- Internal consistency reliability: As a measure of the scale's internal consistency, for the total sample, values for Cronbach's alpha were acceptable (greater than 0.7). Across sites, results were consistently high, with most of the alphas above 0.75, and in the range of 0.51 to 0.77. Alpha analyses showed that all 26 items made a significant contribution to the variance in the WHOQOL-BREF. The universality of the WHOQOL-100 was examined in several ways and was found to be remarkably adept at identifying facets of quality of life that are cross-culturally important.[11,46]
- Test-retest: WHOQOL-100 reliability was excellent in a sample of individuals with multiple diagnoses across seven domains: 1) physical, 2) psychological, 3) independence, 4) social, 5) environment, 6) spiritual, and 7) general health/global quality-of-life facet.[47] Unpublished data show that test-retest reliability is very good.[46]
- Interrater reliability: The WHOQOL-100 US version was shown to be reproducible (ICC range: 0.83 to 0.96 at 2-week retest interval).[47] In a study of 250 veterans, the WHOQOL-100 ICC ranged between 0.59 and 0.86. In a study to test whether a web version of the WHOQOL-BREF is an alternative to the paper version, the ICC coefficients for test-retest reliability ranged from 0.79 to 0.91. Interrater reliability has been shown to be good in studies conducted in a variety of countries with different populations and disorders, such as Dutch adult psychiatric outpatients,[48] older patients with depression,[49] chronic schizophrenics,[50] caregivers, and stroke survivors.[51]
- Parallel-form reliability: no parallel form available
- Discriminant validity: The results of a hierarchical multiple regression demonstrated a small but significant impact by age and gender on domain scores between sick and well people (F = 96.3 [2,7007], P < 0.0001)[52]
- Construct validity: Analysis of correlations showed that in the total population, only seven items had strong correlations (greater than 0.50) with domains other than their intended domain. Summary Pearson correlations (one-tailed test) between domains for the total sample were strong, positive, and highly significant (P < 0.0001), ranging from 0.46 (physical).[43]

Selected References

Bullinger M, , Azouvi P, Brooks N, et al. Quality of life in patients with traumatic brain injury—basic issues, assessment and recommendations. *Restor Neurol Neurosci.* 2002;20(3–4):111.

WHOQOL Group. Development of the WHOQOL: rationale and current status. *Int J Mental Health.* 1994;23(3):24–56.

WHOQOL Group. The World Health Organization Quality of Life Assessment (WHOQOL): position paper from the World Health Organization. *Soc Sci Med.* 1995;41:1403–1409.

THE AMERICAN SPEECH-LANGUAGE-HEARING ASSOCIATION
NATIONAL OUTCOMES MEASUREMENT SYSTEM

Purpose/Description

The ASHA NOMS[12] was designed to develop a national database of functional treatment outcomes for speech-language pathologists and audiologists to use to measure the effects of therapeutic interventions from admission to discharge and compare their outcomes against similar patient populations across the country.

The NOMS consists of 15 disorder-specific Functional Communication Measures (FCMs). Each FCM has a 7-point rating scale ranging from least functional (level 1) to most functional (level 7). The ratings do not depend on particular formal or informal assessment measures, but are determined by clinical observations of the patient's performance in functional contexts. FCMs are scored only if they specifically relate to the patient's individualized treatment plan and goals. The FCMs relevant to c/mTBI include: attention, fluency, memory, pragmatics, problem solving, reading, spoken language comprehension, spoken language expression, and writing.

Recommended Instrument Use: Practice Option

The FCMs were designed to describe changes in abilities over time, from admission to discharge. The ASHA NOMS can be used to examine individual and institution-specific treatment outcomes of patient populations as well as to collect aggregate data from across institutions nationally. FCMs are selected based on the areas targeted in the treatment plan and scored by a certified speech-language pathologist. The ASHA NOMS provide the only functional assessment of cognitive-communication intervention that offers a national database for comparing treatment outcomes of patients with acquired c/mTBI and program outcomes with national outcomes of a similar patient population.

The Centers for Medicare and Medicaid Services classified the NOMS as an approved registry through which eligible speech-language pathologists can report on the quality measures for its Physician Quality Reporting System.

Administration Protocol/Equipment/Time

The FCMs do not depend on other formal or informal test results, but are based on observations of the patient. There are a total of 15 FCMs that can be downloaded from the ASHA website (www.asha.org/members/research/noms). It will take a clinician approximately 2 hours to review the training materials and take the user registration test. There is no cost associated with the training or registration test.

Groups Tested With This Measure

Data collection is ongoing for adults in healthcare settings and includes individuals with mild and moderate TBI.

Interpretability

- Norms: unavailable
- Scoring: Each FCM has a 7-point rating scale ranging from least functional (level 1) to most functional (level 7).
- MDC: Data are being collected; however, patients with c/mTBI can possibly move from level 5 to level 7.

Reliability and Validity Estimates: No information is available.

- Responsiveness: The responsiveness of nine outcomes measurement scales was evaluated with 33 children and adolescents (ages 4–18 years) who had sustained TBI. The ASHA NOMS was sufficient to detect change in each of the children where change occurred.[53]

Selected Reference

American Speech-Language-Hearing Association. *National Outcomes Measurement System (NOMS): Adult Speech-Language Pathology User's Guide.* Rockville, MD: ASHA; 2003.

GOAL ATTAINMENT SCALING

Purpose/Description

Goal attainment scaling (GAS) produces an individualized, criterion-referenced measure of a person's goal achievement that can be aggregated to quantify summary outcomes across patients receiving the same intervention but who have different individual goals.[54,55] Additionally, rather than simply reporting whether or not goals were achieved, GAS provides the clinician information about the degree of goal achievement associated with a given intervention or experimental condition. Some experts recommend GAS as a responsive and reliable metric of cognitive rehabilitation outcomes.[56]

Recommended Method Use: Practice Option

GAS allows clinicians to evaluate the extent to which a group of patients who are receiving the same type of intervention achieve their personal rehabilitation goals. Therefore, use of this method is most appropriate for clinicians who treat a number of service members with c/mTBI. GAS is described as specific to each patient.[57] Therefore, it can be used in heterogeneous populations, including patients with different severity levels of TBI or those with comorbidities. Individual patient goals are set and can be weighted to reflect the opinion of the patient and the therapist or team on the difficulty of achieving the goal.[58] According to Malec,[56(p235)] GAS can be used beneficially for:

- monitoring progress in a time-limited epoch of care;
- structuring team conferences;
- planning and making decisions about ongoing rehabilitation;
- ensuring concise, relevant communication to the client, significant others, referral source, and funding sources;
- guiding the delivery of social reinforcement; and
- evaluating the program.

Used in conjunction with other outcome measures, GAS has been shown to effectively measure outcomes of cognitive-communication intervention. It was one of six main outcome measures used in a randomized controlled trial designed to evaluate the efficacy of a group treatment program addressing social communication skills training for people with TBI.[59] Each goal was expressed objectively in terms of concrete behaviors that can be observed and recorded. Goals were developed with input from the individual participant and assistance from the group leader. The goals were scaled into five steps, so the participant usually fell at the second step, with a chance to achieve one, two, or three steps toward maximum goal achievement as rated by themselves, the group leaders, and a significant other. After setting specific social communication goals in the third week of treatment, goal attainment was evaluated at the end of treatment and at 3-, 6-, and 9-month follow-ups by the TBI subject, significant others, and the group leaders. A sample of the GAS for this study follows:

GOAL: *I will ask more questions in conversations.*

1. I will ask questions in 10% or less of conversations.
2. I will ask questions in 30% of conversations.
3. I will ask questions in 50% of conversations.
4. I will ask questions in 70% of conversations.
5. I will ask questions in 90% or more of conversations.[56(p253)]

Note that GAS requires familiarity with statistical calculations. Therefore, use of this method may only be appropriate in settings in which statistical support or consultants are available.

Administration Protocol/Equipment/Time

See Clinician Tip Sheet: GAS Procedures for a description of the process. Identifying client goals may be incorporated into the interview/evaluation process, adding up to 15 minutes to formalize the five levels of goal achievement used in GAS. No formal materials or equipment are needed.

Groups Tested With This Measure

Originally developed to measure outcomes in mental health,[60] GAS has been used to measure change as a result of cognitive rehabilitation[61] and brain injury rehabilitation,[21,62] including in those with c/mTBI,[55,63] and has been recommended as a useful outcome and planning tool in cognitive rehabilitation after c/mTBI.[59,64]

TABLE 11-1

EXAMPLE GOAL ATTAINMENT SCALE: IMPROVING APPOINTMENT ATTENDANCE

Predicted Attainment	Score	Goal Attainment Levels
Most favorable outcome likely	+ 2	Arrives at medical appointments on time without any reminders from wife.
Greater than expected outcome	+ 1	Arrives at medical appointments on time with occasional reminders from wife.
Expected level of outcome	0	Arrives at medical appointments on time with one morning reminder from wife on the day of the appointment.
Less than expected outcome (and baseline/evaluation performance)	– 1	Arrives at medical appointments on time with multiple reminders from wife on the day of the appointment.
Most unfavorable outcome	– 2	Arrives at medical appointments on time only if driven by wife.

Interpretability

- The goal attainment standardized score has a mean of 50 and a standard deviation of 10. A *t*-score of greater than 50 reflects performance that is above the expected level; less than 50 reflects performance that is lower than the expected level of achievement.[65]
- Responsiveness: Findings from multiple studies suggest that GAS is more sensitive than traditional rehabilitation measures.[61,66,67]

Reliability and Validity Estimates

- Interrater reliability: Various aspects of GAS interrater reliability have been examined.
  - Goal identification: Rushton and Miller reported that 63% of goals were identified by two different investigators in patients with lower extremity amputations.[67]
  - Scale items: Joyce et al[68] reported high levels of agreement when two raters ranked the same scale items (– 2 to + 2; r = 0.92 to 0.94).
  - Outcome goal achievement scoring: Goal scales scores assigned by therapists working with children with cerebral palsy had good correlation (Cohen's kappa = .64) with scores assigned by independent raters.[69]
- Validity: Convergent validity was evaluated in a brain injury rehabilitation program. GAS was highly correlated with global clinical impressions (Pearson correlation = 0.8061) but modestly correlated with other measures (eg, – 0.6162 with the Rappaport Disability Rating).

Selected References

Kiresuk TJ, Sherman RE. Goal attainment scaling: a general method for evaluating comprehensive community mental health programs. *Community Ment Health J.* 1968;4:443–453.

Ottenbacher KJ, Cusick A. Goal attainment scaling as a method of clinical service evaluation. *Am J Occup Ther.* 1990;44(6):519–525.

CLINICIAN TIP SHEET: GAS PROCEDURES

Step 1: Establish competency in GAS.[70]

- Persons experienced in GAS should provide instruction and examples for those new to the method. Novice users of GAS should establish practice GAS levels, which are then reviewed by experts.
- If multiple clinicians at a given site are

developing GAS, procedures should be established for consistency to ensure similar increments for scaling.[70]

- Consult with a statistician to set up data analysis methods.

Step 2: Identify problem areas and related therapy goals.[54,55]

- Via an interactive interview, the patient identifies problem areas of concern and behaviors that should be addressed to resolve the concern.
- Trombly[63,71] used the Canadian Occupational Performance Measure to identify five goal areas, which became the basis for individualized GAS.

Step 3: Specify levels of performance.

- Goal-related behaviors or events are operationalized[54] (Table 11-1).

- Collaborate with the patient in this process to specify goal levels.

Step 4: Ensure there are no overlapping levels, gaps between levels, or more than one indicator in a problem area.[54]

Step 5: Plan a reevaluation strategy and timeframe. Consider revisiting status towards goal achievement with the patient at least once a month.

Step 6: Calculate the GAS score.

GAS is a valuable and rigorous method for evaluating patients' goal achievement. This method allows clinicians to evaluate goal achievement by aggregating GAS across multiple patients to determine if the group experienced statistically significant pre-post changes. Clinicians should collaborate with a statistical expert to set up methods to calculate GAS scores and analyze GAS data.[54]

REFERENCES

1. Resnik LJ, Allen SM. Using International Classification of Functioning, Disability and Health to understand challenges in community reintegration of injured veterans. *J Rehabil Res Dev.* 2007;44(7):991–1006.

2. Daggett V, Bakas T, Habermann B. A review of health-related quality of life in adult traumatic brain injury survivors in the context of combat veterans. *J Neurosci Nurs.* Apr 2009;41(2):59–71.

3. Petchprapai N, Winkelman C. Mild traumatic brain injury: determinants and subsequent quality of life. A review of the literature. *J Neurosci Nurs.* Oct 2007;39(5):260–272.

4. The Center for Outcome Measurement in Brain Injury. http://www.tbims.org/combi. Accessed November 21, 2013.

5. Ware JE, Sherbourne CD. The MOS 36-Item Short-Form Health Survey (SF-36): I. Conceptual framework and item selection. *Med Care.* 1992;30:473–481.

6. Findler M, Cantor J, Haddad L, Gordon W, Ashman T. The reliability and validity of the SF-36 health survey questionnaire for use with individuals with traumatic brain injury. *Brain Inj.* Aug 2001;15(8):715–723.

7. Malec J. *The Mayo-Portland Adaptability Inventory.* The Center for Outcome Measurement in Brain Injury. http://www.tbims.org/combi/mpai. Accessed November 21, 2013.

8. Malec JF, Kragness M, Evans RW, Finlay KL, Kent A, Lezak MD. Further psychometric evaluation and revision of the Mayo-Portland Adaptability Inventory in a national sample. *J Head Trauma Rehabil.* Nov–Dec 2003;18(6):479–492.

9. Malec JF, Lezak MD. *Manual for the Mayo-Portland Adaptability Inventory (MPAI-4) for Adults, Children and Adolescents. Revised with Adaptations for Pediatric Version.* 2008. http://tbims.org/combi/mpai/manual.pdf. Accessed January 7, 2014.

10. Brown M. *Participation Objective, Participation Subjective.* The Center for Outcome Measurement in Brain Injury. http://www.tbims.org/combi/pops. Accessed November 21, 2013.

11. WHOQOL Group. Development of the World Health Organization WHOQOL-BREF Quality of Life assessment. *Psychol Med.* 1998;28(3):551–558.

12. Ylvisaker M, Hanks R, Johnson-Greene D; American Speech-Language-Hearing Association. *Rehabilitation of Children and Adults with Cognitive-Communication Disorders After Brain Injury.* Rockville, MD: ASHA; 2003. Technical Report. http://www.asha.org/policy/TR2003-00146/. Accessed November 21, 2013.

13. Kazis LE, Lee A, Spiro A 3rd, et al. Measurement comparisons of the medical outcomes study and veterans SF-36 health survey. *Health Care Financ Rev.* Summer 2004;25(4):43–58.

14. Kazis LE, Miller DR, Clark JA, et al. Improving the response choices on the veterans SF-36 health survey role functioning scales: results from the Veterans Health Study. *J Ambul Care Manage.* Jul–Sep 2004;27(3):263–280.

15. Quality Metric. SF-36.org: a community for measuring health outcomes using SF tools. Frequently asked questions website. http://www.sf-36.org/faq/generalinfo.aspx. Accessed February 28, 2014.

16. van Baalen B, Odding E, van Woensel MP, Roebroeck ME. Reliability and sensitivity to change of measurement instruments used in a traumatic brain injury population. *Clin Rehabil.* Aug 2006;20(8):686–700.

17. Ware JE Jr. SF-36 health survey update. SF-36.org: a community for measuring health outcomes using SF tools. http://www.sf-36.org/tools/SF36.shtml#VERS2. Accessed November 21, 2013.

18. Finch E, Brooks D, Stratford PW, Mayo N. *Physical Rehabilitation Outcome Measures Second Edition, a Guide to Enhanced Clinical Decision Making.* 2nd ed. Hamilton, Ontario: BC Decker, Inc; 2002.

19. Malec JF. The Mayo-Portland Participation Index: A brief and psychometrically sound measure of brain injury outcome. *Arch Phys Med Rehabil.* Dec 2004;85(12):1989–1996.

20. Malec JF, Thompson JM. Relationship of the Mayo-Portland Adaptability inventory to functional outcome and cognitive performance measures. *J Head Trauma Rehabil.* 1994;9(41):1–15.

21. Malec JF. Impact of comprehensive day treatment on societal participation for persons with acquired brain injury. *Arch Phys Med Rehabil.* Jul 2001;82(7):885–895.

22. Malec JF, Moessner AM, Kragness M, Lezak MD. Refining a measure of brain injury sequelae to predict post-acute rehabilitation outcome: rating scale analysis of the Mayo-Portland Adaptability Inventory. *J Head Trauma Rehabil.* Feb 2000;15(1):670–682.

23. Malec JF, Buffington AL, Moessner AM, Degiorgio L. A medical/vocational case coordination system for persons with brain injury: an evaluation of employment outcomes. *Arch Phys Med Rehabil.* Aug 2000;81(8):1007–1015.

24. Malec JF, Degiorgio L. Characteristics of successful and unsuccessful completers of three postacute brain injury rehabilitation pathways. *Arch Phys Med Rehabil.* Dec 2002;83(12):1759–1764.

25. World Health Organization. *International Classification of Functioning, Disability and Health.* Geneva, Switzerland: World Health Organization; 2001.

26. Gordon WA, Brown M, Hibbard M. Living life after TBI. *RTC on Community Integration of Individuals with TBI.* New York, NY: Mount Sinai School of Medicine; 1998.

27. Curtin M, Jones J, Tyson GA, Mitsch V, Alston M, McAllister L. Outcomes of participation objective, participation subjective (POPS) measure following traumatic brain injury. *Brain Inj.* 2011;25(3):266–273.

28. Brown M, Dijkers MPJM, Gordon WA, Ashman T, Charatz H, Cheng Z. Participation Objective, Participation Subjective: a measure of participation combining outsider and insider perspectives. *J Head Trauma Rehabil.* 2004;19(6):459–481.

29. Orley J, Kuyken W. *Quality of Life Assessment: International Perspectives.* Heidelberg, Ger: Springer Verlag; 1994.

30. Szabo Silvija. The World Health Organisation Quality of Life (WHOQOL) Assessment Instrument. In: Spilker B, ed. *Quality of Life and Pharmaeconomics in Clinical Trials*. 2nd edition ed. New York, NY: Lippincott-Raven; 1996.

31. WHOQOL Group. Development of the WHOQOL: rationale and current status. *Int J Mental Health*. 1994;23(3):24–56.

32. WHOQOL Group. The World Health Organization Quality of Life Assessment (WHOQOL): Position paper from the World Health Organization. *Soc Sci Med*. 1995;41:1403–1409.

33. Bullinger M, Azouvi P, Brooks N, et al. Quality of life in patients with traumatic brain injury-basic issues, assessment and recommendations. *Restor Neurol Neurosci*. 2002;20(3–4):111.

34. Jang Y, Hsieh CL, Wang Y, Wu YH. A validity study of the WHOQOL-BREF assessment in persons with traumatic spinal cord injury. *Arch Phys Med Rehabil*. 2004;85:(1890–1895).

35. Lin MR, Hwang HF, Chen CC, Chiu WC. Comparisons of the brief form of the World Health Organization Quality of Life and Short Form-36 for persons with spinal cord injuries. *AM J Phys Med Rehabil*. 2007;86(2):104–113.

36. Bryant RA, O'Donnell ML, Creamer M, McFarlane AC, Clark CR, Silove D. The psychiatric sequelae of traumatic injury. *Am J Psychiatry*. Mar 2010;167(3):312–320.

37. Chiu WT, Huang SJ, Hwang HF, et al. Use of the WHOQOL-BREF for evaluating persons with traumatic brain injury. *J Neurotrauma*. Nov 2006;23(11):1609–1620.

38. Zalihic A, Markotic V, Mabic M, et al. Differences in quality of life after stroke and myocardial infarction. *Psychiatr Danub*. Jun 2010;22(2):241–248.

39. Zalihic A, Markotic V, Zalihic D, Mabic M. Gender and quality of life after cerebral stroke. *Bosn J Basic Med Sci*. May 2010;10(2):94–99.

40. Lucas-Carrasco R, Skevington SM, Gomez-Benito J, Rejas J, March J. Using the WHOQOL-BREF in persons with dementia: a validation study. *Alzheimer Dis Assoc Disord*. 2011;25(4):345–51.

41. Hsiung PC, Fang CT, Chang YY, Chen MY, Wang JD. Comparison of WHOQOL-BREF and SF-36 in patients with HIV infection. *Qual Life Res*. Feb 2005;14(1):141–150.

42. Struttmann T, Fabro M, Romieu G, et al. Quality-of-life assessment in the old using the WHOQOL 100: Differences between patients with senile dementia and patients with cancer. *Int Psychogeriatr*. 1999;11(3):273–279.

43. Skevington SM, Carse MS, Williams AC. Validation of the WHOQOL-100: pain management improves quality of life for chronic pain patients. *Clin J Pain*. Sep 2001;17(3):264–275.

44. Bonicatto SC, Dew MA, Zaratiegui R, Lorenzo L, Pecina P. Adult outpatients with depression: worse quality of life than in other chronic medical diseases in Argentina. *Soc Sci Med*. 2001;52(6):911–919.

45. von Steinbuchel N, Lischetzke T, Gurny N, Eid M. Assessing quality of life in older people: psychometric properties of the WHOQOL-BREF. *Eur J Ageing*. 2006;3(2):116–122.

46. Power M, Harper A, Bullinger M. The World Health Organization WHOQOL-100: tests of the universality of quality of life in 15 different cultural groups worldwide. *Health Psychol*. 1999;18(5):495–505.

47. Bonomi AE, Patrick DL, Bushnell DM, Martin M. Validation of the United States' version of the World Health Organization Quality of Life (WHOQOL) instrument. *J Clin Epidemiol*. Jan 2000;53(1):1–12.

48. Trompenaars FJ, Masthoff ED, Van Heck GL, Hodiamont PP, De Vries J. Content validity, construct validity, and reliability of the WHOQOL-BREF in a population of Dutch adult psychiatric outpatients. *Qual Life Res*. 2005;14(1):151–160.

49. Naumann VJ, Byrne GJ. WHOQOL-BREF as a measure of quality of life in older patients with depression. *Int Psychogeriatr.* Jun 2004;16(2):159–173.

50. Chan GW, Ungvari GS, Shek DT, Leung Dagger JJ. Hospital and community-based care for patients with chronic schizophrenia in Hong Kong—quality of life and its correlates. *Soc Psychiatry Psychiatr Epidemiol.* 2003;38(4):196–203.

51. Adams C. Quality of life for caregivers and stroke survivors in the immediate discharge period. *Appl Nurs Res.* May 2003;16(2):126–130.

52. World Health Organization. *Programme on Mental Health: WHOQOL Measuring Quality of Life.* Geneva, Switzerland: WHO; 1997.

53. Thomas-Stonell N, Johnson P, Rumney P, Wright V, Oddson B. An evaluation of the responsiveness of a comprehensive set of outcome measures for children and adolescents with traumatic brain injuries. *Pediatr Rehabil.* Jan–Mar 2006;9(1):14–23.

54. Ottenbacher KJ, Cusick A. Goal attainment scaling as a method of clinical service evaluation. *Am J Occup Ther.* 1990;44(6):519–525.

55. Trombly CA, Radomski MV, Trexel C, Burnet-Smith SE. Occupational therapy and achievement of self-identified goals by adults with acquired brain injury: phase II. *Am J Occup Ther.* Sep–Oct 2002;56(5):489–498.

56. Malec JF. Goal attainment scaling in rehabilitation. *Neuropsychol Rehabil.* 1999;9:253–275.

57. Ertzgaard P, Ward AB, Wissel J, Borg J. Practical considerations for goal attainment scaling during rehabilitation following acquired brain injury. *J Rehabil Med.* 2011;43(1):8–14.

58. Turner-Stokes L. Goal attainment scaling (GAS) in rehabilitation: a practical guide. *Clin Rehabil.* 2009;23(4):362–370.

59. Dahlberg CA, Cusick CP, Hawley LA, et al. Treatment efficacy of social communication skills training after traumatic brain injury: a randomized treatment and deferred treatment controlled trial. *Arch Phys Med Rehabil.* Dec 2007;88(12):1561–1573.

60. Kiresuk TJ, Sherman RE. Goal attainment scaling: A general method for evaluating comprehensive community mental health programs. *Community Ment Health J.* 1968;4:443–453.

61. Rockwood KJ, Joyce BM, Stolee P. Use of goal attainment scaling in measuring clinically important change in cognitive rehabilitation patients. *J Clin Epidemiol.* 1997;50:581–588.

62. Malec JF, Smigielski JS, DePompolo RW, Thompson JM. Outcome evaluation and prediction in a comprehensive-integrated post-acute outpatient brain injury rehabilitation programme. *Brain Inj.* Jan–Feb 1993;7(1):15–29.

63. Trombly CA, Radomski MV, Davis ES. Achievement of self-identified goals by adults with traumatic brain injury: phase I. *Amer J Occup Ther.* 1998;52:810–818.

64. Helmick K. Cognitive rehabilitation for military personnel with mild traumatic brain injury and chronic post-concussional disorder: results of April 2009 consensus conference. *NeuroRehabilitation.* 2010;26(3):239–255.

65. Ottenbacher KJ, Cusick A. Discriminative versus evaluative assessment: some observations on goal attainment scaling. *Amer J Occup Ther.* 1993;47(4):349–354.

66. Khan F, Pallant JF, Turner-Stokes L. Use of goal attainment scaling in inpatient rehabilitation for persons with multiple sclerosis. *Arch Phys Med Rehabil.* 2008;89:652–659.

67. Rushton PW, Miller WC. Goal attainment scaling in the rehabilitation of patients with lower-extremity amputations: a pilot study. *Arch Phys Med Rehabil.* 2002;83(6):771–775.

68. Joyce BM, Rockwood KJ, Mate-Kole CC. Use of goal attainment scaling in brain injury in rehabilitation hospital. *Am J Phys Med Rehabil.* 1994;73:10–14.

69. Steenbeek D, Ketelaar M, Lindeman E, Galama K, Gorter JW. Interrater reliability of goal attainment scaling in rehabilitation of children with cerebral palsy. *Arch Phys Med Rehabil.* Mar 2010;91(3):429–435.

70. Mailloux Z, May-Benson TA, Summers CA, et al. Goal attainment scaling as a measure of meaningful outcomes for children with sensory integration disorders. *Am J Occup Ther.* 2007;61(2):254–259.

71. Trombly CA, Radomski MV, Burnett-Smith SE. Achievement of self-identified goals by adults with traumatic brain injury: phase II. *Am J Occupl Ther.* 2002;56:489–498.

APPENDIX A

CLINICAL MANAGEMENT GUIDANCE:
OCCUPATIONAL THERAPY
AND
PHYSICAL THERAPY
FOR
MILD TRAUMATIC BRAIN INJURY

U.S. Army Office of The Surgeon General
Rehabilitation and Reintegration Division

August 2010

Prepared by:

OT/PT MTBI WORK TEAM

Mary Vining Radomski, PhD, OTR/L, FAOTA

Maggie Weightman, PT, PhD

Leslie Freeman Davidson, PhD (Cand), MSEd, OTR/L

Marilyn Rodgers, MS PT

MAJ Robyn Bolgla, MS PT CTRS

Contractor and Subcontractors:

General Dynamics

Sister Kenny Research Center

Riverbend Therapeutics, LLC

Supported and Assisted by:

Expert Panel Members

Advisers and Reviewers

(see Appendix A.1)

Table of Contents

EXECUTIVE SUMMARY

Given the large numbers of Service members sustaining mild traumatic brain injury (MTBI) in OEF/OIF, a group of occupational and physical therapists was tasked by the Proponency Office for Rehabilitation and Reintegration to develop a *Clinical Management Guidance* document that outlines best OT and PT practices for rehabilitation of Service members with MTBI. The *Guidance* in its current form represents a prelude to a final version that includes a toolkit.

Based on reviews of existing guidelines, research literature, and with input from experts, the resultant document includes OT and PT assessment and intervention recommendations related to the following concerns associated with MTBI: Combat Readiness Check, activity intolerance, patient education, vestibular dysfunction, vision dysfunction, headache, temporomandibular disorders, cognitive dysfunction, performance of life roles, participation in exercise. We also provide a brief discussion of outcomes measurement specific to participation.

An expert panel recommended the development of a Combat Readiness Check (CRC) that could be administered by an OT or PT in theater. The CRC, comprised of existing instruments and a dual task test, would provide decision-makers with additional data about safety and readiness to return to duty. Stop-gap assessments were proposed but the dual-task component needs to be developed and validated, along with the entire proposed CRC procedure.

OT and PT have pivotal contributions to the recovery, rehabilitation, and reintegration of Service members with MTBI. Research is needed in every area of practice – presenting opportunities to advance outcomes for Service members and civilians alike.

SECTION I

INTRODUCTION:

The wars in Iraq and Afghanistan - Operation Iraqi Freedom (OIF) and Operation Enduring Freedom (OEF) – have mobilized the civilian and military medical and rehabilitation communities to identify best practices in the care of Service members with mild traumatic brain injury (MTBI). Symptoms of MTBI may have immediate and long term implications for warriors' safe return to duty [31] and veterans' ability to successfully re-establish social relationships and resume productive activities upon discharge from military service [32].

Occupational and physical therapists provide adaptive and remedial interventions to address impairments, activity limitations, and social participation issues associated with MTBI. Occupational therapy (OT) and physical therapy (PT) have played an essential role to the mission of the United States Military and Veteran Affairs for the more than seventy five years. As members of the Army Medical Specialist Corps, occupational and physical therapists contribute to the Corps mission by applying their "...unique skills to maximize the health and enhance the readiness of Warriors across the full spectrum of operational missions and environments" (retrieved December 9, 2007 from https://amsc.amedd.army.mil/ , Army Medical Specialist Corps). Occupational and physical therapists are also members of the United States Veterans Affairs (VA) health care team. As such, they provide rehabilitation Services to military veterans in order to ensure maximum level of functioning and quality of life. This commitment to the health and wellbeing of active duty soldiers (including activated Reservists and National Guard) has helped maintain troop levels, return soldiers to duty, and ensure the best possible recovery and rehabilitation for those who are unable to return to duty. Outcomes of care are optimized as occupational and physical therapists use evidence-based guidelines to inform the assessment and treatment of MTBI across the military and VA eight levels of care – from point of injury to community reintegration.

OVERVIEW:

In September 2007, The Proponency Office for Rehabilitation and Reintegration (PR&R) of the Office of the Surgeon General charged a team of two occupational therapists and three physical therapists (two military and three civilians) to develop OT/PT clinical practice guidance for MTBI by December 31, 2007. Specifically, the MTBI Clinical Management Guidance was to summarize and help establish, "...state-of-the-art rehabilitative care for Soldiers with mild traumatic brain injuries...[by] completing a critical review of current research and clinical rehabilitative care practices in the assessment, treatment and management of mild TBI at all levels of care (from acute theater to long term life care" (Statement of Work, 2007). The work team was further charged to convene a MTBI Rehabilitative Care Summit with OT and PT subject matter experts from the Department of Defense, VA, and the civilian sector to review, refine and reach a consensus on the OT/PT clinical management recommendations. This final document is a result of the above stated charge and is an updated version of two earlier drafts.

This document has eight sections: introduction, background, overview of the OT and PT recommendations, OT and PT recommendations for assessment and intervention for MTBI, references, and appendices.

For convenience, the term "Service member" will be used throughout the Clinical Guidance document – referring generally to active duty, Reservists, National Guard, and veterans of all Services.

METHODS:

The document development process consisted of four phases (see Figure A.1): Phase 1 – Identifying best practices; Phase 2 – Drafting and refining assessment/treatment recommendations for each level of care based on expert input; Phase 3 – Writing a full draft of the document and obtaining expert review; Phase 4 – Finalizing algorithms, references, and recommendations for next steps and submitting the Clinical Management Guidance document. Each phase of development is described below.

Figure A.1

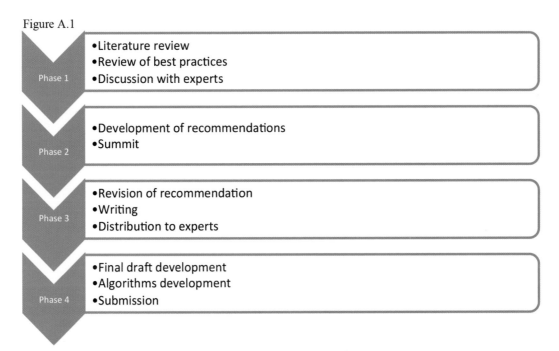

Figure A.1: Overview of Clinical Management Guidance development process.

Phase 1: Identifying best practices

During this phase, the team completed a literature review on the assessment and treatment of MTBI. The literature review consisted of exploring existing evidence-based reviews and research from a variety of rehabilitation disciplines. Disciplines involved in the treatment of MTBI include occupational therapy, physical therapy, speech and language pathology, neuropsychology, counseling psychologists, physicians, nurses, vocational counselors, recreational therapists, and kinesiotherapists. The scope of practice of the various professionals is typically determined by state licensure and practice setting. There was a heavy reliance on literature specific to the MTBI incurred in civilian contexts (e.g., sports or traffic accidents) as little literature exists about rehabilitation after MTBI sustained in combat. The work team also reviewed existing practice guidelines pertinent to MTBI including the following: Practice Management Guidelines for the Management of Mild Traumatic Brain Injury: the EAST Practice Management Guidelines Work Group [33]; Veterans Health Initiative: Traumatic Brain Injury [34]; WHO Collaborating Centre Task Force on Mild Traumatic Brain Injury (see Journal of Rehabilitation Medicine, Supplement 43, February 2004); Guidelines for Field Management of Combat-Related Head Trauma [35]; Traumatic Brain Injury: Diagnosis, acute management, and rehabilitation [36]; Defense and Veterans Brain Injury Center (DVBIC)Working Group on the Acute Management of Mild Traumatic Brain Injury in Military Operational Settings: Clinical Practice Guideline and Recommendations [7]. It should be noted that none of these guidelines specified OT or PT practices. Additionally, team members contacted therapists who are members of the military/VA healthcare system to identify current standards of practice and request information about what may be needed to enhance outcomes. Civilian programs specializing in MTBI and brain injury rehabilitation were also contacted to identify best practices.

Phase 2: Drafting recommended practices

During Phase 2, the team synthesized information obtained from the literature and facility discussions to begin drafting recommendations for OT and PT practice. The draft of assessment and treatment guidelines across the eight levels of care included a number of general assumptions regarding treatment of MTBI as well as assumptions specific to setting and level of care. Overarching goals appropriate for specific settings were also outlined. These recommendations were documented and a multidisciplinary expert panel was identified and invited to participate in a one day Summit (November 15, 2007) to provide feedback on both the process and content of the draft proposal. During the Summit, minutes were taken and a post-Summit meeting was used to summarize and discuss the various suggestions.

Phase 3: Synthesizing feedback and writing a full first draft

During this phase, the OT/PT MTBI work team continued to revisit the literature and utilize their contacts at the various treatment settings to refine and formalize practice recommendations. Writing of the document began at this phase and a revised draft of the complete document was sent to subject matter experts with a feedback form for in-process feedback.

Phase 4: Finalizing and submitting the Clinical Management Guidance document

Feedback from subject matter experts was pooled and modifications were made to the Guidance document. In addition, sample level-of-care algorithms for specific recommendations were developed, references compiled, and the final draft of the Guidance completed. Suggestions for implementation and further work were identified and documented and Draft 1.0 of the Guidance was submitted to the PR&R on January 1, 2008.

In early 2009, Draft 1.0 was further edited, resulting in the current version of the document (Draft 2.0). Draft 2.0 was then updated in May 2010 so that this final version of the Guidance is compatible with the companion OT-PT MTBI Toolkit.

SECTION II

BACKGROUND:

In this section, we discuss definitions of MTBI, outline the typical course of recovery, and describe the implications for MTBI sustained in a military context.

Definitions of Mild Traumatic Brain Injury

There is no consensus on a definition of MTBI, nor is there a symptom complex that demonstrates diagnostic specificity [37]. Three definitions were used to inform this work: the one currently used by the Department of Defense (DoD) (released October 1, 2007); one identified by the World Health Organization (WHO); as well as the definition adopted by the Defense and Veterans Brain Injury Center [7]. While the current DOD definition is the basis of this Clinical Practice Guidance, the literature that has been instrumental in the development of other guidelines often uses alternative definitions for MTBI.

According to the WHO Collaborating Centre for Neurotrauma Task Force on MTBI, MTBI is "… an acute brain injury resulting from mechanical energy to the head from external physical forces. Operational criteria for clinical identification include one or more of the following; confusion, loss of consciousness for 30 min or less, post traumatic amnesia less than 24 hours and other transient neurological abnormalities such as focal signs, seizures, and an intracranial hemorrhage not requiring surgery. Deficits cannot be due to drugs, alcohol, medications, or other injuries or problems (psychological), or by penetrating craniocerebral injury" (Carroll, 2004, p. 114).

The Defense and Veterans Brain Injury Center (2006) developed a definition that incorporated many of the elements outlined in the WHO definition. They stated, " … MTBI is an injury to the brain resulting from an external force and/or acceleration/deceleration mechanism from an event such as a blast, fall, direct impact, or motor vehicle accident (MVA) which causes and alteration in mental status typically resulting in the temporally related onset of symptoms such as: headache, nausea and vomiting, dizziness/balance problems, fatigue, insomnia/sleep disturbances, drowsiness, sensitivity to light/noise, blurred vision, difficulty remembering, and/or difficulty concentrating" (p. 2).

In an attempt to better diagnose and provide treatment to the troops in the theater, the DoD updated the definition of traumatic brain injury and how it classifies severity of injury. According to a memo released by the Assistant Secretary of Defense on October 1, 2007, a traumatic brain injury is "… a traumatically induced structural injury and/or physiological disruption of brain function as a result of an external force that is indicated by new onset or worsening of at least one of the following clinical signs, immediately following the event:

- Any period of loss of or a decreased level of consciousness;

- Any loss of memory for events immediately before or after the injury;

- Any alteration in mental state at the time of injury (confusion, disorientation, slowed thinking, etc.);

- Neurological deficits (weakness, loss of balance, change in vision, praxis, paresis/plegia, sensory loss, aphasia etc.) that may or may not be transient;

- Intracranial lesion" (p. 1).

While acknowledging that cognitive symptoms associated with post traumatic stress may look similar to MTBI, they further characterize MTBI as meeting one or more of the following criteria: loss of consciousness for 0 – 30 minutes; alteration of consciousness/mental state for a moment or up to 24 hours; post-traumatic amnesia for up to one day.

Natural History of Mild Traumatic Brain Injury

Individuals who sustain MTBI typically become symptomatic at the time of incident (McCrea, 2008). Initial symptoms often include headache, dizziness, nausea and vomiting, sleep disturbances, sensitivity to noise and light, slowed thinking and reaction time, memory problems, irritability, depression, and visual changes [38]. During the acute phase of recovery, symptoms are thought to be explained by a short-term neurometabolic process that renders neurons temporarily dysfunctional but not destroyed [39].

Some Service members with MTBI do not report symptoms until later in their medical care (especially if they suffer concomitant life-threatening injuries) or after deployment. In their post-deployment screening study, Terrio and colleagues (2009) reported that for some Service members, memory problems and irritability were first identified after the acute phase, possibly when they are faced with challenging novel tasks and/or feedback from loved ones. Again, MTBI symptoms vary in severity and may or may not impact activity and social participation. In the majority of cases, symptoms resolve within three months of injury [40]. However, for 10-30% of those with MTBI [41-44], problems persist and impact the individual's ability to resume multiple life roles and activity.

The group of individuals who present with persistent problems after three months may have post-concussion syndrome (PCS) [40,45]. A person with possible PCS has a history of head trauma with LOC and experiences symptoms in at least three of the following categories: headache, dizziness, malaise, fatigue, noise intolerance; irritability, depression, anxiety, emotional lability; subjective concentration, memory, or intellectual disabilities without neuropsychological evidence or marked impairment; insomnia; reduced alcohol tolerance; preoccupation with above symptoms and fear of brain damage [45]. There are a number of possible explanations for the difficulties experienced by the subgroup with protracted MTBI symptoms [40]. One explanation is that these people have sustained microscopic brain damage that is responsible (in part) for the physical, cognitive, and emotional sequelae of MTBI [46]. Others suggest that PCS is likely not a neurologic condition stemming from MTBI [39]. PCS may be the result of a vicious cycle in which cognitive inefficiencies, distractions from physical symptoms, and situational stressors interact to compound the challenges presented by the MTBI [47]. As explained by Montgomery (1995), extra effort is required as the person resumes everyday activities and becomes alarmed by inefficiencies and errors in performing premorbidly mundane tasks. The resultant hypersensitivity to error and anxiety mix with misattributions regarding the root cause of deficient performance, further sabotaging self-confidence and subsequent performance. The long term consequences of issues surrounding MTBI and PCS can lead to long term depression, social isolation, behavioral issues, and family burden.

Mild Traumatic Brain Injury in a Military Context

An estimated 10-15% of Service members returning from OEF/OIF may have sustained a MTBI [48]. A critical problem in addressing the needs of Service members with MTBI is that the injury itself is difficult to diagnosis or identify. Unlike that of soldiers who sustain severe TBI, military personnel who, are exposed to single or multiple blast explosions from improvised explosive devices (IEDs) may sustain mild head trauma with no immediate outward signs of injury. Their symptoms may initially present themselves as a brief alteration of consciousness (AOC) or behavioral changes [49]. There is no way of identifying the number of mild traumatic brain injuries at this time as many are initially masked with other more dire diagnoses such as limb loss, burns, spinal cord injury, or fractures.

Service members who present with MTBI fall into one of the following four categories: the warrior who sustained a MTBI only; the warrior who has sustained MTBI and also presents with post traumatic stress disorder (PTSD); the warrior who presents with MTBI and polytrauma; the warrior who presents with all three (MTBI, polytrauma, and PTSD). These multiple variables introduce a number of factors that make initial diagnosis and assessment difficult such that MTBI may often not be detected until well after the incident(s). Furthermore, the concomitant injuries and conditions must be considered in occupational and physical therapy regimens across all levels of care.

Mild Traumatic Brain Injury and Stress Disorders

Similar to MTBI, many Service members experience stress disorders associated with deployment to combat operations and witnessing atrocities [50], with combat injuries increasing the risk for PTSD [51]. The mechanism of injury (over half from a blast) and the combat environment place the Service member who has sustained a MTBI at high risk for an ASR/PTSD overlay [52]. Cognitive symptoms associated with acute stress reaction (ASR) and post traumatic stress disorder mirror many of those apparent in mild traumatic brain injury [53]. These include sleep disturbances, difficulty with attention, concentration, and memory, irritability, and social isolation (Table A.1).

Table A.1 Symptom Comparison MTBI vs ASR/PTSD[7]

Symptom	MTBI	ASR/PTSD
Memory, attention, concentration	X	X
Irritability	X	X
Sleep disturbances	X	X
Visual changes/disturbances	X	
Balance and Vestibular Issues	X	
Psychological distress with cues that symbolize traumatic event		X
"Flashbacks" during day, night or during sleep		X
Impaired functioning limiting participation in activities	X	X
Nausea and/or vomiting (at time of incident)	X	
Chronic headache	X	

Symptoms associated with MTBI are more evident and persistent in individuals who present with PTSD [53,54]. PTSD, like MTBI has become a key issue fore returning OEF/OIF veterans. According to Matthew S. Goldberg, Deputy Assistant Director for National Security, in a report to Congress on October 17, 2007, "Post-traumatic stress disorder (PTSD) is also difficult to diagnose. Among OIF and OEF veterans who have received VA medical care, about 37 percent have received at least a preliminary diagnosis of mental health problems, and about half of those (17 percent) have received a preliminary diagnosis of PTSD. The overall mental health incidence rate may be lower to the extent that OIF and OEF veterans who have not sought VA medical care do not suffer from those conditions. On the other hand, some veterans with PTSD or other mental health problems may not seek care because they fear being stigmatized" (retrieved on 12/8/08 from http://veterans.house.gov/hearings/Testimony.aspx?TID=7260).

In summary, it is clear that many Service members experience a confusing constellation of symptoms associated with MTBI, PCS, ASR, or PTSD. Therapists appreciate that presenting symptoms may have a dual or even multiple underlying causes, especially in those instances where symptoms continue for more than the typical three month period post-injury. Occupational and physical therapists rely on mental health professionals to diagnose the cause of symptoms (MTBI, ASR/PTSD or a combination of both) - information critical for the occupational and physical therapist when they choose their assessment and treatment methods.

MECHANISM OF INJURY:

The mechanisms of injury for deployment-related MTBI include the head being struck by an object, the head striking an object, the brain undergoing an acceleration/deceleration movement without direct external trauma to the head, a foreign body penetrating the brain, forces generated from events such as a blast or explosion.

The most common mechanism of injury in OEF/OIF has been secondary to improvised explosive devices (IED) or mines [55]. IEDs are often placed roadside, hidden within walls, or placed in small confined buildings. When detonated they cause an explosion sending both physical matter and blast waves that travel for hundreds of yards at speeds up to 1,600 feet per second. These blast waves occur in multiple phases with varying injury noted at each phase [56]. The primary phase refers to direct exposure to over pressurized air waves. This may cause diffuse axonal injury and a coup-counter-coup type injury. The secondary phase can be described as the phase where debris follows the air waves often causing penetrating or non-penetrating wounds. The tertiary blast is when the individual is thrown or displaced and hits his or her head on a stationary object, and the quaternary blast injury consists of burns or inhalation of toxic fumes. Many warriors are exposed to multiple blasts and symptoms may or may not be apparent after the first exposure. The minimal neuronal damage that occurs with a single blast is compounded and symptoms may emerge as exposure proximity and frequency increase. To date, there is no way of knowing the risk of MTBI associated with a number of or proximity to blast exposures [56].

Functional Implications for Service Members

As discussed previously, initial symptoms associated with MTBI include headache, dizziness, nausea and vomiting, sleep disturbances, sensitivity to noise and light, slowed thinking and reaction time, memory problems, irritability, depression, and visual changes [38]. These deficits significantly impact the duties of a deployed Service member and may interfere with the veteran's attempts to resume life outside the military system. For example, for warriors, visual disturbances will impact their ability to see the enemy, identify possible IEDs hidden within the brush, read maps and drive safely and effectively in a war zone. Dizziness will hamper use of weapons, negotiating difficult terrain, and tolerating position changes. Decreased processing and reaction time place soldiers and their comrades at risk when quick decisions must be made. If a warrior who has sustained a MTBI remains on duty, the symptoms associated with the injury may place the warrior and their comrades and the mission at risk.

On the home front, persistent symptoms associated with MTBI or PCS often lead to long term activity limitations and social participation restrictions. The long term disability often associated with MTBI may lead to anxiety, stress, depression, and social issues [57], especially if concomitant with other injuries. Activities such as returning to work or school may be challenging or impossible depending on the extent of symptoms. Returning to roles such as a spouse or parent presents challenges as irritability and decreased frustration tolerance impact relationships. Cognitive inefficiencies, such as problems with attention and memory, make seemingly easy daily tasks like medication management a challenge [58]. Given the potential impact of persistent MTBI symptoms on Service members' recovery and reintegration, evidence-informed occupational and physical therapy services are needed at all levels of care.

SECTION III

REHABILITATION AFTER MILD TRAUMATIC BRAIN INJURY WITHIN A MILITARY CONTEXT:

Eight levels of care have been defined to describe medical and rehabilitation resources across the continuum of care – in combat theater through return to community. A Service member may enter the rehabilitation system at any one of the 8 levels or "ports of entry". Furthermore, Service members may enter and exit the Levels of Care multiple times throughout their lifetime.

Rehabilitation Segments of the Levels of Care

The overarching goals of rehabilitation are described within level segments below.

In Combat Theater: Levels I - III

Level I: Buddy Aid to Battalion Aid Station (BAS)

Level II: Forward Support Medical Company/Forward Surgical Team

Level III: Combat Support Hospital (CSH) and Combat Stress Unit

Occupational and physical therapists address symptoms of MTBI for Service members remaining in theater. They may have roles in providing patient education about MTBI and contribute to identifying MTBI symptoms that may interfere with combat readiness. OTs and PTs in theater are advocates for establishing activity tolerance before safe return to duty.

Acute Medical Rehabilitation: Level IV

Level IV: Evacuation Center (Landstuhl Regional Medical Center [LRMAC])

Occupational and physical therapists may begin therapy plans of care during the relatively short episode of care at LRAMC before injured Service members are evacuated to CONUS (continental United States). Therapists continue to evaluate and treat MTBI symptoms, address functional limitations and concomitant impairments, provide education about MTBI, and work with the medical team to identify MTBI.

Single-Service and/or Interdisciplinary Rehabilitation Programming: Levels V - VIII

Level V: Military medical treatment facility (MMTF) - Inpatient and Outpatient

Level VI: Inpatient Rehabilitation

(non-MMTF, such as Veteran's Affairs Medical Center and community partner facilities)

Level VII: Outpatient rehabilitation

(non-MMTF, such as Veteran's Affairs Medical Center and community partner facilities)

Level VIII: Lifetime care

(as Veteran's Affairs Medical Center, a community partner hospital or outpatient facility)

Occupational and physical therapists are part of a larger interdisciplinary team at Levels V – VII, where they work closely with rehabilitation physician, speech pathologist, rehabilitation nurse, therapeutic recreation specialist, chaplain, neuropsychologist, counseling psychologist, and vocational rehabilitation counselor. Occupational and physical therapy specialists (in vision rehabilitation, vestibular rehabilitation, driving) may also be available at these levels.

Inpatient rehabilitation therapies typically focus on helping injured Service members regain basic self-care and mobility skills. They continue to address MTBI-related impairments such as vision, vestibular, and balance problem, provide patient education, and begin to teach Service members with MTBI compensatory techniques. Family members may become involved in the therapy process as well. Therapists provide input regarding return to duty and discharge decisions. Community re-entry readiness will also be addressed, including driving.

Outpatient therapies (at MMTF or VA facilities) tend to address increasingly high-level cognitive, motor, and everyday tasks and functioning. Occupational therapists continue to teach patients to learn to use compensatory cognitive strategies, helping them apply those strategies to home, work, education-related tasks. Occupational therapists are also equipped to help Service members improve communication and emotional control in ways that help with their transition back to family and social life. Physical therapists address MTBI-related symptoms and high-level motor skills needed for return to leisure and fitness activities. Outpatient therapies may be clinic-based or incorporated into the Warrior Transition Units.

SECTION IV

RECOMMENDED OCCUPATIONAL AND PHYSICAL THERAPY PRACTICES:

In this section, we outline recommended OT and PT practices that are supported by the literature and/or by consensus among the work team and advisers. First, assumptions underlying these recommendations are explicated and we then present guiding principles for clinicians treating Service members with MTBI that are applicable across all levels of care. Finally, we orient the reader to the structure and format of the OT and PT recommended practices before describing them according to rehabilitation segment/level of care.

Overarching Assumptions

In order to develop the *Guidance* for occupational and physical therapy across the continuum of care (the military, VA, and lifetime care), the work team made a number of working assumptions about the recipient of therapy services (i.e., Service members) and the potential user of this document (i.e., therapy practitioners).

Assumptions about the Service member receiving OT and/or PT after MTBI (based on DoD definition above):

1) He or she may have suffered a MTBI concomitant with other physical injuries; MTBI may or may not have been identified upon initial medical assessment.

2) Onset and duration of disability associated with MTBI-related symptoms vary across individuals. Sometimes MTBI symptoms may be transient but for some Service members, symptoms are significant enough to impact functioning on the activity level or social participation level, interfering with performance of military duties or civilian life [40].

3) Symptoms of combat stress often mirror that of MTBI, making it difficult to determine which factors are contributing to performance problems. A differential diagnosis is required for accurate treatment.

4) Beyond a possible MTBI, functional performance may be affected by fatigue, stress/mental state, medications, sleep habits, and or other injuries and illnesses.

5) Service members with MTBI may enter the system of rehabilitative care at any level (i.e., in theater, within a formal rehabilitation program, or upon completion of tour of duty). Many individuals may not need or be provided with continuous care over time.

6) Rehabilitation benefits and access to rehabilitation services may vary depending on branch of service, type of warrior (active duty, national guard, reservist), and/or state of residence.

Assumptions about the practitioners using this *Clinical Management Guidance:*

1) **Occupational and physical therapists plan and provide intervention based on an individual Service member's unique set of circumstances, goals, and functional performance problems rather than based primarily on diagnosis.**

2) Recommendations in this document are written for the general practice therapist – that is, licensed occupational and physical therapists that do not have specialty training in various aspects of neurorehabilitation.

3) Scope of practice for the occupational therapist and physical therapist may vary depending on the level of care, the location of the facility, and access to other health care providers and be different from that of civilian practice.

4) Occupational and physical therapists typically work within a larger interdisciplinary team and within such settings, therapists seek out the expertise of other team members including neuropsychologists, counseling psychologists, speech language pathologists, physicians, nurses, therapeutic

recreation specialists, nurses, and other rehabilitation and medical professionals.

Guiding Principles of OT and PT Assessment and Treatment After MTBI

Ruff (2005) outlined a patient-centered approach to rehabilitation for MTBI that informs the recommended guiding principles for delivery of OT and PT services across all levels of care.

1) In their interactions with Service members with MTBI, therapists communicate an optimistic expectation for warriors' full recovery. As stated by Ruff, "...clinicians must avoid fostering the belief that the 'brain damage' subsequent to concussion always leads to permanent deficits" (p. 16).

2) Therapists help Service members identify their strengths and resources as well as their challenges and limitations so that those assets may be harnessed in the rehabilitation and recovery process.

3) Therapists incorporate formal or informal assessment of the Service member's goals and priorities into the evaluation process along with evaluation of MTBI-related symptoms, impairments, and inefficiencies. What does he or she want to be able to do that he or she is unable to do now? Symptoms are treated in the context of realistic goals linked with everyday life.

4) The Service member with MTBI and therapist collaborate on therapy goals and the steps needed to achieve them. That is, interactions with patients are collaborative and not directive.

5) Throughout the treatment process, the therapist "...should gently allow the patient to understand where he or she has misattributed symptoms to the brain injury" [40(p15)] and help him or her see the link between performance problems and personal, situational, or other contributing factors. [47]

Structure and Format of Practice Recommendation Descriptions

Practice recommendations are organized by problem area because typically, this is the manner in which clinicians approach assessment and treatment. Discussions of problem areas loosely follow the sequence in the rehabilitation process in which they might most likely be assessed and/or addressed. Within each problem area, we describe the objective of assessment or treatment, provide background information based on the literature; specify our recommendations; and discuss implications in terms of rehabilitation practices and Service members. We also provide qualifications as to which practitioner(s) and level of care to specific recommendations pertain, along with the strength of our recommendations (and rationale). The strength of a recommendation is characterized as either a Practice Standard or a Practice Option. *Practice Standards* are supported by existing MTBI Guidelines and/or published evidence-based reviews. *Practice Options* do not have such support but are consistent with current theory, literature, and/or expert opinion.

In addition to the above, we indicate the components of the World Health Organization (WHO) International Classification of Functioning, Disability and Health

(ICF) taxonomy [59] that are addressed in assessment and treatment associated with each problem area. The ICF is a framework that depicts how an individual's health condition interacts with other environmental and personal factors to influence his or her physical-emotional status (body structures/function), activity level, and participation in social roles. Similarly, the framework depicts an array of ways in which clinicians may intervene in order to improve patients' health -by removing environmental or social barriers to participation; instruction in compensatory techniques that enable a person to carry out every day activities; or remediating an impairment to restore a functioning of an organ system pertaining to, for example, vision. By including the ICF domains relevant to each problem area, we aim to promote an appreciation of all the possible avenues through which clinicians advance Service members' health and functioning.

Combat Readiness Check

In-Theater Assessment of Combat Readiness after MTBI

Objective: To employ rehabilitation expertise to inform decision-making regarding fitness for return to duty for Service members with possible MTBI.

> Practitioner: Occupational or physical therapist (depending upon setting and availability)
> ICF component(s): Body function & structure and Activity
> Strength of recommendation: Practice Standard (MTBI-symptom based screen); Practice Option (task observation under dual task conditions)
> Rationale: There is evidence to support the clinical relevance and use of standardized tools to identify MTBI-related symptoms but no evidence as yet regarding task observation under dual-task conditions in this context.

Background: It is critically important to identify possible MTBI as early as possible after it occurs. Persons with MTBI need to be monitored for any deterioration in functioning that might indicate a more severe injury or complications [60]. Furthermore, MTBI-related symptoms have the potential to interfere with warriors' safety and competence in executing their responsibilities, putting themselves and their comrades at risk. Symptoms such as dizziness, visual disturbances, and headache may impede reaction time and other aspects of physical performance and also likely interfere with the warrior's concentration, memory, and problem solving [47].

Experts participating in the OT/PT MTBI Summit (11-15-07) suggested that, in order to optimize warrior safety, there is a need for more sophisticated assessments of functional performance related to combat readiness in-theater. Some participants reported that some warriors rehearse elements of the Military Acute Concussion Evaluation (MACE) [7] in advance of possible injury to optimize the likelihood that they can "pass" the test and return to duty, if injured. Experts at the OT/PT MTBI Summit recommended an expanded role for OT and PT in this realm.

Occupational and physical therapists are educated and trained to assess physical, cognitive, and emotional impairments in order to make extrapolations as to how those impairments may impact functioning in everyday life. In theater (Levels I, II, III), therapists have the potential to use their knowledge and skills to help quantify possible MTBI-related symptoms and to observe functional performance to further inform medical decisions about return to duty, evacuation, or rest.

As suggested by the aforementioned expert panel, a brief but comprehensive combat readiness assessment conducted by OT or PT should include the following dimensions: a) a screen for possible MTBI-related symptoms; b) observation of functional performance under dual task conditions; c) a screen for possible stress disorder. This proposed process is referred to as the OT/PT Combat Readiness Check (CRC). Each element of the proposed CRC is described.

A screen for possible MTBI symptoms:

Therapists should identify and quantify MTBI-related symptoms that might present barriers to fitness for duty and inform therapy treatment planning. The following instruments address MTBI-related symptoms and have established reliability and validity (although not all of them have been validated on adults with MTBI):

- *Westmead Post Traumatic Amnesia (PTA) Scale* –Revised . PTA is a widely used index of severity of brain damage and is also an indicator of when concussion is resolved [61]. To administer the Westmead PTA Scale, a clinician asks the patient a series of 7 orientation questions followed by a set of new learning-recall tasks (remembering a face, name, and pictures of objects). It was originally designed to be readministered over a period of days. Ponsford and colleagues [62] modified the procedure such that it is readministered on an hourly basis and found it to be sensitive to MTBI.

- The 5-question subtest of the *Dizziness Handicap Inventory* [63] – see later discussion

- *Dix-Hallpike Test* [64] – see later discussion

- *Dynamic Visual Acuity Test* [64] – see later discussion

- *Balance Error Scoring System (BESS)* [65,66] – see later discussion

Functional performance under dual-task conditions

Members of the Expert Panel suggested that skilled observation of task performance simulating the demands typically placed on warriors could provide critical information for decision-makers about return to duty. Real-life demands could be best simulated by critical common warrior tasks (as specified in the Soldier's Manual of Common Tasks [SMCT]) performed under dual-task conditions. Inclusion of critical common tasks, such as assembling a weapon or donning/doffing gas mask while timed, adds to the face validity of the assessment (to warriors and commanders); inclusion of the dual-task condition assures that warriors are able to perform highly proceduralized tasks while retaining their ability to process information – critical to safety in theater. (See a discussion of dual task procedures ["Attention and Dual Task Performance"] later in the *Guidance*.)

A procedure of this nature should be developed and validated that involves a set of critical common tasks from the SMCT and a set of cognitive tasks (such as counting backward from 100 by 7's, naming all of the states that start with the letters "A" and "M", or reciting the Soldier's Creed [http://www.army.mil/SoldiersCreed/flash_version/] or Army Values [http://chppm-www.apgea.army.mil/co2/CO2_book/Values.htm]). During a CRC with a given soldier, the therapist would select from the sets of common soldier tasks and cognitive tasks, making pre-morbid task learning difficult.

A screen for stress disorder

Because stress is a significant element in combat-related MTBI, the expert panel recommended inclusion of a screen for acute stress reaction and/or post traumatic stress disorder. The specific tool to incorporate into the CRC should be selected by experts this area.

Recommendations:

1) PT and/or OT use standardized instruments to screen for MTBI-related symptoms in theater. This portion of the proposed CRC could be implemented by OT and/or PT in theater immediately (Practice Standard).

2) PT and/or OT use informal methods for evaluating Service members' ability to perform dual cognitive and motor tasks in order to inform return-to-duty decision-making in theater (Practice Option).

Discussion: Based on these recommendations and the ongoing need for a tool to measure progress towards return to duty, a consortium of researchers from the Sister Kenny Research Center, the United States Army Institute of Environmental Medicine, University of North Carolina, University of Minnesota, and Riverbend LLC was awarded funding from the Army Medical Research Materiel Command in September 2009 for Phase I development of a Combat Readiness Check.

Activity Intolerance/Progressive Return to Full Activity

Assessment

Objective: To ensure Service members' safe return to full activity through consistent use the DVBIC assessments and recommendations [7] when evaluating and treating Service members in theater during the acute period following MTBI.

Practitioner: Physical Therapist and Occupational Therapist
ICF components: Activity and Participation
Strength of recommendation: Practice Option
Rationale: Use a symptom checklist and neurocognitive assessment to monitor activity tolerance (DVBIC Guidance 12-06, Prague Consensus: McCrory et al., 2005). This information does not relate specifically to PT and OT interventions.
Applicable level(s) of care: Levels I-III

Background: A review of the issues regarding immediate post concussion management and activity restrictions following MTBI is available in the DVBIC Working Group Clinical Practice Guidelines [7,8]and is not repeated here. A number of neurocognitive assessment tools are described in this guideline including the *Military Acute Concussion Evaluation* (MACE) tool developed by the Defense and Veteran's Brain Injury Center. The purpose of this section of the guidance paper is to encourage the physical and occupational therapists who are evaluating and treating Service members in Levels I-III to remain cognizant of activity and exercise restrictions when designing exercise programs for orthopedic or other morbidities in the presence of a concussion diagnosis. As well, therapists are encouraged to use observation of symptom reoccurrence and neurocognitive assessments when monitoring their patient's tolerance to any therapeutic intervention.

Recommendations:

1) Use observation of symptom reoccurrence, a symptom checklist and neurocognitive assessments when monitoring a Service member's tolerance to any therapeutic intervention in the presence of a concussion co-morbidity.

2) Be aware of the DVBIC guidelines [7,8] with regard to the acute management of mild traumatic brain injury.

Discussion: Updated guidance for the acute management of MTBI in Levels I-III is available from the Proponency Office for Rehabilitation and Reintegration (November 2007).

Intervention

Objective: To promote an awareness of limitations for activity intensity when treating Service members for orthopedic or other injuries requiring Occupational and Physical Therapy intervention when concussion is a co-morbidity. These recommendations are reiterated here only and the reader is referred to the DVBIC guidelines [7,8] for further information.

Practitioner: Physical Therapist and Occupational Therapist
ICF components: Activity and Participation
Strength of recommendation: Practice Option
Rationale: Recommendation is for rest and activity restriction until symptom free at rest with a slow and monitored return to full activity or full duty [7-9].
Applicable level(s) of care: Levels I-III

Background: Therapists are reminded of the recommendation for the slow progression for return to duty as is used for sport [9], which encourages rest until symptom free and then a daily stepwise progression with a regression of the intensity of activity with any symptom return. During the Summit (November 15, 2007) there occurred extensive discussion regarding the need for extreme caution about returning Service members to full activity too soon after mild TBI. No specific information was found regarding restrictions of Physical or Occupational Therapy exercise programs in the presence of acute mild traumatic brain injury.

Studies in rats suggest that exercise in the first 7 days after concussion is detrimental to formation of neurotrophic factors and other molecules that enhance brain plasticity and improve cognitive status after the brain injury [67]. As discussed in Leddy et al. [68], the metabolic and physiologic changes in the brain of an individual post concussion may worsen during physical or cognitive exertion when the cerebral blood flow alters. Exercise in the acute post concussive period may increase brain metabolic requirements when brain metabolism is compromised. Certainly, the activity requirements of full combat duty can be of high intensity with heavy physical loads of rucksacks and safety equipment.

There is much discussion and controversy regarding the issue of post concussion activity and development of post concussion syndrome. A review of that discussion is

beyond the scope of the *Guidance* and the reader is encouraged to review sports concussion literature.

Recommendations:

1) Physical and occupational therapists advocate for early rest following mild TBI or concussion with a slow return to activity.

2) Therapists must be aware of this restriction in making recommendations and treatment plans for post concussion issues alone and when treated orthopedic or other injuries and when designing home programs in the presence of acute concussion.

3) Athletic or other risky activity should not resume until after the physical signs and symptoms of concussion are no longer present at rest or with physical exertion and cognitive deficits are fully resolved.

Discussion: Udated guidance for the acute management of MTBI in Levels I-III is available from the Proponency Office for Rehabilitation and Reintegration (November 2007).

Patient Education about MTBI

Objective: To provide information, counseling, and instruction to Service members who have a history of MTBI so that they a) establish realistic expectations for recovery; b) make correct attributions for temporary changes in performance and c) enact any necessary compensatory strategies.

Practitioner: Occupational and/or physical therapist
ICF component(s): Activity, Participation
Strength of recommendation: Practice standard
Rationale: Supported by evidence reported in Borg et al., 2004
Applicable level(s) of care: All

Background: People with MTBI need information and instruction both early on and throughout their recovery. Immediately after the incident, individuals with suspected MTBI need to be informed of symptoms that might indicate the presence of potentially life-threatening pathology such as intra-cranial hemorrhage or cerebral edema including: vomiting, worsening headache, developing amnesia or evidence of short term memory loss, worsening mental status, neurologic signs such as loss of motor function, vision or speech; seizure [60]. They also need verbal and written information about typical sequelae and likely course of recovery [69]. Most experts recommend the provision of verbal and written educational information about MTBI symptoms (headache, difficulties with memory and/or attention) as well as reassurance that these are likely to recover over a period of weeks or a few months [57,70]. As people are helped to understand their symptoms, they are less likely to overreact to them or misattribute them to significant brain damage [57]. Mittenberg and colleagues demonstrated that patients with mild TBI who reviewed and discussed extensive written instructions with a therapist before leaving the hospital had significantly shorter symptom duration and fewer symptoms than those receiving routine discharge information (written information and an advised period of rest) [71].

People who experience protracted cognitive or neurobehavioral symptoms also appear to benefit from information about how to understand and manage the consequences of MTBI, even those who experience distress and disability for months to years afterwards [40,47]. Experts suggest that PCS may be averted or ameliorated as people with MTBI learn to appreciate how personal and situational factors may interact with typically transient symptoms of brain injury [47] and implement compensatory strategies that optimize their effectiveness. By incorporating a discussion about the influence of stress on performance, survivors of MTBI begin to understand and normalize their own experience [72,73]. Occupational therapy aimed at the patient's acquisition and employment of cognitive compensatory strategies will be discussed later in this section but a therapist-patient conversation about the influence of stress on cognitive functioning might go something like this:

"People can concentrate on or pay attention to a finite number of things at one time. On average and under normal circumstances, people can simultaneously pay attention to between 5 and 9 things at a conscious or semi-conscious level. This capacity is hard-wired from birth. After a MTBI, people may have a variety of distracting physical symptoms (dizziness, headache, musculoskeletal pain) that they can't help but think about. In a sense, these distractions take up space in our thinking process, using up some of our 5 – 9 'slots'. As a result, people with MTBI have a hard time remembering information, concentrating, and even problem solving. Stress and worry can have the same effect. Worry and negative thinking also take up mental space that could otherwise be used in the process of remembering information. This is why we recommend using compensatory strategies like writing things down. If the 'slots' are full (with symptom-related distractions or worries), you can still keep track of information that you need to stay in control of your life."

There are materials available through the VHA, PR&R, and commercial vendors that could be used to provide more in-depth information about consequences of MTBI and what to do about them.

- The PR&R has created a series of downloadable/printable MTBI-related patient education handouts that are available at their website (http://www.armymedicine.army.mil/prr/edtraining.html).

- *"Recovering from Head Injury: A Guide for Patients"* [34] is a 10-page information packet that is incorporated into an Independent Study Course for practitioners designed by the Department of Veterans Affairs. This material was used in the cognitive behavioral intervention described above [74]. Designed as a patient-education resource related to TBI in general, it offers useful information about symptom management specific to TBI. It does not provide information about normal human information processing in ways that fully enable the Service member to both normalize and understand his or her challenges associated with MTBI. A new Quick Series booklet is also available entitled *Recovering from Traumatic Brain Injury* (see http://www.quickseries.com/government/veterans/veterans.asp).

- *The Mild Traumatic Brain Injury Workbook* [75] is a 192 page self-study developed for civilians with MTBI that could be incorporated into therapy. It should be noted that there is no evidence that a more in-depth workbook is any more effective than a handout. Clinicians should be sensitive to unintended messages that are communicated by recommending a workbook to individuals with mild symptoms that are likely to resolve.

Recommendations (Practice Standards):

1) Service members should receive written information and one-on-one instruction with a therapist in theater if MTBI is suspected based on OT/PT Combat Readiness Check or if by other medical personnel. An occupational or physical therapist should review the written description of symptoms that, if present, should prompt the Service member to seek medical attention. The therapist also should review information describing possible short-term consequences of mild TBI, tips and strategies for compensating for these challenges, while emphasizing the fact that most people no longer report symptoms by 3 months post injury [39].

2) As part of their rehabilitation program, Service members with MTBI are helped to normalize brain-injury related challenges by receiving in-depth and individualized information about how personal and situational factors impact

their information processing abilities. The occupational therapist provides information regarding normal human information processing [76] and the finite capacity of working memory [77] in order to help Service members to better understand the how distractions associated with MTBI symptoms make it difficult to concentrate and remember information. Together in therapy, the occupational therapist works with the Service member to identify the physical, emotional, and situational factors that may be interacting with typically short-term symptoms associated with MTBI and contributing to declines in functioning. This educational effort informs the development of compensatory strategies during the treatment process (see discussion later in the Guidance).

Discussion: While patient education is recommended after MTBI, there is nothing published in the literature about the specific roles of OT and PT in doing so.

Vestibular Dysfunction

Complaints of Dizziness/Vertigo, Disequilibrium and Visual Blurring

INTRODUCTION:

Vestibular deficits that arise in conjunction with MTBI can have complex etiologies and so treatment is individualized and specific to the cause. The OT/PT MTBI work group recognized that the types of vestibular damage caused by blast injuries are not yet fully understood. The recommendations in this *Clinical Management Guidance* presume damage similar to that resulting from MTBI in a civilian population. At the 2006 American Physical Therapy Association's Combined Sections Meeting, Laura Morris (Centers for Rehab Services, Pittsburgh, PA) presented a review of causes, assessments and treatment strategies related to MTBI and dizziness. She described eight categories of differential diagnosis for the etiologies of dizziness following MTBI. Hoffer, Gottshall and colleagues categorized the types of dizziness patterns in service personnel with MTBI as one of four categories [23]. These categories include migraine-associated dizziness, spatial disorientation, BPPV or exercise induced dizziness. These categories helped the OT/PT MTBI work group to describe response to treatment.

Obviously, vestibular rehabilitation is complex and an area of specialization within Physical and Occupational Therapy. The OT/PT MTBI work group, in consultation with PT experts at the Minneapolis VA and at the Summit, suggest two of the several types of vestibular deficits resulting from MTBI may be treated by a general practice physical therapist within the military framework in a combat support hospital or similar war zone setting. These two types of vestibular deficits include benign paroxysmal positional vertigo (BPPV) of the posterior canal (and lateral (horizontal) canal as recommended by Bhattacharyya, 2008) and unilateral vestibular hypofunction (UVH). Episodic dizziness that is associated with migraine headache was also considered an appropriate diagnosis for intervention by a general practice therapist when circumstances require it. General practice therapists who have not previously seen vestibular patients may need education in the techniques and assessments beyond what is described in this *Guidance*. For other more complex etiologies such as perilymphatic fistula, bilateral vestibular hypofunction, Meniere's disease, or other etiologies for dizziness complaints, Service members should be referred for further specialty evaluation (ENT/Otolaryngologist) and for treatment by therapists with specialized vestibular training.

The OT/PT MTBI work group assumes that not all Service members with vestibular deficits following a blast or other exposure that results in MTBI-type symptoms are evacuated to higher levels of care. Sometimes Service members reportedly stay with their units in theater, either minimizing their symptoms or allowing space in evacuation vehicles for other more seriously injured persons. However, it would be best for these individuals with exposure to explosion or other incident causing MTBI (dizziness/vertigo, disequilibrium or visual blurring) to be evacuated or allowed to rest until symptom free at rest and with activity. If these Service members remain in theater, the work group and other experts consulted recommended that military PT's (and OT's who are at Combat Stress Units) be encouraged to assess and treat the vestibular diagnoses, as circumstances require. It is further assumed that PT's and OT's in the field are taking a full and appropriate patient history and that they are aware of "red flags" and other precautions that would prompt further questions or referral for neurology evaluation.

Service members at MMTFs or Polytrauma VA's with other serious medical issues may also have vestibular deficits. Medical issues such as burns, fractures, internal injuries or amputations, may prevent easy intervention for the vestibular deficits. Referral to experienced vestibular specialists is recommended in these cases as these specialists may have clinical experience and novel suggestions for interventions that can alleviate the Service member's vestibular symptoms without using standard treatment protocols.

Benign Paroxysmal Positional Vertigo (BPPV) of the posterior semicircular canal

Assessment

Objective: To identify vestibular dysfunction that can be treated by a general practice PT in a war zone or stateside medical facility to reduce complaints of dizziness, imbalance or visual blurring; to screen for BPPV of the posterior or lateral canal; to identify individuals in need of referral to specialists.

Practitioner: Physical Therapist (or Occupational Therapist with specialized training)
International Classification of Functioning: Body Structure/Body Function
Strength of recommendation: Practice Standard
Rationale: Dix-Hallpike test is the most commonly used test to confirm the diagnosis of BPPV of the posterior semicircular canal (SCC) refer to [13,14]. The 5-question subtest of the DHI can be used to determine those persons likely to have BPPV [15]. Use the supine roll test to diagnose lateral (horizontal) canal BPPV [13] is considered a Practice Option.
Applicable level(s) of care: All levels when applicable

Background: Persons including Service members with concussion or MTBI may report the common complaints of imbalance or unsteady walking (postural instability), dizziness or vertigo and blurred vision. These complaints may begin immediately following a MTBI or concussion or may occur after a time delay. Dizziness is a common symptom in patients with post-concussive syndrome. Of 100 patients ages 10-66, 26% reported dizziness on the Rivermead Symptom Scales 3 months after a mild head injury [78].

Benign paroxysmal positional vertigo is the most common cause of vertigo. In a retrospective chart review, Whitney et al. [79](2005) reported that 22.5% of subjects presenting at a balance and falls clinic between September 1998 and March 2003 at the University of Pittsburgh and who had completed the *Dizziness Handicap Inventory* (DHI) were found to have BPPV. Hoffer et al. [23](2004) reported that 28% of 58 active-duty and retired military personnel with dizziness following MTBI had BPPV. The most common semicircular canal involved in BPPV is the posterior canal. Herdman and Tussa [10] reported that of 200 consecutive patients with BPPV seen in their Dizziness and Balance Center Clinic, 76% were found to have posterior canal involvement.

The DHI is a commonly used tool to assess a patient's perception of handicap in the functional, emotional, and physical domains that result from dizziness complaints [63]. This tool has been shown to be reliable, and is frequently used as an outcome measure in persons with dizziness as it has been demonstrated to show change over time with rehabilitation [80]. A higher score on the DHI indicates greater handicap with a maximum score of 100. The DHI has been shown to correlate with *Dynamic Visual Acuity Testing* (DVAT) in active duty military personnel who had suffered a MTBI [19]. It has been used to show improvement in handicap from dizziness in patients with vestibular disorders with and without migraine headaches following a customized physical therapy program including vestibular rehabilitation [81].

Specific questions on the DHI seem to be related to the complaints of persons with BPPV. Typical complaints that characterize BPPV include brief episodes of vertigo that last less than 1 minute and that are triggered by certain movements such as lying down, rolling over in bed, bending over and looking up. Whitney and colleagues [79] looked at a two or 5-question subtest of the DHI. The 2-question subtest asks about dizziness when rolling over in bed and getting out of bed; and the 5-question subtest asks about symptoms when the person is looking up, getting out of bed, making quick head movements, rolling over in bed and bending. The authors found that the five-item subtest of the DHI was a significant predictor of the likelihood of having BPPV. The 5-question subtest of the DHI would be easy to complete quickly and would assist the general practice physical therapist in screening for BPPV.

The *Dix-Hallpike* test is the most commonly used test to confirm the diagnosis of BPPV of the posterior SCC. The specific techniques for this test can be found in the Herdman text (2007) or in the clinical practice guideline for BPPV published by the American Academy of Otolaryngology - Head and Neck Surgery [13]. This clinical practice guideline strongly recommends the diagnosis of posterior canal BPPV using the Dix-Hallpike maneuver. Additionally, a recommendation is made for clinicians to diagnose lateral (horizontal) canal BPPV using a supine Roll Test. Lateral canal BPPV is the second most common type of BPPV with an incidence of approximately 10-15 percent. Lateral canal BPPV can occur as free-floating material migrates from the posterior canal to the lateral (horizontal) canal during a repositioning maneuver (see Bhattacharyya et al., 2008 for a review).

A cervical range of motion screen is done prior to *Dix-Hallpike* testing. The general practice physical therapist should be aware of contraindications to the Dix-Hallpike maneuver, although active duty military personnel are less likely to exhibit some of the contraindicated diagnoses, especially those that are age-related. These contraindications are reviewed by Humphriss et al. [82] and include history of neck surgery, severe rheumatoid arthritis, recent neck trauma and various proximal cervical instabilities and cervical or brainstem pathologies. Modification of the procedure to a sidelying assessment is recommended for those Service members with contraindications to the Dix-Hallpike maneuver [82].

Recommendations:

1) To assist in determining if the Service member's vertigo or imbalance results from BPPV of the posterior SCC, the 5 question subtest of the Dizziness Handicap Inventory (5 questions--looking up, getting out of bed, quick head movements, rolling over in bed and bending) can be a significant predictor of the likelihood of having BPPV. This brief subtest should be used in situations where assessment time is limited such as Levels I-III.

2) The Service member with dizziness complaints in a stateside setting should complete the entire DHI.

3) If BPPV is suspected, the Dix-Hallpike Test, which is commonly used to confirm diagnosis of BPPV of the posterior semicircular canal, is then administered. A positive test results in an upbeat rotational nystagmus (in the direction of the dependent ear) that corresponds with the duration of the

Service member's symptoms of dizziness/vertigo. The Service member with BPPV typically complains of episodic vertigo or dizziness (with associated nystagmus) that lasts less than 1 minute and that occurs specifically with position changes.

4) Nystagmus can be suppressed by visual fixation. Therefore, it is important to have a means of viewing eye movements in darkness or without any visual fixation stimuli present in order to preserve the nystagmus. Ideally, the Dix-Hallpike test is done while the patient is wearing goggles or Frenzel lenses.

5) If the patient has a history compatible with BPPV and the Dix-Hallpike test is negative, a recommendation is made for clinicians to diagnose lateral (horizontal) canal BPPV using a supine Roll Test.

6) Therapists who are unfamiliar with the assessments described and other vestibular issues should obtain a copy of the Herdman [10] and review pertinent sections. Additionally, the Clinical Practice Guideline on BPPV published by the American Academy of Otolaryngology--Head and Neck Surgery [13] provides an explanation of the Dix-Hallpike test as well as the supine Roll Test.

7) When the Service member's condition warrants and when specialized services are available, therapists are encouraged to provide referral for further specialized testing and treatment by therapists with specialized vestibular training.

Discussion: The choice of specific measurement tools to use in evaluating a Service member with dizziness following MTBI depends on the specific clinical presentation of that person. The tools suggested here are for use by a general practice PT. Given the potential scope of this problem among Service members, it is advised that the DoD/VA ensure that therapy specialists are available as resources system-wide.

Intervention

Objective: If the screening evaluation is found to be positive for BPPV of the posterior semicircular canal (posterior canal canalithiasis), the therapist carries out the canalith repositioning procedure (CRP), educates the Service member in precautions and provides home exercises as appropriate. If the supine Roll Test is found to be positive for lateral canal BPPV, the therapist carries out the roll maneuver (bar-b-que roll maneuver), and continues with education and home programming as appropriate. In cases of poor response to initial attempts at intervention, or when the complexities of the vestibular findings warrant, the therapist will provide referral for further specialized testing and for treatment by therapists with specialized vestibular training.

Practitioner: Physical Therapist (or Occupational Therapist with specialized training)
ICF component: Body Structure/Body Function
Strength of recommendation: Practice Standard
Rationale: CRP for posterior canal canalithiasis results in 83-93% rate of remission [1,2]. The effectiveness of the bar-b-que roll maneuver in treating lateral canal BPPV is approximately 75%. See the 2008 Clinical Practice Guideline on BPPV published by the American Academy of Otolaryngology--Head and Neck Surgery [13].
Applicable level(s) of care: All levels when applicable

Background: The CRP is used to treat BPPV of the posterior semicircular canal (posterior canal canalithiasis). An 83% to 93% rate of remission of the BPPV has been reported by several authors following one or multiple CRP treatments depending on the specific positions used [2,83].

Home instructions for precautions following the CRP and instruction in Brandt-Daroff habituation exercises for milder residual complaints of dizziness or vertigo have been suggested [10]. Herdman also suggests instructing patients in the CRP so that they may repeat the treatment on their own as long as they are experiencing vertigo during treatment. It has been suggested that posttraumatic BPPV is different from the idiopathic form. Gordon et al. reported that 67% of patients with traumatic BPPV required repeated treatment before complete resolution of symptoms compared to 14% of patients with idiopathic BPPV. This group also reported that the posttraumatic groups had significantly more frequent recurrences [84].

Yardley et al. [85] conducted a randomized controlled trial with 146 patients with dizziness from a variety of causes and compared a customized home exercise program of vestibular exercises to a control group. This group found a significantly greater improvement in a shortened version of the *Vertigo Symptom Scale* and other measures of symptom severity, on a measure of anxiety, during provocative movements, and on the sharpened Romberg, in the subjects who were on the vestibular habituation program compared to the control group.

The Roll maneuver (bar-b-que roll maneuver) is used to move canaliths from the lateral canal into the vestibule to treat lateral (horizontal) canal BPPV. The effectiveness of this maneuver is approximately 75% according to summary information provided in the Clinical Practice Guideline on BPPV [13].

Recommendations:

1) If assessment results indicate a BPPV of the posterior canal, the canalith repositioning procedure for the posterior semi-circular canal is then administered (see Herdman, 2007, page 243 for specifics or the 2008 Clinical Practice Guideline on BPPV published by the American Academy of Otolaryngology--Head and Neck Surgery [13]).

2) If assessment results indicate a BPPV of the lateral (horizontal) canal, the bar-b-que roll maneuver) is used to move canaliths from the lateral canal into the vestibule (see Herdman, 2007 or see the 2008 Clinical Practice

Guideline on BPPV published by the American Academy of Otolaryngology--Head and Neck Surgery [13]).

3) Therapists who are unfamiliar with the canalith repositioning procedures and vestibular exercises should obtain a copy of Herdman [10] and review pertinent sections.

4) Further home exercise recommendations and activity restrictions are provided to the Service member with follow-up with the physical therapist at approximately one month [10,13].

5) If balance does not improve with the treatment of the BPPV and reduction of dizziness complaints, then further balance and postural stability exercises should be provided (see separate sections of the *Guidance* for information on balance complaints).

6) Service members with MTBI or PCS may also have memory problems along with the dizziness or instability complaints that influence their follow through with exercises. Use of a compliance work sheet or instruction of family members or fellow Service members may enhance adherence to home exercise programs.

Discussion: It is important for the general practice PT to recognize and treat BPPV of the posterior canal as that is the most common canal involved in canalithiasis. While more specialized, the additional assessment maneuvers for the lateral (horizontal) canal are considered important due to the potential for conversion from the posterior to the lateral canal canalithiasis during the CRP. Therapists who are interested in or require further knowledge in vestibular assessment and intervention are encouraged to attend continuing education specialty training in vestibular rehabilitation and to obtain the Herdman, 2007 text. Additionally, therapists are encouraged to review the Clinical Practice Guideline on BPPV [13].

Unilateral Vestibular Hypofunction

Assessment

Objective: To identify vestibular etiologies, specifically unilateral vestibular hypofunction (UVH), that can be treated by a general practice PT in a war zone or stateside medical facility to reduce complaints of dizziness, imbalance or visual blurring; to identify individuals in need of specialized testing and treatment by therapists with specialized vestibular training.

Practitioner: Physical Therapist
ICF components: Body Structure/Body Function, Activity
Strength of recommendation: Practice Standard
Rationale: The DHI and DVAT were described as objective tests as outcome measures for Marines and Navy personnel with concussive injuries [19].
Applicable level(s) of care: All levels when applicable

Background: The vestibulo-ocular reflex (VOR) is a reflex eye movement that stabilizes images on the retina during head movement. The image is maintained on the center of the visual field as the VOR produces an eye movement in the direction opposite to head movement. In order for people to have clear vision, the VOR must be fast and must compensate for head movements almost immediately. The semicircular canals send information as directly as possible to the eye muscles. Damage to one side or the other of the peripheral vestibular apparatus will result in a mismatch of signals and slipping or blurring of the visual image with head movement. Persons with unilateral vestibular hypofunction that is not yet compensated, complain of visual blurring (oscillopsia) because of the decrease in gain of the VOR [1].

One way of assessing the VOR that is used clinically, is the *Dynamic Visual Acuity Test* (DVAT), which compares a person's ability to read a series of letters or detect orientation of a letter (ototypes) in a line chart when the head is stationary to his/her ability to do the same task when the head is moving. Dynamic visual acuity is then calculated by subtracting the number of errors when the head is stable to the number of errors when the head is oscillating [86]. This test was developed clinically with manual oscillation of the head reading an eye chart [87,88]. While there have been a number of design problems with this manual methodology, it is used as a screening tool for dynamic visual acuity as an indication of vestibular hypofunction.

In settings where available, specialized laboratory based measures of vestibular function are used to quantify the extent and location of vestibular loss. Among these assessments are the caloric test, rotary chair test, the vestibular evoked myogenic potential test (VEMP), and a computerized dynamic visual acuity test (DVAT) [10]. In a war zone, the computerized version of the DVAT is likely not available and in such instance, the clinical (manual) DVAT is the best available test to use. Venuto et al. [89] reported that the sensitivity of the clinical DVAT for vestibular deficits is approximately 85% and its specificity is approximately 55%.

Herdman et al. [86] assessed 42 normal subjects (29 with unilateral vestibular hypofunction and 26 with bilateral vestibular hypofunction) between 19 and 87 years of age to assess the reliability, sensitivity and specificity of the computerized DVA test. The sensitivity of the computerized DVA test was 94.5% and the specificity was 95%.

The head-impulse test (also referred to as the head-thrust test) is used to test the function of the vestibular system. It involves an unpredictable, high-velocity, small amplitude head thrust in the horizontal plane. The head-impulse test can assist in confirming the side or sides of the vestibular hypofunction [10].

The Head-shaking Nystagmus (HSN) Test is a clinical test which assesses for dynamic asymmetry in the vestibulo-ocular reflex (VOR). It would be used in a patient with suspected vestibular hypofunction. This is a simple screening evaluation for peripheral vestibular system disease. It is used as part of a vestibular examination for imbalance, dizziness, vertigo and oscillopsia (blurred vision with head movement.) [90,91].

Recommendations:

1) Clinical DVAT is a functional test that can be used to assess Service members with unilateral and bilateral vestibular hypofunction. The Service member is asked to read the smallest possible line on a Snellen chart with the head at rest. This smallest line read is then compared to the smallest line that can be read while the examiner manually oscillates the Service member's head horizontally at 2 Hz for 1-2 inches in either direction. The Service member should be able to read the same line or one line above that read with the head at rest. If the Service member has a greater than two line change from the static to dynamic condition, then he or she likely has a vestibular deficit.

2) If available, a computerized version of the DVAT is the recommended mode of testing.

3) A head impulse test (head thrust test) is administered for confirmation of the side or sides of the vestibular hypofunction. The Head-shaking Nystagmus Test is also used as part of a vestibular examination in a patient with suspected vestibular hypofunction.

4) Specific position and testing instructions for the clinical DVA test and the head-thrust test are found in the Herdman text [10]. Therapists who are unfamiliar with these assessment techniques should obtain a copy of Herdman, 2007 and review pertinent sections.

Discussion: Service members with acute UVH, typically have severe nausea, and spontaneous nystagmus seen in room light during the first several days to a week or two following the onset or causative incident. Service members may also have bilateral vestibular hypofunction with one side more involved than the other.

In a MMTF or VA setting (Level V through Level VIII), specialized equipment such as computerized *Dynamic Visual Acuity Testing* and specific medical specialty personnel (i.e. ENT/Otolaryngology physicians) should be available for more specific and reliable evaluation for persons with complaints of dizziness, vertigo, disequilibrium, and visual blurring or other symptoms of a vestibular nature. The general practice PT should continue to screen via a basic evaluation as described above for BPPV of the posterior SSC and for UVH. If however, findings indicate vestibular pathology that is not responsive to initial treatments or that is complex, the Service member with dizziness/vertigo should receive further specialty evaluation.

Decrements in visual acuity during head movements could potentially contribute to decreased safety in driving, scanning the environment, and other military or job related tasks. When findings indicate visual blurring or acuity issues, therapists in Levels I-III are encouraged to discuss their findings with the Service member in terms of these safety issues.

Intervention

Objective: If the screening evaluation identifies UVH, the therapist provides therapeutic intervention including a vestibular rehabilitation program and home instruction for exercises that reduce the dizziness or visual blurring complaints. In cases of poor response to initial attempts at intervention, or when the complexities of the vestibular findings warrant, therapists provide referral for further specialized testing and for treatment by therapists with specialized vestibular training.

Background: Typically, physical therapy intervention cannot alter the underlying pathology in a case of vestibular hypofunction. Intervention for this disorder includes exercises designed to facilitate central nervous system (CNS) compensation or adaptation rather than alter underlying vestibular disease. Service members can learn to compensate for UVH with appropriate vestibular rehabilitation and gaze stability exercises.

Practitioner: Physical Therapist
ICF components: Body Structure/Body Function, Activity
Strength of recommendation: Practice Standard
Rationale: Vestibular rehabilitation is considered an appropriate treatment approach for patients with vestibular hypofunction [14].
Applicable level(s) of care: All levels when applicable

Vestibular rehabilitation has been shown to be efficacious in the recovery of dynamic visual acuity even if started some time after symptom onset for those with vestibular hypofunction. In a prospective, randomized, double-blind study of 21 patients aged 20-86 years with unilateral vestibular hypofunction, Herdman et al. [1] showed that time since symptom onset and age were not factors in recovery of dynamic visual acuity when vestibular exercises were initiated within 12 months after onset of the vestibular loss. Herdman and colleagues [1] also described the type of gaze adaptation exercises used in a vestibular rehabilitation program and mentioned that non-specific balance and gait activities were part of the rehabilitation program. Additionally, vestibular rehabilitation has been shown to reduce fall risk as measured by the *Dynamic Gait Index* (DGI) in patients with UVH [92].

In a study designed to characterize and classify patterns of dizziness in 58 active duty and retired military personnel with dizziness following a MTBI, Hoffer et al. [23] reported that 84% of patients classified in the posttraumatic vestibular migraines category showed improvement following vestibular rehabilitation. All subjects in their positional (or BPPV) category recovered following treatment. Only 27% of the group categorized as having posttraumatic spatial disorientation improved following vestibular rehabilitation and this group required more than 3 months to return to work. This study is limited by lack of a control group. Hoffer's group does describe a vestibular rehabilitation program that was composed of "individualized programs of vestibulo-ocular reflex, cervico-ocular reflex, and somatosensory exercises combined with aerobic activity" [23].

Most vestibular rehabilitation programs involve exercises to increase the gain of the vestibular system (X1 and X2 exercises), habituation and adaptation exercises, substitution exercises and gait, balance and aerobic components.

Herdman [10] provides descriptions of interventions for the patient with vestibular hypofunction.

Recommendations:

1) If a unilateral vestibular hypofunction is indicated, therapists institute a progressive vestibular rehabilitation program initially including gaze stabilization exercises with progressive postural challenge (sitting, standing, gait), adaptation and compensation exercises, and a progressive aerobic activity program [10].

2) Further home exercise recommendations and activity instructions are provided.

3) Service members who are found to be unresponsive to these adaptation exercises after 10-14 days, are referred for further specialty evaluation and treatment by therapists with specialized vestibular training.

4) The Service member's response to intervention is monitored. DVAT can be used to monitor for improvement in visual stability and decrease in visual blurring for those military personnel who are reticent about admitting their symptoms.

Discussion: Improvement in dizziness following a vestibular rehabilitation program may not alleviate complaints of postural instability. Those Service members with ongoing complaints of imbalance or postural instability will need a progressive balance activity program. The assessment and intervention recommendations for residual postural instability complaints are discussed in another section of the *Guidance*.

Migraine Associated Dizziness

Assessment

Objective: Identify dizziness associated with migraine headache that can be treated by a general practice physical therapist in the combat theater and throughout the higher levels of care to reduce complaints of dizziness associated with migraine.

> Practitioner: Physical Therapist
> ICF components: Body Structure/Body Function, Activity
> Strength of recommendation: Practice Standard
> Rationale: Gottshall and colleagues [21] used standard vestibular assessments for subjects with posttraumatic migraine associated dizziness.
> Applicable level(s) of care: All levels when applicable

Background: Migraine-associated vertigo has been reported to occur in 32% of cases in a retrospective sample of 363 patients presenting with headache to an otology practice [93]. Dizziness by itself has been shown to affect the self-perceived health status of persons with vertigo, but persons with headache (or migraine) associated dizziness have been found to have even lower self –perceived health status scores in the areas of role limitations (emotional), mental health, and social function on the SF-36, [94]. Use of the SF-8 to compare those with migrainous vertigo (MV) with controls also showed lower scores in those with MV [95]. By treating headache associated dizziness, the quality of life of Service members can be enhanced.

Gottshall et al. [21] categorized 34 consecutive patients with migraine-related vestibular symptoms into four groups including patients with idiopathic migraine-associated dizziness (MAD) either with or without BPPV and patients with post-traumatic MAD either with or without BPPV. They used the DHI, the *Activities Specific Balance Confidence Scale* (ABC), the *DGI*, head-thrust test and *Fukuda step test* [21] in their assessment.

Recommendations:

1) A history should be obtained from these Service members confirming dizziness associated with migraine headache. It is assumed that the majority of Service member's with MAD will have received a diagnosis from a physician after appropriate medical assessment.

2) Assessments including the DHI, ABC and the testing for BPPV and UVH should be done. (These assessment tools are described in other sections of this paper.)

Discussion: The therapist is referred to the section on posttraumatic dizziness for further information. Herdman [10] provides further information on migraine-associated dizziness.

Intervention

Objective: If migraine-associated dizziness is identified, provide vestibular rehabilitation to reduce the dizziness associated with the migraine-headache.

Practitioner: Physical Therapist
ICF components: Body Structure/Body Function, Activity
Strength of recommendation: Practice Standard
Rationale: Gotshall et al.'s work [21] demonstrated that a vestibular rehabilitation program produced improvement in patients with post-traumatic dizziness.
Applicable level(s) of care: All levels when applicable

Background: The use of medication and control of dietary triggers is found to be helpful in the control of MAD [96]. Vestibular rehabilitation has also been suggested as an intervention for persons with MAD [96,97]. Whitney et al. [98] concluded that patients with MAD improved with physical therapy intervention. There appeared to be an improved outcome if a patient was taking an anti-migraine medication in conjunction with physical therapy intervention. Gotshall et al. [21] demonstrated that a vestibular rehabilitation program produced improvement in all four groups of patients with migraine-related vestibular symptoms (patients with idiopathic migraine-associated dizziness either with or without BPPV and patients with post-traumatic MAD either with or without BPPV). This group described a rehabilitation strategy that included habituation exercises, balance retraining, and daily aerobic exercises.

Recommendations:

1) Incorporate vestibular rehabilitation program in treatment plan of persons with migraine associated dizziness. Treat for BPPV if identified.

2) Preventatively manage headaches.

3) Refer for specialty vestibular evaluation if the Service member is unresponsive after 10-14 days of vestibular rehabilitation program.

4) If available, and not contraindicated, recommend utilizing anti-migraine medications in conjunction with vestibular physical therapy intervention to improve outcomes of physical therapy.

Discussion: The reader is referred to *Guidance* sections on BPPV and UVH for further information on interventions.

Balance and Functional Activities

Assessment

Objective: To provide assessment for Service members with complaints of postural instability or balance difficulties both immediately following concussion or MTBI and in follow-up.

> Practitioner: Physical Therapist
> International Classification of Functioning: Body Structure/Body Function and Activity
> Strength of recommendation: Practice Standard
> Rationale: Multiple measures including both subjective and objective measures of balance or postural instability are recommended for persons with dizziness and balance issues [10-12].
> Applicable level(s) of care: All levels, specialized equipment used at levels V-VIII

Background: One of the signs of concussion or mild traumatic brain injury is poor balance. Impaired balance following concussion in sport is one of the signs used to restrict return to play for athletes and has been recommended for use as a restrictive sign for return to duty for soldiers ([7,8]; Clinical Guidelines for Primary Care, Proponency Office for Rehabilitation and Reintegration 11-2007). Persons, including Service members, with concussion or MTBI may complain of imbalance (postural instability), or unsteady walking in addition to their complaints of dizziness or vertigo, blurred vision, and/or headache. These complaints may begin immediately following a MTBI or concussion or may occur after a time delay.

Given that the symptoms of vestibular dysfunction can strongly influence a person's quality of life, a measure of confidence in his or her balance and the impact on his or her life is important. The *Activities-Specific Balance Confidence* (ABC) Scale was developed to assess balance confidence in high functioning senior citizens [99]. The ABC has been used to assess balance confidence in patients with vestibular deficits [81,94]. The ABC is a 16 item scale that allows the patient to provide a subjective rating of their balance from 0% as "no confidence" to 100% as "complete confidence". Higher-level tasks are queried such as the person's confidence in stepping off an escalator while holding packages and walking on icy sidewalks. Scores below 50% indicate a low level or homebound level of functioning and those above 80% indicate a normal level of functioning. It is unclear how responsive to change this measure would be in military members undergoing treatment for residual balance deficits; it has been used to describe balance confidence in studies of military personnel with MTBI [19,23].

Williams et al. (2004) developed the *High Level Balance and Mobility Test* (HIMAT) for persons with TBI, to assess high-level mobility important for "participation" in leisure, sporting and social activities [100]. The test is focused on "high-level mobility" rather than "functional mobility". This test measures 13 items using a 0-5 rating scale that is based on time, with a total possible score of 54. To assess validity, 103 patients with TBI were concurrently scored on the HiMAT, motor *Functional Independence Measure* (FIM) and gross function *Rivermead Motor Assessment* (RMA). Correlation between the HiMAT and the motor FIM was only moderately strong due to a substantial ceiling effect of the motor FIM. The motor FIM was unable to discriminate motor performance for 90 (87.4%) of the 103 patients, yet these patients had a mean score on the HiMAT of only 32.6/54 [101]. The HiMAT and gross function RMA had a much stronger correlation (r = .87, p < .01), but the gross function RMA also had a substantial ceiling effect when compared to the HiMAT. Fifty-three patients (51.5%) scored the maximum score of 13/13 on the gross function RMA, yet had a mean score of only 41.7/54 on the HiMAT [101].

The HIMAT can be used to follow change over time. Williams and colleagues (2006b) reported the 95% confidence interval for clinically important change (improvement or deterioration) required improvement by 4 points or deterioration by at least 2 points [102]. Intra-rater and inter-rater reliability were tested and found to be excellent [102]. Full information on the High Level Mobility Assessment Tool can be found on the website for *The Center for Outcome Measurement in Brain Injury* (www.tbims.org/combi/himat).

As mentioned above, one of the signs of concussion post injury is poor balance. The *Balance Error Scoring System* (BESS) was developed to assess balance at the sideline of a game or sports event [103]. "The BESS is a quantifiable version of a modified Romberg test for balance, consisting of 3 tests lasting 20 seconds each, performed on firm and foam surfaces" [104]. Timing of administration of the BESS is important. It has been suggested that the BESS may be useful in determining postural instability problems that would assist clinicians in making return to play decisions when a computerized dynamic posturography system is not available [65]. Clinicians using the BESS should be aware that physical exertion would affect performance on the BESS. Susco et al. [105] found that 20 minutes of rest was required after exertion before performance returned to baseline levels. Clinicians should also be aware of the practice effect that occurs with multiple administrations of the BESS [106]. While this may make it difficult to determine improvement that occurs with recovery versus practice effect, it should be recognized that the practice effect of multiple administrations of an assessment tool has not been routinely studied in assessments used in balance and gait. In general, the BESS has been used as a concussion screening tool, but some therapists report using it clinically. This tool is being recommended for inclusion in a *Combat Readiness Screen.*

The *Functional Gait Assessment* is a 10-item gait assessment based on the *Dynamic Gait Index* with "modifications made to capture those younger patients with vestibular deficits who showed ceiling effects on the DGI and to improve on the ambiguous instructions for some of the DGI items" [107]. The *Dynamic Gait Index* is used in a number of studies that monitor fall risk and functional gait in persons with vestibular diagnoses.

Gait velocity has been demonstrated to be valid and reliable in patients with traumatic brain injury [108]. Gait speed measured in meters per second is an easy measure to obtain and improvements in speed-based classifications are considered meaningful [109]. Comfortable or fast walking speed would be an easy outcome measure to assess for therapists at any of the eight levels of care.

The modified *Clinical Test of Sensory Integration and Balance* (CTSIB) [110] can be included to assess somatosensory and visual contributions to postural stability. The modified test no longer uses the dome to attempt to assess vestibular contributions to stability. Patients with uncompensated vestibular loss will have difficulty maintaining balance when somatosensory and visual inputs are altered. In practice settings where *Computerized Dynamic Posturography* equipment is unavailable, the CTSIB can be used. *Computerized Dynamic Posturography* (CDP) is a quantitative means to assess sensory contributions to postural stability while manipulating directions and forces of externally applied perturbations. This testing system cannot diagnose vestibular disorders, however, it can illustrate common patterns in test performance and the sensory situations that result in these specific patterns of response. CDP incorporates a number of testing situations including the *Sensory Organization Test* (SOT) and the *Motor Control Test* (MCT), which are described in Herdman, 2007.

Patients with mild brain injury often complain of balance impairment and feelings of postural instability when there was no evidence on clinical examination of a neurologic deficit. Computerized posturography has been able to demonstrate abnormalities in postural responses to changing sensory conditions and perturbations that are not detected on clinical examination. Dehail et al. [111] found that center of pressure displacement and area were significantly increased in subjects with brain injury who were enrolling in a vocational program even when they demonstrated no clinical abnormality.

The *Sensory Organization Test* (SOT) was significantly lower for a group of 10 patients with mild TBI who had normal neuromuscular exams and scores on the *Tinetti Balance* Assessment that were not significantly different from a control group [11]. There remain issues of correlating changes or improvements in tests on posturography platforms with changes in clinical tests and patient report of improved functional stability. Again, it has been recommended that multiple assessment tools be combined to fully characterize a person's balance and mobility status and improvement.

The Five-Times-Sit-to-Stand Test (FTSST) is a physical performance test initially developed to measure lower extremity muscle strength [112]. It may be considered as an option to use as a functional strength test in addition to other strength screening manual muscle tests. It has been used to examine functional status, balance, and vestibular dysfunction and to distinguish between fallers and non-fallers [79,113-116] Other versions are Timed Stands Test, Ten Chair Stands Test (10TSTS).

Recommendations:

1) To be consistent with the Defense and Veterans Brain Injury Center Working Group Recommendations [7], the Balance Error Scoring System (BESS) can be used to assess Service members following concussion or MTBI when in a war zone setting. This can be repeated over several days to monitor standing balance changes although a practice effect may occur. This information may be used in part, for determining readiness for return to duty similar to its use in determining readiness for return to sport.

2) In a stateside setting, it is recommended that multiple assessments be used to establish baseline status and follow change over time that occurs from natural recovery and following intervention strategies for Service members with complaints of postural instability or balance difficulties.

3) Assessments should include self-reports of confidence in balance including the *Activities-Specific Balance Confidence* (ABC) Scale for more highly functioning persons such as Service members with MTBI.

4) If a Service member is to be followed over time for high-level balance and mobility skills, the *High-Level Mobility Assessment Tool* (HIMAT) can be used to assess high-level mobility skills. The HIMAT does not require sophisticated equipment beyond a stopwatch, a level 20-meter walkway area, and stairs and could potentially be used in a war zone setting, as well as in stateside medical facilities. Some parts of the HiMAT such as skipping may lack face validity or seem irrelevant to the Service member, however, these items may be useful in assessing coordination and functional strength.

5) Additionally, *Computerized Dynamic Posturography*, can assist the clinician to identify subtle abnormalities in postural control, specific sensory impairments, and can follow change over time for persons with vestibular disorders. Specifically, the SOT measures postural sway under conditions in which the visual and somatosensory feedback is altered. The MCT uses sudden, brief displacements of the support surfaces to measure automatic postural responses that are normally used in the recovery of balance.

6) In settings that lack equipment for computerized Dynamic Posturography, the modified CTSIB (eyes open/closed, with and without foam) can be used to provide some information on sensory contributions to postural instability.

7) The *Functional Gait Assessment* is used to assess gait skills during tasks such as head turns that would challenge the vestibular system and is used to assess postural stability in persons with vestibular disorders. This test was developed to avoid the ceiling effect of the *Dynamic Gait Index* in high functioning patients.

8) Gait velocity should be determined in meters/second for both comfortable and fast walking speeds. This is considered a gold standard assessment in many studies.

9) The therapist is encouraged to incorporate a measure of a Service member's speed in completing an obstacle course. No recommendation for a specific obstacle course assessment is made at this time. Development of an assessment that tests military level tasks would be beneficial.

10)   Repeated testing to monitor change over time is recommended.

Discussion: In a war zone or similar setting, clinical measurement tools that do not require a lot of equipment and time are more reasonable and likely to be done. In a stateside setting, more time, personnel with specialty training, and sophisticated equipment are potentially available.

Intervention

Objective: To provide intervention and instruction in a home exercise program for Service members with complaints of postural instability or balance difficulties both immediately following concussion or MTBI and in follow-up.

Practitioner: Physical Therapist
International Classification of Functioning: Body Structure/Body Function and Activity
Strength of recommendation: Practice Standard
Rationale: Descriptive studies have shown that balance retraining programs improve symptoms in military personnel with dizziness associated with TBI [23]
Applicable level(s) of care: All levels, specialized equipment use at levels V-VIII

Background: Posturography platforms are also used in treatment situations to provide practice in situations with altering platform stability and sensory conditions. Posturography or similar unstable balance platforms have been used as part of an exercise regime for military personnel with balance disorders that are categorized as having posttraumatic spatial disorientation [117].

An extensive discussion of specific suggestions for treatment of postural instability that occurs with dizziness after brain injury can be found in Chapter 28 on Balance and Dizziness in the 2007 edition of Brain Injury Medicine [12]. These types of interventions have been shown to improve symptoms.

Recommendations:

1) Improvement in dizziness following CRP does not always get rid of complaints of postural instability. Those Service members with ongoing balance or postural instability complaints will need a progressive balance activity program. A customized treatment plan is recommended for each patient as appropriate including general strengthening and stretching exercises, habituation exercises, exercises to promote vestibular compensation, gaze stabilization exercises, balance and gait training, endurance exercises and exercises to enhance the use of specific sensory inputs for balance control.

2) Intervention strategies that provide increasing challenge, utilizing a military context, and tasks that are important to the Service member are recommended. Activities could include progressive mobility with head turns, carrying objects, altered terrain, altered speed, and altered base of support.

3) Consider including use of a computerized posturography platform when available.

4) Many sports incorporate balance-related challenges. As well, the military requirements for fitness such as running and obstacle courses, and the common tasks such as position changes with various rucksacks could incorporate progressive challenge. Intervention strategies involving tasks that are part of assessment tools (such as portions of the FGA or the Berg Balance Scale) with progressive postural and functional challenge may also be incorporated.

5) A home exercise program should be provided and updated as appropriate.

Discussion: The therapist is encouraged to develop an individualized treatment program and to use previously mentioned outcome measures consistently to monitor recovery and the Service member's response to interventions.

Vision Dysfunction

Updated March 2012

Assessment

Objective: To identify visual impairments and inefficiencies experienced by Service members with possible MTBI in order to plan treatment and recommendations

---

Practitioner: Occupational therapist or, if not available, physical therapist
ICF components: Body structure/function, activity
Strength of recommendation: Practice option
Rationale: While clinical experts advise screening for vision symptoms after MTBI, no such recommendations are included in published evidence-based guidelines.
Applicable level(s) of care: III (Combat Stress Unit), IV, V, VI, VII, VIII

Background: Many Service members with TBI, polytrauma, and/or blast exposure experience vision difficulties and impairments [118,119]. Although visual disturbances post-TBI are commonly associated with moderate and severe brain injury, evidence supports similar deficits in those patients who present with mild traumatic brain injury [120]. In a retrospective analysis of medical records of individuals referred to optometry for vision-based symptoms, Ciuffreda and colleagues found that 90% of patients with MTBI manifested oculomotor dysfunction including accommodation dysfunction, deficits of saccades, and/or convergence insufficiency [121,122]. Almost 40% of these individuals also presented with visual field deficits [123]. These vision disturbances likely explain patient complaints of decreased reading ability, reduced reading duration, inability to track printed materials, or photosensitivity [118].

TBI-associated vision problems are not well understood. Visual problems evident in Service members who have sustained MTBI may be secondary to the head injury, polytrauma such as eye injury associated with projected shrapnel, and/or blast waves [119]. Because vision problems may interfere with performance of everyday tasks and confound efforts to identify and treat other problems (e.g., cognition), Service members with possible MTBI are screened for vision complaints and receive a comprehensive low vision and visual perceptual evaluation, if appropriate.

The occupational therapist is a member of a larger team concerned with vision. Team members include, but are not limited to occupational therapists, low vision specialists, neuro-optometrists and ophthalmologists, low vision specialists, and physical therapists. Occupational therapists have expertise in the area of vision and understand the functional consequences of visual changes, critical for return to life tasks. The occupational therapist uses symptom checklists, dynamic observation, and standardized assessments to gain insight into the specific and global implications of deficits [124].

Occupational therapy vision screening

Because of the relatively high incidence of vision disturbances associated with MTBI, occupational therapists incorporate a vision screen into their initial occupational therapy evaluation. Occupational therapists perform vision screens in order to identify unrecognized visual deficits that interfere with daily life but not to diagnose [125]. The vision screen has two elements: a self-reported symptom inventory and observation of functional performance.

Self-report of vision symptoms: A screen for visual changes should include an interview or questionnaire specific to vision disturbances experienced by the Service member after MTBI. While there are no gold standards described in the literature, symptom inventories generally involve a series of yes/no questions regarding the patient's everyday experiences. Some patients can independently read and complete a questionnaire; others will need the therapist to read the questions aloud and to take note of responses. Here are some examples of questions asked to inventory symptoms [126]:

- Do you wear glasses?
- Do your glasses work as well now as before your injury?
- Do you have blurry vision? Is the difficulty at far or near?
- Do your eyes feel tired?
- Do you ever see double?
- Do you ever have to close one eye?
- Do you experience eyestrain, headaches when using your eyes?
- Do you find yourself losing your place or skipping lines when reading?
- Do you bump into chairs, objects?

Consider using a standardized self-report such as the *COVD QOL Assessment* (Daugherty et al., 2007).

Dynamic assessment of functional performance: An individual's occupational performance in any given situation is shaped by many internal and external variables including his or her innate capacities, the strategies he or she uses, the nature of the task, and characteristics of the environment [127]. When observing functional performance based on a dynamic investigative approach, the occupational therapist methodically manipulates task and environmental variables as the patient performs a selected everyday activity in order to determine under what conditions that individual functions at his or her best [128,129]. To observe the impact of possible vision disturbances, the occupational therapist asks the Service member to perform familiar tasks that involve the following components: moving around a room to find and retrieve items under variety of lighting conditions; reading; visually attending during mobility; bending and reaching; and visually scanning. The occupational therapist makes note of behaviors such as squinting, over-reaching for items, difficulty reading, missing items placed in the periphery, inability to visually attend when ambulating or changing position, complaints of dizziness with position changes, or complaints of visual changes over time. Service members wear their glasses or contact lenses during functional performance, as they would in any other everyday activity. Occupational therapists often use a checklist of the aforementioned behaviors and/or a stopwatch as they observe performance.

Occupational therapy comprehensive vision assessment

If potential vision disturbances are evident during either component of the vision screen, the occupational therapist performs a comprehensive vision assessment using an array of existing standardized tools and methods. The purpose of the comprehensive vision assessment is two-fold: 1) to specify components of vision dysfunction requiring occupational therapy intervention; 2) to identify individuals needing referral to vision specialists (e.g., optometrist with expertise in TBI). In general, an occupational therapy comprehensive vision assessment includes the following elements: visual acuity (distance); accommodation; convergence; eye alignment; saccades/pursuits; visual fields; binocular vision; glare/photophobia. We now describe a number of evaluation options reflect that standard assessment methods used in occupational therapy for visual impairment. Note that occupational therapy comprehensive vision assessment is not intended to replace a comprehensive vision evaluation by a neuro-optometrist/opthamalogist. We now describe a number of evaluation options reflect that standard assessment methods used in occupational therapy for visual impairment. (Readers are referred to Zoltan [2007] and Scheiman [2002] for excellent discussions of evaluation and treatment of vision problems in occupational therapy.)

Practice Options include the following:

- Distance visual acuity using Chronister Pocket Acuity Chart
- Accommodation using the Accommodative Amplitude Test (Chen & O'Leary, 1998)
- Convergence using the Near Point Convergence (Scheiman, 2011)
- Eye alignment and binocular vision using the Eye Alignment Test (Scheiman, 2011)
- Saccades using the Developmental Eye Movement Test – Adult (Sampedro, Richman, & Sanchez Pardo, 2003)
- Pursuits using the Northeastern State University College of Optometry Oculomotor Test (Maples & Ficklin, 1988)
- Visual fields using confrontation testing (Scheiman, 2011)
- Binocular vision using the Viewer-free Random Dot Test (Scheiman, 1997)
- Brain Injury Visual Assessment Battery for Adults (biVABA) (Warren, 1998)

Recommendations

1) Occupational therapists provide a vision screen consisting of vision symptom inventory and dynamic assessment of function on all Service members with diagnosed or suspected MTBI (Practice Option).

2) If vision symptom inventory and/or observations of function suggest possible vision disturbances, occupational therapists conduct a comprehensive vision assessment using standardized batteries (such as the biVABA) or individual tests of visual acuity (distance); accommodation; convergence; eye

alignment; saccades/pursuits; visual fields; binocular vision; glare/photophobia (Practice Option).

3) If comprehensive vision assessment in occupational therapy suggests vision deficits, the Service member is referred to the optometrist and/or vision specialist on the rehabilitation team for further diagnostic testing (Practice Option).

Discussion: Visual changes are a common complaint post MTBI. They may be mild such as blurred vision or difficulty focusing in high or low light or they may be severe such as visual field cuts, diplopia, or total vision loss. The functional consequences of visual changes for soldiers in-theater are particularly significant as they may be unable to see hazards that place themselves and others at risk for injury or attack. The occupational therapist is educated to evaluate visual changes, identify potential activity limitations associated with visual dysfunction and provide strategies to compensate and exercises to remediate problems. The findings from an occupational therapy vision assessment may result in referrals to other specialized vision Services and contribute to the diagnostic process. While many of the symptoms associated with MTBI mirror PTSD, this is not the case with visual changes. Therefore, findings from an assessment of visual functioning may help the Service member's physician rule out combat stress and PTSD in the Service member's symptom presentation.

Intervention

Objective: To provide remedial training or adaptive strategies in order to restore premorbid level of functioning and decrease symptoms associated with visual deficits.

> Practitioner: Occupational therapist
> ICF components: Body structure/function, activity, participation
> Strength of recommendation: Practice option
> Rationale: Existing guidelines and evidence reviews do not specify interventions for vision problems after MTBI.
> Applicable level(s) of care: III (Combat Stress Unit), IV, V, VI, VII, VIII

Background: Efficacy of treatment for visual disturbances associated with MTBI is limited, although there is some evidence that interventions may improve convergence and visual scanning [130]. Treatment methods may be restorative or adaptive and the strategies employed will vary depending on the underlying issue as well as the individual's needs and goals. In general, occupational therapists work with optometrists/opthalmologists who have TBI expertise to develop an intervention plan (incorporating the treatment suggestions described above) based on the individual Service member's vision deficits, specific goals, and level of care. The Service member's treatment plan should be coordinated across the rehabilitation team. For example, everyone on the team should work to reinforce adaptive vision strategies to help the Service member master the strategies and build new habits. Open communication between team members will help to provide this continuity of care.

An array of vision-related intervention strategies are described below. Note that the biVABA also provides a number of suggested treatment strategies, both adaptive and remedial for visual attention, scanning, and low vision.

Visual acuity

In the case of visual acuity deficits, occupational therapists refer patients to eye specialists for appropriate prescription for corrective lenses. Additionally, occupational therapists provide patient education associated with use of compensatory strategies such as increased illumination and contrast; decreasing background pattern and clutter; using magnification.

Visual scanning and tracking

Scanning deficits may be secondary to a number of underlying issues including saccadic eye movement problems, balance issues, hyperactive nystagmus, or weak extraocular musculature. Intervention strategies must address the underlying issue. For example, intervention for deficits secondary to saccadic eye movements may include pointing to letters that have been written on opposing sides of a page, engaging in activities that require gross motor movements such as looking over left shoulder then right and identifying objects or visual targets, as well as computer retraining software [131]. Other compensatory techniques include use of visual anchors while reading and decreasing the amount of visual stimuli that may be present during task engagement [131].

The Dynavision has been used to address visual scanning and reaction time and also as a tool to advance driver rehabilitation in an occupational therapy setting. Once again there is no empirical support for these intervention strategies but have been suggested by experts in the field of brain injury rehabilitation.

Accommodation

Individuals with impaired accommodation may complain of discomfort and eye strain with near tasks and difficulty changing focus from near to far and far to near. Patients are referred to staff optometrist/ophthalmologist with expertise in TBI and vision. Occupational therapists provide education, compensatory intervention, and if recommended by vision specialist, support performance of eye exercises (Scheiman, 2011).

Convergence

Kapoor and colleagues [132] described the use of visual exercises to increase oculomotor control and improve convergence. These exercises may include the use of a Brock string or exercises that promote visual fixation and identification of objects placed close to the nose (at the end of a spoon placed in the mouth) [131]. As supervised by vision specialist, patients may benefit from patching and/or exercises such as pencil push-ups.

Diplopia

Individuals who present with diplopia should be referred to a vision specialist for suggestions regarding use of full eye occlusion, partial occlusion or use of prisms. The occupational therapist shares information with the specialist regarding the Service member's functional performance associated with vision changes [131]. If the therapist is in-theater and no vision specialist is available, patching one eye should remediate diplopia but this is a "quick fix" only. Additionally, occupational therapists instruct patients in compensatory strategies including increasing illumination and contrast; decreasing clutter and background pattern; using visual markers or anchors; limiting time doing visual tasks that take concentration and taking frequent breaks.

Recommendations (Practice Options):

1) Occupational therapy-based interventions for vision consist of both remedial and adaptive approaches and must occur in the context of a larger team.

2) Occupational therapists refer patients with vision impairments to eye specialists and collaboratively develop the treatment plan.

3) Rehabilitation for visual deficits should use activities that are of interest and need for the Service member. This may help to provide motivation and reinforcement.

4) Restriction of activities may be necessary as part of the treatment program. For example, driving restrictions or restrictions on some sports may be recommended for safety.

5) Therapy should take place in multiple environments including the home and community whenever possible at the higher levels of care or in theater in the case of the deployed Service member. Practice in multiple contexts will assist with generalization of newly-acquired skills.

Discussion: Visual disturbances associated with MTBI potentially have a significant impact on the Service member's ability to resume military activity safely and efficiently. More research is needed to both identify the nature of vision disturbances after MTBI as well as to identify the most effective intervention methods for this population.

Post Traumatic Headache (PTH)

Assessment

Objective: Identify headache etiologies secondary to mild TBI that can be treated by a general practice physical therapist. Monitor progress and response to treatment of contributing factors.

Practitioner: Physical Therapist
ICF component(s): Body structure/Body function, (if HA becomes chronic may include Activity and Participation)
Strength of recommendation: Practice standard
Rationale: Recommended assessment tools suggested here have been shown to be reliable and valid for their specified conditions, such as neck pain, TMJ disability, or pain. None of the assessment tools recommended have been developed specifically for patients with MTBI. The numeric pain scale or visual analog pain scale is used to classify headache pain levels [24,25]. A visual analog scale may be used to monitor limitation resulting from headache. If cervical spine or TMJ issues are contributing to headache pain, assessments including the *Neck Disability Index* [26,27], the *Jaw Functional Limitation Scale* (JFLS) [20,28], the *Temporomandibular Index* (TMI) [29] may be used. Use of the *Patient-specific Functional Limitation Scale* should be considered [30].
Applicable level(s) of care: All

Background: Post traumatic headache (PTH) is defined as a headache that occurs 1 week after regaining consciousness, or within 1 week of head trauma [133]. Most of these resolve within 6-12 months and are associated with cervical muscle tenderness and postural abnormalities. Lew et al. (2006) found that many patients with PTH presented clinically with symptoms similar to tension headache (37%), migraine (29%), and cluster headaches (6-10 %).

The number of individuals who develop PTH following a MTBI usually ranges from 30% to 50% [134]. In a recent survey of army infantry soldiers, 3-4 months after return from a yearlong deployment in Iraq, about 30%, who had been injured with loss of consciousness, also described headache as a disability affecting their overall health [48]. Paradoxically, many researchers have found that the milder the brain injury, the more "frequently severe" is the post traumatic headache [134,135]. These authors also conclude that PTSD may mediate chronic pain but that traumatic brain injury has an independent association with chronic pain. Based on a retrospective review of the literature, the prevalence of chronic pain after brain injury for veterans is 43.1% (95% CI, 39.9%-46.3%) [135].

In situations where patients sustain whiplash injuries, 82% will experience headache immediately following the injury [134]. These headaches have a higher association with light and sound and are aggravated by movement [133]. Whiplash injury may also aggravate the temporomandibular joint (TMJ) due to tearing and stretching of ligamentous structures. TMJ injury is unlikely a sole cause of headache, but may be a contributor to overall discomfort and disability [134].

Direct trauma to the face, head, or neck can also result in supraorbital, infraorbital or occipital neuralgias. Structures innervated by C1/C2 cervical segments including sternocleidomastoid, trapezius, structures of the atlantoaxial and atlanto-occipital joint, prevertebral and paravertebral cervical muscles as well as the vertebral arteries may contribute to headache. According to Packard (1999), these types of neuralgias are often mistakenly attributed to trigeminal nerve injuries. Identification of trigger points in upper cervical region is a key clinical sign of these types of neuralgias.

Cervicogenic headache overlaps with whiplash and cervical strain injuries. The trigeminal nociceptive system converges with upper cervical pain pathways and may play a role in PTH. A proposed set of guidelines to describe cervicogenic headache has been published. A main criterion is that neck movement exacerbates headache or that sustained movement or awkward postures cause headache symptoms [17].

The clinical presentation of the various types of headache disorder can mimic or co-exist with each other, making it difficult to distinguish between the different types of headache. High levels of muscle tenderness, postural and mechanical abnormalities all have been reported in tension headaches, migraine, whiplash syndromes and cervicogenic headaches [17,134].

The heterogeneity of clinical presentations for disability due to neck and jaw pain, and headache is large. The diversity of clinical presentation also makes it difficult to include all possible functional items that can be impacted by patients' injuries or conditions that can result in headache. As mentioned, neck pain, temporomandibular joint disorders (TMD), and shoulder pain are three common complaints reported in conjunction with MTBI, all of which contribute to PTH. Measurement tools used to assess headache include both general measures of the frequency, severity, and limitations caused by headache pain, as well as condition-specific measures that are used to determine the disability and severity of that disability related to the neck, jaw and headache.

Given the overlapping nature of headache and TMD following MTBI, it is important for the therapist to distinguish disability related to the physical and biomechanical factors that contribute to the origins of headache. This distinction will guide the clinical decision-making process to develop a specific and therefore, effective treatment program. The main criterion involves an assessment of how neck and jaw movements exacerbate headache. For the appropriate assessment tools for the TMD contribution to headache pain, see that section of the *Guidance.*

In the gathering of basic PT clinical measures of headache, consideration should be given to a standardized approach. Typically the numeric pain scale or visual analog pain scale is used to classify headache pain levels [24]. For example, a numeric pain scale that assesses two dimensions of pain within a consistent time frame may be used. These dimensions include pain limitation of activity over the last 24 hours or last week, and the pain intensity in the last 24 hours, last week, or other specific time frame. Additionally, a standardized approach includes recording of the number and type of headaches within a consistent time frame. This may be expanded to include the recording of the amount and type of headache-related medications under a standard context such as within the last 24 hours, or the amount needed to complete a worked day or any context associated with pain management.

The *Headache Disability Inventory* (HDI) is a 25-item patient self-report that measures the impact of headache on daily living [136]. This inventory includes assessment of daily living issues with both functional and emotional scales that combine for a total score. The HDI can also be used to monitor the effect of therapeutic intervention for headache. The HDI has high internal consistency, reliability, content validity and good test-retest stability [136,137].

The *Neck Disability Index* (NDI) is a patient self-report questionnaire that measures clinical change in individuals that have acute or chronic neck pain of musculoskeletal or neurogenic origin [138]. This questionnaire is designed to help understand how neck pain affects an individual's ability to manage everyday-life activities. The NDI has been studied in both acute and chronic neck pain (including those with traumatic etiology) in a variety of settings (hospital, rural clinics, urban settings, tertiary care). A recent systematic review of the studies on the NDI indicate that there are important limitations [27], although the NDI is considered the gold standard for assessment of the impact of neck pain and for following change resulting from treatment interventions.

The *Patient Specific Functional Scale* (PSFS) is a patient-specific outcome measure, which investigates functional status [30]. Patients are asked to nominate up to five activities with which they have difficulty due to their condition and then rate the functional limitation associated with these activities. The PSFS is intended to complement the findings of generic or condition-specific measures. The PSFS has been shown to be valid and responsive to change in musculoskeletal conditions such as neck pain, cervical radiculopathy, knee pain, and low back pain [26,139,140]. When compared to other fixed-item instruments, the PSFS has been shown to be more responsive than the *Neck Disability Index* [26], the *Pain Rating Index*, and the *Roland Morris Questionnaire* [139]. In pain-focused patients, the PSFS is useful to redirect questioning towards function and ability rather than pain and disability. In a patient population of workman's compensation patients the PSFLS was associated with timely recovery. Use of the PSFLS would be appropriate in the condition of headache resulting from MTBI.

Recommendations:

1) Basic PT clinical measures of PTH should involve a standardized approach, including:

   a. A numeric or visual analog pain scale that assesses two dimensions of pain within a consistent time frame:

   b. Pain limitation due to activity during the last 24 hours or last week, etc.

   c. Pain intensity in the last 24 hours or last week etc.

   d. Recording the number /type of headaches within a consistent time frame.

   e. Recording the amount and type of headache related medications under a standard context such as within the last 24 hours; or the amount and type of medication needed to complete a worked day or any context associated with pain management.

2) The PSFLS is a unique tool to assist with an individualized approach by the PT and should be considered for patients with headache resulting from MTBI. It is a patient-specific outcome measure, which investigates functional status [30].

3) Condition specific measures should be used to determine disability and severity of disability related to the neck/jaw/headache. These measures can be administered before and after an episode of care to determine the degree of significant improvement. Data can be aggregated to inform overall treatment program effectiveness. These condition specific measures may include the *Neck Disability Index, Jaw Functional Limitation Scale* and/or the *Headache Disability Inventory*.

4) A standard musculoskeletal evaluation of the head and neck and related structures should be included.

Discussion: Therapists are encouraged to complete a thorough initial evaluation that includes evaluation of any orofacial pain, TMJ disorders, cervical spine, thoracic spine and upper quadrant to include upper extremities. Frequently headache pain is caused by dysfunction and referred pain from another area of dysfunction. Neck pain, back pain, or upper extremity pain are all areas that may affect a Service member's ability to perform duties safely in a field environment. The Service member's primary military occupation and duty requirements must be taken into consideration when determining fitness for duty.

Intervention

Objective: To alleviate pain and minimize activity limitations due to headache after MTBI.

Practitioner: Physical Therapist
International Classification of Functioning: Body structure/body function
Strength of recommendation: Practice option
Rationale: Physical therapy appears to have at least a modest impact on outcome in patients experiencing headache [17]. Multimodal approaches that include manipulation and/or mobilization in combination with exercise are generally more effective. Patient education on medication management and avoidance of headache triggers is considered essential.
Applicable level(s) of care: All

Background: Pharmacologic treatment is common for headache, as is its use preventatively. This type of treatment is not typically within the scope of civilian physical therapy practice. In a field environment with no access to imaging, the initial medical treatment for headache is acetaminophen ONLY until intracranial bleeding has been ruled out through appropriate imaging. Physical therapists at this level should advocate to Service members of the need to avoid other headache-related medication, as Service members often "self-medicate" and do have access to over-the-counter pain medications. Medication reconciliation and notation of medication changes during an episode of care are important considerations for PTs, especially with the increasing use of alternative and complimentary therapies.

Reconciliation of medication can also assist in the overall management of analgesic rebound headache. This is a situation where patients that have used medications to manage their chronic daily headache, become dependent on these medications such that once medications are stopped the patient can experience a rebound headache [134].

As with other joint dysfunction, patient education regarding PTH and appropriate exercise program handouts are effective intervention techniques. Unique to headache, is the inclusion of environmental triggers for headache that include sleep patterns, use of caffeinated beverages, stress, inconsistent exercise and irregular diet [141]. All of the above listed "triggers" are present in the combat environment.

A structured review of the literature that examined physical treatment for headache [17] concluded that physical therapy appears to have a modest impact on outcome in patients experiencing headache. This review included studies that examined headache etiologies that were both traumatic and non-traumatic. The quality of the studies was generally low and the author emphasizes that individualized evaluation and intervention is the best approach. Bondi (2005) notes that these conclusions are in the context of common clinical presentations that include pronounced muscle tenderness of neck, face and shoulder associated with neck pain and headache.

PT interventions with the strongest evidence include specific training in exercise, stretching and ergonomics at home and in the workplace. Multimodal approaches that include manipulation and/or mobilization in combination with exercise are generally more effective [142]. In a case series of 20 patients whose headache pain was of muscular origin, treatment included posture training at home/workplace, isotonic home exercise, massage, stretching of cervical muscle. The patients were seen once a week for six weeks. [143]. In a case report on cervicogenic headache, interventions including exercise and functional instruction were successful in improving functional and work related activities as well as improving sleep and decreasing the number of pain medications. Outcomes for this case report included headache frequency/intensity and the *Neck Disability Index* [144].

Recommendations:

1) Physical Therapists in theater educate Service members with MTBI about the dangers associated with taking over-the-counter medications NOT prescribed

by medical personnel.

2) Physical Therapists provide education and handouts regarding "red flags" [7,34], triggers for headache, and exercise programs (to include postural re-education).

3) Individualized goal setting (as with the Patient-specific Functional Limitation Scale) has shown promise in developing a more positive tone to the PT episode of care, focusing on change in function that is most important to an individual patient.

4) Symptom management of head/neck pain is best applied using a multimodal approach that includes self-care instruction, stretching /strengthening exercise, manual therapy and application of therapeutic modalities.

5) The general overall approach should be to address physical deficits (including movement related disabilities, postural deficits and muscle tenderness) that result in increased head/neck and jaw pain.

6) Monitor response to treatment using assessment tools such as the NDI, TMI, pain scale, and other pain and disability indexes to track recovery and effectiveness of treatment techniques used.

7) Develop well-designed randomized controlled trials in the treatment of post traumatic headache in those with mild TBI or concussion to establish definitive treatment standards for both Service members and the civilian patient population.

Discussion: Therapists are encouraged to design individualized intervention strategies based on findings in the evaluation. It is assumed that general practice physical therapist's in military settings have a strong knowledge base in orthopedic and pain-related assessments and interventions.

Temporomandibular Disorders (TMD)

Assessment

Objective: Identify temporomandibular joint (TMJ) disorders with etiologies that can be treated by a general practice physical therapist in the combat theater and throughout the higher levels of care to reduce complaints of TMJ pain and dysfunction.

Practitioner: Physical Therapist
ICF component(s): Body structure/Body function
Strength of recommendation: Practice standard
Rationale: The assessment tools recommended were not
specifically developed for patients with MTBI. The *Jaw
Functional Limitation Scale* (JFLS) measures functional
limitations that is independent of pain related behaviors [20]. The
Temporomandibular Index (TMI) is a physical assessment of the
TMJ joint and surrounding musculature that provides
information regarding the severity of TMD [29]. Use of the
Patient-specific Functional Limitation Scale should be considered
[30].

Applicable level(s) of care: All

Background: Temporomandibular Disorders (TMD) are defined as a subgroup of
craniofacial pain problems that involve the temporomandibular joint (TMJ), muscles
of mastication, and associated head and neck musculoskeletal structures. Common
symptoms can include ear pain and stuffiness, tinnitus, dizziness, neck pain, and
headache. TMD disorders, as well as neck and shoulder pain complaints, are
commonly seen in conjunction with concussion, and may be contributing to the
headaches that the person is experiencing [134]. Common impairments found in
persons with TMD include joint mobility restrictions, muscle length limitations, as
well as postural limitations and neuromuscular deficits.

The prevalence of at least one sign of TMD is reported in 40-75% of adults in
the United States [5]. Temporomandibular joint sounds and deviation on opening the
jaw occur in approximately 50% of otherwise asymptomatic persons and usually do
not require treatment. Other signs such as decreased mouth opening and occlusal
changes occur in 5% of the population. The TMD are most commonly reported in
persons aged 20-50 years of age, affecting females in proportionately greater
numbers [5].

Epidemiological studies conclude that despite the high prevalence of TMD, up
to 40 % of those who experience signs/symptoms of TMD dysfunction resolve
spontaneously [5]. It should be noted however, that some studies that show that
patients with post traumatic TMD "mildly" differ from those with nontraumatic
disorders on reaction time testing, neuropsychological testing, clinical testing of TMJ
and on results from single-photon emission computerized tomography (SPECT) [145].
Packard (1999) discusses the epidemiology of headache in the US population that
experience PTH and states that there is evidence that TMJ disorders may contribute
to PTH. Packard further concludes that TMD disorders are not a causative but
rather an associated factor in mild TBI headaches.

Given the high prevalence of TMD in the general population, the impact of
PTH in mild brain injury and the association between the two, implementation of a
physical therapy program by a general practice PT requires a focused assessment
and evaluation of the severity of TMD.

The *Jaw Functional Limitation Scale* (JFLS) and the *Temporomandibular Index* (TMI) are clinical assessment tools that provide information regarding the severity of TMD. The JFLS is a relatively simple patient report that measures functional limitation (related to body structure/function) that is independent of pain related behaviors. It is a new tool and requires pencil and paper administration. It is easy to use, responsive to change [28], but has not been used extensively in outcome studies.

The TMI is an extensive measurement protocol grounded in epidemiological data and associated with the Research Diagnostic Criteria (RDC/TMD) (see [146] for information on international research consortiums and reliability). The benefit of this system is that it determines levels of severity for TMD that separates patients with physical disability from patients that experience chronic pain and pain-related behaviors (see [147] for outcomes following comprehensive care; and definitions of levels of severity).

The TMI is a physical assessment of the TMJ joint and surrounding musculature. The tool has the added advantage that it is used by the dental community at large and would facilitate communication and referral between the general practice PT and chronic pain teams [29]. The use of the TMI does require training (studies report 30-50 hours) to achieve reliability between testers. The TMI has also been responsive to change following typical interventions employed by physical therapists in patients with chronic pain [148].

Recommendations:

1) Conduct a standard assessment of TMJ joint mechanics, muscle tenderness, and symptom occurrence. The most comprehensive tool available is the *Temporomandibular Index.* Use of this tool requires training of up to 30 hours and helps to define the type and severity of TMJ dysfunction.

2) Use the *Jaw Functional Limitation* scale to determine how TMD is affecting the patient's daily activity. This tool would also be useful to determine functional goals.

3) Use of the *Patient-specific Functional Limitation Scale* should be considered (see Headache section of this Guidance document for more information). This tool is easy to use, clinically relevant as well as sensitive to change. It is not a good tool to gather aggregate data on patient outcomes, however is useful for the individual patient.

4) Refer to dental services when needed and if available.

Discussion: It is assumed that general practice physical therapists in a military setting may or may not be experienced in working with Service members with specialty issues such as TMD. They are encouraged to use a team approach.

Intervention

Objective: Provide interventions that address TMJ dysfunction and pain issues; to encourage referral for dental services and specialty treatment for complicated cases. The interventions must fit into the skill set of the general practice physical therapist.

Practitioner: Physical Therapist
ICF component(s): Body structure/Body function, Activity
Strength of recommendation: Practice standard
Rationale: No studies specifically address TMJ disorders that occur as a result of MTBI. Several systematic reviews of TMD interventions are available [3-6]. Symptom management of TMD is best applied using a conservative and multimodal approach. Evaluation and treatment should also include other areas of the head, neck and upper trunk that demonstrate any deficits in posture or function or pain. The majority of TMD respond to symptom management techniques but for those who experience chronic pain, referral and collaboration with dentists and/or a multidisciplinary chronic pain center may be needed.
Applicable level(s) of care: All

Background: In randomized controlled trials (RCT) that have controlled for severity, TMD patients with mostly physical limitations have shown improvement with patient education on self-care. This approach included use of heat/cold packs, jaw exercises, guidance in activities to avoid (i.e. chewing gum, eating hard candy) and progressive muscle relaxation [6].

Systematic reviews of the literature, indicate that the majority of TMD can be treated with noninvasive interventions [3,5]. Medlicott & Harris [4] reviewed 30 articles, noting many methodological limitations to the studies, and made the following recommendations:1) active exercises and manual mobilizations may be effective, 2) postural training may be used in combination with other interventions, 3) programs involving relaxation techniques and biofeedback, electromyography training and proprioceptive re-education may be more effective than placebo treatment and occlusal splints, 4) combinations of active exercises, manual therapy, postural correction, and relaxation techniques may be effective.

Wright and colleagues [149] studied patients with a primary muscle disorder of the TMJ and used a combination of self-care and posture training compared to a group that did self-care management only. The recommended exercise protocols included neck and upper trunk stretching activities in supine and in sitting. Self-care instructions included education on resting masticatory muscles; avoiding parafunctional habits that increase pain (chewing hard candy/gum); applying heart/cold to most painful areas and the use of anti-inflammatory medications. This group found that posture training and TMD self-management instructions were significantly more effective than TMD self-management instructions alone for reducing TMD and neck symptoms.

Au and Klineberg [150] examined the use of isokinetic exercise in patients with clicking of the TMJ joint. The recommended exercises include jaw movements performed at a constant speed with moderate resistance applied by the patient's hand, over a study period of 6 months. Eighty-two percent (18/22) of subjects in the intervention group had resolution of clicking as measured by a Doppler auscultator. There were no changes in the control group reporting neither increased clicking nor development of clicking. Further, at the 2-year follow-up, 72% (16/22) remained symptom free.

Furto and colleagues [151] published a nonrandomized study that did not control for TMD severity. The interventions included manual therapy by therapists trained under the American Physical Therapy Association and the American Academy of Orthopedic Manual Physical Therapy Fellowship Program. Intervention consisted of manual therapy techniques and exercise that included the Rocabado condylar remodeling exercise program and iontophoresis for those patients with limited range of motion. Of the 15 patients treated, 13 showed improvement on patient self-report functional measures. The discussion of this paper provides an informative description of the clinical rational of a multimodal approach. These researchers also used patient self-report measures that have less rigor than JFLS, and TMI, (do not control for patient severity) but require less training than the TMI.

There are no published guidelines based on a consensus review process. One published guideline, based on current evidenced–based practice as implemented by one university setting, has been documented by Decker and Bromaghim, PTs at the TMD, Orofacial Pain and Oral Medicine Clinic at the University of Minnesota. The guideline is a comprehensive summary that links temporomandibular joint dysfunction with indications and contraindications for therapeutic modalities, exercise for the jaw and neck including indications for manual therapies, and treatment goals for three groups of disorders including hypomobility (myofascial pain, joint inflammation, post surgery) and hypermobility (clicking, arthralgia, muscle pain).

Recommendations:

1) Symptom management of TMD is best applied using a multimodal approach that includes self-care instruction, stretching exercise, manual therapy and application of therapeutic modalities.

2) Evaluation and treatment should also include other areas of the head, neck and upper trunk that demonstrate any deficits in posture or function or pain.

3) The majority of TMD responds to conservative, symptom management techniques but those who experience chronic pain may benefit from referral and collaboration with dentists (occlusal spints, evaluation of intracranial sources of pain) and/or a multidisciplinary chronic pain center.

Discussion: The majority of TMD can be treated with noninvasive interventions. It is important to utilize a team approach in treating TMD disorders where available.

Cognitive Impairments and Inefficiencies

Assessment

Objective: To identify cognitive inefficiencies and impairments experienced by Service members with MTBI in order to plan treatment.

> Practitioner: Occupational therapist
> ICF component(s): Body functions and structure; Activity
> Strength of recommendation: Practice Option
> Rationale: Existing guidelines provide little guidance as to the optimal timing or composition of cognitive assessment, although there appears to be general agreement that cognitive assessment can be of value for individuals who experience persistent cognitive complaints [18]. Existing guidelines do not mention cognitive assessment performed by occupational therapists.
> Applicable level(s) of care: III (Combat Stress Unit), IV, V, VI, VII, VIII

Background: As discussed earlier, some people describe decrements in their memory, attention, and information processing speed for three or more months after MTBI [45]. These cognitive symptoms may, in part, be explained by a bottleneck in terms of the brain's limited processing capacity as he or she attempts to manage distractions associated with symptom-management [47]. While highly practiced skills may be preserved, activities requiring new learning, problem solving, and self-control may be more difficult or problematic [47]. Unlike those with moderate – severe traumatic brain injury, persons with MTBI tend to be aware of decrements in cognitive performance; their self-reports of functioning are consistent with that of the appraisal of family members throughout their recovery [152]. However, they may be unaware of the influence of situational factors on their performance and are at risk for misattributing symptoms and cognitive inefficiencies that most everyone experiences to the MTBI [153]. They also may have limited awareness of when and how to use compensatory cognitive strategies to optimize their performance.

Occupational and physical therapists are concerned with the impact of cognitive impairments and inefficiencies on everyday functioning, with occupational therapists typically assuming formal roles related to cognitive assessment and treatment. The primary purpose of cognitive assessment from an occupational therapy perspective is to identify (and ultimately address) possible cognitive barriers to functioning, not to diagnose neuropsychological impairment. Cognitive assessment in occupational therapy involves the evaluation of everyday functioning in order to make inferences about cognition (using dynamic investigative approach) and/or the evaluation of cognitive processes in order to make inferences about functioning (using standardized tests) [154].

Interpretation of findings is as important to occupational therapists as test administration. Because cognitive assessment involves more than observation checklists and score assignment, occupational therapists consider other factors such as the patient's level of pain, fatigue, and stress and presence of environmental distracters as they interpret and document the results or findings. In fact, many experts suggest that it is impossible to obtain a true picture of the Service members' cognitive functioning until these other factors are resolved [55].

Examples of functional assessments of cognition

Dynamic assessment of functional performance.

As discussed in the Vision section, an individual's cognitive functioning in any given situation is shaped by many internal and external variables including his or her innate capacities, the strategies he or she uses, the nature of the task, and characteristics of the environment [127]. When assessing cognition based on a dynamic investigative approach, the occupational therapist methodically manipulates task and environmental variables as the patient performs a selected everyday activity in order to determine under what conditions that individual functions at his or her best [128,129]. Semi-familiar, multi-step and/or unstructured tasks (such as money-management, meal preparation, household, construction, or simulated work tasks) tend to approximate the problem solving demands of everyday performance. Typically, therapists use observation worksheets that help them track qualitative aspects of the patient's performance of an unstructured self-care, household, leisure, or work task such as number of reminders or redirections required; response to visual or auditory distractions; ability to self-monitor; speed and efficiency of performance; ability to multi-task; response to feedback; initiation of compensatory techniques; evidence of planning and/or strategy use (versus trial and error approach). See Appendix B for an example of an observation worksheet that could be used when employing this approach to assessment.

Self-reflection/self-awareness analysis.

There are no formalized procedures described in the literature specific to assessing patients' awareness of situational factors impacting performance after MTBI. However, occupational therapists may incorporate self-awareness assessment into a dynamic assessment of functional performance by adding the following elements:

- The therapist selects an assessment task that is likely to present a challenge to the patient based on suspected areas of inefficiency, impairment, or concern. Assessment tasks typically involve specific, detailed procedural instructions (memory demands), incorporate both structured and unstructured elements (problem solving demands); require at least 20-30 minutes of sustained effort (energy, concentration demands). Clerical, kitchen, craft or assembly tasks are well-suited to dynamic assessment with a self-assessment component.

- After describing the to-be-performed task, the therapist asks the patient to predict how well/easily he or she will perform the assigned task (e.g., performance time, percent accuracy, number of off-task responses to distractions, number of rest breaks required).

- The therapist establishes a plan to measure these parameters during actual task performance (with measurement/tracking performed by either the patient or therapist or both).

- The patient performs the task.

- Upon completing the task, the therapist provides actual task performance data to the patient and asks him or her to a) compare the predicted to the actual performance; b) describe situational, environmental, personal, or strategy factors that enhanced or deterred performance; and c) determine how to approach the task differently next time.

The process of task prediction and performance analysis can be incorporated into a wide array of therapy tasks and structures a process wherein the patient actively engages in self-reflective learning rather than passively receiving feedback from the therapist.

Mortera Cognitive Screening Measure- M-CSM [155-157].

The M-CSM also involves observing functional performance. It was developed as a means to assess seven selected cognitive processes - sustained attention, shifting attention, visual attention-scanning, awareness of disability, judgment relative to safety, recall, planning/problem solving - during the completion of two functional tasks (preparation of a bowl of soup and sandwich). The therapist assigns one of three scores (0 – no problem; 1 – a potential problem; 2 - evidence of a problem) to observable behaviors that objectively and operationally describe each of the seven cognitive processes underlying the functional tasks. Content validity was addressed, in part, by validating the seven cognitive processes relative to adequacy for inclusion and appropriate use of content domain and the accuracy of the cognitive descriptors or observable behaviors that indicate on what level the cognitive processes are impaired. Inter-rater reliability is very good (intraclass correlation coefficient = .83) [156,157].

Examples of standardized assessments of specific cognitive domains with established reliability and validity for use with traumatic brain injury

Cognistat (Neurobehavioral Cognitive Status Examination [NCSE]) [158] – a microbattery comprised of 10 subtests in areas of orientation, attention, comprehension, repetition, naming, construction, memory, calculation, similarities and judgment. The NCSE profile and process observations have been used as a cognitive screen with patients with MTBI in an acute medical setting to identify deficits and ensure patient education and treatment in patients with MTBI [159].

Contextual Memory Test [129] – test of visual memory that examines immediate and delayed recall, awareness of memory capacity, and memory strategy in which the patient tries to remember 20 objects associated with 1 of 2 themes.

Rivermead Behavioral Memory Test (RBMT) [160,161] – involves memory skills used in everyday life such as remembering names, faces, routes, appointments. Wills and colleagues [162] combined two of the four parallel versions of the RBMT to create an extended version (RBMT-E) which is more sensitive to subtle memory problems, as may be experienced by persons with MTBI.

Test of Everyday Attention [163] – means of evaluating various dimensions of attention in the context of everyday tasks such as Map and Telephone Search, Elevator Counting, and Telephone Dual Task.

Recommendations (Practice Options):

1) For Service members with MTBI, occupational therapists assess cognition in the context of functional task performance in order to detect possible cognitive impairments or inefficiencies.

2) Occupational therapists coordinate their cognitive assessment efforts with other team members. In general, in-depth cognitive-behavioral assessment is deferred to neuropsychologists on the rehabilitation team, if available within rehabilitation setting/level of care.

3) If the results of the functional cognitive assessment suggest possible cognitive impairments/inefficiencies, the occupational therapist administers standardized assessments of memory, attention, and/or executive functions (and/or corroborating data are obtained from tests administered by clinicians from other disciplines).

Discussion: Occupational therapists within the DoD and VA systems will best serve individuals with MTBI as they are familiar with administering cognitive assessments related to everyday functioning, sophisticated in selecting the type of assessment methods to employ in specific situations, and skilled as observers who are able to link elements of functional performance to hypotheses about cognitive processes. Observations of functional performance could be formalized by creating fill-in-the-blank worksheets and/or checklists that specify the cognitive processes involved in various everyday tasks and that prompt the therapist to make note of task and environmental variables that may be affecting performance.

<u>**Intervention**</u>

Objective: To help the Service member improve his or her cognitive functioning and as a result, performance of everyday tasks

---

Practitioner: Occupational therapist
ICF component(s): Body functions and structure; Activity; Participation
Strength of recommendations: Practice Standard
Rationale: In their State of the Science literature review of empirical literature published between 1998 - 2004, Gordon and colleagues (2006) concluded that "training in the use of compensatory strategies seems to be effective for the remediation of attention and mild memory impairments after TBI" (p. 355). This is consistent with recommendations from resulting from two evidence-based reviews conducted by Cicerone and colleagues (2000, 2005).
Applicable level(s) of care: III (Combat Stress Unit), IV, V, VI, VII, VIII

Background: Cognitive rehabilitation involves two approaches: the effort to retrain impaired or deficient cognitive processes and the effort to help people acquire compensatory cognitive strategies that circumvent the problem [164]. A retraining approach involves repeatedly exposing the patient to structured, graded cognitive challenges (via work sheets and computer programs) in order to stimulate presumably damaged areas of the brain in the hope that resultant neuronal changes that will yield improved functional performance [165]. There is little evidence to support this approach [166]. However, many experts recommend cognitive compensatory strategy training for persons with MTBI specific to attention, memory, and executive function difficulties [47,57,167]. It should be noted that most of the research in the area of cognitive rehabilitation has been conducted by neuropsychologists or speech language pathologists and involved subjects with moderate to severe traumatic brain injury.

Strategy training to address attentional deficits is recommended for outpatients in the post acute phase of rehabilitation [168-170]. Attentional strategies might include the following:

- single task completion [171];
- initiating the removal of visual or auditory distractions [171];
- learning to consciously monitor activities to avoid lapses in attention [172];
- performing challenging tasks during high-energy times of the day;
- pacing, planning breaks, and self-monitoring of fatigue/attention levels [172];
- using an "ideas log" so that people can capture good ideas that come to mind but want to address later [172];
- routinely double-checking work for accuracy.

Instruction in the use of memory aids (notebooks, diaries, personal digital assistants [PDAs],and internal memory strategies) is also supported by evidence [168-170]. Radomski and Davis (2008) described a training hierarchy that proceeds as follows: information retrieval (patient learns to find information in function-specific sections); basic planning (patient learns to use checklists to carry out daily and weekly planning routines that involve creating daily to-do lists); basic information entry (patient learns to record appointments, to-do's, lists in the correct sections of the planner or device as well as to take notes on step by step tasks); complex information entry (patient learns to take notes during conversations, meetings, classes); complex planning (patient learns project management techniques). Some people also benefit from learning to use alarm prompts for time-specific action items and/or internal memory strategies such as visual imagery and first-letter mnemonics [173], although such strategies are time- consuming to learn and effortful to employ.

Training in the use of problem solving and organization strategies as applied to real life tasks is also supported by evidence [170]. Here are some examples of strategies that, if effectively learned and employed, may help people circumvent difficulties with executive functions:

- establishing a routine for daily and weekly planning;
- breaking multi-step or complex tasks into step-by-step checklists;

- using a problem solving mnemonic to proactively and systematically think through many aspects of the problem before initiating action. (The IDEAL Problem Solver [174] outlines a five-step process – Identify the problem; Define the problem; Evaluate all possible solutions; Act; Look back.)

Finally, occupational therapists use a wide array of ongoing activities as opportunities to

help patients with MTBI become more aware of the influence of situational/environmental and strategy factors on their performance. While designed to improve self-awareness for patients with moderate to severe TBI, features of the Toglia-Kirk self awareness training model [175] may have utility in advancing self-reflection after MTBI. After receiving instruction to the task at hand, Service members are asked to restate their understanding of the task procedures; predict their performance; anticipate possible errors; select strategies that might avert the errors; perform the tasks; reflect on performance.

The following principles can be applied to any area of compensatory cognitive strategy training.

- Patients who are aware of their cognitive impairments or inefficiencies are most likely to benefit from compensatory strategy training [176]. People tend to be engaged in the training process if they expect that it will enable them to carry-out tasks of personal significance.

- The training process should involve both supervised rehearsal and real-life application. Sohlberg and Mateer [177] described a three phase approach that includes acquisition, application, and adaptation phases of training. During the acquisition phase, therapists teach patients how to carry-out the new strategy or technique. During the application phase, patients practice the new strategy while performing an array of therapy tasks. During the adaptation phase, individuals actually use the strategy to perform real-life activities of personal relevance.

- While therapists always individualize the cognitive compensatory strategies that are recommended to patients, the training process may be conducted within a one-on-one or group setting.

- The more abstract the cognitive strategy, the longer the training time needed [178]. Learning a concrete skill or routine (such as setting alarm prompts each morning to avoid missing medications) takes less training time than learning to use the IDEAL Problem Solver in one's daily life.

- Compensatory cognitive strategies are described to patients as cognitive energy saving techniques that buoy their everyday functioning as the symptoms of MTBI (which may derail information processing) continue to resolve. Patients are reminded that many people without MTBI use similar strategies to optimize their performance on a routine basis.

- The men and women who join the Armed Forces are conditioned to work in group environments. The feedback they receive from their comrades carries significant weight and may be a strong motivator. Therefore, therapy should take place in both 1:1 environments with the therapist and the Service member as well as in a small group milieu. The groups should be both topical (discussion based) and task oriented and use of group activities and materials should be presented in such a way as to challenge participants. Time for group process at the end of the session is essential for self-reflection and improving awareness of situational and environmental factors that impact their performance.

Recommendations (Practice Standards):

1) If Service members with MTBI report or demonstrate problems with attention and concentration during everyday activities, occupational therapists incorporate attention strategy training into their treatment plans. These strategies may be rehearsed in the context of computer or videogames, crafts, leisure activities, or work tasks. Homework assignments in which the Service member uses the strategy in personally-relevant activities are recommended as this may facilitate the generalization of newly-acquired skills and strategies [171].

2) If Service members with MTBI report or demonstrate problems with memory, occupational therapists incorporate compensatory memory training into their treatment plans. In general, Service members learn to routinely write notes about appointments and intended tasks in calendars or input the information into electronic devices such as PDAs rather than trying to remember the information. As above, homework assignments are provided so that Service members practice initiating notetaking or data entry and then use these prompts in the context of personal activities outside of the clinical setting.

3) If Service members with MTBI report or demonstrate difficulties with problem solving and organization, occupational therapists help them learn to use related compensatory strategies. Given the abstract nature of these strategies, therapists must provide ample opportunity for rehearsal and personal application (over a period of weeks).

4) Occupational therapists precede compensatory cognitive strategy training with an assessment of the Service member's central concerns and performance priorities as well as his or her preferences in terms of compensatory cognitive strategies (i.e., high tech versus low tech). Structured opportunities for self-reflection on performance (what went well, what to do differently next time) are woven into the training process.

Discussion: Occupational therapists within the DoD and VA system will best serve individuals with MTBI as they are familiar with an array of cognitive compensatory strategies and how to match those strategies to specific performance problems. DoD/VA clinicians might consider identifying a limited number of memory aids (notebook and electronic) that will be used with Service members for which formal training toolkits could then be developed.

Attention and Dual Task Performance Deficits

Assessment

Objective: To provide an assessment of how impairments of attention or cognitive deficits affect balance, walking or other mobility tasks in Service members with MTBI or concussion.

Practitioner: Physical therapist   (Occupational therapists as appropriate)
ICF components: Activity and Participation
Strength of recommendation: Practice Option
Rationale: A specific assessment tool for assessment of dual-task costs or a decrement of physical task performance resulting from cognitive deficits in persons with MTBI is not available. Recommendations of potential tools and formulas for calculating dual-task costs are found in [16].
Applicable level(s) of care: V-VIII (also part of a Combat Readiness Screen)

Background: Persons with concussion or MTBI frequently complain of imbalance, unsteady or slow walking, which may become even more pronounced when they attempt to do more than one task at a time. They may report a problem with speed and/or accuracy when they attempt simultaneous tasks. These complaints may begin immediately following a MTBI or concussion or may occur after a time delay.

Persons with traumatic brain injury and specifically with concussion have been shown to have a significantly slower gait speed and stability under dual task conditions [179,180]. For example, Parker et al. (2006) demonstrated significantly slower walking speeds and greater sway than controls, in subjects with concussion for up to 4 weeks post injury. Persons with brain injury, whether mild or moderate, have been anecdotally reported by physical therapists to show decrements in their balance function when their attention wanders during formal assessments of balance or gait such as with the *Berg Balance Scale* or the *Functional Gait Assessment.*

A comprehensive review of the issues related to the assessment and intervention for attention issues specifically in dual-task conditions has recently been published [16]. Suggestions are provided in this thorough review for assessment tools that are considered feasible in a population with acquired brain injury such as the *Walking and Remembering Test* [181]. The reader is referred to the McCulloch (2007) article for detailed information on available assessment tools and for formulas for calculating relative dual-task costs when combining mobility, cognitive and/or manual tasks.

There is a clear need for development of valid and reliable assessment tools to assess recovery and the effects of intervention of these common problems involving cognitive deficits affecting physical task performance after MTBI in order to establish definitive therapy assessment and treatment standards for both Service members and the civilian patient population.

Recommendations:

1) An assessment of dual-task performance is recommended. A specific and appropriate dual-task test that is clearly relevant for Service members with mild TBI cannot be recommended at this time. Some options are available. *The Functional Gait Assessment* is a clinical test of walking that contains items that require performance of more than one task such as walking while turning the head or walking around objects. Anecdotally, therapists report using a number of dual-task assessments such as the manual Timed Up and Go Test (TUG) which involves comparing time differences when a patient completes the TUG and the TUG while carrying a cup of water. *The Walking and Remembering Test* has been shown to be reliable and feasible in persons with acquired brain injury and can be considered for use.

2) Ideally, calculation of relative dual-task cost should be done. The therapist and the Service member should determine tasks that are relevant to the Service member. In order to determine dual-task costs, a baseline assessment (for example, walking time) is determined, and a cognitive task baseline is also obtained (for example serial 7 subtractions from 100 measured in time and number of errors). The relative dual-task cost is determined with a formula that takes into consideration the baseline performance (so that the patient's performance can be followed over time and can be compared to others) [16].

3) It is recommended that an effort be made to develop a dual-task assessment tool that is relevant to Service members, likely involving common soldiering tasks, and is feasible, valid, reliable and responsive to change so that it can be used to monitor natural recovery and response to therapeutic intervention.

Discussion: Therapists are encouraged to assess dual-task costs in Service members with mild TBI with a tool that fits their practice environment and the Service member's deficits. Cognitive issues during difficult physical tasks could seriously affect the Service member's safety and ability to carry out his/her duties or life tasks.

Intervention

Objectives: To provide interventions that involve a progression of task difficulty and that include dual tasks involving motor, manual and cognitive tasks for those Service members who demonstrate a decrement in motor or cognitive function in dual task conditions; to assist the Service member in improving his/her ability to perform everyday tasks in complex environments.

Practitioner: Physical therapist   (Occupational therapist as appropriate)
ICF components: Activity and Participation
Strength of recommendation: Practice Option
Rationale: A number of dual task training strategies have been employed with manipulation of the environment (closed versus open), task, and the instructional set for the subject. See McCulloch, 2007 for a comprehensive review of intervention approaches.
Applicable level(s) of care: V-VIII (also part of a Combat Readiness Screen)

Background: Balance during functional tasks is affected by attention. High-level mobility skills can be affected by shifting or dividing attention in persons with MTBI. A decrement in performance during tasks in complex environments that involve the interaction of attention and mobility would severely affect the safety of Service members in combat roles, driving, work and other environments.

In a case series involving older adults with balance deficits and issues with falling, Silsupadol et al. [182] describe that the adults were able to improve their balance under both single and dual task conditions, with improvements tending to be condition specific. That is, those subjects who trained under dual-task conditions showed greater improvement in dual-task assessment. This report describes a number of intervention strategies and tasks that can be used to train dual task skills [182]. A Defense and Veterans Brain Injury Center paper has described the design of an ongoing clinical trial that looks at two ways of approaching rehabilitation for persons with TBI and cognitive impairment. These approaches termed "cognitive-didactic" and "functional experiential" provide and attempt to understand the most effective treatment methods for persons with TBI and cognitive issues [183]. Again, McCulloch provides a comprehensive review of the issues related to intervention for attention issues specifically in dual-task conditions for persons with acquired brain injury [16].

Recommendations:

1) If Service members with MTBI demonstrate deficits in dual-task conditions, interventions should include tasks in progressively more complex environments and progressively more difficult multi-tasking conditions.   For example, the therapist may begin with simple interventions such as walking while carrying a cup of water in a quiet environment and progress to packing and carrying a rucksack through rough terrain while looking for specific items or signs.

2) Recreational sport activities often involve multiple task performance while maintaining a Service member's attention and motivation.   Common military tasks required of Service members also often involve multiple task performance with accuracy and speed and would be relevant and motivating to the Service member. Incorporation of these types of dual tasks as therapeutic interventions is recommended.

3) There is a need for well-designed randomized controlled trials in the treatment of these common problems of cognitive deficits affecting physical task performance after MTBI in order to establish definitive physical therapy assessment and treatment standards for both Service members and the civilian patient population.

Discussion: Therapists are encouraged to design individualized intervention strategies for Service members with deficits in dual-task conditions that begin with simple interventions and move to more complex tasks as appropriate. Tasks that are relevant to the Service member are encouraged. Again, "cost" or decrement in skill level or time to complete a task when two or more tasks are done simultaneously, should be monitored in order to assess recovery and the effect of intervention.

Performance of Self-Management, Work, and Social Roles

Assessment

Objective: Identify the Service member's concerns about and specify any barriers to his or her performance of life roles.

> Practitioner: Occupational therapist
> ICF Component(s): Activity, Participation
> Strength of recommendation: Practice Options
> Rationale: Existing guidelines provide little guidance as to the optimal timing or composition of life role assessment after MTBI
> Applicable level(s) of care: III (Combat Stress Unit), IV, V, VI, VII, VIII

Background: Trombly [184,185] characterized three domains of personal roles that are essential to being in control of one's life: self-maintenance roles, self-advancement roles, and self-enhancement roles. Self-maintenance roles pertain to the maintenance of oneself and care of the family and home, comprising basic activities of daily living (BADL) (e.g. dressing, grooming, eating) and instrumental activities of daily living (IADL) (e.g., meal preparation, household tasks, bill paying) [186]. Self-advancement roles have to do with education and work-related tasks while self-advancement roles are associated with leisure and social participation [186].

Self-management roles after MTBI

While most people recover from concussion/MTBI within three months of injury [40], some experience symptoms that interfere with performance of life roles. For example, people who sustain a MTBI without other concomitant injuries or conditions typically do not experience disability related to performance of highly-automatic basic self-care tasks. That is, they retain their ability to independently put on their clothing, feed, and bathe themselves, albeit with greater concentration and effort [47]. However, the efficiency of performance may suffer because of difficulties with attention/concentration, decision-making, and disruption in his or her daily routine. After MTBI people may experience errors and inefficiencies during IADL because these tasks tend to involve less automatization, more steps, and therefore, place greater demands on higher order thinking abilities (planning, prioritizing, self-monitoring)[187].

Similarly, some Service members report difficulties resuming personal roles after deployment, especially those with polytrauma [188]. In Resnik and Allen's qualitative study, researchers conducted semi-structured interviews with 14 injured veterans. The veterans (some polytrauma that included MTBI and others had orthopedic injuries) described difficulty initiating self-care tasks (even though they were able to perform the tasks) along with challenges in health maintenance. For example, they reported challenges taking medications as prescribed, not keeping medical appointments, changes in health habits including weight gain.

Work and social roles after MTBI

As discussed in the previous sections, some people with MTBI are not able to resume life roles that are important to their independence and full participation in social and community roles. In their long term follow-up study of Vietnam veterans, Vanderploeg and colleagues found that compared to uninjured controls, those with self-reported MTBI had increased likelihood of depression and poorer psychosocial outcomes including under-employment and marital problems [189]. Therefore, occupational and physical therapists aim to identify possible concerns regarding work, social relationships, transportation, and leisure during early stages of recovery and at any time in life long care in order to provide therapy intervention and optimize Service members' functioning in these realms.

Successful return to work and school is often a priority and concern of Service members who are returning from OEF/OIF and have sustained a MTBI. Although little research has been conducted in the area of MTBI and post-secondary education, challenges have been observed. These include difficulty with information processing, memory, problem solving, and visual-spatial ability [190], all skills necessary for success in the classroom and at work. These issues may not emerge until Service members face the novel challenges and multi-tasking demands of the work or education environments. Difficulty may indicate the need for a comprehensive occupational therapy evaluation as well as specialized vocational and educational assessments.

The ability to return to many of life roles and occupations (including work or school) depends on access to transportation and for most people that means driving. Driving is one of the predictors of life satisfaction with individuals with brain injury [58] and it is an area of concern for many returning Service members. Service members returning from OEF/OIF have been driving in combat zone conditions which require aggressive, fast driving often on sidewalks and down small alleys; these skills do not translate to safe driving on the roads of Chicago, or rural Texas. Returning veterans have reported panic attacks and hypervigilence that cause them to be overly aggressive during driving [188]. In fact, driving behaviors of Service members at home on leave, or home after multiple deployments, is dangerous when compared with those that did not serve in a combat zone (E. Stern, personal communication on December 11, 2007). In addition, MTBI-related symptoms can impact driving performance including visual disturbances, attention, decreased frustration tolerance, memory and executive functioning deficits, vertigo, seizures, and fatigue. Therefore, driving evaluations, pre-screens, simulator, as well as on-the-road evaluation may be indicated for returning Service members with MTBI.

Family functioning is often a primary concern after MTBI. Testa et al. (2006) reported issues of somatic complaints, memory and attention deficits, communication difficulties, and episodes of aggression being issues for family life one year after injury. High stimulations levels associated with busy households and the demands for multi-tasking make it difficult for some Service members to easily resume parenting responsibilities [188]. For some Service members, problems with anger, irritability, depression, and/or anxiety creates a climate in the household that prevents family members from doing things together [188]. Furthermore, post-deployment roles of family members change as those on the home front become responsible for household tasks that were typically delegated to the spouse. Family wellbeing, happiness of couples, and relationships can be impacted by MTBI [191-193], PTSD, and/or post-deployment readjustment to home life. As with problems in other life roles, once identified, occupational therapy intervention may be beneficial.

Performance of life roles are assessed through structured observation and self-report. While some researchers question the validity of self-report measures, formal and informal inquiries as to those issues that most concern the patient will most certainly optimize his or her engagement in the therapy process and adherence to therapy recommendations [194].

- The *Canadian Occupational Performance* Measure (COPM) is a semi-structured interview that provides the therapist with information about the tasks that the patient most wants and needs to do [195,196]. Patients rate their skill level and their degree of satisfaction with their performance of tasks that are important to them. The COPM has construct and criterion validity [197] as well as good to strong inter-rater reliability [198]. It was used to organize treatment and for outcomes measurement in two studies involving outpatients with mild to moderate TBI who received occupational therapy [199,200]. However, the COPM may not be useful in planning care for individuals with severe TBI who tend to be less aware of deficits [199]. The COPM is a Practice Standard for overall assessment of role performance and satisfaction.

Here are other assessment options specific to the performance of various life roles.

- The *Occupational Self Assessment Version* 2.2 (OSA) is somewhat more structured approach to identifying the patient's primary concerns and priorities [201]. Rather than asking the patient to generate a list of his or her concerns within broad categories of self-care, productivity, and leisure, the OSA is comprised of 21 statements regarding functioning ("concentrating on tasks", "taking care of myself", "expressing myself to others", "having a satisfying routine"). First, the patient rates his or her competency specific to each statement and then rates how important the area is. Finally, the patient chooses up to 4 areas/statements that he or she would like to change, which inform the treatment plan. Kielhofner and colleagues [202] found that the OSA can be used as a valid, sensitive, and reliable measure of occupational competence and preferences.

- Asking a patient to provide an hour-by-hour detailing of his or her typical day is another way to identify problem areas that may be helped by therapy, especially for outpatients [203]. It also catalyzes patient-therapist conversations about how the individual spends his or her time and satisfaction levels with daily activities. Patients who describe no semblance of routine may benefit from habit re-instatement (re-establishing patterns of everyday activities so they become increasingly automatic, accurate and effortless).

- The *Epworth Sleepiness Scale* (ESS) [204] is a self-administered, 8-item questionnaire to measure daytime sleepiness in adults. The total ESS score provides an estimate of a person's sleepiness in daily life but does not specify what factors contribute to sleepiness or diagnose specific conditions.

- The *Fatigue Severity Scale* (FSS) [205] is designed to measure the impact of fatigue on a person and may be useful when Service members indicate that fatigue is a barrier to their performance of everyday tasks. The FSS has good psychometric properties and detects change over time [206].

- The *Assessment of Communication and Interaction Skills* [207] is a structured observation rating scale that explores the interaction of an individual during occupational engagement or in a group setting. It may be a helpful inclusion in occupational therapy evaluation when the patient or others indicate that communication and social functioning interfere with task performance.

- The *Activity Co-engagement Self-Assessment* (ACeS) [208] is a self-report tool designed to help the occupational therapist better understand the patient's engagement in activities with loved ones including types of activities performed together, potential barriers to activity engagement; perceived self-characteristics as related to engaging in activities with others.

Respondents may specify the relationship at issue (with children, spouse/significant other, or friends/siblings).

- The *Dyadic Adjustment Scale*(DAS) [209] is a standardized 32-question self-report questionnaire exploring adjustments in partner relationships. It is administered via paper-pencil or interview to married or partnered couples to gain understanding of activity engagement and social roles.

- Return to duty/work performance may occur via structure observation of task performance.

- *Drivers screening and testing* - In preliminary studies of driver evaluation outcomes, one of the best predictors of safe driving is the report of general driving performance from family members (D. Warden personal communication, April, 2003). However, there are currently no standardized pre-driving screens or driving screening for individuals post MTBI at this time. The pre-driving screenings typically contain components of motor skills, reaction time, visual screening and cognition. Driver simulators are used to evaluate safe return to the road as well as reaction time, visual attention, and general driving skill even before patients demonstrate competence for on-the-road driving. Evaluation of skills needed for driving should be completed by occupational therapists because of their expertise in understanding impact of impairment on activity performance. On-the-road assessments are also completed by a therapist with specialized knowledge and training. The VA has a comprehensive initiative for returning our veterans to the road and detailed information can be found at the following URL:
http://www1.va.gov/vhapublications/ViewPublication.asp?pub_ID=435

Finally, in order to proceed to plan intervention, the findings from above-mentioned assessment should be further informed by other assessment data specific to the Service member's cognitive, physical, and emotional status.

Recommendations:

1) Occupational therapists use a combination of interview and observational methods to assess competence in self-maintenance roles.

2) Occupational therapists directly observe the Service member's performance in key ADL and IADL, if at all possible, noting level of independence/competence as well as qualitative aspects of performance (i.e., number of reminders or redirections required; response to visual or auditory distractions; ability to self-monitor; speed and efficiency of performance; ability to multi-task; response to feedback; initiation of compensatory techniques; evidence of planning and/or strategy use versus trial and error approach) as per the earlier discussion of a dynamic assessment.

3) If it is not possible to directly observe the Service member's performance on a given self-maintenance activity, the therapist solicits input from the Service member's family regarding their observations.

4) Occupational therapists ask Service members with MTBI who are outpatients to describe their "typical day" and also ask specific questions about sleep-wake hygiene (i.e., presence and nature of wind down routine), especially if the Service member is having problems with sleep and rest.

Discussion: Because there are few standardized methods for assessing ompetence/independence in self-maintenance tasks after MTBI, observation of functional performance, particularly the qualitative aspects of performance, become of central importance. Worksheets/tools with operational definitions of various qualitative aspects of performance would likely help therapists use a consistent rubric for objectifying and interpreting observations of functional performance. Tools of this nature could improve the sophistication of observational skills for clinicians who are relatively unfamiliar with the functional manifestations of cognitive impairments and inefficiencies that often accompany MTBI.

Intervention

Objective: Provide intervention that optimizes the Service member's competence, efficiency, and self-confidence in performing life roles after MTBI.

> Practitioner: Occupational therapist
> ICF component(s): Activity and Participation
> Strength of recommendation: Practice Option
> Rationale: Existing guidelines provide little guidance as to the optimal timing or composition of intervention specific to life roles after MTBI
> Applicable level(s) of care: III (Combat Stress Unit), IV, V, VI, VII, VIII

Background: There is little empirical literature that specifies intervention to enable the patient with MTBI to quickly and fully return to his or her self-maintenance roles. In general, patients with MTBI who are seen in the Emergency Department are told to return to their everyday activities (non-jarring, non-contact) as they feel able to do so [210]. One could correctly assume that this includes resuming activities associated with life roles.

As previously mentioned in the assessment discussion, unless the individual experiences other concomitant injuries or conditions, MTBI in and of itself typically does not impact a person's ability to perform self-care activities. MTBI-symptoms (such as dizziness, headache, or vision changes) may distract the patient during these typically mundane activities, making the individual less efficient and more error-prone. Intervention, then, focuses on helping the individual understand the impact of potentially-transient MTBI sequelae on performance so that he or she does not erroneously misattribute performance inefficiencies to brain damage and thereby suffer further assaults to self-confidence and helping the patient figure out ways to perform everyday activities despite these issues.

Intervention associated with self-management roles

Patients may also benefit from help to reboot various aspects of her or her daily self-care habits and routines. Patients with MTBI are vulnerable to habit disruption because related symptoms may at least temporarily prevent them from carrying out previously routinized everyday activities in the manner most familiar to them. As a result, patients find themselves having to think through and organize each step of many self-maintenance tasks, increasing the energy demands and decreasing the performance efficiency on relatively mundane tasks [211].

Patients may realize improvements in their efficiency and accuracy as they re-establish a consistent sequence of task performance which, with enough repetition, will once again become automatic [212]. Giles [213] recommended performing a task analysis on a potentially disrupted habit sequence and then with the patient, deciding on an optimal chain of steps [214]. These steps are recorded on a checklist so that the individual does not have to rely on memory/recall in order to correctly adhere to the sequence each time the task is performed. Therapists reinforce the everyday use of the checklist past the point of competence to that of overlearning [215] so that over time, performance of one step prompts the patient to initiate the next step on an automatic basis [216]. In the meantime, patients find themselves more successfully able to carry-out everyday tasks despite the presence of distracting MTBI symptoms. Checklists to re-establish automatic routines may prove beneficial for a variety of self-maintenance activities that are typically performed with a consistent sequence of steps including: morning self-care activities (grooming, bathing, dressing sequence); pre-sleep wind-down (to promote improved sleep-wake hygiene); leaving the house/office/barracks (to ensure that the individual has what he or she needs to take with, has turned off lights and locked the doors).

IADLs that comprise self-maintenance roles tend to involve more problem solving than routinization. Therefore, therapists help patients design and employ compensatory cognitive strategies that lessen the demands of IADLs (see the discussion of Cognitive Interventions).

For example, prompts to initiate various household or work tasks might be incorporated into a weekly planning procedure involving a memory aid. For unstructured multi-step home repair projects, the patient can be taught to use a project planning technique such as the IDEAL Problem Solver to break the task into a sequence of steps before beginning work. Intervention may also involve teaching patients new strategies to improve financial management including the following:

- Service members learn/re-learn basic math skills necessary for personal finance tasks;

- Service members establish routines for bill paying, bank account management and organizational systems to maintain personal paperwork;

- Service members and spouses learn to set-up cooperative systems for money management.

Intervention associated with work, social, leisure roles

As with resumption of personal roles, there is relatively little empirical literature that specifies intervention and outcomes associated with occupational therapy and community re-entry after MTBI. However, Trombly et al. (2002) reported that individualized outpatient OT contributed to goal achievement for persons with mild to moderate TBI; many of those goals pertained to resumption of work, social, leisure, and parenting roles. Occupational therapy to improve study and job skills for persons with mental health concerns [217] may be similarly beneficial to those with MTBI.

In general, occupational therapists use assessment data (related to specific community re-entry concerns and current cognitive, physical, and emotional status) to inform the intervention plan. The following examples typify occupational therapy intervention specific to community re-entry and lifelong care. Note that intervention may occur in one-on-one or group formats and take place in the clinical or community settings.

Occupational therapy for return to work or school:

- Service members learn to use compensatory cognitive strategies to improve task follow-through, task planning, recall of verbal or written information, how to optimize performance by minimizing distracting variables. See the Cognition section of the *Guidance*.

- Service members establish habits and routines for frequently-performed work tasks to improve efficiency (such as the series of tasks that take place at the beginning or end of each day.) See discussion of habit formation in the Performance of Self-Maintenance Roles section of the *Guidance*.

- Service members establish personal habits and routines that maximize their accuracy and efficiency in getting to work and/or school on time. See discussion of habit formation in the Performance of Self-Maintenance Roles section of the *Guidance*.

- Service members learn how to request and employ feedback from superiors and co-workers.

Occupational therapy for driving and transportation

- Occupational therapists may intervene to improve driving if there are no other concerns that would prevent legal driving in the Service member's home state. Some of these medical issues may include presence of a seizure disorder, significant visual impairment, vertigo, and anger management issues.

- Intervention involves remediation of deficits such as activities specifically designed to improve reaction time, visual scanning, attention, range of motion, as well as adaptive strategies. The latter include adaptations to the vehicle for easy reaching, only driving during the day, driving with another in the car, or restricted highway driving.

- Driving simulation may be used to desensitize Service members to anxiety-provoking elements of driving situations as well as to promote self-awareness of driving safety issues.

Occupational therapy for leisure

- Service members learn new leisure outlets to replace those they are no longer able to perform.

- Service members learn cognitive, communication, coping, and pacing strategies that enable them to engage in leisure activities with family members.

- Service members learn planning strategies that enables them to consistently schedule time for leisure by themselves or with others and to budget resources for these stress-relieving activities.

Occupational therapy for family and social relationships

- Service members learn pacing/fatigue management, communication, and/or planning strategies to enable them to routinely engage in activities with family or friends.

- Service members acquire new household or parenting skills to optimize their engagement in family roles.

- Service members and spouses learn and employ information management systems (calendars, bulletin boards, etc.) to improve communication and planning.

Occupational therapy for health and wellness

- Service members learn to identify and modify situational factors that are linked to alcohol use or abuse and smoking.

- Service members learn to compensatory cognitive strategies to routinely perform daily exercise to prevent weight gain and other consequences of a sedentary lifestyle.

Recommendations:

1) Service members' input regarding tasks of personal importance and self-report of performance status should be important drivers of the intervention plan, especially when the Service member is an outpatient who has had exposure to real-life challenges after MTBI.

2) Occupational therapists should facilitate the early resumption of ADLs by helping the Service member to identify the conditions under which he or she is most successfully able to perform the tasks and/or by setting up a checklist to promote the reinstatement of related habit sequences.

3) To that end, occupational therapists help Service members with MTBI learn to use individualized compensatory cognitive strategies that will enable them to successfully resume self-maintenance roles.

4) The therapist may also consider working with the employer to suggest modifications for environment, length of day, and changes to duties. Education to both the employee and the employer reduce attrition levels [218]. The occupational therapist should would closely with the vocational counselors to insure adopted strategies and modifications facilitate successful employment.

5) Interventions aimed at helping the Service member or veteran return to school should emphasize cognitive skills training, pacing, insight, stress reduction strategies, and load reduction. Acquisition of cognitive compensatory strategies (discussed earlier in the *Guidance*) may also be important for return to school success. Educators and University administrators must be educated on the significance of MTBI on the performance of their students.

6) If Service members or veterans describe difficulties resuming roles within their families, OT intervention should include activity-based family group work like cooking or use of games. Videotaping and discussion post-activity can provide insight into elements of the task that were problematic. These types of activities can be done with spouses and veteran, with child and veteran or with the family. Activities should take place in multiple contexts to offer opportunity for generalization of skills. It is further recommended that group work be done with groups of families. Feedback from peers, especially in the military culture, may carry greater weight than from a therapist.

7) Activities such as role playing, skills training, and education regarding communication may also be beneficial in the area of family roles and associated occupations.

8) Intervention regarding driving should be client-specific involving remediation of driving-related subskills and/or provision of adaptive strategies. Recommendations should be made in conjunction with a driving rehabilitation specialist, if such a resource is available within the setting.

9) If the Service member is concerned about leisure or finances, incorporate skill-building specific to these areas into the OT intervention plan.

10) Health and wellness should be addressed though education seminars, individual coaching, leisure coaching, and nutritional supports.

11) Use of a buddy system and incorporation of physical fitness program will assist with many of the issues associated with health and wellness.

Discussion: Service members with MTBI run the risk of trivializing the importance of resuming self-maintenance activities. Therefore, it is important that occupational therapists frame the resumption of self-maintenances activities (ADL and IADL) as work hardening activities that are important prerequisites for return to duty, work, or education.

The concept of habit formation and reinstatement may have expanded importance for soldiers receiving rehabilitation as outpatients in the Warrior Transition Units. With larger blocks of unstructured time, Service members with MTBI would likely benefit from occupational therapy intervention aimed at structuring daily routines around balanced and therapeutic use of self-care, work, and leisure activities in ways that are both satisfying and advance recovery. Research about the effectiveness of such interventions is needed.

Participation in Exercise

Assessment

Objective: To identify the frequency and duration of the Service member's participation in aerobic and strengthening exercise; to determine the Service member's ability to monitor his/her response to exercise using heart rate or Rate of Perceived Exertion Scale, or for the Service member to determine the intensity of exercise using a metabolic equivalent (MET) table.

Practitioner: Physical therapist (or Occupational therapist if PT not available)
ICF component: Activity and Participation
Strength of recommendation: Practice Option
Rationale: No specific information has been located that specifies the type of self-monitoring during exercise that is the easiest to use for persons with MTBI. The American Heart Association website includes information for determining target heart rate (www.americanheart.org).
Applicable level(s) of care: VII, VIII (also V, VI at therapist's discretion)

Background: The American College of Sports Medicine and the American Heart Association have published updated guidelines on the frequency and duration of exercise for all healthy adults [219]. There are a number of ways to determine the intensity of exercise. These include such measures as heart rate, rate of perceived exertion, and metabolic equivalents. Target heart rate zones may be calculated in many ways. One means to monitor exercise intensity is to use the guideline of 50-85% of age-predicted maximum heart rate as the target zone for exercise (see the American Heart Association's website information on target heart rates). Other means to measure exercise intensity may be more accurate for various individuals and the reader is referred to sports medicine literature for further information on recommendations for this.

The *Rate of Perceived Exertion Scale* (RPE) uses a subjective numeric rating (range 6-19) of exercise intensity based on how a subject feels in relation to level of fatigue. For example, RPE of 13 or 14 (exercise that feels "somewhat hard") coincides with an exercise heart rate of about 70% maximum. The Haskell et al. guideline [219] provides a table using metabolic equivalent (MET) level to classify common physical activities as light, moderate or vigorous in intensity.

Graded exercise testing of persons after moderate to severe traumatic brain injury has been shown to be reliable for both submaximal and peak exercise testing [220]. Information on this level of exercise testing was not found for persons with MTBI. At this point formal exercise testing does not appear to be necessary for Service members who are otherwise able to monitor their exercise intensity and response.

Recommendations:

1) Therapists use an oral or written question format that asks the Service member's current participation in aerobic and strengthening exercises, including specifically the frequency and duration of their participation. This can be a simple question and answer or take the form of a survey or questionnaire using a Likert-type scale.

2) Therapists determine if Service members can accurately take their own resting heart rate and also determine their heart rate following an exercise bout.

or

3) Therapists determine if Service members can accurately use the Rate of Perceived Exertion Scale to determine their perception of exercise intensity.

Discussion: Physical therapists within the DOD and VA systems should choose the type of exercise monitoring system that fits their practice setting and knowledge base as well as the easiest system for the particular Service member to learn and provide instruction in that monitoring system.

Intervention

Objective: To provide the Service member with recommendations and support for lifetime participation in fitness activities to enhance their well-being and to potentially improve cognitive status.

Practitioner: Physical therapist (or Occupational therapist if PT not available)
ICF components: Activity and Participation
Strength of recommendation: Practice Standard
Rationale: All healthy adults aged 18 to 65 yr need moderate-intensity aerobic physical activity for a minimum of 30 minutes on 5 days each week and activities to increase muscular strength and endurance for a minimum of two days each week. (Haskell et al., 2007;ACSM and AHA Guidelines). Exercise may improve mood and aspects of health status in individuals with TBI [22].
Applicable level(s) of care: VII, VIII (also V, VI at therapist's discretion)

Background: As discussed above, the American College of Sports Medicine and the American Heart Association have published updated guidelines on the frequency and duration of exercise for all healthy adults [219]. These guidelines are specifically that: "All healthy adults ages 18 to 65 years need moderate-intensity aerobic physical activity for at least 30 minutes on 5 days each week or vigorous-intensity aerobic physical activity for at least 20 minutes on 3 days each week" (p. 1423). Additionally, recommendations are made for healthy adults to participate in activities that increase muscular strength and endurance in order to promote and maintain good health and physical independence. A thorough review of the guidelines and the various combinations of exercises that meet these recommendations are found in the special report by Haskell et al. (2007).

Physical activity has been shown to improve quality of life and other factors in older adults [221] and persons with traumatic brain injury [22]. In a retrospective review, Gordon et al. (1998) examined the benefits of exercise in a community-based sample of persons with traumatic brain injury compared to persons without disabilities. The findings of this review indicated that the persons with TBI who were exercisers reported less depression, fewer symptoms and a better self-reported health status than the non-exercising individuals with TBI. Gordon's group has developed a "TBI Consumer Report" that is available on their website (www.mssm.edu/tbinet/resources/publications/tbi_consumer_reports.shtml#issue2) which can be used to provide education about exercise following TBI. Persons with traumatic brain injury have been shown to improve their cardio-respiratory fitness after a 12-week circuit-training program although they did not show any significant reductions in percent body fat [222].

Physical activity that resulted in increased cardiovascular fitness may improve cognitive status, including attentional control in older adults [223] as well as learning and memory [224]. In animal studies, voluntary exercise after traumatic brain injury resulted in an upregulation of brain-derived neurotrophic factor (BDNF) when it was implemented at an appropriate time [67]. This BDNF can improve cortical plasticity, neuronal survival and growth, all factors that are important in cognitive enhancement. Studies are beginning that are investigating the effect of aerobic exercise on cognition and brain activity following traumatic brain injury in humans (J. Lojovich, personal communication, 12/18/07 dissertation proposal University of Minnesota). Given the enhancement in cognitive performance in the animal model and older adults, it would be expected that participation in a consistent aerobic exercise program could enhance the cognitive status of Service members with MTBI cognitive symptoms that haven't resolved.

Certainly, a screening of health risk factors prior to beginning or resuming an exercise or fitness routine is important in the general public and in Service members with MTBI [225]. As appropriate to other populations, Service members with risk factors should be referred for medical clearance before beginning an exercise program. It is noted that the ACSM and the AHA have made a companion recommendation to the one for adults, specifically applied to adults age 65 and older, and adults age 50-64 with chronic conditions or physical functional limitations that affect movement ability or physical fitness [226]. The American Physical Therapy Association (APTA) has developed a web-based resource called the APTA's Physical Fitness for Special Populations (PFSP) web resource that provides information on participation in fitness activities for persons with disabilities. As yet this resource does not provide specific information for persons with traumatic brain injury although it does have recommendations for persons post stroke and other disabilities.

Recommendations:

1) Physical therapists provide instruction to the Service member on the frequency and duration of aerobic and strengthening exercise based on the updated physical activity guidelines recently released by the American College of Sports Medicine (ACSM) and the American Heart Association while recognizing any person-specific limitations or residual MTBI-related symptoms.

2) Therapists provide instruction on the rationale for lifetime exercise to the Service member including information on wellness, alleviation of co-morbidities, etc.

3) Therapists provide suggestions and/or specific means for Service member to monitor their own exercise frequency, duration and exercise response including a log or calendar.

4) Therapists provide training in self-monitoring techniques such as heart rate and/or exertion. They consider teaching Service members to use the Rate of Perceived Exertion Scale to allow the Service members to determine their exercise intensity and tolerance or provide information on MET levels of specific types of exercise.

Discussion: Exercise is important for all adults to maintain health status and well-being. It may be additionally important for Service members with deficits following MTBI to reduce co-morbidities and potentially enhance cognitive status. Therapists should screen for factors that may affect exercise prescription for the Service member. Tolerance to activity and symptoms such as increased dizziness should be monitored and appropriate adjustments made to an exercise program per individual Service member's needs and presentation. Structured exercise programs may be important elements to build into the regimen of Warrior Transition Units.

Outcome Assessment-Participation

Objective: To identify long term outcomes and participation or restriction of participation issues in Service members and veterans who have sustained a MTBI during active service in the OEF/OIF campaigns.

> Practitioner: Physical Therapist or Occupational Therapist
> ICF component: Participation
> Strength of recommendation: Practice Option
> Rationale: Long-term outcomes measuring participation provide information on individual patient and program evaluation outcomes. No recommendation for a specific evaluation of participation is made at this time.
> Applicable level(s) of care: Level VIII

Background: As paraphrased by Resnik and Allen [188], participation (from an ICF perspective) has to do with the extent to which an individual takes part in the life areas or situations of his or her own choosing and do so in a manner that is expected of a person without restrictions. Both occupational and physical therapy view participation as an overarching outcome of intervention.

A number of outcome measures designed to assess outcome or participation in persons following brain injury are available. These include both generic and disease-specific type outcomes. The Center for Outcome Measurement in Brain Injury (http://www.tbims.org/combi, accessed December 30, 2007) describes measurement tools for all levels of the International Classification of Functioning (ICF) Model for persons with moderate to severe traumatic brain injury. For example, *The Mayo-Portland Adaptability Inventory* (MPAI) was primarily designed to "…assist in the clinical evaluation of people during the postacute (post-hospital) period following acquired brain injury (ABI), and to assist in the evaluation of rehabilitation programs designed to serve these people" (COMBI website). The *Participation Objective, Participation Subjective* (POPS) was developed in 2004 at Mount Sinai School of Medicine, New York NY. This instrument consists of a list of 26 elements of participation (e.g., going to the movies, housework, opportunities to meet new people). Another instrument used to assess participation is the *Community Integration Questionnaire* which looks at long- term community participation outcomes in persons with brain injury [227]. However, use of these instruments to measure participation after MTBI has not been established.

As an example of a generic outcome measure, the *SF-36 Health Survey* was developed for the Medical Outcomes Study and its psychometric properties extensively evaluated. This short-form was constructed to survey health status and was designed for use in clinical practice, research, health policy evaluations and general population surveys [228]. A version of the SF-36 is available to assess health outcomes for veterans [229,230]. Given the need to consider their health status over the prior 4 weeks, memory impairment in a Service member with concussion/mTBI may hinder their ability to answer the questions appropriately. There is a 1-week acute version of the SF-36 with requires recall of health status over the preceding 1 week only.

Recommendations:

1) A participation level outcome measure should be given to Service members and veterans to monitor their individual situations and to allow evaluation of programs designed to serve these individuals.

2) Further work needs to be done to identify appropriate participation level outcome measures for this DOD-VA population with mild traumatic brain injury.

Discussion: Extensive information on outcome measures in persons with brain injury can be obtained from *The Center for Outcome Measurement in Brain Injury.* http://www.tbims.org/combi (accessed December 30, 2007). A group should be tasked to identify the optimal measurement strategy for program evaluation and long term management of Service members with MTBI.

REFERENCES

1. Herdman SJ, Schubert MC, Das VE, Tusa RJ. Recovery of dynamic visual acuity in unilateral vestibular hypofunction. *Archives of Otolaryngology--Head & Neck Surgery.* 2003;129(8):819-824.

2. Wolf JS, Boyev KP, Manokey BJ, Mattox DE. Success of the modified Epley maneuver in treating benign paroxysmal positional vertigo. *The Laryngoscope.* 1998;109(6):900-903.

3. McNeely ML, Armijo Olivo S, Magee DJ. A systematic review of the effectiveness of physical therapy interventions for temporomandibular disorders. *Physical therapy.* May 2006;86(5):710-725.

4. Medlicott MS, Harris SR. A systematic review of the effectiveness of exercise, manual therapy, electrotherapy, relaxation training, and biofeedback in the management of temporomandibular disorder. *Physical therapy.* 2006;86(7):955-973.

5. Scrivani SJ, Keith DA, Kaban LB. Temporomandibular disorders. *New England Journal of Medicine.* 2008;359(25):2693-2705.

6. Truelove E, Huggins KH, Mancl L, Dworkin SF. The efficacy of traditional, low-cost and nonsplint therapies for temporomandibular disorder: A randomized controlled trial. *Journal of the American Dental Association.* 2006;137(8):137, 1099-1107.

7. Defense and Veterans Brain Injury Center. DVBIC working group on the acute management of mild traumatic brain injury in military operational settings: Clinical practice guideline and recommendations. Silver Springs, MD2006.

8. Defense and Veterans Brain Injury Center. Clinical Guidance for Evaluation and Management of Concussion/mTBI - Acute/Subacute (CONUS)2008.

9. McCrory P, Johnston K, Meeuwisse W, et al. Summary and agreement statement of the 2nd International Conference on Concussion in sport. *British Journal of Sports Medicine.* 2005;39:196-204.

10. Herdman SJ. *Vestibular Rehabilitation.* Vol 3. Philadelphia: FA Davis Company; 2007.

11. Kaufman KR, Brey RH, Chou LS, Rabatin A, Brown AW, Basford JR. Comparison of subjective and objective measurements of balance disorders following traumatic brain injury. *Medical Engineering & Physics.* 2006;28(3):234-239.

12. Zasler ND, Katz DI, Zafonte RD. *Brain Injury Medicine Principles and Practice.* Vol 1. New York: Demos Medical Publishing; 2007.

13. Bhattacharyya N, Baugh RF, Orvidas L, et al. Clinical practice guideline: Benign paroxysmal positional vertigo. *Otolaryngology - Head and Neck Surgery.* 2008;139:S47-S81.

14. Herdman SJ, Hall CD, Schubert MC, Das VE, Tusa RJ. Recovery of dynamic visual acuity in bilateral vestibular hypofunction. *Arch Otolaryngol Head Neck Surg.* Apr 2007;133(4):383-389.

15. Whitney SL, Wrisley DM, Marchetti GF, Gee MA, Redfern MS, Furman JM. Clinical measurement of sit-to-stand performance in people with balance disorders: validity of data for the Five-Times-Sit-to-Stand Test. *Physical therapy.* Oct 2005;85(10):1034-1045.

16. McCulloch K. Attention and dual-task conditions: physical therapy implications for individuals with acquired brain injury. *Journal of Neurologic Physical Therapy.* 2007;31(3):104-118.

17. Biondi DM. Physical treatments for headache: a structured review. *Headache.* 2005;45(6):738-746.

18. Peloso PM, Carroll LJ, Cassidy JD, et al. Critical evaluation of the existing guidelines on mild traumatic brain injury. *Journal of Rehabilitation Medicine : Official Journal of the UEMS European Board of Physical and Rehabilitation Medicine.* 2004(43):106-112.

19. Gottshall K, Drake A, Gray N, McDonald E, Hoffer ME. Objective vestibular tests as outcome measures in head injury patients. *The Laryngoscope.* 2003;113(10):1746-1750.

20. Ohrbach R, Granger C, List T, Dworkin S. Preliminary development and validation of the Jaw Functional Limitation Scale. *Community Dentistry and Oral Epidemiology.* 2008;36(3):228-236.

21. Gottshall KR, Moore RJ, Hoffer ME. Vestibular rehabilitation for migraine-associated dizziness. *International Tinnitus Journal.* 2005;11(1):81-84.

22. Gordon WA, Sliwinski M, Echo J, McLoughlin M, Sheerer MS, Meili TE. The benefits of exercise in individuals with traumatic brain injury: a retrospective study. *Journal of Head Trauma Rehabilitation.* 1998;13(4):58-67.

23. Hoffer ME, Gottshall KR, Moore R, Balough BJ, Wester D. Characterizing and treating dizziness after mild head trauma. *Otology & Neurotology.* 2004;25(2):135-138.

24. Bijur PE, Silver W, Gallagher EJ. Reliability of the Visual Analog Scale for measurement of acute pain. *Academy of Emergency Medicine.* 2001;8:1153-1157.

25. Huskisson EC. Measurement of pain. *Lancet.* 1974;2(7889):1127-1131.

26. Cleland JA, Fritz JM, Whitman JM, Palmer JA. The reliability and construct validity of the Neck Disability Index and patient specific functional scale in patients with cervical radiculopathy. *Spine.* 2006;31(5):598-602.

27. MacDermid JC, Walton DM, Avery S, et al. Measurement properties of the neck disability index: a systematic review. *Journal of Orthopaedic and Sports Physical Therapy.* 2009;39(5):400-417.

28. Ohrbach R, Larsson P, List T. The Jaw Functional Limitation Scale: Development, reliability, and validity of 8-item and 20-item versions. *Journal of Orofacial Pain.* 2008;22(3):219-230.

29. Pehling J, Schiffman E, Look J, Shaefer J, Lenton P, Fricton J. Interexaminer reliability and clinical validity of the Temporomandibular Index: A new outcome measure for temporomandibular disorders. *Journal of Orofacial Pain.* 2002;16(4):296-304.

30. Stratford P. Assessing disability and change on individual patients: A report of a patient specific measure. *Physio Canada.* 1995;47:258-263.

31. Helmick LF, Parkinson GW, Chandler LA, Warden DL. Mild traumatic brain injury in wartime. *Federal Practitioner.* 2007;October:58-65.

32. Stalnacke BM. Community integration, social support and life satisfaction in relation to symptoms three years after mild traumatic brain injury. *Brain Injury.* 2007;21(9):933-942.

33. Cushman JG, Agarwal N, Fabian TC, et al. Practice management guidelines for the management of mild traumatic brain injury: The EAST practice management guidelines work group. *Journal of Trauma.* 2001;51(5):1016-1026.

34. Department of Veterans Affairs. Traumatic Brain Injury. In: Initiative VH, ed. Washington DC2004.

35. Brain Trauma Foundation. Guidelines for field management of combat-related head trauma. New York, NY: Brain Trauma Foundation; 2005.

36. New Zealand Guidelines Group. *Traumatic brain injury: Diagnosis, acute management and rehabilitation.* Wellington, New Zealand: AAC;2006.

37. Dikmen S, Machamer J, Temkin N. Mild head injury: facts and artifacts. *Journal of Clinical and Experimental Neuropsychology.* 2001;23(6):729-738.

38. Carroll LJ, Cassidy JD, Peloso PM, et al. Prognosis for mild traumatic brain injury: Results of the WHO Collaborative Center Task Force on Mild Traumatic Brain Injury. *Journal of Rehabilitative Medicine.* 2004b;43:84-105.

39. McCrea MA. *Mild Traumatic Brain Injury and Post Concussion Syndrome.* New York: Oxford University Press; 2008.

40. Ruff RM. Two decades of advances in understanding of mild traumatic brain injury. *The Journal of head trauma rehabilitation.* Jan-Feb 2005;20(1):5-18.

41. Alves W, Colohn A, O'Leary T, Rimel R, Jane J. Understanding posttraumatic symptoms after minor head injury. *Journal of Head Trauma Rehabilitation.* 1986;1.

42. Edna TH, Cappelen J. Late postconcussional symptoms in traumatic head injury: An analysis of the frequency and risk factors. *Acta Neurochirurgica.* 1987;86:12-17.

43. Ponsford J, Willmott C, Rothwell A, et al. Factors influencing outcome following mild traumatic brain injury in adults. *Journal of the International Neuropsychological Society.* 2000;6(5):568-579.

44. Ruff RM, Camenzuli L, Mueller J. Miserable minority: Emotional risk factors that influence the outcome of a mild traumatic brain injury. *Brain Injury.* 1996;10(8):551-565.

45. Mittenberg W, Strauman S. Diagnosis of mild head injury and the postconcussion syndrome. *The Journal of head trauma rehabilitation.* Apr 2000;15(2):783-791.

46. Cohen BA, Inglese M, Rusinek H, Babb JS, Grossman RI, Gonen O. Proton MR spectroscopy and MRI-volumetry in mild traumatic brain injury. *American Journal of Neuroradiology.* 2007;28(5):907-913.

47. Montgomery GK. A multi-factor account of disability after brain injury: implications for neuropsychological counseling. *Brain Injury.* 1995;9(5):453-469.

48. Hoge CW, McGurk D, Thomas JL, Cox AL, Engel CC, Castro CA. Mild traumatic brain injury in U.S. Soldiers returning from Iraq. *The New England Journal of Medicine.* 2008;358(5):453-463.

49. Warden D. Military TBI during the Iraq and Afghanistan wars. *Journal of Head Trauma Rehabilitation.* 2006;21(5):398-402.

50. Sareen J, Cox BJ, Afifi TO, et al. Combat and peacekeeping operations in relation to prevalence of mental disorders and perceived need for mental health care: Findings from a large representative sample of military personnel. *Archives of General Psychiatry.* 2007;64(7):843-852.

51. Schneiderman AI, Braver ER, Kang HK. Understanding sequelae of injury mechanisms and mild traumatic brain injury incurred during the conflicts in Iraq and Afghanistan: Persistent postconcussive symptoms and posttraumatic stress disorder. *American Journal of Epidemiology.* 2008;167(12):1446-1452.

52. Kennedy JE, Jaffee MS, Leskin GA, Stokes JW, Leal FO, Fitzpatrick PJ. Posttraumatic stress disorder and posttraumatic stress disorder-like symptoms and mild traumatic brain injury. *Journal of rehabilitation research and development.* 2007;44(7):895-920.

53. Bryant RA, Harvey AG. Relationship between acute stress disorder and posttraumatic stress disorder following mild traumatic brain injury. *American Journal of Psychiatry.* 1998;155(5):625-629.

54. Bryant RA, Harvey AG. Acute stress disorder: A critical review of diagnostic issue. *Clinical Psychology Review.* 1997;17:757-773.

55. Terrio H, Brenner LA, Ivins BJ, et al. Traumatic brain injury screening: Preliminary findings in a U.S. Army Brigade Combat Team. *Journal of Head Trauma Rehabilitation.* 2009;24(1):14-23.

56. DePalma RG, Burris DG, Champion HR, Hodgson MJ. Blast injuries. *New England Journal of Medicine.* 2005;352(13):1335-1342.

57. Ponsford J. Rehabilitation interventions after mild head injury. *Current Opinion in Neurology.* 2005;18(6):692-697.

58. Steadman-Pare D, Colantonio A, Ratcliff G, Chase S, Vernich L. Factors associated with perceived quality of life many years after traumatic brain injury. *Journal of Head Trauma Rehabilitation.* 2001;16(4):330-342.

59. World Health Organization. *International classification of functioning, disability and health.* Geneva, Switzerland: World Health Organization; 2001.

60. Fung M, Willer B, Moreland D, Leddy JJ. A proposal for an evidenced-based emergency department discharge form for mild traumatic brain injury. *Brain Injury.* 2006;20(9):889-894.

61. Wilson BA, Evans JJ, Emslie H, Balleny H, Watson PC, Baddeley AD. Measuring recovery from post traumatic amnesia. *Brain Injury.* 1999;13(7):505-520.

62. Ponsford J, Willmott C, Rothwell A, Kelly AM, Nelms R, Ng KT. Use of the Westmead PTA scale to monitor recovery of memory after mild head injury. *Brain Injury.* 2004;18(6):603-614.

63. Jacobson GP, Newman CW. The development of the Dizziness Handicap Inventory. *Arch Otolaryngol Head Neck Surg.* Apr 1990;116(4):424-427.

64. Herdman SJ, Blatt PJ, Schubert MC. Vestibular rehabilitation of patients with vestibular hypofunction or with benign paroxysmal positional vertigo. *Current Opinion in Neurology.* 2000;13(1):39-43.

65. Riemann BL, Guskiewicz KM. Effects of mild head injury on postural stability as measured through clinical balance testing. *Journal of Athletic Training.* 2000;35(1):19-25.

66. Riemann BL, Guskiewicz KM, Shields E. Relationship between clinical and forceplate measures of postural stability. *Journal of Sports Rehabilitation.* 1999;8:71-82.

67. Griesbach GS, Hovda DA, Molteni R, Wu A, Gomez-Pinilla F. Voluntary exercise following traumatic brain injury: brain-derived neurotrophic factor upregulation and recovery of function. *Neuroscience.* 2004;125(1):129-139.

68. Leddy JJ, Kozlowski K, Fung M, Pendergast DR, Willer B. Regulatory and autoregulatory physiological dysfunction as a primary characteristic of post concussion syndrome: implications for treatment. *NeuroRehabilitation.* 2007;22(3):199-205.

69. Borg J, Holm L, Peloso PM, et al. Non-surgical intervention and cost for mild traumatic brain injury: results of the WHO Collaborating Centre Task Force on Mild Traumatic Brain Injury. *J Rehabil Med.* Feb 2004(43 Suppl):76-83.

70. Ponsford J, Willmott C, Rothwell A, et al. Impact of early intervention on outcome following head injury in adults. *Journal of Neurology, Neurosurgery, and Psychiatry.* 2002;73(3):330-332.

71. Mittenberg W, Tremont G, Zielinski RE, Fichera S, Rayls KR. Cognitive-behavioral prevention of postconcussion syndrome. *Arch Clin Neuropsychol.* 1996;11(2):139-145.

72. Mateer CA, Sira CS, O'Connell ME. Putting Humpty Dumpty together again: the importance of integrating cognitive and emotional interventions. *Journal of Head Trauma Rehabilitation.* 2005;20(1):62-75.

73. Ownsworth T, Fleming J. The relative importance of metacognitive skills, emotional status, and executive function in psychosocial adjustment following acquired brain injury. *Journal of Head Trauma Rehabilitation.* 2005;20(4):315-332.

74. Mittenberg W, Tremont G, Zielinski RE, Fichera S, Rayls KR. Cognitive-behavioral prevention of postconcussion syndrome. *Archives of Clinical Neuropsychology.* 1996;11(2):139-145.

75. Mason DJ. *The Mild Traumatic Brain Injury Workbook.* Oakland, CA: New Harbinger Publications; 2004.

76. Atkinson RC, Shiffrin RM. The control of short-term memory. *Scientific American.* 1971;225(2):82-90.
77. Miller GA. The magical number seven, plus or minus two: Some limits on our capacity for processing information. *Psychological Review.* 1956;63:81-97.
78. Ingebrigtsen T, Waterloo K, Marup-Jensen S, Attner E, Romner B. Quantification of post-concussion symptoms 3 months after minor head injury in 100 consecutive patients. *Journal of Neurology.* 1998;245(9):609-612.
79. Whitney SL, Marchetti GF, Morris LO. Usefulness of the dizziness handicap inventory in the screening for benign paroxysmal positional vertigo. *Otol Neurotol.* Sep 2005;26(5):1027-1033.
80. Brown KE, Whitney SL, Wrisley DM, Furman JM. Physical therapy outcomes for persons with bilateral vestibular loss. *Laryngoscope.* Oct 2001;111(10):1812-1817.
81. Wrisley DM, Whitney SL, Furman JM. Vestibular rehabilitation outcomes in patients with a history of migraine. *Otology & Neurotology.* 2002;23(4):483-487.
82. Humphriss RL, Baguley DM, Sparkes V, Peerman SE, Moffat DA. Contraindications to the Dix-Hallpike manoeuvre: a multidisciplinary review. *International Journal of Audiology.* 2003;42(3):166-173.
83. Herdman SJ, Tusa RJ, Zee DS, Proctor LR, Mattox DE. Single treatment approaches to benign paroxysmal positional vertigo. *Archives of Otolaryngology--Head & Neck Surgery.* 1993;119(4):450-454.
84. Gordon CR, Levite R, Joffe V, Gadoth N. Is posttraumatic benign paroxysmal positional vertigo different from the idiopathic form? *Archives of Neurology.* 2004;61(10):1590-1593.
85. Yardley L, Beech S, Zander L, Evans T, Weinman J. A randomized controlled trial of exercise therapy for dizziness and vertigo in primary care. *British Journal of General Practices.* 1998;48(429):1136-1140.
86. Herdman SJ, Tusa RJ, Blatt P, Suzuki A, Venuto PJ, Roberts D. Computerized dynamic visual acuity test in the assessment of vestibular deficits. *The American Journal of Otology.* 1998;19(6):790-796.
87. Burgio DL, Blakley RW, Myers SF. The high-frequency oscillopsia test. *Journal of Vestibular Research.* 1992;2:221-226.
88. Longridge NS, Mallinson AI. The dynamic illegible E (DIE) test: a simple technique for assessing the ability of the vestibulo-ocular reflex to overcome vestibular pathology. *The Journal of Otolaryngology.* 1987;16(2):97-103.
89. Venuto PJ, Herdman SJ, Tusa RJ. Interrater reliability of the clinical dynamic visual acuity test. *Physical therapy.* 1998;78:S21.
90. Fife TD, Tusa RJ, Furman JM, et al. Assessment: vestibular testing techniques in adults and children: report of the Therapeutics and Technology Assessment Subcommittee of the American Academy of Neurology. *Neurology.* Nov 28 2000;55(10):1431-1441.
91. Schubert MC, Minor LB. Vestibulo-ocular physiology underlying vestibular hypofunction. *Physical therapy.* Apr 2004;84(4):373-385.
92. Hall CD, Schubert MC, Herdman SJ. Prediction of fall risk reduction as measured by dynamic gait index in individuals with unilateral vestibular hypofunction. *Otol Neurotol.* Sep 2004;25(5):746-751.
93. Savundra PA, Carroll JD, Davies RA, Luxon LM. Migraine-associated vertigo. *Cephalalgia.* 1997;17(4):505-510.
94. Wrisley DM, Whitney SL. The effect of foot position on the modified clinical test of sensory interaction and balance. *Arch Phys Med Rehabil.* Feb 2004;85(2):335-338.
95. Neuhauser HK, Radtke A, von Brevern M, et al. Migrainous vertigo: prevalence and impact on quality of life. *Neurology.* 2006;67(6):1028-1033.
96. Cass SP, Furman JM, Ankerstjerne K, Balaban C, Yetiser S, Aydogan B. Migraine-related vestibulopathy. *The Annals of Otology, Rhinology, and Laryngology.* 1997;106(3):182-189.
97. Johnson GD. Medical management of migraine-related dizziness and vertigo. *Laryngoscope.* 1998;108(Supplement 85):1-28.
98. Whitney SL, Wrisley DM, Brown KE, Furman JM. Physical therapy for migraine-related vestibulopathy and vestibular dysfunction with history of migraine. *The Laryngoscope.* 2000;110(9):1528-1534.
99. Myers AM, Fletcher PC, Myers AH, Sherk W. Discriminative and evaluative properties of the activities-specific balance confidence (ABC) scale. *J Gerontol A Biol Sci Med Sci.* Jul 1998;53(4):M287-294.
100. Williams G, Robertson V, Greenwood K. Measuring high-level mobility after traumatic brain injury. *American Journal of Physical Medicine & Rehabilitation.* 2004;12:910-920.
101. Williams GP, Greenwood KM, Robertson VJ, Goldie PA, Morris ME. High-Level Mobility Assessment Tool (HiMAT): Interrater reliability, retest reliability, and internal consistency. *Physical therapy.* 2006a;86(3):395-400.

102. Williams G, Robertson V, Greenwood K, Goldie P, Morris ME. The concurrent validity and responsiveness of the high-level mobility assessment tool for measuring the mobility limitations of people with traumatic brain injury. *Archives of Physical Medicine and Rehabilitation.* 2006b;87(3):437-442.

103. Guskiewicz KM. Postural stability assessment following concussion: one piece of the puzzle. *Clin J Sport Med.* Jul 2001;11(3):182-189.

104. Oliaro S, Anderson S, Hooker D. Management of Cerebral Concussion in Sports: The Athletic Trainer's Perspective. *J Athl Train.* Sep 2001;36(3):257-262.

105. Susco TM, Valovich McLeod TC, Gansneder BM, Shultz SJ. Balance recovers within 20 minutes after exertion as measured by the balance error scoring system. *Journal of Athletic Training.* 2004;39(3):241-246.

106. Valovich TC, Perrin DH, Gansneder BM. Repeat administration elicits a practice effect with the balance error scoring system but not with the standardized assessment of concussion in high school athletes. *Journal of Athletic Training.* 2003;38(1):38, 51-56.

107. Wrisley DM, Marchetti GF, Kuharsky DK, Whitney SL. Reliability, internal consistency, and validity of data obtained with the functional gait assessment. *Physical therapy.* 2004;84(10):906-918.

108. van Loo MA, Moseley AM, Bosman JM, de Bie RA, Hassett L. Inter-rater reliability and concurrent validity of walking speed measurement after traumatic brain injury. *Clinical Rehabilitation.* 2003;17(7):775-779.

109. Schmid A, Duncan PW, Studenski S, et al. Improvements in speed-based gait classifications are meaningful. *Stroke.* 2007;38(7):2096-2100.

110. Shumway-Cook A, Horak FB. Assessing the influence of sensory interaction of balance. Suggestion from the field. *Physical therapy.* Oct 1986;66(10):1548-1550.

111. Dehail P, Petit H, Joseph PA, Vuadens P, Mazaux JM. Assessment of postural instability in patients with traumatic brain injury upon enrolment in a vocational adjustment programme. *Journal of Rehabilitation Medicine.* 2007;39(7):531-536.

112. Csuka M, McCarty DJ. Simple method for measurement of lower extremity muscle strength. *Am J Med.* Jan 1985;78(1):77-81.

113. Belgen B, Beninato M, Sullivan PE, Narielwalla K. The association of balance capacity and falls self-efficacy with history of falling in community-dwelling people with chronic stroke. *Arch Phys Med Rehabil.* Apr 2006;87(4):554-561.

114. Chandler JM, Duncan PW, Kochersberger G, Studenski S. Is lower extremity strength gain associated with improvement in physical performance and disability in frail, community-dwelling elders? *Arch Phys Med Rehabil.* Jan 1998;79(1):24-30.

115. Lord SR, Murray SM, Chapman K, Munro B, Tiedemann A. Sit-to-stand performance depends on sensation, speed, balance, and psychological status in addition to strength in older people. *J Gerontol A Biol Sci Med Sci.* Aug 2002;57(8):M539-543.

116. Meretta BM, Whitney SL, Marchetti GF, Sparto PJ, Muirhead RJ. The five times sit to stand test: responsiveness to change and concurrent validity in adults undergoing vestibular rehabilitation. *J Vestib Res.* 2006;16(4-5):233-243.

117. Hoffer ME, Balough BJ, Gottshall KR. Posttraumatic balance disorders. *International Tinnitus Journal.* 2007;13(1):69-72.

118. Goodrich GL, Kirby J, Cockerham G, Ingalla SP, Lew HL. Visual function in patients of a polytrauma rehabilitation center: A descriptive study. *Journal of rehabilitation research and development.* 2007;44(7):929-936.

119. Weichel ED, Colyer MH, Bautista C, Bower KS, French LM. Traumatic brain injury associated with combat ocular trauma. *Journal of Head Trauma Rehabilitation.* 2009;24(1):41-50.

120. Hellerstein LF, Freed S, Maples WC. Vision profile of patients with mild brain injury. *Journal of the American Optometric Association.* 1995;66(10):634-639.

121. Ciuffreda KJ, Kapoor N, Rutner D, Suchoff IB, Han ME, Craig S. Occurrence of oculomotor dysfunctions in acquired brain injury: a retrospective analysis. *Optometry.* 2007;78(4):155-161.

122. Ciuffreda KJ, Rutner D, Kapoor N, Suchoff IB, Craig S, Han ME. Vision therapy for oculomotor dysfunctions in acquired brain injury: a retrospective analysis. *Optometry.* 2008;79(1):18-22.

123. Suchoff IB, Kapoor N, Ciuffreda KJ, Rutner D, Han E, Craig S. The frequency of occurrence, types, and characteristics of visual field defects in acquired brain injury: A retrospective analysis. *Optometry.* 2008;79(5):259-265.

124. Abreu BC, Seale G, Podlesak J, Hartley L. Development of critical paths for post-acute brain injury rehabilitation: lessons learned. *American Journal of Occupational Therapy.* 1996;50(6):417-427.

125. Bryan VL. Management of residual physical deficits. In: Ashley MJ, Krych DK, eds. *Traumatic Brain Injury: Rehabilitative Treatment and Case Management.* 2 ed. Boca Raton: CRC Press; 2004:455-508.

126. Scheiman M. *Understanding and Managing Vision Deficits: A Guide for Occupational Therapists.* Thorofare, NJ: Slack Inc.; 2002.

127. Toglia JP. A dynamic interactional approach to cognitive rehabilitation. In: Katz N, ed. *Cognition & Occupation Across the Life Span -2nd Edition.* Bethesda, MD: American Occupational Therapy Association; 2005:29-72.

128. Dougherty PM, Radomski MV. *The Cognitive Rehabilitation Workbook.* Gaithersburg, MD: Aspen Publishers; 1993.

129. Toglia JP. Approaches to cognitive assessment of the brain injured adult. *Occupational Therapy Practice.* 1989;1:36-55.

130. Barrett BT. A critical evaluation of the evidence supporting the practice of behavioral vision therapy. *Ophthalmic and Physiological Optics.* 2009;29:4-25.

131. Zoltan B. *Vision, Perception, and Cognition: A Manual for the Evaluation and Treatment of the Adult with Accquired Brain Injury - 4th Edition.* Vol 4. Thorofare, NJ: Slack Inc.; 2007.

132. Kapoor N, Ciuffreda KJ, Han Y. Oculomotor rehabilitation in acquired brain injury: a case series. *Archives of Physical Medicine and Rehabilitation.* 2004;85(10):1667-1678.

133. Lew HL, Lin PH, Fuh JL, Wang SJ, Clark DJ, Walker WC. Characteristics and treatment of headache after traumatic brain injury: a focused review. *American Journal of Physical Medicine & Rehabilitation / Association of Academic Physiatrists.* 2006;85(7):619-627.

134. Packard RC. Epidemiology and pathogenesis of posttraumatic headache. *Journal of Head Trauma Rehabilitation.* 1999;4:9-21.

135. Nampiaparampil DE. Prevalence of chronic pain after traumatic brain injury: a systematic review. *Journal of the American Medical Association.* 2008;300(6):711-719.

136. Jacobson GP, Ramadan NM, Aggarwal SK, Newman CW. The Henry Ford Hospital Headache Disability Inventory (HDI). *Neurology.* 1994;44(5):837-842.

137. Jacobson GP, Ramadan NM, Norris L, Newman CW. Headache disability inventory (HDI): short-term test-retest reliability and spouse perceptions. *Headache.* 1995;35(9):534-539.

138. Vernon HT, Mior SA. The Neck Disability Index: A study of reliability and validity. *J Manip Physiol Therapy.* 1991;14:409-415.

139. Pengel LH, Refshauge KM, Maher CG. Responsiveness of pain, disability, and physical impairment outcomes in patients with low back pain. *Spine.* 2004;29(8):879-883.

140. Westaway MD, Stratford PW, Binkley JM. The patient-specific functional scale: Validation of its use in persons with neck dysfunction. *Journal of Orthopaedic and Sports Physical Therapy.* 1998;27(5):331-338.

141. Bell KR, Kraus EE, Zasler ND. Medical management of posttraumatic headaches: pharmacological and physical treatment. *Journal of Head Trauma Rehabilitation.* 1999;14(1):34-48.

142. Pho C, Godges J. Management of whiplash-associated disorder addressing thoracic and cervical spine impairments: A case report. *Journal of Orthopaedic and Sports Physical Therapy.* 2004;34(9):511-523.

143. Hammill JM, Cook TM, Rosecrance JC. Effectiveness of a physical therapy regimen in the treatment of tension-type headache. *Headache.* 1996;36(3):149-153.

144. McDonnell MK, Sahrmann SA, Van Dillen L. A specific exercise program and modification of postural alignment for treatment of cervicogenic headache: a case report. *Journal of Orthopaedic and Sports Physical Therapy.* 2005;35(1):3-15.

145. Goldberg MB, Mock D, Ichise M, et al. Neuropsychologic deficits and clinical features of posttraumatic temporomandibular disorders. *Journal of Orofacial Pain.* 1996;10(2):126-140.

146. John MT, Dworkin SF, Mancl LA. Reliability of clinical temporomandibular disorder diagnoses. *Pain.* 2005;118(1-2):61-69.

147. Dworkin SF, Turner JA, Mancl L, et al. A randomized clinical trial of a tailored comprehensive care treatment program for temporomandibular disorders. *Journal of Orofacial Pain.* 2002;16(4):259-276.

148. Fischer MJ, Reiners A, Kohnen R, et al. Do occlusal splints have an effect on complex regional pain syndrome? A randomized, controlled proof-of-concept trial. *The Clinical Journal of Pain.* 2008;24(9):776-783.

149. Wright EF, Domenech MA, Fischer JR, Jr. Usefulness of posture training for patients with temporomandibular disorders. *Journal of the American Dental Association.* 2000;131(2):202-210.

150. Au AR, Klineberg IJ. Isokinetic exercise management of temporomandibular joint clicking in young adults. *Journal of Prosthetic Dentistry.* 1993;70(1):33-39.

151. Furto ES, Cleland JA, Whitman JM, Olson KA. Manual physical therapy interventions and exercise for patients with temporomandibular disorders. *Cranio.* 2006;24(4):283-291.

152. Dirette DK, Plaisier BR. The development of self-awareness of deficits from 1 week to 1 year after traumatic brain injury: preliminary findings. *Brain Injury.* 2007;21(11):1131-1136.

153. Davis CH. Self-perception in mild traumatic brain injury. *American Journal of Physical Medicine & Rehabilitation / Association of Academic Physiatrists.* 2002;81(8):609-621.

154. Radomski MV. Assessing abilities and capacities: Cognition. In: Radomski MV, Trombly Latham CA, eds. *Occupational Therapy for Physical Dysfunction.* Philadelphia: Lippincott Williams & Wilkins; 2008:260-283.

155. Mortera MH. The development of the Cognitive Screening Measure for individuals with brain injury: Initial examination of content validity and interrater reliability. *Dissertation Abstracts International.* 2004;65:906.

156. Mortera MH. Instrument development in brain injury rehabilitation: Part I. *Physical Disabilities Special Interest Section Quarterly.* 2006a;29(3):1-4.

157. Mortera MH. Instrument development in brain injury rehabilitation: Part II. *Physical Disabilities Special Interest Section Quarterly.* 2006b;29(4):1-2.

158. Kiernan RJ, Mueller J, Langston JW, Van Dyke C. The Neurobehavioral Cognitive Status Examination: a brief but quantitative approach to cognitive assessment. *Ann Intern Med.* Oct 1987;107(4):481-485.

159. Blostein PA, Jones SJ, Buechler CM, Vandongen S. Cognitive screening in mild traumatic brain injuries: analysis of the neurobehavioral cognitive status examination when utilized during initial trauma hospitalization. *J Neurotrauma.* Mar 1997;14(3):171-177.

160. Wilson B, Cockburn J, Baddeley A, Hiorns R. The development and validation of a test battery for detecting and monitoring everyday memory problems. *J Clin Exp Neuropsychol.* Dec 1989;11(6):855-870.

161. Wilson BA, Cockburn J, Baddeley A. *The Rivermead Behavioral Memory Test.* Gaylord, MI: National Rehabilitation Services; 1985.

162. Wills P, Clare L, Shiel A, Wilson BA. Assessing subtle memory impairments in the everyday memory performance of brain injured people: exploring the potential of the extended Rivermead Behavioural Memory Test. *Brain Inj.* Aug 2000;14(8):693-704.

163. Robertson IH, Ward T, Ridgeway V, Nimmo-Smith I. The structure of normal human attention: The Test of Everyday Attention. *Journal of the International Neuropsychological Society.* 1996;2(6):525-534.

164. Radomski MV. Cognitive rehabilitation: Advancing the stature of occupational therapy. *American Journal of Occupational Therapy.* 1994;48(3):271-273.

165. Wilson BA. Cognitive rehabilitation: How it is and how it might be. *Journal of the International Neuropsychological Society.* 1997;3(5):487-496.

166. Ylvisaker M, Hanks R, Johnson-Greene D. Perspectives on rehabilitation of individuals with cognitive impairment after brain injury: Rationale for reconsideration of theoretical paradigms. *Journal of Head Trauma Rehabilitation.* 2002;17(3):191-209.

167. Gordon WA, Zafonte R, Cicerone K, et al. Traumatic brain injury rehabilitation: state of the science. *American Journal of Physical Medicine & Rehabilitation / Association of Academic Physiatrists.* 2006;85(4):343-382.

168. Cappa SF, Benke T, Clarke S, Rossi B, Stemmer B, van Heugten CM. EFNS guidelines on cognitive rehabilitation: Report of an EFNS Task Force. *European Journal of Neurology.* 2003;10:11-23.

169. Cicerone KD, Dahlberg C, Kalmer K, et al. Evidence-based cognitive rehabilitation: Recommendations for clinical practice. *Archives of Physical Medicine and Rehabilitation.* 2000;81:1596-1615.

170. Cicerone KD, Dahlberg C, Malec JF, et al. Evidence-based cognitive rehabilitation: updated review of the literature from 1998 through 2002. *Arch Phys Med Rehabil.* Aug 2005;86(8):1681-1692.

171. Tiersky LA, Anselmi V, Johnston MV, et al. A trial of neuropsychologic rehabilitation in mild-spectrum traumatic brain injury. *Archives of Physical Medicine and Rehabilitation.* 2005;86(8):1565-1574.

172. Michel JA, Mateer CA. Attention rehabilitation following stroke and traumatic brain injury. A review. *Europa Medicophysica.* 2006;42(1):59-67.

173. Parente R, DiCesare A. Retraining memory theory, evaluation and applications. In: Kreutzer JS, Wehman PH, eds. *Cognitive rehabilitation for persons with traumatic brain injury: A functional approach.* Baltimore: Paul H. Brooks; 1991:147-162.

174. Bransford JD, Stein BS. *The IDEAL Problem Solver: A guide for improving thinking, learning and creativity.* New York: W.H. Freeman; 1984.

175. Groverover Y, Johnston MV, Toglia J, Deluca J. Treatment to improve self-awareness in persons with acquired brain injury. *Brain Injury.* 2007;21(9):913-923.

176. Dirette DK. The development of awareness and the use of compensatory strategies for cognitive deficits. *Brain Inj.* Oct 2002;16(10):861-871.

177. Sohlberg MM, Mateer CA. *Introduction to Cognitive Rehabilitation.* New York: Guilford Press; 1989.

178. Kirby JR. Educational roles of cognitive plans and strategies. In: Kirby JR, ed. *Cognitive Strategies and Educational Performance.* Orlando, FL1984:51-88-51-88.

179. Parker TM, Osternig LR, P VAND, Chou LS. Gait stability following concussion. *Med Sci Sports Exerc.* Jun 2006;38(6):1032-1040.

180. Vallee M, McFadyen BJ, Swaine B, Doyon J, Cantin JF, Dumas D. Effects of environmental demands on locomotion after traumatic brain injury. *Archives of Physical Medicine and Rehabilitation.* 2006;87(6):806-813.

181. McCulloch K, Blakeley K, Freeman L. Clinical tests of walking dual-task performance after accquired brain injury: Feasibility and dual-task cost compared to a yound adult group. *Journal of Neurological Physical Therapy.* 2005(29):213.

182. Silsupadol P, Siu KC, Shumway-Cook A, Woollacott MH. Training of balance under single- and dual-task conditions in older adults with balance impairment. *Physical therapy.* Feb 2006;86(2):269-281.

183. Vanderploeg RD, Collins RC, Sigford B, et al. Practical and theoretical considerations in designing rehabilitation trials: The DVBIC cognitive-didactic versus functional-experiential treatment study experience. *Journal of Head Trauma Rehabilitation.* 2006;21(2):179-193.

184. Trombly CA. Anticipating the future: Assessment of occupational function. *American Journal of Occupational Therapy.* 1993;47(3):253-257.

185. Trombly CA. Occupation: Purposefulness and meaningfulness as therapeutic mechanisms. *American Journal of Occupational Therapy.* 1995;49(10):960-972.

186. Latham Trombly CA. Conceptual foundations for practice. In: Radomski MV, Latham Trombly CA, eds. *Occupational Therapy for Physical Dysfunction - 6th edition.* Philadelphia: Lippincott; 2008.

187. American Occupational Therapy Association. Occupational therapy practice framework: Domain and process. *American Journal of Occupational Therapy.* 2002;59:609-639.

188. Resnik LJ, Allen SM. Using International Classification of Functioning, Disability and Health to understand challenges in community reintegration of injured veterans. *Journal of rehabilitation research and development.* 2007;44(7):991-1006.

189. Vanderploeg RD, Curtiss G, Luis CA, Salazar AM. Long-term morbidities following self-reported mild traumatic brain injury. *Journal of Clinical and Experimental Neuropsychology.* 2007;29(6):585-598.

190. Beers SR, Goldstein G, Katz LJ. Neuropsychological differences between college students with learning disabilities and those with mild head injury. *Journal of Learning Disabilities.* 1994;27(5):315-324.

191. Eriksson G, Tham K, Fugl-Meyer AR. Couples' happiness and its relationship to functioning in everyday life after brain injury. *Scandinavian Journal of Occupational Therapy.* 2005;12(1):40-48.

192. Hall KM, Karzmark P, Stevens M, Englander J, O'Hare P, Wright J. Family stressors in traumatic brain injury: a two-year follow-up. *Archives of Physical Medicine and Rehabilitation.* 1994;75(8):876-884.

193. Testa JA, Malec JF, Moessner AM, Brown AW. Predicting family functioning after TBI: Impact of neurobehavioral factors. *Journal of Head Trauma Rehabilitation.* 2006;21(3):236-247.

194. Schonberger M, Humle F, Teasdale TW. Subjective outcome of brain injury rehabilitation in relation to the therapeutic working alliance, client compliance, and awareness. *Brain Injury.* 2006;20(12):1271-1282.

195. Law M, Baptiste, S., McColl, M., Opzoomer, A., Polatajko, H., Pollock, N. The Canadian Occupational Performance Measure: An outcome measure for occupational therapy. *Canadian Journal of Occupational Therapy.* 1990;57(2):82-87.

196. Law M, Polatajko H, Pollock N, McColl MA, Carswell A, Baptiste S. Pilot testing of the Canadian Occupational Performance Measure: clinical and measurement issues. *Can J Occup Ther.* Oct 1994;61(4):191-197.

197. McColl MA, Paterson M, Davies D, Doubt L, Law M. Validity and community utility of the Canadian Occupational Performance Measure. *Canadian Journal of Occupational Therapy.* 2000;67(1):22-30.

198. Law M, Baptise S, McColl MA, Carswell A, Polatajko H, Pollock N. *Canadian Occupational Performance Measure.* Toronto: CAOT Publications ACE; 1994a.

199. Trombly CA, Radomski, M.V., Davis, E.S. Achievement of self-identified goals by adults with traumatic brain injury: Phase I. *American Journal of Occupational Therapy*. 1998;52:810-818.

200. Trombly CA, Radomski MV, Burnett-Smith SE. Achievement of self-identified goals by adults with traumatic brain injury: Phase II. *American Journal of Occupational Therapy*. 2002;56:489-498.

201. Baron K, Kielhofner G, Iyenger A, Goldhammer V, Wolenski J. *A user's manual for the Occupational Self Assessment (OSA)*. Chicago, IL: University of Illinois at Chicago; 2006.

202. Kielhofner G, Forsyth K, Kramer J, Iyenger A. Developing a client self report measure, Part I: Assuring internal validity and sensitivity. *British Journal of Occupational Therapy*. 2007.

203. Radomski MV. There's more to life than putting on your pants. *American Journal of Occupational Therapy*. 1995;49(6):487-490.

204. Johns MW. Reliability and factor analysis of the Epworth Sleepiness Scale. *Sleep*. Aug 1992;15(4):376-381.

205. Krupp LB, LaRocca NG, Muir-Nash J, Steinberg AD. The fatigue severity scale. Application to patients with multiple sclerosis and systemic lupus erythematosus. *Arch Neurol*. Oct 1989;46(10):1121-1123.

206. Whitehead L. The measurement of fatigue in chronic illness: a systematic review of unidimensional and multidimensional fatigue measures. *J Pain Symptom Manage*. Jan 2009;37(1):107-128.

207. Forsyth K, Lai J, Kielhofner G. The assessment of communication and interaction skills (ACIS): Measurement properties. *British Journal of Occupational Therapy*. 1999;62:69-74.

208. Davidson LF. *Activity Co-engagement Self-assessment*. Winchester, VA: Shenandoah University; 2009.

209. Spanier GB. Measuring dyadic adjustment: New scales for assessing the equality of marriage and similar dyads. *Journal of Marriage and the Family*. 1976;38:15-28.

210. Vos PE, Battistin L, Birbamer G, et al. EFNS guideline on mild traumatic brain injury: Report of an EFNS task force. *European Journal of Neurology*. 2002;9(3):207-219.

211. Wallenbert I, Jonsson H. Waiting to get better: A dilemma regarding habits in daily occupations after stroke. *American Journal of Occupational Therapy*. 2005;59(2):218-224.

212. Radomski MV, Davis ES. Optimizing cognitive abilities. In: Radomsk MV, Trombly Latham CA, eds. *Occupational Therapy for Physical Dysfunction*. Philadelphia: Lippincott Williams & Wilkins; 2008:748-773.

213. Giles GM. A neurofunctional approach to rehabilitation following severe brain injury. In: Katz N, ed. *Cognition and Occupation Across the Life Span*. Bethesda, MD1998:139.

214. Giles GM, Ridley JE, Dill A, Frye S. A consecutive series of adults with brain injury treated with a washing and dressing retaining program. *American Journal of Occupational Therapy*. 1997;51:256-266.

215. Giles GM. A neurofunctional approach to rehabilitation following severe brain injury. In: Katz N, ed. *Cognition and Occupation Across the Life Span*. Bethesda, MD: American Occupational Therapy Association; 2005.

216. Davis ES, Radomski MV. Domain-specific training to reinstate habit sequences. *Occupational Therapy Practice*. 1989;1:79-88.

217. Gutman SA, Schindler VP, Furphy KA, Klein K, Lisak JM, Durham DP. The effectiveness of a supported education program: The Bridge Program. *Occupational Therapy in Mental Health*. 2007:23, 21-38.

218. O'Neill J, Hibbard MR, Brown M, et al. The effect of employment on quality of life and community integration after traumatic brain injury. *Journal of Head Trauma Rehabilitation*. 1998;13(4):68-79.

219. Haskell WL, Lee IM, Pate RR, et al. Physical activity and public health: Updated recommendations for adults from the American College of Sports Medicine and the American Heart Association. *Medicine and Science in Sports and Exercise*. 2007;39(8):1423-1434.

220. Mossberg KA, Green BP. Reliability of graded exercise testing after traumatic brain injury: submaximal and peak responses. *American Journal of Physical Medicine*. 2005;84(7):492-500.

221. Elavsky S, McAuley E, Motl RW, et al. Physical activity enhances long-term quality of life in older adults: efficacy, esteem, and affective influences. *Annals of Behavioral Medicine*. 2005;30(2):138-145.

222. Bhambhani Y, Rowland G, Farag M. Effects of circuit training on body composition and peak cardiorespiratory responses in patients with moderate to severe traumatic brain injury. *Archives of Physical Medicine and Rehabilitation*. 2005;86(2):268-276.

223. Colcombe SJ, Kramer AF, Erickson KI, et al. Cardiovascular fitness, cortical plasticity, and aging. *Proceedings of the National Academy of Sciences of the United States of America*. 2004;101(9):3316-3321.

224. Lojovich JM. The relationship between aerobic exercise and cognition: is movement medicinal? *The Journal of head trauma rehabilitation*. May-Jun 2010;25(3):184-192.

225. Vitale AE, Sullivan SJ, Jankowski LW, Fleury J, Lefrancois C, Lebouthillier E. Screening of health risk factors prior to exercise or a fitness evaluation of adults with traumatic brain injury: A consensus by rehabilitation professionals. *Brain Injury.* 1996;10(5):367-375.
226. Nelson ME, Rejeski WJ, Blair SN, et al. Physical activity and public health in older adults: Recommendations from the American College of Sports Medicine and the American Heart Association. *Medicine and Science in Sports and Exercise.* 2007;39(8):1435-1445.
227. Dijkers M. Measuring long-term outcomes of traumatic brain injury: a review of Community Integration Questionnaire studies. *Journal of Head Trauma Rehabilitation.* 1997;12:74-91.
228. Ware JE, Sherbourne CD. The MOS 36-Item Short-Form Health Survey (SF-36): I. Conceptual framework and item selection. *Medical Care.* 1992;30:473-481.
229. Kazis LE, Lee A, Spiro A, 3rd, et al. Measurement comparisons of the medical outcomes study and veterans SF-36 health survey. *Health Care Financ Rev.* Summer 2004;25(4):43-58.
230. Kazis LE, Miller DR, Clark JA, et al. Improving the response choices on the veterans SF-36 health survey role functioning scales: results from the Veterans Health Study. *J Ambul Care Manage.* Jul-Sep 2004;27(3):263-280.

Appendix A.1: Summit Expert Panel and Guidance Advisers and Reviewers

Expert Panel Members Participating in the 11-15-07 OT/PT MTBI Summit

Carla Alexis, PT

Walter Reed Army Medical Center (WRAMC)

Allen Brown, MD

Mayo Clinic

TBI Model System of Care

Alison Cernich, PhD

Neuropsychologist

Baltimore VA

CPT Yadira DelToro, PT

Bethesda Navy Hospital

COL Mary Erickson, OTR

OTSG

COL Melissa Jones, PhD OT

WRAMC

Catherine Trombly Latham, ScD, OTR, FAOTA
Boston University

LTC Lynne Lowe, PT, DPT, OCS
OTSG

Karen McCulloch, PT, PhD, NCS
University of North Carolina

MAJ Matthew St. Laurent, OT
WRAMC

Ronald Tolchin, MD
Miami VA

Content Advisers and Reviewers

Betty Abreu, PhD, OTR/L, FAOTA
University of Texas Galveston
AOTA Representative

COL Robinette Amaker, PhD, OTR/L, CHT, FAOTA

Anne Armstrong, OT
Rehabilitation Institute of Chicago

Alison Cernich, PhD
Neuropsychologist
Baltimore VA

Rose Collins, PhD
Neuropsychologist
Minneapolis VA

Barbara Darkangelo, PT, DPT, NCS
Tampa VA

COL Mary Erickson, OTR
OTSG

Sharon Gutman, PhD, OTR/L
Columbia University, NY

COL Melissa Jones, PhD OT
WRAMC

Catherine Trombly Latham, ScD, OTR
Boston University

Lynnette Leuty, MSPT, NCS
Sister Kenny Rehabilitation Institute

Jeanne Lojovich, PT, PhD (cand), NCS
University of Minnesota

Karen McCulloch, PT, PhD, NCS
University of North Carolina

Pam Millington, PT, DPT, MS
Zablocki VA Medical Center
Milwaukee, WI

Marianne Mortera, PhD, OTR/L
Columbia University, NY

Melissa Oliver, MS OTR/L
Richamond VA

Michelle Peterson, PT, DPT, NCS
Minneapolis VA

Mandyleigh Smoot, MOT, OTR/L
Minneapolis VA

Jill Storms, OTR/L
Palo Alto VA

Deborah Voydetich, OTR/L
Minneapolis VA

Tammy Wagner, OTR/L
VAMC
Mountain Home, TN

APPENDIX B

Speech-Language Pathology

Clinical Management Guidance

Cognitive-Communication Rehabilitation

**For Combat-Related
Concussion/Mild Traumatic Brain Injury**

05 March 2012

Working Group to Develop Speech-Language Pathology Clinical Guidance for Cognitive-Communication Rehabilitation for Combat-Related Concussion/Mild Traumatic Brain Injury

Micaela Cornis-Pop, Ph.D., CCC-SLP
Richmond VA Medical Center

Shari Y. S. Goo-Yoshino, M.S., CCC-SLP
Tripler Army Medical Center

Don L. MacLennan, M.A., CCC-SLP
Minneapolis VA Medical Center

Linda M. Picon, M.C.D., CCC-SLP
Tampa VA Medical Center

Maile T. Singson, M.S., CCC-SLP
VA Pacific Island Healthcare System

Elaine M. Frank, Ph.D., CCC-SLP
University of South Carolina

Emi Isaki, Ph.D., CCC-SLP
Northern Arizona University

Pauline A. Mashima, Ph.D., CCC-SLP
Tripler Army Medical Center

Carole R. Roth, Ph.D., CCC-SLP
Naval Medical Center San Diego

Carol Smith Hammond, Ph.D., CCC-SLP
Durham VA Medical Center

Reviewers:

MAJ Beau Hendricks, USA
Ft. Hood, TX

Henry L. Lew, M.D., Ph.D.
Defense and Veterans Brain Injury Center

Diane R. Paul, Ph.D., CCC-SLP
Rockville, MD

McKay Moore Sohlberg, Ph.D., CCC-SLP
University of Oregon

Lyn S. Turkstra, Ph.D., CCC-SLP
University of Wisconsin-Madison

With support from: Rehabilitation and Reintegration Division, Health Policy and Services, Office of The Army Surgeon General.

Acknowledgements: Ms. Lei T. Colon-Yoshimoto, MAJ Sarah Goldman, COL William J. Howard, III (USA, Ret), LTC Christopher Klem (USA, Ret), LTC Lynne Lowe (USA, Ret), COL Suzanne D. Martin (USA, Ret), Dr. Lisa A. Newman, Ms. Gwen S. Niiya, COL Joseph C. Sniezek (USA), SGT Samuel Teague (USA

Table of Contents

1. Development of Clinical Management Guidance (CMG)

1.1 Objective

This document was developed to provide speech-language pathologists (SLPs) with clinical guidance for cognitive-communication interventions for Active Duty (AD) Service Members and Veterans (SMs/veterans) with cognitive-communication deficits after concussion/mild traumatic brain injury (mTBI).

A clinical toolkit with resources and examples of educational, assessment, and treatment materials accompanies this document.

1.2 Scope/Target Population

This Clinical Management Guidance (CMG) is intended to address the cognitive-communication needs of SMs/veterans who: a) are 18 years or older, b) have a history of concussion/mTBI, and c) are three months or more post injury with persistent cognitive-communication symptoms.

This guidance does NOT address: a) interventions for moderate or severe traumatic brain injury (TBI) managed in an inpatient setting, or b) concussion/mTBI in the acute phase (<3 months post injury). The VA/DoD Clinical Practice Guideline for Management of Concussion/Mild TBI (April, 2009) recommends that, between 7 days and 3 months post-injury, concussion/mTBI symptoms be addressed through education and by setting expectations for full resolution of symptoms.

1.3 Approach

This document is offered as guidance for clinical decision-making. Recommendations are based upon reviews of: a) research literature; b) existing guidelines and documents; c) consensus recommendations of experts with clinical experience in cognitive-communication rehabilitation within the Department of Defense (DoD), Department of Veterans Affairs (VA), and academia; and d) feedback from patients who participated in cognitive-communication interventions.

A Working Group comprised of subject matter experts from the DoD, VA, and the civilian sector convened in three face-to-face meetings in September 2008, November 2008, and September 2009, and met biweekly via WebMeeting from February through August 2009 to discuss the charge, define the scope of work, formulate a plan to meet the charge, develop an outline of the SLP CMG, assign writing sections, discuss and refine drafts of the document, and finalize recommendations based upon suggestions from an expert review panel. The SLP CMG was revised in January 2011 and January 2012 based upon feedback from the Proponency Office for Rehabilitation and Reintegration, Health Policy and Services, Office of The Army Surgeon General (OTASG). In 2010, the SLP Working Group was invited by OTASG to collaborate with occupational and physical therapists to develop the cognitive-communication section of the companion mTBI rehabilitation toolkit. The final draft of the toolkit was completed in March 2012.

1.4 Evidence-Based Practice

Evidence-based practice is an integration of: 1) best available current evidence, 2) clinical expertise, 3) clinical judgment, and 4) patient/family preferences and values with the goal of providing high-quality services reflecting the interests, needs, and choices of the individuals served (ASHA, 2005; Montgomery & Turkstra, 2003). References in this CMG, were shaped by the consensus conference on cognitive rehabilitation conducted by the Defense Center of Excellence for Psychological Health and Traumatic Brain Injury (DCoE) and the Defense and Veterans Brain Injury Center (DVBIC) (Helmick, 2010), and the "VA/DoD Clinical Practice Guideline for Management of Concussion/Mild Traumatic Brain Injury" (April 2009). The literature review was inclusive of research on moderate and severe TBI since studies specific to the mTBI population are sparse. Likewise, research on concussion/mTBI incurred in civilian settings (e.g., from sports injuries or motor vehicle crashes) was included in the review because literature on combat-related concussion/mTBI is still emerging. Despite differences between mTBI and moderate-to-severe TBI, as well as between concussion/mTBI sustained in combat versus civilian life, crossover of effectiveness of intervention strategies is reasonably expected. Recommendations also evolved through a consensus process for areas where research does not exist, is not sufficient, or is not of high quality. It is important to appreciate that insufficient evidence for the efficacy of cognitive-communication intervention with the mTBI population should not be interpreted as evidence for the lack of efficacy of such treatments (Ruff & Jamora, 2009; Institute of Medicine, 2011).

The SLP CMG document was reviewed by a panel of experts including: a) three SLPs with distinguished research careers, clinical expertise, and publications as subject matter experts in cognitive-communication rehabilitation for individuals with brain injury, b) a physiatrist/audiologist/researcher who serves as chair of an academic program in Communication Sciences and Disorders and as a consultant to the Defense and Veterans Brain Injury Center, and, c) a U.S. Army S3 Operations Officer who earned advanced degrees at the Command and General Staff College and the School of Advanced Military Studies after completing cognitive-communication rehabilitation and treatment for polytrauma injuries sustained during his deployment in Iraq.

1.5 Overview of Process

The following describes the process of developing and disseminating this CMG:

Phase 1: Define scope of work; identify best practices based on review of literature; solicit expert advice; conduct focus group with SM/veteran stakeholders; draft outline of document; determine the need for and identify additional subject matter experts; assign writing tasks and determine timeline for task completion.

Phase 2: Draft recommendations for each aspect of care based on review of literature and expert opinion; request funding for face-to-face meeting to finalize document.

Phase 3: Integrate feedback from external subject matter experts; finalize recommendations; explore avenues for continued support for project development and dissemination of outcomes; submit CPG document to the Office of the Surgeon General (OTSG) and the Veterans Health Administration (VHA).

Phase 4: Develop clinical toolkit; develop educational and mentoring programs to disseminate CPG; survey impact of CPG.

1.6 Overview of Format

This SLP CMG provides: 1) background of the target population including mechanisms of injury, co-morbidities, special aspects of mTBI in the military population; 2) overview of cognitive-communication deficits, and assessment and treatment modules for SMs/veterans with mTBI. Modules include background information (introduction/rationale), an "Action Statement" (summary/charge), recommendations, and discussion (literature synopsis to support recommendations).

2. Key Elements Addressed in the CMG

The following statements provide a summary of the key elements covered in this guidance. The CMG will provide the rationale, references, and more information for each of these statements.

2.1 Background of Mild Traumatic Brain Injury (mTBI) and the Military Experience

- Mild TBI, also known as concussion, is the most frequent type of brain injury in the civilian population. It is also one of the "invisible injuries" experienced by SMs who served the two theaters of operation in Iraq [Operation Iraqi Freedom (OIF)] which ended in December 2011, and Afghanistan [Operation Enduring Freedom (OEF)].
- Blasts are a leading cause of TBI for AD military personnel in war zones. The mechanisms of blast-related TBI may include both high-force blast waves and external force application.
- The diagnosis of mTBI is based on the injury event and the alteration of mental state immediately following the event.
- The recovery trajectory from mTBI sustained in combat may be different from that of the civilian cohort. The high incidence of blast-related mTBI, multiple injuries, and co-morbidities, particularly the psychologically traumatic component, complicate recovery from wartime mTBI.
- Symptoms associated with concussion are not specific to mTBI. They can occur in persons with other conditions such as chronic pain or depression, and can also be found in healthy individuals.
- DoD and VA have implemented TBI screening processes to help identify persons with possible TBI and provide appropriate services.

2.2 Cognitive-Communication Sequelae of mTBI and the Role of Speech-Language Pathologists (SLPs)

- Persistent mTBI symptoms may include cognitive-communication deficits that can cause significant functional disability.
- Cognitive-communication difficulties related to mTBI persisting beyond the acute phase of injury (3 months) should be assessed and treated symptomatically regardless of the time elapsed since injury or the confirmed etiology of the complaint.
- SLPs have a unique role in assessing and treating cognition as manifested through spoken and written communication (i.e., cognitive-communication symptoms).
- SLPs who provide cognitive-communication services to SMs/veterans with mTBI should be competent in brain injury rehabilitation and military/veteran culture and capable of developing a therapeutic alliance with their patients.
- It is essential that DoD and VA medical facilities recruit, train, and retain SLP providers with specific TBI expertise. Additionally, continued professional education in the areas of assessment and treatment of TBI and associated conditions is an ongoing need.

2.3 Assessment of Cognitive-Communication Disorders in the Target Population

- Speech-language pathology (SLP) screenings are used to identify individuals with potential cognitive-communication symptoms.
- A comprehensive assessment helps to determine the nature of the problem, establish the clinical indications for rehabilitation, and develop a treatment plan.
- Assessment tools should include standardized performance and self-report measures. These tools serve to determine the level of cognitive-communication functioning of the individual and to develop measurable treatment goals.
- To the extent possible, the cognitive-communication screening and evaluation should be incorporated into a comprehensive assessment process conducted by an interdisciplinary rehabilitation team.
- Upon completion of the assessment, the SLP (or interdisciplinary team, when available) should be able to determine the following:
  - o What is the nature of the cognitive-communication deficits, if present?
  - o Is cognitive rehabilitation needed? Warranted?
  - o What kinds of rehabilitation interventions are recommended?
  - o What are the short- and long-term goals (functional and measurable)?
- If, at any time after cognitive-communication problems are identified, the SM/veteran does not choose to engage in treatment, information should be made available to enable him/her to contact the appropriate DoD or VA medical facility for follow-up in the future.

2.4 Treatment of Cognitive-Communication Disorders in the Target Population

- Cognitive-communication rehabilitation should be grounded in scientific evidence including theoretical foundations of brain-behavior relationships, cognition, communication, neuroplasticity, learning theories, behavioral modification, and counseling.
- Clinical experience in treating SMs/veterans suggests that a comprehensive holistic approach that integrates treatment of cognitive-communication, emotional, and interpersonal skills is a "best practice model" for the rehabilitation of mTBI sequelae.
- Cognitive-communication rehabilitation is most effective when provided as part of an interdisciplinary team (IDT) approach. Alternatively, cognitive treatment can be offered as a discrete therapy, often assigned to SLP.
- Group treatment, in addition to individual treatment, provides a supportive context for rehabilitation and reinforces the concept of unit cohesion in military and veteran culture.
- The following are identified as potential areas for cognitive-communication interventions:
  - o Education about mTBI symptoms and recovery patterns that should target normalizing symptoms and recommending techniques to manage stress;
  - o Direct attention training;
  - o Selection and training of assistive technology for cognition, including devices to compensate for memory deficits;
  - o Metacognitive strategy training;
  - o Social communication training;
  - o Environmental modification and strategy training to support re-entry into community and vocational/educational activities.

- Treatment should address the unique needs of military and veteran populations with reference to returning to duty or work, balancing military and family relationships, readjusting to civilian life, and considering risk for post-traumatic stress and other co-morbidities.
- Cognitive-communication treatment goals, strategies, intensity, and duration of treatment should be based on the individual functional needs of the SM/veteran and reasonable expectations of improvement with treatment.
- Involvement of family members and the SM's Command is highly encouraged to optimize treatment outcomes.

2.5 Return to Duty and Community Re-entry

- Across each phase of treatment, identifying, assessing, and addressing community reintegration needs are key to successful transition and community reintegration.
- Discharge from cognitive-communication rehabilitation should be considered when the SM/veteran no longer requires the facilities, skills, and therapeutic intensity of SLP interventions to make progress and meet his/her cognitive-communication needs for social, vocational, and avocational activities.
- Follow-up visits should be scheduled, whenever possible, to monitor the transfer of treatment gains into the community environment, to refine strategies established in therapy, and to provide additional support, as necessary.
- Use of telehealth technologies can facilitate transition of care and treatment follow-up, and return of Reservists and National Guardsmen to their local communities.

3. Background of mTBI/Target Population

3.1 Definition of Traumatic Brain Injury (TBI)

Traumatic brain injury (TBI) refers to a traumatically induced structural injury and/or physiological disruption of brain function as a result of an external force that is indicated by new onset or worsening of at least one of the following clinical signs, immediately following the event (VA/DoD, 2009):

- Any period of loss of or a decreased level of consciousness (LOC);
- Any loss of memory for events immediately before or after the injury (post-traumatic amnesia [PTA]);
- Any alteration in mental state at the time of the injury (confusion, disorientation, slowed thinking, etc.) (Alteration of consciousness/mental state [AOC]);
- Neurological deficits (weakness, loss of balance, change in vision, praxis, paresis/plegia, sensory loss, aphasia, etc.) that may or may not be transient;
- Intracranial lesion.

External forces may include any of the following events:

- The head being struck by an object, the head striking an object,
- The brain undergoing an acceleration/deceleration movement without direct external trauma to the head,
- A foreign body penetrating the brain,
- Forces generated from events such as a blast or explosion, or other forces yet to be defined.

TBI severity is divided into mild, moderate, and severe categories, based on the length of LOC, AOC, or PTA, and the Glasgow Coma Scale results. Table B.1 summarizes the classification of TBI severity (VA/DoD, 2009).

Table B.1. Classification of TBI Severity (VA/DoD Clinical Practice Guideline for Management of Concussion/mTBI, 2009)

Criteria	Mild	Moderate	Severe
Structural imaging	Normal	Normal or abnormal	Normal or abnormal
Loss of Consciousness (LOC)	0-30 min	>30 min and <24 hrs	>24 hrs
Alteration of consciousness/ mental state (AOC)*	a moment up to 24 hrs	>24 hrs Severity based on other criteria	
Post-traumatic amnesia (PTA)	0-1 day	>1 and <7 days	>7 days
Glasgow Coma Scale (best available score in first 24 hrs)	13-15	9-12	<9

Alteration of mental state must be immediately related to the trauma to the head. Typical symptoms would be looking and feeling dazed and uncertain of what is happening, confusion, difficulty thinking clearly or responding appropriately to mental status questions, and being unable to describe events immediately before or after the trauma event.

A TBI resulting from an object passing through the skull into the brain, such as a bullet or fragments from an explosion, is called a penetrating brain injury. Penetrating brain injuries are classified as severe.

Each year in the United States, approximately 1 to 2 million people sustain a TBI (Thurman, Alverson, Dunn, Guerrero, & Sniezek, 1999); approximately 75% of patients who sustain TBI have mild TBI (Centers for Disease Control and Prevention (CDC), 2003).

3.2 mTBI or Concussion

The terms *mild TBI (mTBI)* and *concussion* are used interchangeably in this and other DoD and VA guidance documents (VA/DoD, 2009). Concussion/mTBI may result when injury triggers a pathologic neurochemical cascade but is insufficient to produce widespread neuronal dysfunction or the diffuse axonal disruption that characterizes more severe brain injuries (Silver, McAllister, & Arciniegas, 2009). In mTBI, there is often an absence of structural injury that can be reliably detected with conventional clinical neuroimaging. The formal definition of mTBI by the American Congress of Rehabilitation Medicine (1993) is presented in Table B.2.

Table B.2. Diagnostic Criteria for Mild Traumatic Brain Injury (American Congress of Rehabilitation Medicine, 1993)

I. Traumatically induced physiologic disruption of brain function as indicated by at least one of the following:

    A. Any period of loss of consciousness
    B. Any loss of memory for events immediately before or after the accident
    C. Any alteration in mental state at the time of the accident
    D. Focal neurologic deficits that may or may not be transient

II.   Severity of the injury does not exceed:
    A. Loss of consciousness of 30 min
    B. GCS score of 13–15 after 30 min
    C. Post-traumatic amnesia of 24 hr

3.3 Mechanisms of Injury in TBI

For the general population, the most common means of sustaining a TBI is through falls. Data from the CDC indicate that falls account for 28% of all reported TBIs. Following falls are motor vehicle-related incidents (20%). These include all incidents involving motor vehicles, bicycles, pedestrians, and recreational vehicles. Firearm use is the leading cause of death related to TBI (CDC, 1999). Blasts in combination with other mechanisms are a leading cause of TBI for AD military personnel in war zones (Warden, 2006).

Brain injuries can be classified as focal, diffuse, or mixed depending on the mechanism of injury and the host response. Focal damage, such as contusion or hematoma, can be appreciated by standard neuroimaging studies such as computed tomography (CT) or magnetic resonance imaging (MRI). Widespread disruption of neuronal circuitry or *diffuse axonal injury* (DAI) can be difficult to detect on standard neuroimaging. It is possible to have both focal and diffuse injuries from a single traumatic incident.

Focal lesions are usually the result of direct impact of the brain against the cranium, most often from impact with the frontal and temporal bones or the occipital bone. Focal injuries may also occur in penetrating TBI resulting from gunshot wounds, fragments, or missiles. The anterior and inferior frontal and temporal areas of the brain are those most commonly and most severely affected by impact forces (Bigler, 2007). Inertial and particularly rotational forces stretch and strain white matter in these and other areas (the upper brainstem, the parasagittal white matter of the cerebrum, the corpus callosum, and the gray-white matter junctions of the cerebral cortex), resulting in diffuse (or, more accurately, multifocal) axonal injury (Meythaler, Peduzzi, Eleftheriou, & Novack, 2001).

Traumatic brain injury is a frequent injury among U.S. military and civilian personnel who served in Iraq and Afghanistan (Hoge et al., 2008; Tanielian & Jacox, 2008; Terrio et al., 2009; Warden, 2006). The DoD and VA have implemented TBI screening procedures to help identify persons with possible TBI and to ensure that SMs/veterans receive appropriate follow-up services. The TBI screen consists of identifying any injury that resulted in an alteration of consciousness and determining current symptoms. SMs/veterans with positive TBI screens are then evaluated with a clinical interview to establish the TBI diagnosis and to make appropriate referrals. For OEF/OIF veterans entering the VA system of care, similar screening occurs upon presentation for medical care, regardless of entry portal. The purpose of this screening is to identify those in need of ongoing TBI related services.

Points to Remember

- Falls and motor vehicle crashes (MVCs) are the most common causes of TBI in the general population.
- Brain injuries can result in diffuse axonal injuries, focal lesions, or both depending on the mechanism of injury and the host response.
- Diffuse axonal injury results from inertial (rotational acceleration-deceleration) forces.
- Focal injuries are typically due to a direct blow to the head or penetrating head injury.
- DoD and VA have implemented TBI screening processes to help identify persons with possible TBI and initiate appropriate services.

3.3.1 Blast-Related mTBI

Blast-related mTBI is among the most common injuries experienced by U.S. military and civilian personnel who served in Iraq and Afghanistan. Data based on self-reports indicate that approximately 15% to 22% of troops deployed in OIF/OEF may have suffered a mTBI as a result of exposure to improvised explosive devices (IED) (Hoge et al., 2008; Tanielian & Jacox, 2008; Terrio et al., 2009; Warden, 2006).

Explosive mechanisms (e.g., IEDs, landmines, rocket-propelled grenades) account for 78% of injuries in servicemen and women injured in Afghanistan and Iraq, which is the highest proportion seen in any large-scale conflict (Owens et al., 2008). While blast-related injuries are not new, it is the use of IEDs with ever-increasing amounts of explosive (and sometimes toxic) materials that have become the hallmark of OEF/OIF.

IEDs and other explosive munitions can cause injury via high-force blast waves (primary blast injuries); or by penetration of expelled missile fragments (secondary injuries); or by being forcefully thrown against hard surfaces, or being crushed by collapsing objects (tertiary injuries); or from inhalation of gases and vapors or from anoxic injuries (quaternary blast injuries) (DePalma, Burris, Champion, & Hodgson, 2005; Taber, Warden, & Hurley, 2006). As such, exposure to blast-level forces can result in a multitude of injuries, including damage to internal organs, multiple fractures, amputations, burns, and TBI.

The effects of the high-force blast waves in the brain have received increased scrutiny in recent years. Primary blast most often damages air-filled organs, such as the lungs, colon, and the ear; or those filled with fluid, such as the eyes (DePalma et al., 2005). The effect of blast on the brain is more uncertain. The Institute of Medicine (2008), weighed on the side of accepting "biologic plausibility" of blast induced neurotrauma, and concluded that rigorous human studies are needed to examine the consequences of these injuries, their recovery trajectory, and factors that determine their outcome. In contrast to injury from the primary blast, secondary and tertiary blast injuries are mechanical injuries and would therefore likely be physiologically similar to brain injuries sustained from falls or MVCs.

The potential neuropsychological implications of exposure to blast are still uncertain. The existing TBI literature was created almost exclusively using data from individuals having sustained TBIs from blunt force trauma. Preliminary studies seem to indicate that neuropsychological consequences of blast related TBI are not very different from those of non-blast related TBI. Sayer et al. (2008) found that the mechanism of injury did not predict outcomes, such as changes in motor or cognitive functioning, as measured by the Functional Independence Measure. More pointedly, Belanger et al. (2009) suggest that cognitive sequelae following TBI are determined by severity of injury rather than the mechanism of injury. Overall, current literature does not provide strong evidence that blast is categorically different from other mechanisms of TBI, at least with regard to cognitive sequelae.

Points to Remember

- Blast exposure is one of the common causes of TBI in combat zones.
- The mechanisms of blast-related TBI can include both high-force blast waves and external force application.
- Preliminary data indicate that the neuropsychological effects of blast related TBI are not categorically different from those of non-blast related TBI.

3.3.2 Multiple mTBIs

A study of the Navy-Marine Corps Combat Trauma Registry revealed that the battle-injured were more likely than those injured outside of battle to have multiple TBIs (Galarneau, Woodruff, Dye, Mohrle, & Wade, 2008).

Most of the data regarding the impact of multiple concussions is derived from the sports literature, which suggests a possible cumulative effect of multiple concussions (De Beaumont, Lassonde, Leclerc, & Theoret, 2007; Pontifex, O'Connor, Broglio, & Hillman, 2009). With regard to long-term outcomes, the threshold for frequency and severity of concussion has yet to be established. There is concern that a second concussion prior to complete recovery from the first injury may pose increased risk for poorer eventual functional and vocational outcome and greater symptoms than would be expected from either of the injuries separately (Macciocchi, Barth, Littlefield, & Cantu, 2001).

Finally, the cumulative effect of two or more TBIs that occur well after full recovery from the initial injury may still result in worsened outcomes and greater symptoms than would otherwise have been expected with either injury in isolation (Iverson, Gaetz, Lovell, & Collins, 2004). Multiple mTBIs are of particular concern in the veteran population and current military cohorts given their exposure to multiple combat-related events that can result in brain injury.

Points to Remember

- Incidence of multiple concussions is higher in combat-injured veterans than in those injured outside battle.
- There is growing evidence of negative effects of multiple concussions on long-term neuropsychological outcomes.

3.4 The Natural History of mTBI

Immediately following mTBI, cognitive, emotional, behavioral, physical, and psychosocial problems are frequent and may be a source of temporary disability and stress for TBI survivors. The overwhelming majority of people who sustain mTBI recover fully in a matter of days to a couple of months (Dikmen, Machamer, & Temkin, 2001). Some, however, may develop chronic neuropsychological problems and significant disability

(Vanderploeg, Curtiss, Luis, & Salazar, 2007). It is not clear how long it takes to recover from mTBI, what the predictors of positive or negative outcomes are, and what treatments best promote recovery.

A large number of studies and several recent meta-analyses have shown that trauma patients and athletes often report extensive symptoms and perform poorly on neuropsychological tests in the initial days and up to the first month following the mTBI (McCrea et al., 2003; Carroll, Cassidy, Holm, Kraus, & Coronado, 2004; Belanger & Vanderploeg, 2005). Headache is the most commonly reported symptom in mTBI, with dizziness also frequently reported. Immediate symptoms such as nausea, vomiting, and drowsiness are typically short-lived. Other possible symptoms include decreased concentration, slowed information processing speed, fatigue, and irritability. Most severe symptoms occur immediately after the injury. Within a week to one month from injury, the vast majority of people with mTBI return to baseline level on neuropsychological testing (McCrea et al., 2003).

A small minority of people, estimated at approximately 5% (McCrea, 2008) to 15% (Helmick, 2010; Ruff & Jamora, 2009) continue to exhibit physical, cognitive and/or behavioral symptoms for more than three to six months after injury. These are known as post-concussive symptoms (PCS). If symptoms continue beyond 12 months post-injury, the term *persistent* post-concussion symptoms can apply. When distant from the time of the injury, PCS tend to be non-specific and the etiology is not always clear. It is important to note that mTBI is not the only predictor of PCS. Multiple factors including demographic, psychiatric, and social support variables, and mTBI co-morbidities and their interactions all contribute to ongoing PCS in persons with mTBI (Vanderploeg, Belanger, & Curtis, 2009).

The most common system for defining and diagnosing post-concussion syndrome comes from the 10th edition of the International Classification of Diseases (ICD-10). See Table B.3.

Table B.3. ICD-10 Diagnostic Criteria for Post-Concussion Syndrome

A. A history of head trauma with loss of consciousness precedes symptom onset by maximum of four weeks.

B. Symptoms in three or more of the following symptom categories:
    - Headache, dizziness, malaise, excessive fatigue, noise intolerance
    - Irritability, depression, anxiety, emotional lability
    - Subjective complaints of concentration or memory difficulty
    - Reduced alcohol tolerance
    - Preoccupation with above symptoms and fear of brain damage

Several points related to the ICD-10 criteria warrant further discussion. First, it is not clear what the minimum threshold for injury is that would result in post-concussion syndrome. There is general acceptance in clinical practice and research that mTBI can occur without loss of consciousness. In such cases, it becomes difficult to determine whether a "being dazed and confused" episode is causally related to PCS occurring many months after the injury. At the same time, there is now substantial literature showing that PCS are not specific to brain injury. Rather, PCS occur among individuals with various medical and psychological disorders (Hoge et al., 2008) and even in the healthy population (Vasterling et al., 2006).

The nature of treatment for concussion/mTBI symptoms depends on the time post-injury when the patient enters clinical care. In the acute phase of uncomplicated TBI (<3 months), treatment typically includes education, counseling, and a period of rest and observation. Education regarding fatigue, irritability, and mood lability that may occur during recovery has been shown to facilitate improvement and lessen the likelihood that the patient develops persistent PCS (Mittenberg, Tremont, Zielinski, Fichera, & Rayls, 1996). Recommendations regarding return to partial or full-time work are tailored to the individual depending on the speed of recovery.

Symptomatic interventions for cognitive-communication difficulties related to PCS (>3 months post injury) can be effective in lessening the functional impact of the disability. There is increasing evidence that functional improvements may continue years post-injury and that SMs/veterans can be effectively supported through active treatment (Draper & Ponsford, 2008). Additionally, interventions to reduce the level of functional disability caused by cognitive-communication symptoms should be considered irrespective of whether the etiology of the symptoms can be teased out among presenting co-morbidities (Cornis-Pop, 2008).

Points to Remember

- The overwhelming majority of people who suffer mTBI recover fully in a matter of days to months.
- Approximately 5% to 15% of all individuals who sustain mTBI may experience prolonged symptoms and require ongoing medical care.
- PCS typically are not specific to brain injury, and therefore are difficult to assess and treat.
- Educational intervention in the acute phase of mTBI can significantly reduce the extent of post-concussive symptoms.
- Cognitive-communication difficulties related to PCS should be assessed and treated symptomatically regardless of the time elapsed since injury or the etiology of the complaint.

3.5 Co-Morbidities of mTBI – The Military Experience

The same combat exposure that causes mTBI may also result in other co-morbidities. In contrast to civilian settings, recovery from combat-related concussion/mTBI is complicated by at least four factors:

1. The physically and emotionally traumatic circumstances in which injuries are sustained;
2. The potentially repetitive and cumulative nature of concussions sustained over a tour (or multiple tours) of combat duty;
3. The high incidence of co-morbid mental health conditions (Tanielian & Jacox, 2008; Hoge et al., 2008);
4. The difficulty in following typical recommendations for post-concussion care (e.g., rest) in the deployed setting.

Common post-deployment co-morbid conditions, such as post-traumatic stress disorder (PTSD), pain conditions, amputations, acute stress reactions, and substance use also can result in symptoms overlapping with TBI. Mental health co-morbidities are common in the SM/veteran population including PTSD, depression, anxiety, and somatoform disorders. Other complications include frequent auditory and visual dysfunction and exacerbations of pre-existing conditions.

In addition to the co-morbid conditions, returning SMs/veterans presenting to military or VA healthcare facilities often have numerous psychosocial and financial stressors. The normal psychological adaptations that occur in a theatre of war are referred to as "battlemind." Readjustment from a "battlemind" state to a civilian mind-set and environment is neither instantaneous nor easy for individuals returning home (Munroe, 2005).

It is reasonable to assume that the overall recovery process is more complicated and prolonged in OEF/OIF veterans with mTBI and co-morbid conditions than in veterans without these conditions, or than in civilians.

3.5.1 mTBI and Post Traumatic Stress Disorder (PTSD)

Recent combat service is frequently associated with TBI, PTSD, and depression. In the RAND study (Tanielian & Jacox, 2008), 37.4 percent of those individuals with an mTBI history also had either PTSD or depression. Similar findings are reported in a VA study in which 42 percent of OEF/OIF veterans with an mTBI history also had PTSD symptoms (Lew, Poole, et al., 2007). Hoge et al. (2008) also found that more than 40% of soldiers who had symptoms associated with mTBI with loss of consciousness also met criteria for PTSD.

Overlapping symptoms impede understanding of the relationship between PTSD and mTBI (Hoge et al., 2008). Because cognitive impairments such as decreased memory and attention/concentration can occur in mTBI, depression, and PTSD, it can be difficult to determine the presence or absence of an independently recognizable, "pure" post-concussion syndrome. The symptoms of co-morbid PTSD (associated with intrusive thoughts, concentration difficulty, and poor sleep) interfere with normal cognitive functioning. On the other hand, the cognitive impairment and emotional dyscontrol associated with mTBI are detrimental to the resilience essential to overcoming PTSD (Vanderploeg et al., 2009).

For individuals with co-morbid mTBI and PTSD, studies have shown that established treatments for PTSD may need to be modified given the potential interference of TBI-related cognitive compromise. Vanderploeg et al., (2009) showed that the combination of mTBI and PTSD is associated with more complicated and prolonged recovery and that there are no empirically validated treatments for this population. The appropriate timing of treating either co-morbidity is a matter of clinical judgment - one size does not fit all (Knight, 2008). When symptoms of PTSD and mTBI co-exist, they can be addressed sequentially or concurrently. If a determination is made to address them sequentially, arguments can be made to treat one first over the other. The choice will depend in large measure on the amount of distress experienced and the person's tolerance within sessions and between sessions. A "best practice model" would require engaging the SM/veteran in coordinated treatment of both PTSD and mTBI sequelae (Vanderploeg et al., 2009).

3.5.2 mTBI and Depression

After mTBI, as individuals attempt to return to their prior roles, physical and cognitive difficulties may become more apparent and, consequently, psychological adjustment problems may develop leading to depression. Estimates of post-traumatic depression range from 10%

to 77% (Alderfer, Arciniegas, & Silver, 2005). The risk of developing depression is higher in the first year after TBI, but it remains elevated in later years.

As with mTBI and PTSD, the interaction between co-morbid mTBI and depression is bi-directional. Depression has been shown to be associated with an increase in the number and perceived severity of mTBI symptoms. Co-morbid depression may also increase anger, aggression, the risk of suicide, and cognitive dysfunction (Fann, Katon, Uomoto, & Esselman, 1995). Alternatively, impaired daily functioning and the experience of other psychosocial changes after mTBI may exacerbate depressive symptoms (Pagulayan, Hoffman, Temkin, Machamer, & Dikemen, 2008).

Other factors such as sleep disturbance, fatigue, problems with concentration, and apathy may produce apparent depressive symptoms. However, when there are sufficient symptoms to merit a diagnosis of depression—regardless of the possible causes—treatment should be promptly initiated both to improve mood and to mitigate its adverse effects on cognitive, behavioral, physical, and psychosocial functioning (Fann, Uomoto, & Katon, 2001).

3.5.3 mTBI and Headaches/Pain

Pain is common in SMs/veterans with mTBI. Headache is the most frequent pain complaint, but other pain sources, either musculoskeletal or neuropathic, also occur. Post-traumatic headaches develop within seven days of head trauma in up to 90% of all individuals who sustain a concussion (Lew et al., 2006). Most post-traumatic headaches resolve within three to six months following injury. However, chronic headaches beyond one year post-injury may be present in 50 to 93% of OEF/OIF SMs/veterans with mTBI (Hoge et al., 2008; Ruff, Ruff, & Wang, 2008).

Evaluating pain and treating it symptomatically is important as pain is associated with poor outcomes in TBI. Treatment depends on the etiology of the pain and should focus on interventions that are least likely to cause cognitive side effects and abuse. Specific treatment options include short-term use of medication, conventional physical therapy, biofeedback, and psychotherapy for the development of coping techniques. The use of cognitive behavioral therapy may be effective, but more difficult to use in SMs/veterans with TBI due to cognitive demands (Scholten & Walker, 2009). With such individuals, a holistic approach to rehabilitation, where cognitive behavioral therapy is provided in the broader context of a team based cognitive rehabilitation, could be a "best practice model."

3.5.4 mTBI and Substance Abuse

Substance use disorders and TBI may occur together. Alcohol use may be a cause and also a consequence of TBI. Alcohol use is a recognized risk factor for motor vehicle injuries, falls, and violence, all of which are frequent causes of TBI. Studies have shown that one-third to one-half of persons with TBI are intoxicated at the time of their injuries (Parry-Jones, Vaughan, & Cox, 2006). Alcohol use may also persist after TBI. While drinking may initially decrease after the TBI event, it has been shown to increase by two years post-injury in many individuals (Ponsford, Whelan-Goodinson, & Bahar-Fuchs, 2007). Neurological deficits associated with TBI may explain the increased susceptibility of individuals with TBI to substance use disorders.

The goals of therapy for TBI and substance use disorders may be viewed as complementary. Enhancing the ability of SMs/veterans to cope with cognitive and emotional impairments associated with TBI is also critical for managing the patterns of behavior that sustain addiction. The complexity of co-occurring TBI and substance use disorders may necessitate the development of new treatment concepts to address these combined disorders (Corrigan & Cole, 2008).

3.5.5 mTBI and Sensory Impairments

Visual impairments occur in up to half of all individuals who sustain mTBI. Typical symptoms include sensitivity to light, diplopia, blurring of vision and other difficulties in visual acuity. In turn, these can cause pain, headache and eye ache. Visual symptoms of mTBI tend to resolve within a month from the time of the injury (Goodrich, Kirby, Cockerham, Ingalla, & Lew, 2007).

The visual impairments of mTBI may negatively impact the individual's ability to engage in education, employment, and activities of daily living. SLPs who provide services for individuals with mTBI should be observant for visual impairments and facilitate referrals to specialists. Treatments of visual difficulties generally target symptom management: reassurance, pain management, controlling environmental light, sunglasses, and intermittent patching for double vision (Brahm et al., 2009).

Hearing difficulties resulting from head trauma with damage to the auditory system can occur anywhere from the outer ear, middle ear, and inner ear to the auditory cortex. In studies of SMs/veterans with TBI, hearing impairments were reported in approximately 30% of SMs/veterans, and complaints of tinnitus were reported in approximately 25% {Jury, 2001 #101;Lew, 2007 #100}.

Injuries to the auditory system are common in individuals who sustained a blast-related concussion. Up to three-quarters of those with a blast-related concussion experience altered acuity and sensitivity to noise during the first month following the injury. The majority of those symptoms resolve, though complaints of hearing loss may persist well beyond the acute phase of the injury (Lew, Jerger, et al., 2007).

When hearing loss is suspected in an individual with a blast-related concussion, referrals should be initiated for complete otologic and hearing examinations. Recommended treatments include controlling environmental noise, using white noise generators, prescribing assistive listening devices and hearing aids, and counseling/education. The collaboration between SLPs and audiologists can be particularly effective when providing auditory training and rehabilitation services for SMs/veterans with hearing difficulties due to mTBI.

Points to Remember

- The same combat exposure that causes mTBI may also result in other co-morbidities, particularly PTSD.
- Common post-deployment issues, such as PTSD, pain conditions, acute stress reactions, depression, and substance use also can result in numerous symptoms overlapping with mTBI.
- It is reasonable to assume that the overall recovery process will be more complicated and prolonged in the OEF/OIF veterans with mTBI and co-morbid conditions.
- SLPs should be particularly vigilant for signs of vision, hearing, and vestibular impairments in the SM/veteran with TBI.

4. Special Aspects of mTBI in the Military Experience

4.1 Environment of Care – Echelons of Care

BACKGROUND

The United States has been engaged in military conflict in Afghanistan and Iraq since 2001. Improvements in body armor and advances in medical care have resulted in the highest survival rate of wounded SMs from any previous conflicts in U.S. history (Gawande, 2004). A study (Murray et al., 2005) found that 88% of military personnel treated at a medical unit in Iraq had been injured by IEDs or mortar. A VA-based study found that 56% of its war-injured sample had been injured by blasts (Sayer et al., 2008). Survival of the wounded SM has highlighted issues of TBI and PTSD in returning troops.

The true incidence of mTBI among military troops remains largely unknown, as many either do not seek immediate medical care or receive a diagnosis long after the injury, when the details of the event are more difficult to establish. There is no question, however, that mTBI is one of the most common injuries sustained by our Warriors (Helmick, 2010). Data from combat-exposed military personnel returning from Afghanistan and Iraq since 2001 report a 15% to 22% mTBI incidence rate (Hogue et al., 2008; Terrio et al., 2009).

Neurocognitive assessment is an important part of a comprehensive approach to care for mTBI in the theater of operations. Medics in the field screen troops for TBI using the Military Acute Concussion Evaluation (MACE) tool developed by DVBIC. The history component of this measure can confirm the diagnosis of mTBI and provide further assessment data by utilizing the Standardized Assessment of Concussion (SAC) (McCrea, Kelly, & Randolph, 2000) to preliminarily document neurocognitive deficits. The four cognitive domains tested are: orientation, immediate memory, concentration, and delayed recall.

The MACE is the recommended tool for use in theater at Levels I, II, and III. Level I is the Battalion Aide Station staffed by a Combat Medic and provides immediate treatment and transport. Both the medic and the casualty are still under fire and there is limited medical equipment available. Triage outcome at this level is either return to duty with minimal treatment, or evacuate to Level II echelon of care that ideally is less than one hour away.

Level II echelon of care generally comprises a Forward Surgical Team (FST) ranging from 5 to 20 personnel, including orthopedic and general surgeons, nurse anesthetists, critical care nurses and technicians. The team is able to perform life-saving resuscitative surgery. Evacuation to Level III echelon of care is up to 24 hours after injury and may take several hours of transport to access, depending on mode of travel and distance.

Level III is defined by a Combat Support Hospital (CSH), Navy ships, or Air Force Theater Hospitals which is capable of further definitive care, still rendered within the combat zone. The Level III team is capable of providing resuscitation, initial surgery, definitive and re-constructive surgery, post-operative care, and intensive care for either return to duty in theater or stabilization for further evacuation. Some facilities are quite large, accommodating up to 300 patients in their full complement of intensive care unit (ICU) beds, intermediate care beds, ward care, and up to eight surgical tables. Within 48 to 72 hours, a strategic evacuation can be underway to the next level of care out of the combat theater.

When injuries are extremely severe, requiring Level IV echelon of care, evacuation can occur within 12 hours or less from the time of injury. Level IV is the definitive care stop at the general hospital that is en route to the continental United States (CONUS). For OEF/OIF this is Landstuhl Regional Medical Center (LRMC) in Germany. Level IV echelon of care treats complex injuries. The hospital is staffed and equipped for general and specialized medical and surgical care. Those SMs not expected to return to duty within the theater are stabilized and evacuated to CONUS. Those SMs who will be returned to duty within the theater are provided reconditioning and rehabilitative services. Virtually 100% of U.S. troops injured in OEF/OIF pass through LRMC before returning to duty or being transferred to CONUS medical facilities. When it is determined that the SM needs further evaluation and/or intervention and is not able to remain in combat, he/she is medically evacuated to one of four military treatment facilities (MTF) in the United States: Walter Reed Army Medical Center, Naval Medical Center Bethesda, Brooke Army Medical Center, or Naval Medical Center San Diego.

A recent advancement in the medical care provided at the front is the establishment of several Level 2 TBI Centers in theater that have the capacity to rehabilitate casualties who experience events associated with TBI. A group of specially trained experts evaluates blast injury patients within 24 hours of the injury to assess for indications of TBI with a battery of tests including hearing, vestibular function, and cognition. Cognitive exercises include memory quizzes and timed maze completion (Hoffer, 2009).

Early detection of the symptoms of mTBI has been promoted at all levels of military medical care, resulting in more immediate evaluation and treatment than ever before. All SMs with multiple injuries are screened for concussion and military medics and corpsmen are now being trained to assess for TBI on the battlefield.

4.2 Veterans Administration (VA) Polytrauma/Traumatic Brain Injury System of Care

BACKGROUND

Department of Veterans Affairs (VA) facilities may provide health care to SMs and their beneficiaries on a referral basis under the auspices of a sharing agreement. All VA facilities have been directed to become TRICARE network providers. This action has been taken to ensure VA's ability to meet its responsibility to provide timely care to SMs returning from theaters of war.

Additionally, there has been a long-standing Memorandum of Agreement (MOA) between VA and DoD for the provision of specialized care for SMs sustaining spinal cord injury (SCI), TBI, and blindness. VA is known for its integrated health care system for the treatment of these conditions. The MOA provides opportunities for AD military personnel to receive timely and high quality specialty care within a continuum of health care services dedicated to the needs of persons with SCI, TBI, and blindness.

VA receives referrals for health care services from MTFs or TRICARE Service Centers through clinical orders or authorization for care. The point of contact (POC) for VA-DoD issues at each VA facility receives and expedites referrals and transfers of care and ensures that the appropriate linkage is made for the requested clinical services. It is VA policy that injured and ill SMs are transitioned seamlessly from MTFs to VA facilities and that the care of all SMs/veterans treated at VA facilities is coordinated, monitored, and tracked.

4.2.1 VA Polytrauma/TBI System of Care (PSC)

The VA Polytrauma/TBI System of Care (PSC) is a nationwide integrated system of more than 100 facilities with specialized rehabilitation programs for veterans and SMs. The mission of the PSC is to ensure that veterans and SMs have access to the full continuum of specialized rehabilitation services, case management, family education and support, psychosocial services, and community re-integration assistance.

PSC is organized into a four-tier system of hub and spokes facilities that include four Polytrauma Rehabilitation Centers (PRC) serving as regional referral centers for acute medical and rehabilitation care. They provide national leadership in clinical research, education, and training. The four PRCs are located at the medical centers in Richmond, Tampa, Minneapolis, and Palo Alto.

Polytrauma Network Sites (PNS) (22 sites) serve veterans/SMs in each of the Veterans Integrated Service Networks (VISN) and provide key components of post-acute rehabilitation care and case management. Services may be provided in inpatient, outpatient, and community-based settings.

Polytrauma Support Clinic Teams (PSCT) (82 programs) are responsible for managing veterans/SMs with TBI and polytrauma within their geographical catchment area. These teams address chronic and emerging medical and psychosocial problems that affect community re-integration.

Polytrauma Points of Contact (PPOC) (48 POCs) are designated at VA facilities without specialized rehabilitation capabilities. Their role is to manage referrals for TBI and polytrauma rehabilitation and to coordinate such services.

PSC either directly provides, or formally links with, key components of rehabilitation care including, but not limited to, inpatient rehabilitation, outpatient rehabilitation, emerging consciousness programs, transitional rehabilitation, day programs, and community re-entry programs. The hallmark of rehabilitative care in PSC is interdisciplinary team (IDT) interventions by specialists who work collaboratively to identify veterans' rehabilitation needs and to develop treatment plans to meet those needs. SLPs are core members of the IDT in PSC and provide a full range of services including swallowing, voice, language, and cognitive-communication interventions.

Cognitive rehabilitation for TBI sequelae is a well-established area of practice in the VA. These services are delivered by IDTs of rehabilitation specialists in a variety of settings including acute, transitional, outpatient, and re-integrated in the community. Cognitive rehabilitation can take many forms, including modeling, guided practice, distributed practice, errorless learning, direct instruction with feedback, neurofeedback (EEG biofeedback), computer-assisted retraining programs, and use of memory aids. The interventions can be provided in either one-on-one or in a small group setting. SLPs in the VA are active providers of cognitive-communication services and receive ongoing education and training to support them in this role.

4.2.2 TBI Screening and Evaluation in the VA

Since April 2007, all OEF/OIF veterans who come to the VA for health care services are screened for possible TBI. Veterans who screen positive are offered referral for a comprehensive medical evaluation and follow-up services, as indicated. Veterans who already have a TBI diagnosis may also be referred for further specialized evaluation and follow-up, depending on their established needs.

The TBI screening tool consists of four sections that address: (a) identification of events that increase the risk of TBI, (b) alteration of consciousness related to the event, (c) symptoms immediately following this event, and (d) current symptoms associated with TBI. If a person responds positively to one or more questions in each of the four sections, the screen is positive. Veterans who screen positive for TBI are offered referral for a comprehensive evaluation to confirm a diagnosis and to provide treatment and follow-up for associated symptoms. Completion of the comprehensive evaluation determines the presence of a TBI (vs. other causes for their symptoms) and assists with developing a treatment plan.

5. Cognitive-Communication Deficits in mTBI

BACKGROUND

Cognitive-communication deficits are observed when changes in cognition adversely affect communication and language abilities (ASHA, 2005). Cognitive deficits often result in communication impairment because of the complex, dynamic interactions among cognition, language, and speech. Linguistic processes are critical to the acquisition of knowledge and mediate cognitive processes (ASHA, retrieved 14 Jun 2009; Cicerone et al., 2000).

A pilot study was conducted with injured veterans, caregivers, and clinicians using semi-structured interviews to identify challenges faced by OEF/OIF veterans as they transition and reintegrate into their communities. Findings highlighted specific difficulties across three functional domains of the World Health Organization's International Classification of Functioning, Disability and Health (Resnik & Allen, 2007).

- Challenges in *communication* included: difficulties with word finding, sustaining a conversation, recalling conversations because of memory impairments, social pragmatics;
- Challenges in the areas of *learning and applying knowledge* included: acquiring complex skills, focusing attention, remembering important information, solving problems, reading lengthy and complex material, planning, participating and succeeding in learning activities and decision making, generating alternative solutions;
- Challenges in the areas of *general tasks and demands* included: undertaking multiple tasks, organizing and managing time.

The following is a summary of cognitive-communication domains. Refer to Table 4 for a list of cognitive changes in mTBI and potential effects on function and communication.

5.1 Attention

Attention impairments are common after mTBI. Problems with attention are likely to affect other cognitive processes including memory and executive functions (Cicerone, 2002; Lezak, 2004).

Attention problems after TBI are seen particularly with novel and timed tasks. Difficulties are due, in part, to slowed information processing speed associated with diffuse axonal injury (Stuss et al., 1989) and problems with controlling and allocating attention resources resulting from injury to the dorsolateral aspects of the frontal lobes. Common functional complaints related to attention problems include:

- Difficulty completing tasks, reading lengthy materials, or following the plot line of a movie (may indicate problems with <u>sustained attention</u>);
- Distractibility or poor concentration when other activities are occurring in the immediate environment (may be related to impaired <u>selective attention</u>);
- Decreased ability to shift from task to task or to multitask (may indicate impaired <u>alternating attention</u>).

5.2 Speed of Processing

Information processing speed refers to the ability to perceive, attend to, organize, analyze, integrate, retain, and apply information in an efficient manner. Rather than a cognitive function in itself, speed of processing refers to how well incoming information can be processed through the various linguistic and non-linguistic components of the cognitive system to result in a desired output. A conceptual model of cognitive processing (Vanderploeg, 2000), shows speed and efficiency as dependent on the integrity of underlying cognitive functions and their connections. From reflexive responses that go directly from sensory-perceptual functions to motor responses, to those that require higher order abstraction and reasoning, disruptions in necessary aspects of the feedback loop will result in cognitive impairment and/or compromised speed and efficiency of processing. Increased complexity of information to be processed is directly related to speed (Tombaugh, Rees, Stormer, Harrison, & Smith, 2007) given the greater number of interrelated cognitive components that must be employed.

Individuals who experience difficulty at any of the levels of cognitive processing will have problems responding appropriately to incoming information during daily functioning. Slowing of information processing capacity has been shown to affect various cognitive and communication processes such as encoding information, verbal comprehension, and adaptive responding to novel situations (Felmingham, Baguley, & Green, 2004). Functionally, individuals may report experiencing problems with a wide range of daily tasks such as processing information over the telephone, processing verbal or written instructions at work or at school, learning and integrating new information, and effectively participating in social communication and "reading" other people's feelings, opinions and intentions.

These problems may become more prominent when tasks require more mental control and are less automatic. People who have sustained mTBIs often report that their thinking is less automatic and that it requires more effort to respond appropriately (Cicerone, 1996). As such, cognitive fatigue may occur at a lower threshold of mental effort than it did prior to the injury, and trigger symptoms such as headaches or irritability that, in turn, may further tax the speed and capacity of the information processing system.

Problems with speed of processing or problems related to a reduced capacity for information processing may be difficult to capture in the clinical setting, as individuals with mTBI tend to perform adequately under structured, single-task testing conditions and for finite periods of time. To best identify efficient and sustained processing skills, it is necessary to use measures that require higher levels of sustained effort than are typically associated with standardized tests or measures that most resemble the multi-faceted demands of the workplace. In fact, it is measures of complex speed of processing (e.g., conceptual/semantic processing), along with working memory and attention that show the most potential for being sensitive to cognitive dysfunction after mTBI (Frencham, Fox, & Mayberry, 2005; Tombaugh et. al., 2007).

5.3 Memory

Memory deficits are a common consequence of mTBI that affect working memory (the ability to hold information in mind and manipulate it), episodic recall (remembering information that is linked to a specific time and place), and new learning of episodic and semantic (fact) information. Individuals identified with attention problems frequently also exhibit difficulties on memory tasks (Mateer & Sira, 2006).

Based on clinical experience, SMs/veterans with concussion/mTBI frequently report forgetting appointments, directions/instructions, names of individuals, and losing or misplacing items such as keys, cell phones, and identification badges/cards. These problems present significant barriers for many SMs/veterans at work or school, and in activities of daily living.

5.4 Executive Functions

The prefrontal cortex, which is likely to be injured during blunt force trauma, is associated with the processes of executive function. Cicerone et al. (2000) define executive functions as "cognitive processes that determine goal-directed and purposeful behavior and are super-ordinate in the orderly execution of daily life functions. These processes include the ability to: a) establish goals; b) initiate behavior; c) anticipate consequences of actions; d) plan and organize behaviors according to spatial, temporal, topical or logical sequences; and e) monitor and adapt behavior to fit a particular task or context" (p. 1605).

Executive functions are comprised of a set of skills rather than a single skill. An integration of these skills is necessary to complete complex activities successfully (Kennedy & Coelho, 2005). Executive function disorders following mTBI are heterogeneous (Kennedy et al., 2008); resulting in different profiles of executive function strengths and weaknesses.

5.5 Social Communication

Social communication refers to verbal and nonverbal communication skills necessary to be successful in social situations (Turkstra, 2009). It involves integration of linguistic (Cummings, 2007), cognitive (Godfrey & Shum, 2000; Moran & Gillon, 2005), and behavioral (Ylvisaker, Turkstra, & Coelho, 2005) processes and requires speed and agility in formulating comments that directly address the topic at hand, controlling utterance length to avoid monopolizing the conversation, taking the perspective of others, and using both verbal and non-verbal methods to convey stated and implied meaning (Burgess & Turkstra, 2006). Impairments in social communication may result from both cognitive and behavioral changes associated with concussion/mTBI and co-morbid conditions such as PTSD.

5.6 Acquired Stuttering and Other Speech Dysfluencies

Starkweather (1987) defined fluency as "the ability to talk with normal levels of continuity, rate, and effort" (p. 12). Fluency is recognized by the ease and rapidity with which words are produced. It is having words at one's command and producing them easily and smoothly. This latter definition encompasses aspects of both speech and language. Perkins (1971) suggested that when observers judge the fluency of a speaker they are probably judging the "adequacy of performance of the semantic, syntactic, morphemic, and prosodic dimensions of speech" (p. 92).

Table B4. Cognitive Changes in mTBI and Potential Effects on Function and Communication

Cognitive Domain	Changes Due to mTBI	Effects on Function and Communication
Attention	Lapses in sustained attention Highly distractible Decreased concentration Poor performance on competing tasks or stimuli	Difficulty responding appropriately to incoming information Difficulty learning new information Difficulty filtering out irrelevant stimuli Difficulty conversing in situations with distractions, background noise, and multiple participants Difficulty managing the demands of high-level activity Difficulty sustaining attention when reading complex and/or lengthy material Difficulty shifting attention as needed Difficulty maintaining or changing topics in conversation Tangential discourse Social avoidance to compensate for sense of overstimulation (Because attention is the foundation of other cognitive processes, problems in attention are likely to result in or compound impairment in other processes including memory and executive functions)
Speed of Processing	Slowness in processing information	Delayed response time Difficulty making decisions Difficulty comprehending rapid rate of speech Slowness when interacting in social situations Difficulty staying on topic Long pauses within discourse

Memory	Impaired memory Problems with new learning	Difficulty recalling instructions or messages Difficulty learning new information Difficulty remembering names of individuals, appointments, directions, location of personal effects (e.g., keys, cell phones, identification cards, head gear) Difficulty recalling details when reading complex and/or lengthy material Difficulty maintaining topic or remembering purpose of conversation Repetition of ideas, statements, questions, conversations or stories Failure to use compensatory strategies to improve performance on everyday tasks
Executive Functions	Disorganized thoughts and actions Ineffective planning Reduced initiation Decreased insight Ineffective reasoning, judgment, and problem solving Decreased mental flexibility Difficulties in self-monitoring performance and assessing personal strengths and needs Impulsivity and disinhibition	Lack of coherence in discourse Lack of organization in planning daily activities Difficulty implementing plans and actions Difficulty initiating conversations Problems recognizing and repairing conversational breakdowns Inability to determine the needs of communication partners Difficulty making inferences or drawing conclusions Difficulty assuming another person's perspective Difficulty interpreting the behavior of others Difficulty evaluating validity of information Verbose; lack of conciseness in verbal expression Decreased comprehension of abstract language, humor, indirect requests Difficulty meeting timelines Difficulty formulating realistic goals Difficulty recognizing complexity of tasks and need for simplification Difficulty anticipating consequences of actions Inappropriate comments

Hartley (1995); Sohlberg (2009); Sohlberg & Mateer (2001)

Fluency includes the ability to formulate and express thoughts by retrieving words, sequencing words into phrases and sentences according to grammatical rules and standards of practice for the speaker's cultural-linguistic community. Two aspects of fluency typically are considered in evaluation of communication ability: verbal fluency, which relates to word-finding ability and the fluent expression of ideas; and speech fluency, which refers to the articulation of speech sounds (vs. stuttering).

Fluency problems may also occur as a result of word-finding difficulties associated with cognitive impairments of attention and speed of information processing (Canter 1971). Motor speech disorders including stuttering may result from neurologic diagnoses. The nature and characteristics of communication dysfluencies require an examination of language, cognition and motor speech abilities as well as an astute perceptual assessment and analysis for differential diagnosis and intervention. Stuttering as it impacts conversational fluency will be discussed in section 6.5.7.

There is limited research that has systematically investigated the existence and nature of word retrieval deficits in naming and discourse contexts after mTBI (King, Hough, Walker, Rastatter, & Holbert, 2006).

5.7 The Role of SLPs in Cognitive-Communication Rehabilitation Services

Speech-language pathologists (SLPs) are uniquely qualified to provide rehabilitation services for individuals with cognitive-communication disorders, due to their specialized knowledge and skills in the following areas:

- Cognition and its relationship to language and communication in normal development and aging as well as in neurogenic and psychogenic disorders;
- Clinical tools and methods for assessing cognitive-communication disorders;
- Evidence-based interventional approaches and methods for cognitive-communication disorders across the life span;
- Effects of pharmacological interventions on cognition and communication;
- Counseling, collaboration, education, and advocacy;
- Responsivity to cultural and linguistic diversity of SMs, veterans, and their family members;
- Research principles.

A broad spectrum of cognitive-communication impairments may result from TBI. As a member of the IDT of professionals who collaborate to evaluate and treat individuals with TBI, the role of the SLP includes evaluation and treatment of all aspects of communication as well as the communication implications of cognitive deficits (ASHA, 1987, 1991).

Intervention for cognitive-communication disorders involves not only direct therapy but also environmental modifications. Modifying contextual factors can reduce barriers and facilitate successful communication and community participation. SLPs also serve as advocates for persons with language, socio-communicative, and cognitive-communication impairments. Through education of the Command and supervisors, SLPs and members of the IDT advocate for adaptations and environmental modifications when appropriate, to improve a SM's/veteran's job performance (ASHA, 1991, 2004a, 2005).

Counseling and consultation are essential components of SLP interventions that address the nature and impact of cognitive-communication symptoms and engage the SM/veteran, family/caregiver, SM's Command, and others (e.g., teachers, employers, peers) in the clinical process, as appropriate. Services may include instruction of communication partners in how to facilitate functioning, remove communication barriers, and enhance community participation.

6. Clinical Pathway

6.1 Interdisciplinary Team (IDT)

BACKGROUND

Care for SMs/veterans with concussion and cognitive-communication deficits is complex and may require the intervention of multiple medical, mental health, social work and rehabilitation specialties. Integration of medical, psychosocial, financial, educational, and vocational resources will support optimal outcomes for TBI and polytrauma survivors.

An interdisciplinary team (IDT) should be used to reduce the risk of missing potential complicating factors that may negatively influence rehabilitation outcomes. Members of the team may have complementary roles in cognitive intervention. For example, cognitive-communication deficits may adversely affect progress in the treatment of behavioral and emotional problems and the SLP can offer important information to assist mental health professionals to optimize treatment of SMs/veterans with mTBI. At the same time, the mental health professional can provide a more nuanced understanding of the influence of cognitive and behavioral processes on communication.

The IDT should develop a patient-centered treatment plan that incorporates the results of the comprehensive assessments from each discipline and formulates treatment goals in collaboration with the SM/veteran and his/her family, as appropriate.

The IDT may include medical and rehabilitation professionals such as physician, nurse, social worker, neuropsychologist, rehabilitation psychologist, SLP, audiologist, occupational therapist (OT), physical therapist (PT), and vocational counselor. Membership in the team should be adjusted based on the SM's/veteran's individual needs.

ACTION STATEMENT

Cognitive-communication rehabilitation is most effective when provided by an interdisciplinary team (IDT).

RECOMMENDATIONS

1. Ideally, an IDT should be formed at medical facilities charged with the care of SMs/veterans with mTBI and cognitive-communication deficits.
2. The IDT should be integrated and supportive to provide a strong rehabilitative framework, and should meet at appropriate intervals throughout the rehabilitative process.
3. The IDT should include the SM/veteran and, upon the SM's/veteran's consent, his/her family.
4. The SM/veteran and family should be invited to team meetings during active rehabilitation.
5. SLPs should educate the IDT regarding the results of speech, language, and cognitive-communication assessment and progress in treatment.

6. Members of the IDT should be available to the SLP for consultation during the course of rehabilitation.

DISCUSSION

The development of IDT in rehabilitation has been central to the emergence of creative approaches and innovative strategies to provide comprehensive and collaborative care (Strasser, Uomoto, & Smits, 2008). Behavioral, cognitive, communication, and physical issues may be addressed without unnecessary duplication or fragmentation of services. While each discipline contributes unique perspectives, collaboratively the team can provide integrated services and advocacy with joint planning, goal setting, strategy selection, and implementation (Joint Committee on Interprofessional Relations between the American Speech-Language-Hearing Association and Division 40 [Clinical Neuropsychology] of the American Psychological Association, 2007).

Patients with stroke (Strasser et al., 2008) and TBI (Sarajuuri et al., 2005) have shown improved outcomes when an IDT was a key component in the rehabilitation process. Strasser et al. (2005) found characteristics of team functioning that predicted improvement in stroke rehabilitation in a VA project. Forty-six VA rehabilitation teams including 530 rehabilitation team members from six disciplines (medicine, nursing, social work, SLP, and physical and occupational therapy) and 1,688 veterans with stroke participated in the study. Task orientation, order and organization, and utility of quality information were significantly associated with functional improvement in the stroke patients. Team effectiveness was associated with decreased length of stay. The authors concluded that improving team activities and relationships, including collaborative planning and problem solving and the use of feedback information may enhance rehabilitation treatment effectiveness (Strasser et al., 2005).

A non-randomized controlled trial compared "productivity" at two years post TBI between a conventional rehabilitation program in which physicians made referrals to the general health care system, and an intensive, interdisciplinary rehabilitation program. Patients' and significant others' reports of "productivity" were defined as employed, in school, or participating in volunteer activities. Eighty-nine percent of those patients who participated in the comprehensive, interdisciplinary rehabilitation program were productive, compared to 55% of the conventional care group (Sarajuuri et al., 2005).

In the current healthcare environment, patients and families have high expectations regarding their input into daily and long-term clinical care decisions. Family members can be effective advocates for services and resources that may benefit the SM/veteran. This trend presents a growing challenge for rehabilitation professionals to help families through a recovery process that may be frustrating and life-long (Strasser et al., 2008). Care should be taken to provide a supportive atmosphere for the family and medical caregivers to reach optimal rehabilitation outcomes.

6.2 Referral

Concussion or mTBI is a common combat-related injury, yet it is often overlooked when more obvious physical injuries must take precedence in the medical care of the individual. Identification of injuries that result in subtle cognitive deficits is difficult, particularly when those deficits are masked by the overwhelming complexity of other medical problems.

In cases where there are no apparent physical injuries, subtle cognitive deficits may be also be overlooked when they are attributed to pre-injury factors, combat-related stress, or other mental health factors, and do not receive appropriate follow up. Logistical problems of proper identification and follow-up of SMs/veterans may result in delayed referrals and underutilization of potentially effective services.

Referral for SLP evaluation may be initiated at the MTF or the VA upon identification of possible cognitive-communication problems. Common referral sources include primary care providers, physiatrists, neurologists, psychiatrists, psychologists, neuropsychologists, social workers, and case managers.

6.3 Cognitive-Communication Screening and Evaluation

When evaluating a SM/veteran with confirmed or suspected mTBI, it is important to recognize that acute symptoms will typically resolve within 90 days following trauma (Levin, Goldstein, & Mackenzie, 1997; Helmick, 2010). During this time of natural recovery, symptoms quickly evolve in a positive direction and comprehensive evaluation is generally not recommended. At the same time, education about the symptoms and risk communication that conveys reassurance about expected positive recovery have been shown to prevent or reduce the development of persistent symptoms (Mittenberg et al., 1996).

Comprehensive evaluation of persistent cognitive-communication symptoms (post 90 days) should take into account the fact that these symptoms are probably multi-factorial with regard to presentation and etiology. The evaluation should be based on a thorough history and include standardized instruments; patient (and family, and Command when appropriate) report of symptoms and the impact of symptoms on function; and problem-focused, hypothesis-based, and ecologically valid assessments (e.g., that consider military occupational specialties or work demands and environment). (Note: Refer to clinical toolkit that accompanies this CMG for examples of assessment instruments.)

6.3.1 Case History and Intake Interview

BACKGROUND

Assessment, including screening and evaluation of cognitive-communication impairments following mTBI, begins with review of records and case history. A case history is information gained by asking specific questions of the SM/veteran and other corroborative sources, with patient consent, such as family, friends, and/or the SM's Command. The case history and interview provide valuable information in determining a diagnosis and treatment strategy.

Records review and case history should be used to obtain information on the following (ASHA 2004a; Nolin, Villemure, & Heroux, 2006; VA/DoD, 2009):

- Medical status and timelines regarding injury(ies);
- Medical and surgical treatment since injury;
- Medical history including review of prescribed and over-the-counter medications, supplements, caffeine, tobacco, other stimulants such as energy drinks, alcohol/drug use (for potential causative or exacerbating influences);
- Presence and progression of the following:
  - affective symptoms: irritability, anger, depression, anxiety, and altered social functioning;
  - cognitive symptoms: poor concentration, loss of memory, reduced attention, slowness in processing information, and altered problem-solving skills;

- o physical symptoms: headaches, sleep problems, fatigue, dizziness, nausea, visual difficulties, auditory difficulties;
- Educational history;
- Vocational and recreational history;
- Socio-economic, cultural, and linguistic background;
- Communication history;
- Social history including family and support systems;
- SM/veteran reports of goals and preferences, as well as domains and contexts of concern.

ACTION STATEMENT

A screening and/or diagnostic assessment of cognitive-communication disorders should begin with a relevant case history and patient interview (and/or with patient consent, interview with a corroborative source, such as family, friends, or the SM's Command).

RECOMMENDATIONS

1. A case history and interview are essential components of the initial screening and/or assessment of cognitive-communication disorders following mTBI to identify the symptoms that may affect cognitive-communication status (e.g., headaches, sleeping problems) as well as the SM's/veteran's perception of his/her difficulties.

2. The interview should include detailed questioning about the frequency, intensity, and nature of symptoms and their impact on social and occupational functioning.

3. Open-ended questions should be used to allow the SM/veteran to describe his/her difficulties. While symptom checklists may be useful in documenting symptoms and their intensity, it is not recommended that these checklists be presented to patients.

4. The intake should include detailed description/inventory of the SM's Military Occupational Specialty (MOS)/veteran's occupation, including roles, responsibilities, type of transactions, work environment, and stressors.

DISCUSSION

The persistence of complaints or symptoms after mTBI is used to diagnose PCS (McCrea, 2008). The interview process is necessary to get a complete picture of the symptoms. The clinician's interview method may impact the symptoms reported by the patient. Specifically, patients who have suffered mTBI may report a greater number of symptoms when presented with a list of symptoms versus an open-ended question about symptoms experienced (Nolin et al., 2006; VA/DoD, 2009).

Personal contact during the initial interview sets the stage for patient-centered care. The two most common methods of obtaining a case history are interviews and questionnaires (Tomblin, Morris, & Spriestersbach, 2000). Although questionnaires may be effective and useful, an initial interview can facilitate trust and rapport between the SM/veteran and clinician and between the caregiver and clinician.

The following are additional benefits of a case history and interview: a) beginning the assessment with an interview as opposed to formalized testing helps the clinician to understand and gain insight into the effects of the mTBI on the SM/veteran; b) the clinician can learn about other symptoms which may affect cognitive-communication status (e.g., pain, sleep disorders, hypervigilance); and c) will help identify the need for referrals to other specialists.

6.3.2 Cognitive-Communication Screening

BACKGROUND

Cognitive-communication screening of individuals with mTBI is conducted to identify individuals with potential cognitive-communication symptoms.

- Screening is a pass/fail procedure to identify individuals who require further assessment.
- Screening may result in recommendations for re-screening, comprehensive cognitive-communication assessment, or referral for other services.
- Screening typically focuses on body structures/functions, but may also address activities/participation, and contextual factors affecting communication.
- Individuals who fail screenings are seen by SLPs for further comprehensive evaluations.

SMs/veterans with mTBI may be referred for SLP services for concerns other than cognitive-communication issues (e.g., dysphagia, dysphonia, dysarthria, stuttering). In such cases, screening of cognitive-communication problems may still be considered based on patients' symptoms.

ACTION STATEMENT

Screening of cognitive-communication abilities may be conducted prior to a comprehensive evaluation.

RECOMMENDATIONS

1. Group or individual screenings of cognitive-communication abilities may precede more comprehensive evaluation to identify the need for further assessment or referral to other services.
2. Screening is indicated when an individual presents with cognitive-communication symptoms related to a concussive event or with a recent history (<90 days) of loss of or altered consciousness related to an acute physically traumatic event such as a blast explosion or MVC.
3. It is recommended that screening include:
   - Information on the SM's/veteran's cognitive-communication symptoms and concerns;
   - History of the injury event including mechanism of injury, duration and severity of alteration of consciousness, immediate symptoms, symptom course and prior treatment;
   - Information about pre-morbid intellectual functioning, level of education, previous speech-language diagnosis or services received, and other neuropsychological, psychiatric, or social factors that may affect current communication;
   - Patient self-ratings of symptoms or concerns, a written and/or verbal intake questionnaire and informal interaction/conversation with the SM/veteran;

- Identification of health care concerns that may be contributing to cognitive-communication symptoms and may warrant referral for further evaluation or management.

4. Referral to primary care or case management may be warranted following the initial cognitive-communication screening if there are co-occurring concerns (e.g., PTSD, pain or sensory deficits, medication side-effects).

6.3.3 Cognitive-Communication Evaluation

BACKGROUND

Cognitive-communication screenings with positive results should be followed by comprehensive evaluations that include formal (i.e., standardized) and informal (i.e., non-standardized) instruments that assess impairment as well as activities/participation, and contextual factors affecting communication. It is important to evaluate cognitive-communication abilities in real-life contexts, including the use of language in social and vocational contexts.

Many authors recommend a combination of standardized and non-standardized assessments to document real world functioning (Coelho, Ylvisaker, & Turkstra, 2005; Milton, 1988; Sohlberg & Mateer, 1989; Turkstra, Coelho, & Ylvisaker, 2005). According to Turkstra and McCarty (2006), communication competence, including the use of language within vocational and social contexts, is best assessed in real-world situations, which may be more sensitive to communication breakdowns than standardized tests or clinical tasks such as monologic discourse.

It is important that information regarding cognitive-communication skills is gathered from individualized tasks that test the upper limits of the person's resources. Cognitive-communication problems may be difficult to capture in the clinical setting as individuals with concussion tend to perform adequately under structured conditions.

Comprehensive evaluations are conducted for one or more of the following purposes:

- Diagnosing a cognitive-communication disorder;
- Documenting clinical characteristics of the cognitive-communication disorder; specifically, identifying underlying strengths and weaknesses related to cognitive, and linguistic factors, including social skills that affect communication performance;
- Measuring the effects of cognitive-communication impairments on the SM's/veteran's activities (capacity and performance in everyday communication contexts) and participation (ability to assume pre-injury roles in employment, education, and social and community life);
- Identifying contextual factors that serve as barriers to or facilitators of successful communication and participation for individuals with cognitive-communication impairment;
- Formulating recommendations for intervention and support;
- Assessing prognosis for change;
- Testing intervention hypotheses;
- Measuring the effectiveness of intervention and supports;
- Assessing change in a SM's/veteran's cognitive-communication symptoms or status;
- Determining the need for referral to other assessments or services;

- Supporting medical or neurological diagnoses;
- Generating epidemiologic or other research data.

ACTION STATEMENT

A comprehensive cognitive-communication evaluation is conducted to diagnose the impairment, make a prognosis for outcome, formulate treatment recommendations, and identify appropriate referrals.

RECOMMENDATIONS

1. Comprehensive cognitive-communication evaluation is not recommended in the first 90 days following an mTBI as full recovery is expected although current performance may be depressed. Education about possible cognitive-communication problems during this time, using the Mittenberg model (Mittenberg et al., 1996) and emphasizing positive expectations of recovery, have been shown to decrease the odds of developing persistent PCS.

2. Evaluation of cognitive-communication abilities includes the domains of:
   - Language
   - Attention
   - Memory
   - Processing speed
   - Executive functions
   - Self-awareness
   - Social communication.

3. Results of the comprehensive evaluation should be cross-referenced with test results from other rehabilitation team members (e.g., neuropsychologist, OT, audiology, vision) involved in cognitive assessments and with findings obtained on different days or at different times of the day (Malia et al., 2004).

4. Persistent cognitive-communication symptoms (post 90 days) are probably multi-factorial with regard to etiology and should not be labeled without careful consideration. It is recommended that interpretation of results of comprehensive evaluation of cognitive-communication impairments should also take into consideration other factors such as pain, sleep disturbance, or psychological factors.

5. Referral to mental health providers may be indicated when post-traumatic stress, anxiety, or other psychological health concerns may be contributing to depressed cognitive-communication performance.

DISCUSSION

SLPs are one of several rehabilitation disciplines that contribute to defining the nature of the cognitive deficits resulting from TBI. The focus of the SLP evaluation is on the underlying cognitive impairments that impact an individual's communication functioning (NIH, 1999). Comprehensive evaluation provides the basis for determining the nature, severity, and characteristics of cognitive-communication disorders. Effective evaluation of cognitive-communication abilities is a prerequisite to designing and implementing an effective treatment program with baseline/pre-treatment measures, functional goals, and required supports.

The number of assessment tools designed specifically for cognitive-communication impairments resulting from TBI is limited. The Academy of Neurologic Communication Disorders and Sciences (ANCDS) reviewed 127 standardized assessments recommended by SLPs and test publishers or distributers for use with TBI patients (Turkstra, Coelho et al., 2005). The review focused on tests that were designed or administered to patients with TBI and met reliability and validity measures established by the Agency for Health Care Policy Research. Findings indicated a "striking absence of a test developed for the evaluation of individuals with cognitive-communication disorders, versus tests of basic neuropsychological functions that may be administered by SLPs or tests borrowed from other populations, such as aphasia" (p. 219).

Whelan, Murdoch, and Bellamy (2007) emphasized the importance of assessing higher-level language skills dependent on the integrity of the frontal lobes. Higher-level language skills appear to be particularly vulnerable to TBI and include summarization of written text, ability to persuade and debate, and comprehension of implied information (e.g., metaphors, sarcasm, or humor). They recommended that valid and reliable measures be used to assess language function, attention, word retrieval, and executive functions.

Assessment of the cognitive-communication challenges of SMs/veterans with concussion/mTBI should also address issues central to real-life situations, different family roles, social /community participation, and return to duty, work or school (Ylvisaker & Feeney, 1996).

A combination of standardized and non-standardized assessments, including functional and context-sensitive assessments, is required to address and document real-world functioning (Coelho et al., 2005; Turkstra, Ylvisaker, et al., 2005). For the military population, real-life demands include performing military operational specialties (MOS) and carrying out missions with potential emotional, physical, and environmental stressors. For the veteran population, challenges are related to community re-integration after discharge from the military and adjustment to disability.

6.4 Treatment

6.4.1 Principles of Cognitive-Communication Rehabilitation

BACKGROUND

Cognitive rehabilitation is a systematic, functionally-oriented treatment program based upon assessment and understanding of a patient's brain-behavioral deficits (Cicerone et al., 2000). Neuroplasticity is believed to be the mechanism by which the intact brain encodes experience and learns new behavior, and by which individuals with TBI re-learn lost behavior in response to environmental demands and rehabilitation. Understanding the nature of neuroplasticity can improve rehabilitation strategies to optimize functional outcomes (Kleim & Jones, 2008). Instructional practices that enhance neuroplasticity include providing intensive, repetitive practice of functional targets with careful consideration of salience, potential for generalization, and personal factors (Sohlberg & Turkstra, 2011).

The goals of therapeutic interventions for cognitive-communication sequelae of TBI are to enhance the individual's capacity to process and interpret information, to foster independence, and to improve the individual's ability to function in all aspects of family and community life (Cicerone, et al., 2008; NIH, 1999; Tsaousides & Gordon, 2009).

Cognitive-communication treatments for SMs/veterans should address their unique needs with reference to returning to duty or work, balancing military and family relationships, readjusting to civilian life, and considering risk for post-traumatic stress and other co-morbidities including pain, headache, irritability, sleep disturbances, and poor anger management (Trudel, Nidffer, & Barth, 2007).

The presence of co-morbidities has been found to be a significant predictor of physical, cognitive, and emotional symptoms post-deployment, including those associated with concussion/mTBI (Hoge et al., 2008; Vanderploeg et al., 2009). As such, caution must be exercised when assuming that cognitive-communication difficulties are the direct result of neurological deficits.

Cognitive-communication rehabilitation goals, strategies, scope, intensity, duration, and interval of treatment should be based upon diagnosis, prognosis, individual functional needs of the SM/veteran, and reasonable expectations of continued progress with treatment (Katz, Ashley, O'Shanick, & Connors, 2006).

Individuals with mTBI respond positively to appropriate information and reassurance given shortly after injury (Comper et al., 2005). While education and support seem to benefit patients with respect to somatic and psychological complaints (Comper, Bisschop, Carnide, & Tricco, 2005), a recent review of trials incorporating educational and supportive treatment for mTBI identified a proportion of patients who demonstrated intractable disability (Snell, Surgenor, Hay-Smith, & Siegert 2009).

Cognitive-communication rehabilitation domains include attention, memory, comprehension, social communication, reasoning, problem solving, judgment, initiation, planning, and self-monitoring. Specific interventions may be directed at:

*   Reinforcing, strengthening, or reestablishing previously learned patterns of behavior;
*   Establishing new patterns of behavior through compensatory mechanisms;
*   Enabling persons to adapt to their cognitive disability to improve their overall functioning and quality of life (Cicerone et al., 2000).

A paradigm shift has occurred in cognitive-communication therapy from repetitive decontextualized drills in the clinic to training of compensatory and metacognitive strategies that can be directly applied in naturalistic situations to address functional recovery goals using supports available within the individual's personal interactions and communication environments (ASHA, 2003). Training/education in the use of compensatory strategies has been shown to be effective in decreasing the functional impact of cognitive-communication impairments related to non-degenerative neurological and mental health conditions (NIH, 1999). Comprehensive-holistic rehabilitation programs provide individual- and group-based treatment of cognitive, emotional, and interpersonal skills within an integrated therapeutic environment to remediate impairments and promote meaningful and satisfactory life, even in the presence of existing limitations (Cicerone et al., 2008).

ACTION STATEMENT

Cognitive-communication rehabilitation is recommended to optimize functional recovery from mTBI.

RECOMMENDATIONS

1. Cognitive-communication rehabilitation should be grounded in scientific evidence including theoretical foundations of brain-behavior relationships, cognition, communication, neuroplasticity, learning theories, behavioral modification, and counseling.

2. Intervention programs should be based upon results of thorough individualized assessments to identify cognitive strengths and weaknesses and changes in cognitive-communication function following brain injury.

3. Co-morbidities should be addressed as appropriate to optimize recovery and rehabilitation.

4. Rehabilitation plans should be developed with consideration for the time frame available, realistic discharge criteria, and skills and abilities that the SM/veteran brings to the rehabilitation process.

5. Rehabilitation programs should focus on retraining previously learned skills, reinforcing residual abilities, teaching compensatory strategies, developing functional skills, modifying the environment, and increasing awareness and acceptance of disability in order to facilitate successful adaptation or adjustment.

DISCUSSION

Patient and family education are important components of early intervention and should continue throughout the continuum of care (Mittenberg, Canyock, Condit, & Patton, 2001; Ponsford et al., 2002). Clinical management of patients with mTBI symptoms typically has focused on (a) prevention of "excess disability" through education to promote expectations of rapid and complete recovery, (b) providing a "timeout" period to permit recuperation, (c) avoidance of dangerous activities that could lead to secondary injury, and (d) using aggressive medical treatment to improve symptoms (e.g., headache, sleep disturbance, dizziness) that can interfere with optimal recovery (Comper et al., 2005). This period of recovery should include increased rest hours that are interspersed within the workday, reduced daily demands and expectations, simplification of work schedule and work-load, and reinforcement of successes.

The recovery trajectory from combat-related mTBI is complicated by the physically and emotionally traumatic circumstances in which many concussions are sustained, multiple co-morbidities, the potentially repetitive and cumulative nature of concussions sustained during combat duty, and the difficulty in following typical recommendations for post-concussion care (e.g., rest) in the deployed setting.

Post-acute neurologic rehabilitation is based upon concepts of brain plasticity and evidence that brain reorganization is possible even years after brain damage occurs (Bach-y-Rita, 2003). Cognitive-communication intervention should be supported by sound theory with clear conceptualization of dysfunction caused by the brain injury, and cogent understanding of normal information processing and learning as well as dimensions of everyday communication (Hartley, 1995).

Although directly aimed at improving cognitive and psychosocial functioning, cognitive-communication rehabilitation may indirectly result in enhanced physical functioning. For example, improvement in memory may facilitate compliance with a medication regimen, improvement in attention and comprehension may increase understanding of instructions from healthcare providers, and improvement in executive function may foster better decision-making with respect to treatment options (Tsaousides & Gordon, 2009).

Comprehensive-holistic programs provide individual and group rehabilitation treatments to improve cognitive function, increase awareness, and address interpersonal, social, and emotional concerns. Involvement of significant others is highly encouraged, and community activities and vocational trials should be incorporated when appropriate to promote generalization (Cicerone et al., 2008; Tsaousides & Gordon, 2009).

Clinical experience with military and veteran populations suggests that a comprehensive-holistic approach supports the rehabilitation of cognitive and emotional sequelae of chronic symptomatic mTBI. Group therapy in addition to individual therapy promotes unit cohesion and recovery within a supportive context. Involvement of family members, the SM's Command, or the veteran's employer can optimize rehabilitation outcomes.

Rehabilitation of cognitive processes and functional skills training should be combined to facilitate application of compensatory strategies to real life situations (Hartley, 1995). Treatment should be embedded in meaningful contexts and individualized to fulfill the unique needs of each SM/veteran and ensure generalizability from controlled situations in therapy to natural environments and daily routines (Cicerone et al., 2008).

Clinicians should be systematic in their treatment planning and should realize that every SM/veteran learns differently and requires individually-tailored instructions or strategies (Ehlhardt et al., 2008). Methods involved in selecting instructional targets and presenting and reinforcing target information can facilitate learning and directly influence learner outcomes. Sohlberg, Ehlhardt, and Kennedy (2005) formulated a checklist for deliberate, systematic treatment planning for individuals with cognitive impairments with instructional practices supported by research, including direct instruction combined with strategy instruction and errorless learning techniques.

Instructional practices that have been experimentally validated and are key to promoting learning for individuals with memory impairments include:

- Clearly delineating intervention targets with use of task analyses when training multi-step procedures;
- Limiting errors when teaching or re-teaching information and procedures;
- Providing sufficient practice;
- Distributing practice within sessions and across sessions;
- Using stimulus variation or multiple exemplars;
- Using strategies to promote more effortful processing (e.g., verbal elaboration, imagery);
- Selecting and training ecologically valid targets (Ehlhardt et al., 2008).

Structuring or modifying the individual's environment and generating management strategies can be helpful in reducing the load on attention, memory, and organizational abilities. Strategies include:

- Organizing and labeling storage cabinets
- Setting up filing systems
- Creating message centers
- Establishing bill payment systems

- Reducing clutter
- Eliminating distractions
- Posting signs to inform others in the environment about management strategies (Sohlberg & Mateer, 2001).

6.4.2 Therapeutic Alliance

BACKGROUND

Cognitive-communication rehabilitation is a dynamic process that involves a collaborative relationship between clinician and patient. The World Health Organization (WHO, 2008) strongly recommends patient-centered care with continuity and an enduring relationship of trust between patients and their providers. A detailed case history including information about physical, emotional, and social concerns, the SM's/veteran's past and future, and environment contribute to understanding the individual and the disorder, and can positively affect the therapeutic relationship.

A patient-centered approach that integrates goal-directed counseling for eliciting behavior change can promote positive health outcomes and improved quality of life for patients and their families. Aspects of supportive counseling include (a) caring and empathy (e.g., perceived sincerity, ability to listen, viewing issues from the perspectives of others); (b) competence and expertise (e.g., perceived intelligence, training, experience, professional attainment, knowledge); (c) dedication and commitment (e.g., perceived altruism, involvement, diligence in pursuit of health goals); and (d) honesty and openness (e.g., perceived truthfulness, candidness, fairness, objectivity) (VA/DoD, 2009).

While the prognosis after mTBI is favorable and the overwhelming majority of individuals with mTBI are expected to experience complete recovery of cognitive symptoms within the first several months after injury (Lannsjo, Geifjerstam, Johansson, Bring, & Borg et al., 2009; McCrae, 2008), persisting symptoms may result from neurologic abnormality or inefficiency related to the injury (Sohlberg & Mateer, 2001). Persistent cognitive symptoms may also arise from a variety of secondary factors including pre-injury psychiatric history (Vanderploeg, Belanger, & Curtiss, 2006), misattribution of pre-injury characteristics to the injury (Mittenberg et al., 2001), expectation of significant symptoms after concussion that may be amplified by subsequent stress and anxiety (Mittenberg, DiGiulio, Perrin, & Bass 1992), and the influence of compensation for symptoms (Hoge, Goldberg, & Castro, 2009). These factors may contribute to an exaggeration of symptoms in individuals with mTBI.

While engaging in intervention for cognitive-communication symptoms, it is important to emphasize expectancy of recovery by providing education regarding positive outcomes in mTBI, highlighting skills and abilities shown by the SM/veteran with mTBI, and engaging in risk communication whereby, the language used in delivering treatment creates the expectation for recovery (e.g., avoiding terms such as brain damage, impairments, post-concussion syndrome) (Borg et al., 2004).

The challenges in mTBI management, including the difficulties of determining the etiology for the symptoms or most effective treatment, reinforce the need to build strong alliances based upon trust and credibility among the clinician, the SM/veteran, and their family. Patient's concerns and experiences should be validated by allowing adequate time for building a clinician-patient alliance and applying an effective risk communication approach (VA/DoD, 2009).

ACTION STATEMENT

A strong therapeutic alliance should be established with patients to optimize rehabilitation outcomes.

RECOMMENDATIONS

Establishing a therapeutic alliance and employing risk communication techniques are essential to effectively address the emotional and psychosocial needs of patients and families. Strategies include:

1. Demonstrating a commitment to understanding the patient's concerns and symptoms,
2. Encouraging an open and honest transfer of information to capture a comprehensive representation of the patient's concerns and medical history,
3. Presenting information regarding a positive outcome and symptom remission to create an expectation of recovery,
4. Avoiding open skepticism or disapproving comments in discussing the patient's concerns (VA/DoD, 2009).

DISCUSSION

Therapeutic working alliance refers to the partnership between clinician and patient in their efforts to achieve change through the therapy process. The alliance is built upon agreement on the goals of therapy, agreement of tasks to achieve these goals, and the development of a personal bond between the clinician and the SM/veteran. A strong therapeutic working alliance can positively influence outcomes in post-acute brain injury rehabilitation (Bordin, 1979; Schonberger, Humle, & Teasdale, 2006, 2007; Sherer et al., 2007).

Sherer et al. (2007) surveyed 69 patients with acute brain injury, their families, and medical caregivers to identify factors influencing the strength of therapeutic alliance for patients with TBI enrolled in post-acute brain injury rehabilitation, and to examine the association of therapeutic alliance with outcome. Higher levels of family discord were associated with poorer therapeutic alliance. Greater discrepancies between family and clinician ratings of patient functioning were associated with poorer therapeutic alliance and poorer effort in therapies. Productivity status at discharge was predicted by functional status at admission and degree of therapeutic alliance. The authors concluded that family perceptions and family functioning are important determinants of therapeutic alliance for patients in post brain injury rehabilitation.

6.4.3 Individual Treatment

BACKGROUND

Individual therapy is a critical component of cognitive-communication rehabilitation programs for SMs/veterans with mTBI. The cognitive consequences of mTBI are complex, and effects on individuals are variable. Therefore, intervention must be individualized to address the myriad of functional problems that emerge as a result of the mTBI.

Cognitive-communication rehabilitation at the post-acute stage is focused on enabling SMs/veterans to resume a productive life based on individualized goals, functional needs, and personal interests and preferences.

ACTION STATEMENT

Individual therapy is a keystone of cognitive-communication rehabilitation.

RECOMMENDATIONS

1. Cognitive-communication intervention must be individually tailored to achieve short-term objectives and long-term functional outcomes.
2. Individual therapy provides the environment for clinicians to develop a strong working alliance with SMs/veterans that can optimize the process and outcomes of therapy.

DISCUSSION

Individual therapy provides a milieu for developing functional goals to address cognitive-communication deficits and for implementing an individualized, patient-centered program. The goals of cognitive rehabilitation are to enhance the SM's/veteran's capacity to process and interpret information and to improve his/her ability to function in all aspects of life. Instructional methodologies can be implemented to establish targets in a structured environment to minimize errors, control stimuli and responses, and provide repetitive practice. There is strong evidence to support the effectiveness of individualized systematic instruction (e.g., errorless learning, method of vanishing cues, spaced retrieval/spaced presentation) (Elhardt et al., 2008; NIH, 1999).

Treatment should be matched to the functional needs, strengths, and capacities of each SM/veteran and modified as those needs change over time. As SMs/veterans attempt to resume their usual daily activities, additional challenges may emerge with increasing environmental demands. Intervention strategies must be individualized to reestablish appropriate and adaptive behaviors within functional contexts and actual life situations to address these challenges (Hartley, 1995; NIH, 1999).

Individual therapy provides the context to address factors that influence a SM's/veteran's cognitive-communication functions such as physiological state, perceptual skills, emotional status, motivation, and social skills. Cognitive-communication rehabilitation is most effective when the focus is on the subsystems that are assumed to be important in cognition (e.g., attention, comprehension, learning, memory, social communication, problem-solving, creative thinking) as well as aspects of an individual's life that can affect cognition such as emotions, nutrition, health, stress, and social functioning (Parente & Herrmann, 2002).

6.4.4 Group Treatment

BACKGROUND

Group therapy is a valuable component of cognitive-communication rehabilitation programs for SMs/veterans with mTBI. Group sessions provide a forum to practice skills in real-life situations, and opportunities for peer interaction, feedback and support. Treatment outcomes may include social and emotional benefits in addition to improvement in cognitive-communication skills.

Group therapy may focus on reinforcing and generalizing strategies and techniques established in individual therapy to improve skills such as concentration/attention, memory, organization, planning, goal setting, decision making, problem solving, reading comprehension, test-taking, and social communication.

Group therapy enables participants to learn from other participants' prior experiences and their proposed solutions to problems. Participants have an opportunity to give advice to each other and practice strategies suggested by their peers.

The group context may be effective in teaching executive function and problem-solving skills because participants have an opportunity to apply strategies and processes in challenging situations and to other participants' problems as well as their own.

Interactions within the group provide a meaningful context for improving social communication skills, including opportunities to apply strategies and practice conversational skills with multiple communication partners.

ACTION STATEMENT

Group therapy should be considered as an integral component of cognitive-communication rehabilitation.

RECOMMENDATIONS

1. Group intervention should be considered throughout the rehabilitation process when appropriate and available.
2. Group therapy may be particularly helpful in generalizing skills established in individual therapy, practicing social communication skills, receiving feedback from other participants, and providing peer support when addressing psychosocial issues.
3. The group format may be more effective than individual therapy when presenting general patient education information.

DISCUSSION

Group therapy can serve as a forum for education to develop the SM's/veteran's understanding of brain injury and rehabilitation, cognitive and emotional problems following brain injury, and how to cope with and compensate for changes (Malia et al., 2004).

A pilot study was conducted with survivors of brain injury to evaluate the effectiveness of group cognitive skills training as a precursor to vocational placement and re-entry into the workforce. Data indicated that 76% of those patients who completed training and group therapy were placed into competitive employment compared with the overall rehabilitation rate of 58% for patients who received comparable services but did not participate in the cognitive skills group (Parente & Stapleton, 1999).

In a study that examined the efficacy of a structured group memory rehabilitation program for adults following brain injury, participation significantly increased the use of memory aids and strategies, increased knowledge of memory and memory strategies, and reduced self-rated behaviors indicative of memory impairment (Thickpenny-Davis & Barker-Collo, 2007).

A randomized treatment and deferred treatment controlled trial design was used to evaluate the efficacy of a group intervention program to improve social communication skills following TBI. Results indicated that although overall social participation measures did not demonstrate improvement, specific individual communication deficits and overall satisfaction with life measures showed improvement over baseline (Dahlberg et al., 2007).

The group format has been used effectively in treating veterans with other neurogenic communication disorders. A study involving five VA Medical Centers compared individual with group treatment for veterans with aphasia. Results indicated that both individual and group treatment yielded positive outcomes, with veterans in both groups demonstrating significant improvement in language abilities (Wertz et al., 1981).

The therapeutic power of group psychotherapy is considerable and may be a critical component in post-acute brain injury rehabilitation. The group milieu can enhance self-awareness of deficits and provide a place where safe confrontation can occur (Peppings, 1998).

6.4.5 Cognitive-Communication Interventions for Active Duty Service Members and Veterans

BACKGROUND

Comprehensive, integrated, and collaborative efforts of the IDT are directed toward enabling and empowering SMs to return to duty – able, confident, and competitive to meet the challenges of their vocational ambitions. These efforts support the ideals of the Warrior in Transition Battalion:

"I am a Warrior in Transition. My job is to heal as I transition back to duty or continue serving the nation as a Veteran in my community.

This is not a status, but a mission. I will succeed in this mission because...I am a Warrior and I am Army strong."

In preparation for return to duty or work, treatment must consider and include personal and contextual factors that can enhance or hinder job performance. Contextual factors include the physical, social, and attitudinal surroundings in which SMs/veterans function (e.g., work space, perceptions and expectations of the unit or place of employment, Command climate). Personal factors include features of the individual that are not part of a health condition or functional state (e.g., coping styles, social background, education, past and current experiences) (Cornis-Pop et al., 1998).

For SMs/veterans with disabilities, the process of transition and community reintegration is vital to return successfully to college and the workforce, and critical for financial independence and quality of life (Ruh, Spicer, & Vaughan, 2009).

Assessment for community reintegration may include the following:

- Social and support systems (e.g., immediate and extended family, friends, co-workers, supervisors; spiritual, religious, and cultural beliefs and networks);

- Availability of medical, mental health, and rehabilitation services and support;
- Co-existence of psychological or physical conditions that may influence or preclude ability to participate in rehabilitation (e.g., PTSD, depression, anxiety, sleep deprivation, headaches, pain, vertigo, tinnitus, decreased vision);
- Home/family role expectations and responsibilities;
- Career/employment goals, responsibilities, and demands including assessment of actual work tasks;
- Job-site environmental challenges (e.g., noise, distractions, lighting, distance, position in room);
- Geographic location (e.g., access to and distance from resources and assistance);
- Driving or transportation needs (e.g., restrictions, safety, anxiety related to driving);
- Financial stress or hardship that may impact participation in rehabilitation.

To the extent possible, SLPs should assess functional cognitive-communication skills in simulated complex tasks to:

- Validate (or invalidate) and augment test findings;
- Identify the impact of strengths and weaknesses that can support or compromise rehabilitative, social, educational, and vocational activities and participation, all critical to successful return-to-unit and duty;
- Generate hypotheses on the SM's/veteran's ability to fulfill his/her MOS or school and work requirements;
- Identify underlying processes or contextual variables that contribute to successes or failures in activities or participation;
- Identify functional and critical needs and develop functional objectives to perform duties safely and competently;
- Determine generalization and effectiveness of intervention procedures including strategies, supports, and environmental modifications.

SMs/veterans with persistent mTBI symptoms may require accommodations to facilitate return to duty or work place. These may include:

- Gradual work re-entry,
- Flexibility in time and length of the work shift,
- Adjustment of job responsibilities or conditions,
- Environmental modifications (VA/DoD, 2009).

Treatment principles to prepare SMs/veterans for return-to-duty and vocational success include:

- Individualized interventions that target personally meaningful real-world goals;
- Training that begins with existing strengths or needed support to ensure success (as skills and performance improve, supports are faded and complexities of tasks are increased to maintain level of challenge);
- Training with different stimulus modalities;
- Strategies using strengths to compensate for weaknesses;
- Coaching and feedback to shape, chain, and reinforce use of compensatory strategies;
- Environmental modifications (e.g., quiet work environment, highly organized work space);
- To the extent possible, complex and functional tasks in real-world settings and simulations that create a meaningful context for skill and strategy development;

- Coordinated and integrated services with other providers addressing complementary issues (e.g., joint OT and SLP sessions to plan, organize, and prepare for a group outing).

Counseling and consultation are essential components that address the nature and impact of the disorder or difference, and engage the SM/veteran, family/caregiver, and others (e.g., Command, employers, teachers, peers) in the clinical process, as appropriate. Vocational interventions may be beneficial, including working with the SM's Command or veteran's employer.

Services may include: (a) advocacy and information on legal rights against discrimination on the basis of cognitive disability including academic adjustments and reasonable accommodations to facilitate success in educational and work settings (Americans with Disabilities Act, 2008), and (b) instruction of key individuals interacting with the SM/veteran on how to facilitate functioning, remove communication barriers, and enhance participation.

The impact of persistent cognitive-communication symptoms can be addressed by including spouses/partners in individual and/or group sessions to promote better understanding and offer opportunities to discuss challenges. A support group or spouse session within a cognitive-communication rehabilitation group provides a forum for families to receive information and advice, and learn strategies for coping with day-to-day difficulties (VA/DoD, 2009).

ACTION STATEMENT

During all phases of recovery, intervention is directed at maximizing the SM's/veteran's potential to attain real-world goals including successful return to duty, employment, academic achievement, and community reintegration. The determination of duty status is based on the recommendations of the IDT members following a period of patient assessment, education, and intervention.

RECOMMENDATIONS

1. If combined assessments of the IDT suggest that the SM/veteran is cognitively, emotionally, and physically fit for duty/return to work, a trial-of-duty/work should be considered before return-to-full duty/work. Ideally, this trial is structured, supervised, supported, and modeled after a "community services only" reintegration program (Helmick, 2010).

2. During this trial period, SMs/veterans should continue to have access to the SLP and other team members for on-going support and intervention until it is determined that discharge from treatment is indicated.

3. Intermittent follow-up visits should be scheduled as warranted. At this phase of recovery, the individual should be empowered to control his or her own activity by means of effective decision-making, strategic thinking, self-regulation of behavior, and self-regulated control over environmental contingencies (Cornis-Pop et al., 1998).

4. If a trial of duty is not recommended, alternative considerations should include continued treatment, referral for other specialty care, change in MOS, or the Medical Evaluation Board (MEB).

DISCUSSION

The emphasis of SLP intervention at this phase is to reduce the disability associated with cognitive-communication symptoms that restrict functioning in home, social, and career roles. Treatment focuses on both improving patient function while modifying and adjusting the environment in which he/she is expected to function (VA/DoD, 2009).

During this transition, it is key for the SLP to collaborate and coordinate services on an on-going basis with mental health providers, social work/case managers, vocational rehabilitation counselors and others involved in treatment to facilitate optimum attainment of the SM's/veteran's potential (Malia et al., 2004).

6.4.6 Assistive Devices

BACKGROUND

The effectiveness of assistive technology, including cognitive aids for improving the daily function and independence of persons with cognitive impairments is well documented in the scientific literature (Cicerone et al., 2000 & 2005; Quemada et al., 2003; Sohlberg & Mateer, 2001; Sohlberg et al., 2005 & 2007; Wilson, Emslie, Quirk, & Evans, 2001).

Assistive devices discussed in the early TBI literature included low-tech or no-tech devices such as memory notebooks, checklists and planners, or cueing devices such as pagers and alarms for single-task guidance (Burke et al., 1994; Schmitter-Edgecome, Fahy, Whelan, & Long, 1995; Zencius, Wesolowski, & Burke, 1990). Since then, a number of specialized devices have been designed specifically to address the problems encountered by people with cognitive disabilities.

Simultaneously, the use of electronic memory and organization devices designed for the general population has grown exponentially. This has resulted in more individuals having familiarity and expertise in the use of these devices. The development of more sophisticated assistive devices that help with the complex array of activities encountered in work and school settings and the advantage of pre-injury experience with technology have led to the use of electronic cognitive aids as a practical and functional intervention in cognitive rehabilitation.

In working with SMs/veterans with mTBI, the goal of cognitive interventions is to minimize the negative impact of cognitive symptoms on daily living and work settings with an emphasis on return to normal function. Whether the person is a candidate for a direct treatment approach or more indirect services for residual cognitive symptoms, cognitive aids can offer the necessary support to encourage independence and promote positive experiences in the recovery process.

ACTION STATEMENT

The use of cognitive assistive technology is recommended to facilitate compensation for cognitive symptoms, including problems with attention, memory, initiation, planning, organization and execution that may be associated with mTBI. Training and use of cognitive aids may take place in the context of direct treatment for confirmed cognitive deficits, or as a component of an education-based intervention to support functional activity and promote successful return to duty and community re-entry.

RECOMMENDATIONS

1. An individualized assessment is the first step in determining need for cognitive assistive technology.
2. Device selection and prescription is a complex process that forms an integral component of cognitive rehabilitation for mTBI.
3. All SMs/veterans receiving cognitive assistive devices must be involved in a training program that is systematic, goal-oriented, and designed to help them use the cognitive aids as a strategy to optimize function in daily activities.
4. The benefit of cognitive aids must be measurable and should show functional improvement in day-to-day functioning, including the ability to achieve a desired level of productive life while using the device.

DISCUSSION

No single assessment of cognitive functioning can serve as a prescriptive guideline for cognitive assistive devices. Generally, the evaluation should include a combination of global cognitive measures and domain-specific assessments. However, the lack of ecological validity of standardized cognitive tests creates a need for additional evaluation methods that expand beyond the clinical presentation.

Assessment in the form of history/intake interview and self-report and/or questionnaire adds relevant information for determining the needs of the SM/veteran with mTBI. Scherer and Craddock (2002) describe the Matching Person & Technology (MPT) process, a systematic approach to the cognitive aids needs assessment. The MPT includes measures that match abilities and needs of the individual, with the various vocational and avocational contexts in which the device may be used, and ensures that the evaluation and selection process is an objective and collaborative effort between the individual and the provider. Ultimately, the combined results of standardized and non-standardized methods of the individualized needs assessment will drive prescription for the cognitive aid.

There are many special considerations when determining what device or devices may best benefit the person with mTBI. Single and multi-function devices can be beneficial in certain situations or for certain individuals, but not everyone can benefit from the same device in the same way. Devices that offer multiple features may offer the benefit of meeting multiple needs within an all-encompassing system, but may be too cognitively demanding for individuals with high levels of anxiety or that have trouble multi-tasking.

Aspects of current and expected cognitive functioning, and the settings in which the device will assist the individual now and in the future, need to be considered. Special considerations, such as low vision, upper limb amputations or paresis/paralysis and hearing loss also must be taken into account to ensure that the selected device will be effective. Prior experience with cognitive aids also should be considered to take full advantage of pre-injury familiarity and exposure to electronic systems.

Device selection can be time consuming. To facilitate this process, the SM/veteran should be encouraged to become involved in the search for an appropriate device, as this will also promote a sense of ownership and involvement in treatment.

SMs/veterans with mTBI, who are likely to present with minimal learning challenges or who have previous expertise with cognitive aids, may require very little or no training in the use of a particular cognitive device. In fact, many SMs/veterans with mTBI can become a skilled user of cognitive aids in a short amount of time.

However, even people who are familiar with the technology will need training in the effective use of cognitive aids as a strategy for daily living in the face of cognitive disability. This training may be implemented simultaneously with other cognitive therapies or as part of an educationally-oriented program.

Scientific evidence suggests that training procedures must be goal-oriented, systematic, and individualized to the situation and learner's characteristics (Sohlberg, 2005). The general training sequence described by Sohlberg and Mateer (1989) provides a useful framework to guide training in the use of cognitive aids. In their three-step training process, the individual must first become familiar with all aspects of the device, followed by analysis of how and when the device may be most effective as a cognitive strategy, and finally by practicing and gradually moving into systematic use in real-life situations.

The first phase of the training is likely to be completed quickly, while the emphasis is placed on strategy development and functional use of the cognitive device in real-life situations. Initial treatment sessions should be scheduled regularly, with a focus on strategic planning (i.e., statement of the problem, development of an action plan and outcomes measurement). In the final phase of the training program, it is appropriate for sessions to decrease in frequency to allow opportunities for the SM/veteran to test action plans and identify any obstacles to goal achievement in his/her own situation. To reduce the chances of failure, follow-up sessions are a necessary part of the final phase of cognitive aid training.

The ultimate measure of the benefit of a cognitive aid is a demonstration of the ability to return to a previous level of productive life while using the device. Review of the initial needs-assessment and plan of care may serve as an objective basis for outcomes measurement. Perceived satisfaction with goal achievement may be just as significant for the SM/veteran, as is evidence of improved daily functioning. This can be determined with the use of questionnaires, by self-report, and by report of family, friends, co-workers, and superiors. For the SM/veteran who may perceive residual cognitive symptoms, concrete evidence of improvements in daily functioning with cognitive assistive technologies using pre and post comparisons, and comparisons of self and others' reports may be useful.

Cognitive assistive technologies can provide viable treatment options to facilitate return to everyday functions.

6.5 Treatment by Specific Domain

6.5.1 Attention

BACKGROUND

Attention impairments can impact outcomes in a variety of ways. The moderate-severe TBI literature indicates that patients with attention impairments have diminished participation in rehabilitation (Novack, Caldwell, Duke, Bergquist, & Gage, 1996), and are less likely to return to driving (Lengenfelder, Schultheis, Al-Shihabi, Mourant, & DeLuca, 2002), work (Brooks, McKinlay, Symington, Beattie, & Campsie, 1987), and school (Melamed, Stern, Rahmani, Groswasser, & Najenson, 1985). SMs/veterans with persisting attention impairments characterized by slow processing, distractibility, and impairment in working memory, present with similar challenges in achieving positive functional outcomes.

Direct attention training as an intervention strategy is based on the premise that attention abilities can be improved by activating particular aspects of attention through a stimulus drill approach. Repeated stimulation of attentional systems with hierarchically organized remediation exercises is hypothesized to facilitate changes in attention functioning. Current evidence suggests that this type of treatment is most appropriate for people with moderate-severe TBI (post-acute) and people with mild TBI, who have intact vigilance. Furthermore, treatment is most effective when provided in context with functionally meaningful tasks and in conjunction with metacognitive strategy training in which feedback is provided to develop self-monitoring and strategy development (Sohlberg et al, 2003).

ACTION STATEMENT

Attention impairment is highly prevalent in mTBI and has a negative impact on functional outcomes. Attention impairment should be a target for treatment in SMs/veterans with mTBI.

RECOMMENDATIONS

1. Treatment may focus on compensatory strategies to improve attention skills in functional contexts.
2. Direct treatment techniques may be employed in the context of functional tasks to improve performance on these tasks.

Strength of Recommendation: Attention training has been the subject of well-designed research and numerous studies have confirmed its benefit (Helmick, 2010). Recent evidence-based reviews recommend treatment of attention using direct and metacognitive training to promote development of compensatory strategies and foster generalization to real world tasks during post-acute recovery from mild or moderate TBI. Repeated use of computer-based tasks without intervention by a clinician is not recommended (Cicerone et al., 2011).

DISCUSSION

Positive results of treatments for attention skills have been reported for people with mTBI.

- Mateer (1992) reported on the impact of a post-acute treatment program designed specifically for people with mTBI. Components of the program included cognitive rehabilitation, psychosocial counseling, and vocational services. Results were reported for five cases of mTBI with symptoms persisting beyond one year. Subjects made significant improvements on 60% of the neuropsychological measures of attention, memory and general intellectual functioning used for clinical assessment.

- Cicerone (2002) investigated attention treatment in four individuals with mTBI and persisting attention impairment 7 to 8 months post injury. Treatment focused on strategies to better allocate attentional resources (e.g., rehearsal, self-pacing) as well as strategies to minimize anxiety and frustration related to high-level working memory demands. Results indicated that individuals who received treatment demonstrated improvements in neuropsychological measures (Continuous Performance Test; Paced Auditory Serial Addition Test) as well as a subjective self-report measure of functional attention skills whereas a similar control group did not show such improvement.

The larger cognitive rehabilitation literature that includes moderate-severe TBI provides support for the efficacy of treatment for both direct treatment procedures (Sohlberg, McLaughlin, Pavese, Heidrich, & Posner, 2001) as well as development of compensatory strategies to cope with time pressure and overstimulation (Cicerone et al., 2000; Fasotti, Kovacs, Eling, & Brouwer, 2000) and distractibility (Webster & Scott, 1983).

6.5.2 Speed of Processing

BACKGROUND

While cognitive dysfunction for individuals with mTBI tends to be partial, even in the acute recovery period (Lange, Iverson, & Franzen, 2009), one of the most frequent complaints is slowed thinking and difficulty concentrating (Cicerone, 1996). Speed of processing of complex information (semantic processing) yielded significant differences between mTBI and control groups on measures of reaction time (Tombaugh et al., 2007). Slowness of information processing has been found to account for most of the attention deficits present after TBI (Gentilini, Nichell, & Schoenhube, 1989). Cicerone (1996) found that processing speed was related to acquisition and recall ability in neuropsychological measures six months after mTBI, which may reflect the underlying contribution of information processing speed to memory functioning.

Contrary to approaches that aim at increasing processing capacity and speed through practice by gradually increasing the amount and complexity of information to be processed, the types of intervention for SMs/veterans that experience these difficulties after mTBI should focus on emotional and social adjustment. Development of educational tools, compensatory strategies specific to limitations and situations, environmental modifications, and coping mechanisms for managing changes in processing speed may be needed (Vanderploeg et al., 2009).

ACTION STATEMENT

Treatment for deficits in capacity and efficiency of information processing should address the use of compensatory techniques for the underlying cognitive and emotional symptoms.

RECOMMENDATIONS

1. Identification and assessment of information processing deficits after mTBI should include formal evaluations and informal data gathering during tasks that require effortful cognitive processing and that exceed the SM's/veteran's available cognitive resources.
2. Underlying language impairments and/or impairments in attention, organization, working memory and new learning, reasoning, and visuo-spatial skills, may contribute to perceived changes in speed of information processing and should be examined concurrently. Hearing, auditory processing, and vision deficits should be ruled out.
3. Interventions for the management of deficiencies in speed and capacity of information processing in most cases will take the form of counseling, education, and the development of and training in appropriate compensatory strategies that are specific to the SMs/veteran's situation and limitations.

DISCUSSION

Difficulty with efficiency of the information processing loop can have a negative impact on lower order functions of the cognitive processing system such as arousal and attention to higher order functions such as abstraction and problem solving (Vanderploeg, 2000). As these cognitive functions are interrelated and impossible to separate, problems with any of the cognitive functions will inevitably result in deficits in the efficiency of the information processing loop. For example, while the expected relationship between information capacity for complex information and working memory is well understood, difficulties with information processing and speed also have significant negative effects on new learning ability (Chiaravalloti, Christodoulou, Demaree, & DeLuca, 2003). Studies have also reported subtle, long-term cognitive symptoms after TBI on measures of attention targeting complex information that may impact speed (Vanderploeg, Curtiss, & Belanger, 2005).

In addition to the underlying cognitive functions that impact processing speed, careful consideration must be given to other contributing factors to cognitive slowing such as stress, sleep deprivation, PTSD and other mental health conditions (Belanger, Kretzmer et al., 2009), and pain (Etherton, Bianchini, Heinly, & Greve, 2006). Reading and writing skills, pre-injury psychosocial and educational factors, and integrity of vision and hearing systems must also be considered. Collaborative evaluation and treatment with audiologists, vision specialists, psychologists and neuropsychologists, and vocational rehabilitation specialists may be needed.

Brief psychoeducational interventions with an emphasis on reducing the presence of functional limitations caused by difficulties with information processing speed are recommended to reduce the severity and duration of symptoms (Belanger, Uomoto, & Vanderploeg, 2009; Cicerone, 2002). The aim is to promote better understanding of the cognitive demands of high-level everyday tasks, the impact of contributing factors on cognitive stamina, and awareness of techniques that may ease their complexity and temporal demands.

Early intervention in the form of education and support with suggested coping strategies for problems in processing speed contributes to reducing anxiety and ongoing problems after mTBI (Ponsford et al., 2002). Education should include helping the individual to identify and eventually anticipate situations likely to result in cognitive overload so that they can be modified. Minimizing distractions, preparing for situations ahead of time, allowing ample time to complete tasks, taking rest breaks and reducing simultaneous demands may be beneficial strategies in some situations. A variety of cognitive assistive technologies also is available to facilitate fast-paced activities such as note taking in a classroom (e.g., digital audio recorder, smartpen).

The pre-existing use of strategies, as well as modality strengths and preferences (auditory and/or visual) will also influence the selection of compensatory strategies and the amount of training that will be required to employ them successfully. Although education and training in these techniques should only take a few sessions for the SM/veteran with mTBI, some individuals may require a more direct strategy training in order to achieve mastery of the techniques. Using role-play related to work or school, and rehearsing use of appropriate strategies in the clinical setting may be necessary for some to carry over the techniques into their target environments.

6.5.3 Memory

BACKGROUND

The ability to retain and learn new information can be inhibited due to deficits in working, episodic, and semantic memory. Baddeley (1992) describes working memory as the temporary storage and maintenance of information. Giovanello and Verfaellie (2001) describe episodic memory as the conscious recollection of experiences from one's personal past, and semantic memory as the acquisition and retention of generic factual information that is not referenced to a specific learning context. Therefore, if any of these memory systems is impaired, the information cannot be accurately retained for long-term storage.

Internal memory strategies such as mnemonics, visual imagery, and repetition may be used to encode information and improve retrieval. There is evidence that imagery may be helpful to patients by teaching them to elaborate and expand on the information that is to be recalled (Kaschel et al., 2002).

External memory aids include daily planners, calendars, memory books, use of environmental anchors (designated areas at home or work to keep specific items or lists), and electronic devices. Cicerone et al. (2005) reported that external devices could require extensive training before they are used effectively. However, if the memory aid is used consistently, procedural (motor) memory skills will be utilized to assist the SM/veteran in using the device(s) routinely.

ACTION STATEMENT

Memory impairments must be addressed during cognitive-communication therapy in support of functional everyday activities.

RECOMMENDATIONS

1. Techniques and compensatory strategies to improve memory should be selected to accommodate the individual needs of the SM/veteran.
2. SMs/veterans are encouraged to identify, individualize, and generalize the use of techniques and compensatory strategies that are most beneficial to functional everyday activities.
3. Sufficient training opportunities for the use of techniques and strategies should be provided during therapy sessions.
4. These techniques and strategies should be constantly evaluated and incorporated in a variety of functional situations and environments for successful generalization.

Strength of Recommendation: Training in the use of memory compensation strategies as applied to real-life tasks is supported by empirical evidence {Cicerone, 2000 #817;Cicerone, 2005 #818}. According to guidance provided by members of the DCoE/DVBIC consensus conference (Helmick, 2010), "efficacy has been demonstrated for memory training techniques derived from cognitive neuroscience" (p. 245) particularly for patients with mTBI and mild memory impairment.

DISCUSSION

Memory strategy training that assists patients in developing techniques to enhance registration and encoding of information and to improve memory retrieval has been shown to be successful. External memory aids in combination with strategy training resulted in improvement that extended into patients' everyday memory function, while repetitive memory drills (e.g., memorizing word lists, faces or designs without explicit strategy training) have been shown to have little or no efficacy (Helmick, 2010).

Visual imagery may be helpful to patients with mTBI. However, the use of internal memory techniques may actually require more cognitive effort to retain items and need to be taught systematically (Ehlhardt et al., 2008).

External devices are often used for memory impairment. However, certain memory aids can require extensive training and practice for everyday use (Cicerone et al., 2005).

The SM/veteran and clinician should complete continual on-going assessment and feedback of the effectiveness and adequacy of the memory techniques and strategies. Additional feedback can also be obtained from the SM's/veteran's co-workers, Command or supervisors, and friends and family to determine if the SM's/veteran's memory skills are adequate for duty, job, school, social, and daily living requirements.

6.5.4 Executive Functions

BACKGROUND

Executive functions refer to the set of skills related to the achievement of goal-oriented activity. Intervention in this domain often focuses on two subskills commonly impaired after TBI: metacognition (self-monitoring and control of one's own cognitive functions) and problem solving.

Metacognitive strategy training focuses on teaching the SM/veteran to self-regulate thoughts and actions, and self-monitor his/her performance during an activity, in order to control and optimize his/her learning and behavior (Sohlberg & Turkstra, 2011). Individuals with mTBI typically have good self-awareness to self-monitor their performance. Therefore, direct treatment for unawareness of impairment, as conceptualized in the cognitive rehabilitation literature, is typically not indicated. In fact, treatment for unawareness in mTBI may be contraindicated as it may foster an expectation of poor recovery, resulting in iatrogenic occurrence of persisting cognitive symptoms.

A systematic review of studies indicated that step-by-step metacognitive strategy instruction with young to middle aged adults with TBI improved problem solving skills, planning, and organization for personally relevant activities or problem situations (Kennedy et al., 2008). Although various sets of skills were emphasized across studies, immediate positive changes were reported in functional activities, and to a lesser extent in impairment-level outcomes (e.g., standardized test scores). The most frequent approaches used for the remediation of metacognition and problem solving deficits included: (a) acknowledging and/or generating goals, (b) self-monitoring and self-recording performance, and (c) making strategy decisions based on performance-goal comparisons in which individuals adjusted or modified a plan based on self-assessment and/or external feedback.

ACTION STATEMENT

Deficits in executive functions should be addressed in cognitive-communication therapy since they are likely to affect functional activities and participation in everyday life events.

RECOMMENDATIONS

1. The clinician and SM/veteran should consider step-by-step metacognitive strategy instruction to improve executive function skills.
2. Step-by-step intervention procedures can include: (a) acknowledging and/or formulating goals related to the everyday needs of the SM/veteran, (b) determining how to initiate the goals, (c) self-monitoring and self-recording of performance, (d) choosing and revising strategies based on goals and performance, (e) reformulating decisions or plans based on self-assessment, and (f) reviewing what was successful and what was unsuccessful (Kennedy et al., 2008; Kennedy & Coelho, 2005).
3. Remediation of executive functions should initially include external strategies and explicit instruction and feedback, but gradually shift to the internalization of self-regulation strategies through self-instruction and self-monitoring (Cicerone et al., 2005; Kennedy & Coelho, 2005).

Strength of Recommendation: Training in the use of problem solving and organization strategies as applied to real life tasks is supported by empirical evidence {Cicerone, 2000 #817;Cicerone, 2005 #818}. According to guidance provided by members of the DCoE/DVBIC consensus conference (Helmick, 2010), "a robust literature supports the use of metacognitive strategy training as an intervention for executive function impairments due to TBI" (p. 246).

DISCUSSION

Kennedy et al. (2008) reported that in the studies they reviewed, results from using the step-by-step intervention procedures indicated positive changes in executive function skills for everyday activities. However, these changes were not identified on standardized testing.

Rath, Simon, Langenban, Sherr, and Diller (2003) used a similar therapy approach to target problem solving in group therapy. Groups consisted of patients with mild to severe brain injuries. Patients were taught problem-orientation and problem solving skills. Group members were taught to accept the increased time needed to solve daily functional problems and use systematic structured choices to formulate solutions (Rath et al., 2003). Results from this study indicated significant changes in standardized test scores in the areas of memory and perseveration of responses using the Wisconsin Card Sorting Test.

If unrealistic self-appraisal exists in which an individual overestimates his/her skills, a brief period of awareness training using a "predicted vs. actual performance" paradigm may be helpful (MacLennan & MacLennan, 2008; Rebmann & Hannon, 1995). For example, a SM/veteran presenting with poor awareness of difficulties involving concentration and prospective memory, may overestimate his/her learning capacity and risk failure by enrolling in a full time college course load. Having the SM/veteran predict his/her ability to learn information in a classroom-like setting, and then compare the predicted vs. actual performance may serve to highlight difficulties in learning new information. Where cognitive difficulties are confirmed, compensatory cognitive strategies can be developed that will maximize the potential for success.

6.5.5 Social Communication

BACKGROUND

Social communication involves a complex interaction of cognitive abilities, awareness of social rules and boundaries, and emotional control (Dahlberg et al., 2007). For individuals with concussion/mTBI, impairment in attention, concentration, memory, speed of information processing, judgment, abstract thinking and executive control can interfere with language and communication (VA/DoD, 2009).

Social communication impairments may be appropriately viewed as one of the common consequences of behavioral impairment after TBI. Persisting irritability and anger may manifest as negative self-talk, verbal abusiveness to others, or physical aggression that can negatively impact social interactions (Raskin & Mateer, 2000). Post-deployment military personnel may be especially vulnerable to the effects of anger as this is a symptom of "battlemind" (Munroe, 2005), a set of psychological changes that are adaptive in a theater of war but maladaptive when returning to non-combat contexts.

Individuals with mTBI may show high levels of stress and anxiety (Ponsford et al., 2000) which have been associated with social phobia and an avoidance of social situations (Moore, Terryberry-Spohr, & Hope, 2006; Raskin & Mateer, 2000). Anxiety may be compounded by overstimulation related to significant demands on working memory (Cicerone, 2002; MacLennan & Petska, 2008) and by co-morbid PTSD (Brady, Killeen, Brewerton, & Lucerini, 2000).

ACTION STATEMENT

Problems with social communication may have a negative effect on functional outcomes and should be targeted for treatment by SLPs.

RECOMMENDATIONS

1. Social communication treatment may focus on: a) affective-behavioral impairments such as anger and anxiety that result in socially disruptive behavior or social avoidance; b) maladaptive behaviors arising from cognitive-communication impairments (e.g., diminished attention, memory, and impulsivity); and c) direct training of family and friends (who provide the circle of support) on techniques that facilitate improved communication skills for the SM/veteran with mTBI.

2. When unawareness of poor interpersonal skills is demonstrated, review of video recordings of social interactions can provide immediate feedback regarding the appropriateness of communication and can facilitate the adoption of positive communication strategies (Helffenstein & Wechsler, 1982). .

3. Treatment directed at modifying patterns of social communication in the partners of the patient with TBI may also serve to improve the communication skills of the patient (Togher, McDonald, Code, & Grant, 2004; Ylvisaker, Jacobs, & Feeney, 2003).

4. Group treatment provides a more natural communication context and should be considered as a strategy to facilitate generalization.

Strength of Recommendation: According to guidance provided by members of the DCoE/DVBIC consensus conference (Helmick, 2010) social skills training has shown effectiveness in improving problems in comprehending and responding to nonverbal social cues. Clinical experience with the military population with concussion/mTBI has supported the need to address impairments in social communication, particularly in light of co-morbidities such as PTSD.

DISCUSSION

Social communication treatment may focus on affective-behavioral impairments.

- Treatment may be directed at managing anger.

○ Medd and Tate (2000) describe the effects of an anger management protocol on 16 subjects with acquired brain injury, 13 who had closed injury with severity ranging from mild to severe. Treatment involved: a) psychoeducation regarding the relationship between brain injury and anger and a model of anger; b) awareness-building exercises to explore the cognitive, physical, and emotional changes that may be contributing to anger; and c) development and rehearsal of strategies to deal with anger, including relaxation, self-talk, cognitive challenging, assertiveness training, distraction, and time-out methods. Participation in the program resulted in a significant decrease in anger on objective test measures.

○ Uomoto and Brockway (1992) describe an anger management program involving two subjects with brain-injury and their families. The subjects with brain injuries were taught to use self-talk as a means of defusing tension when angry and to execute a time-out procedure when aware of significant anger escalation. Family members were trained to identify antecedent conditions to anger outbursts and to modify their communication style so as to reduce irritability in their family member with a brain injury. Both subjects showed diminished episodes of angry outbursts, and one subject showed improved social participation after treatment.

- Treatment may be directed at reducing anxiety and social avoidance.
  ○ Anxiety disorders, independent of TBI, may result in social discomfort and avoidance of social situations. A number of social skills treatments have been described for this population (Hambrick, Weeks, Harb, & Hemiberg, 2003; Van Dam-Baggen & Kraaimaat, 2000; Norton & Price, 2008). Cognitive therapies (e.g., cognitive-behavioral treatments) and exposure therapy alone, in combination, or combined with relaxation training, have been found to be efficacious across a variety of anxiety disorders. These techniques are likely to provide benefit for SMs/veterans with mTBI, particularly when they present with co-morbid PTSD and anxiety for specific situations that may result in social withdrawal.
  ○ MacLennan and Petska (2008) describe a social skills group run by SLP and psychology in which people with mTBI and co-morbid PTSD first develop relaxation strategies, then use the relaxation strategies during systematic exposure to increasingly stressful social situations.

- SLPs who possess the skill set to apply behavioral techniques in the treatment of communication are encouraged to do so. Clinicians who are not comfortable with practicing in this area, may elect to partner with psychologists and other mental health professionals to provide treatment in which behavioral change improves communication (e.g., exposure based communication group cited in MacLennan and Petska, 2008).

Where significant cognitive-communication impairments exist, most likely in patients with complicated mTBI, techniques described in the traditional treatment of social communication may be of benefit (see Struchen, 2005 for review). However, for best results, this treatment should be intensive, make extensive use of videotaped feedback, and deliberately incorporate strategies that will facilitate generalization to meaningful contexts (Ylvisaker, Turkstra, & Coelho, 2005). These strategies include use of group treatment sessions, treatment of social skills interactions in the community, and training family and other community members to communicate with the patient with brain injury.

Use of videotaped feedback should be considered as a powerful technique for behavioral change. Video review of social interactions can provide relatively immediate feedback regarding the appropriateness of communication and allow SMs/veterans to identify problems in social interactions. This technique has been used to effect positive change in social communication that can generalize to untrained situations (Helffenstein & Wechsler, 1982). Aron and colleagues (1997) provided videotaped feedback of conversations to people with orbitofrontal brain damage who consistently engaged in inappropriate personal disclosure and showed no awareness or embarrassment for inappropriate self-disclosure. Videotaped review of such interactions was shown to heighten awareness of inappropriate disclosure resulting in feelings of social embarrassment. Such use of videotaped review of conversational interactions to improve awareness can be the first step in developing strategies to modify that behavior.

Effective treatment may target everyday support people that interact with the person with brain injury. This includes family, friends, employers, and coworkers (Ylvisaker, et al., 2003; Togher, et al., 2004). Strategies directed at modifying social communication skills in the communication partners of the person with TBI often serve to improve the communication skills of the person with brain injury.

6.5.6 Acquired Stuttering and Other Speech Dysfluencies

BACKGROUND

SLPs working in the DoD and VA are reporting increasing numbers of referrals for fluency problems in SMs with suspected blast-related mTBI. While stuttering is not a symptom typically associated with mTBI, SLPs need to be mindful of the complex interaction of emotional and neurological consequences of combat injuries on communication and provide the most appropriate individualized services that address the SM's functional needs. The information below reviews the types and causes of adult-onset dysfluencies or stuttering as discussed in the literature and provides the SLP a starting point for conceptualizing his/her services for this unique population.

Stuttering

Speech dysfluency is typically referred to as stuttering. Stuttering is characterized by repetition of sounds, syllables, and whole monosyllabic words; prolongation of sounds; interjections; interruptions of word; silent or audible freezing or blocking; avoidance of difficult words by the use of different phrasing; and excessive physical tension accompanying the production of words.

The majority of adults who stutter have a developmental history of stuttering that began shortly after they learned to speak. There is believed to be a genetic predisposition to stuttering of childhood-onset as well as a similar predisposition to recovery from developmental stuttering that has been estimated to be as high as 80%. The majority of preschool children with stuttering-like speech dysfluencies recover before kindergarten (Ambrose, Cox, & Yairi, 1997).

Acquired Stuttering

Acquired stuttering, or speech dysfluencies that begin in adulthood may result from neurologic changes due to injury, disease, medication or in reaction to psychosocial-emotional stressors. Neurogenic stuttering typically appears following injury or disease to the central nervous system (i.e., the brain and spinal cord, including cortex, subcortex, cerebellar, and even the neural pathway regions). Drug-related side effects of some medications also can cause stuttering. In the majority of cases, the injury or disease that caused the stuttering can be identified. In a small number of cases, however, the individual may only show evidence of speech disruption without any clear evidence of neurological damage or drug effect. Psychogenic stuttering typically begins after a prolonged period of stress or after a traumatic event. Determining the etiology of adult onset stuttering can be challenging, especially when it occurs in the context of emotionally and physically traumatic events such as combat injury.

Neurogenic Stuttering

Speech dysfluencies of neurogenic etiology are common in individuals with diagnosis of stroke, TBI, Parkinson's disease, epilepsy, Alzheimer's disease, Multiple Sclerosis, and Huntington's disease. Neurogenic stuttering can occur in isolation or in conjunction with other motor speech and language disorders (e.g., aphasia, apraxia, dysarthria). Neurogenic stuttering should be distinguished from other dysfluent behaviors that are associated with neurologic problems such as palalalia (word and phrase repetitions produced with increasing rate and decreasing loudness) (Rosenbek, 1984); and repetitions that some individuals make as they try to correct their motor speech or linguistic errors.

Acquired neurogenic stuttering differs from developmental stuttering in a number of ways: neurogenic stuttering usually has a sudden onset in adulthood; stuttering may not be restricted to initial syllables and may include context as well as function words; repeated readings of the same passage have less of an adaptation effect; many fluency-inducing conditions do not reduce stuttering; there is often awareness but without the typical anxiety, fear, or struggle evident in adults with a childhood history of stuttering. Helm-Estabrooks (1999) suggested that neurogenic stuttering also applies to adults with pre-existing history of childhood stuttering that either worsens or recurs as a result of an acquired neurological disorder.

Drug-Related Stuttering

It is common for drugs active in the central nervous system to cause changes in speech as part of a symptom complex resulting from adverse cognitive effects of the drug (Fayen, Goldman, Moulthrop, & Lurchins, 1988; Miller et al., 1988). Speech impairment including slurred speech, dysfluency, and word unintelligibility are used to describe the dysarthria reported to be related to medication usage (Bond, Carvalho, & Foulkes, 1982). Dysarthria, aphonia, mutism, and speech blockage have all been associated with administration of drugs, with various degrees of severity and duration (Bond et al., 1982).

Drugs that have been implicated in causing speech dysfluencies include: neuroleptics or antipsychotic agents including fluphenazine or chlorpromazine, benzodiazepines, antidepressants including amitriptyline, desipramine, fluoxetine, sertraline, and metrazamide, a radiopaque contrast medium used in positive contrast myelography. Other drugs that have been associated with stuttering include theophyline, prochlorperazine, methylphenidate and pemoline, and alprazolam. It has been speculated that these drugs interact with neurochemical, neurotransmitter function in the central nervous system resulting in cognitive and/or extrapyramidal symptoms that interrupt speech fluency (Adler, Leong, & Delgado, 1987; Bertoni, Schwartzman, Van Horn, & Partin, 1981; Guthrie & Grunhaus, 1990; Lee et al., 2001; Meghji, 1994; Nurnberg & Greenwald, 1981).

Psychogenic Stuttering

Sudden-onset stuttering in adults is sometimes attributed to malingering (the conscious feigning of an illness to benefit the individual, such as avoidance of work or financial reward). However, it is more likely a form of psychogenic stuttering, a conversion symptom or a somatoform disorder in which physical symptoms occur where there is no organic or physiological explanation found, and for which there is a strong likelihood that psychological factors are involved (Lazare, 1981; Roth, Aronson, & Davis, 1989).

Psychogenic stuttering may occur alone or in combination with other signs of psychological or neurological involvement. Baumgartner and Duffy (1997) suggested that people may be predisposed by personality, social or cultural bias, early learning, or visceral structure. If predisposed and then exposed to trauma or interpersonal difficulties, conflict and stress may then be channeled into musculoskeletal tension. Speech and laryngeal muscles are known to be susceptible to emotional stress as seen in muscle tension dysphonia and conversion aphonia (Aronson & Bless, 2009); stuttering-like behavior, infantile speech, pseudo-foreign dialect, and other speech and resonance disorders (Darley, Aronson, & Brown, 1975; Duffy, 2005).

Several authors have described the manifestations, diagnosis and treatment of psychogenic stuttering (Baumgartner, 1999; Lazare, 1981; Mahr & Leith, 1992; Roth, Aronson, & Davis, 1989). Similar to neurogenic stuttering, the stuttering pattern of psychogenic stuttering resembles developmental stuttering in terms of core behaviors, with sound and word repetitions, prolongations and blocks. In some cases, however, secondary behaviors may be unusual and occur independently of core stuttering behaviors.

ACTION STATEMENT

It is important to acknowledge and validate for the SM/veteran the presence of speech dysfluencies and to address this communication disorder through evaluation of its nature and severity, followed by therapeutic interventions to improve symptoms.

RECOMMENDATIONS

1. SMs/veterans with sudden onset of stuttering following combat-related concussion/mTBI should be seen by a SLP for evaluation and treatment.
2. A multidisciplinary approach involving neurology, psychiatry, and SLP is recommended.
3. The evaluation should include:
   - Complete case history
   - Motor speech exam
   - Speech samples under traditional fluency-enhancing conditions
   - Trial therapy
   - Analysis of stuttering behaviors to establish baseline measures of stuttering patterns and severity.
4. Treatments that have been suggested are similar to those used with developmental stuttering including: prolonged speech, fluency-shaping, easy onset, light contact, easy repetitions; diminishing extra motor behaviors and reducing physical tension associated with efforts to speak; providing education, support and reassurance; desensitization combined with vocal control therapy emphasizing adequate respiratory support, and optimal vocal resonance with gentle onsets; and finally following a hierarchy of easy to difficult situations to transfer learned skills outside of therapy (Baumgartner, 1999; Duffy, 2005; Roth et al., 1989; Weiner, 1981).

Strength of Recommendation: Acquired stuttering related to TBI is more common in individuals who sustained moderate to severe brain injuries. An early case description of combat-related acquired stuttering involved an individual diagnosed with combat-psychoneuroses (Dempsey & Granich, 1978). Other more recent case studies have described acquired stuttering in the presence of TBI and PTSD (Duffy, 2009; Duffy, Manning & Roth, 2011; Roth & Bibeau, 2011; Roth & Manning, 2009). Review of existing studies and expert consensus endorse the effectiveness of SLP involvement in cases of adult onset stuttering.

DISCUSSION

Adult-onset stuttering can have several etiologies that need to be considered: purely neurogenic, purely psychogenic, neurogenic with psychogenically-based neurologic symptoms, psychogenic accompanied by psychogenically-based neurologic signs, and psychogenic with coexisting but unrelated neurologic disease (Baumgartner & Duffy, 1997; Roth et al., 1989).

One of the first aims of an evaluation of adult-onset stuttering is to rule out a neurologic etiology. An interdisciplinary approach involving neurology, psychiatry and SLP may be the best option for assessment especially if a SM/veteran has other neurological symptoms such as headache, dizziness, or other cognitive-communication problems.

It can be difficult at times to determine etiology of dysfluencies as individuals with neurologic disease can experience depression, stress, and/or adjustment disorder. Organic disease may precede psychogenic response. It may "direct the somatization of psychodynamic conflict" (e.g., mTBI preceding psychogenic stuttering). Some individuals may be hypervigilant concerning their internal body environment ("spectatoring"). They may perceive ambiguous sensory changes in their speech (voice) mechanism as a result of trauma or emotional states as threatening or cause for alarm. Following a traumatic event, an individual may sustain motor inhibition without appropriate release leading to unnecessarily high muscular tonus, leading to partial or complete stuttering (Duffy, 2008).

Individuals who are able to decrease their stuttering in trial therapy and whose psychological adjustment is adequate are often good candidates for stuttering therapy.

An individual who is unable to improve fluency during trial therapy and/or who is dysfunctional because of psychological issues may benefit from psychotherapy concurrently with stuttering therapy. Even though an individual may need supportive or interventional psychotherapy, speech therapy may start immediately. Treatment of psychogenic stuttering can be successful with limited intervention. An individual who resists the idea that his/her stuttering may have a stress-related basis and who does not improve with trial therapy may not be a candidate for treatment or may need extended treatment.

An individual taking medications that may contribute to the onset of stuttering may respond well when the medication is eliminated or adjusted.

6.6 Discharge from Cognitive-Communication Treatment

6.6.1 Planning for Discharge

BACKGROUND

Discharge planning begins with the development of the treatment plan and long-term goals following the initial evaluation. It is a documented sequence of tasks and activities designed to achieve, within projected time frames, stated goals that lead to the timely transfer of SMs/veterans back to their Commands, into the community, to the VA System of care, to other providers in local communities, or to civilian facilities with specialized rehabilitation programs or services.

Discharge planning is undertaken in collaboration with the IDT, including the SM/veteran and family, to ensure that SMs/veterans receive health-care services, including rehabilitation therapies, for as long as medically necessary (Joint Commission on Accreditation of Healthcare Organizations, 2004).

ACTION STATEMENT

Discharge planning is conducted to ensure successful transition of the SM/veteran from the rehabilitation setting to their Commands or into the community.

RECOMMENDATIONS

1. Planning for return to AD status or transition to the VA System, and to the community involves the IDT, Command, SM/veteran and family, and includes the following:
   - Assessing the discharge destination environment and supports available;
   - Providing equipment and adaptations as needed;
   - Communicating with the interdisciplinary treatment team, the Command, the VA, or social services to ensure that appropriate follow up services are available as needed;
   - Establishing a monitoring process for tracking the SM's/veteran's progress and outcomes and providing follow-up, as appropriate;
   - Providing information about appropriate services and self-help groups in the discharge community that may be beneficial to the SM/veteran and family.

2. Discharge planning includes a written care plan outlining current needs and follow-up recommendations including:
   - Key contacts, responsible services/professionals, sources of continued information, support and advice;
   - Potential future problems and how to manage them, follow-up arrangements, the responsible service/person to contact if problems arise;
   - Services that address the SM's/veteran's and family's preferences, goals, and special needs to enhance participation and improve functioning in life activities.

3. SMs/veterans with persistent symptoms may need to proceed through the medical or disability evaluation processes. This process follows national and local regulations.

DISCUSSION

The SLP should insure that the following factors have been addressed for successful discharge planning: (a) appropriate interventional goals and objectives were specified; (b) sufficient instructional time was provided; (c) current and suitable intervention methods or materials were used; (d) meaningful and functional performance data were collected and analyzed on an ongoing basis to monitor and evaluate progress; (e) appropriate assistive technology or other supports were provided, when necessary; (f) a plan was designed and implemented as needed to address the needs and concerns of culturally/linguistically diverse families as they affect participation in communication services (e.g., use of interpreter or translator) (ASHA, 2004b); (g) relevant and accurate criteria were used to evaluate intervention; and h) health, educational, environmental, or other supports relevant to cognitive-communication interventions were provided.

Discharge planning is best conducted through IDT collaboration including, when appropriate, the SM/veteran and family member, Command, or whoever the SM/veteran chooses to include. The goal of discharge planning is to transition the SM/veteran into the setting where there is the greatest probability of performing successfully. When planning the discharge, it is the clinician's ethical responsibility to review and analyze all aspects of past services and to make recommendations for follow up.

Recommendations may include: (a) discontinuation from therapeutic services and return to Active Duty/work/community in pre-injury roles and responsibilities; (b) return to Active Duty/work/community in a new or modified position of responsibility; or (c) continuation of therapeutic services in another facility or at a different level of care.

6.6.2 Criteria for Discharge

BACKGROUND

Criteria for discharge from cognitive-communication therapy are based on the individualized treatment plan for each SM/veteran. There are no established thresholds on standardized testing that can substitute for clinician judgment, and the SM's/veteran's goals, perceptions, and preferences.

Discharge from cognitive-communication treatment ideally occurs when the SM/veteran, family, and SLP, as a team, conclude that the cognitive-communication disorder is remediated and/or compensatory strategies enable the individual to function adequately in his/her environment.

ACTION STATEMENT

Discharge from cognitive-communication rehabilitation should be considered when the SM/veteran no longer requires the facilities, skills, and therapeutic intensity of SLP services to meet the cognitive-communication challenges of their social, vocational, and avocational goals.

RECOMMENDATIONS

1. Discharge from cognitive-communication rehabilitation is recommended when one or more of the following criteria are met:
   - Cognitive-communication abilities are within normal limits or are consistent with the SM's/veteran's pre-morbid status;
   - Therapeutic goals have been met;
   - Cognitive-communication abilities are functional and no longer interfere with the SM's/veteran's ability to participate in home and community activities to their satisfaction;
   - No progress is demonstrated toward the next level of cognitive-communication independence despite repeated efforts and different treatment approaches;
   - There is a change in the SM's/veteran's medical, psychological, or other conditions preventing further benefit from therapeutic intervention at the current time.

2. Recommendations for reassessment or follow-up in the MTF, VA system, or in the community, or a referral for other services may be made at the time of discharge.

3. Discharge is also appropriate in the following situations, provided that the SM/veteran is advised of the likely outcomes of discontinuation:
   - SM/veteran is unwilling or chooses not to participate in treatment;
   - Treatment attendance has been inconsistent or poor, and efforts to address these factors have not been successful;
   - SM/veteran requests to be discharged or requests continuation of services with another provider;
   - SM/veteran is transferred or discharged to another location where ongoing service from the current provider is not reasonably available, in which case efforts should be made to ensure continuation of services at the new locale;
   - Treatment no longer results in measurable benefits. There does not appear to be any reasonable expectation for improvement with continued treatment. Reevaluation should be considered at a later date to determine whether the SM's/veteran's status has changed or whether new treatment options are available.
   - SM/veteran is unable to tolerate treatment because of a serious medical, psychological, or other condition;
   - SM/veteran demonstrates behavior that interferes with improvement or participation in treatment (e.g., noncompliance, malingering), providing that efforts to address the interfering behavior have been unsuccessful.

DISCUSSION

The restoration of quality of life after TBI is a primary endpoint of recovery and rehabilitation (Cicerone & Azulay, 2007). Treatment is expected to result in deficit reduction, and measurably enhanced functioning and participation.

In the majority of cases, a patient with mild cognitive-communication impairments may require a very limited period of intervention defined as education, counseling, and provision of functional accommodations and compensatory or support strategies with discharge occurring within a few weeks of initial contact.

In those SMs/veterans with persisting cognitive-communication deficits associated with PCS, a lengthier period of intervention may be required. In this small percentage of cases, discharge planning may benefit from collaboration of the SLP, SM/veteran/family, case manager, and other IDT members to ensure the most successful outcomes.

6.7 Follow-Up

BACKGROUND

Each program should have established policies and procedures for following the SM/veteran after discharge. Follow-up is necessary for a variety of reasons, including the fact that circumstances may change in the SM's/veteran's environment, new treatment options may become available, or the SM/veteran may respond differently due to maturational or motivational changes or new life transitions. The discharge plan should stipulate a follow-up schedule and long-term goals that promote recovery from cognitive symptoms and prevent harm due to their persistence.

To date, evidence is not available on how long blast-related cognitive-communication symptoms typically persist. However, preliminary studies suggest that, while a single mTBI or concussion is a transient neurological event with a relatively rapid and spontaneous recovery, recurrent mTBI may be associated with longer recovery time and persistent symptoms, and may potentially increase the lifetime risk of psychiatric and neurological problems (McCrae, 2008).

ACTION STATEMENT

Follow-up interventions should be planned after discharge from cognitive-communication services with goals and on a schedule that are appropriate to the community re-integration needs of the individual.

RECOMMENDATIONS

Follow up services for cognitive-communication problems of mTBI should be considered under the following conditions:

1. SMs/veterans who present with cognitive-communication problems in the acute phase of mTBI should be seen at three months from the most recent injury event to determine if symptoms have resolved or to initiate evaluation, as necessary;
2. Follow-up interventions following discharge from treatment should be scheduled as prescribed in the discharge plan, and at times that are least disruptive for the SM/veteran so that employment and academic status are not compromised;
3. Telephone follow-up should be used to provide additional support;
4. If cognitive-communication problems are identified and the SM/veteran does not choose to engage in treatment at that time, information should be made available to facilitate contact with the appropriate VA or DoD facility for follow-up in the future;
5. The SLP should advocate for case management for SMs/veterans with complicated histories, co-morbidities, and lack of social support.

DISCUSSION

Guskiewicz et al. (2005) studied the association between prior TBI and long-term mild cognitive impairment and Alzheimer's disease in a group of retired professional football players. Results of surveys obtained from 758 retired athletes and spouses or immediate caregivers focused on memory and other cognitive problems. More than half (61%) reported sustaining at least one concussion and 24% sustained three or more previous concussions. There was a significant association between recurrent concussions and clinical diagnosis of mild cognitive impairment and

Mild TBI Rehabilitation Toolkit

self reported memory impairments. Those with three or more concussions had a five-fold prevalence of cognitive disorder and a three-fold prevalence of reported significant memory problems compared with subjects who had no prior history of concussion. There was an earlier onset of Alzheimer's disease in retired professional football players than in the general American male population. The authors concluded that the onset of dementia-related syndromes may be initiated by repetitive cerebral concussions in professional football players.

Results of the Neurobehavioral Symptom Inventory (Cicerone & Kalmar, 1995) administered at the Durham VAMC to veterans (n=162), who screened positive to exposure to blast or blunt head trauma, indicated some level of cognitive problems, with forgetfulness (96%), concentration (95%), organization (93%), and decision making (85%) being most frequently represented. Most of these veterans were employed, seeking employment, or were students, and reported problems at work/school or in their family and social life due to cognitive problems. A significant number was over five years post exposure to multiple blast and blunt head trauma. Follow-up to address these problems and improve quality of life is imperative, although visits are difficult to schedule because these veterans are employed or seeking employment and fulfilling their responsibilities to their family and community.

7. Outcome Measurement

BACKGROUND

In an era of emphasis on evidence-based clinical practice, the employment of outcome measures is essential for validating the efficacy of cognitive-communication interventions. When appropriately used, outcome measures allow SLPs to communicate to the individuals served, persons with administrative oversight, and the public at large about the value of the services provided.

The gold standard of outcome measurement is pre- vs. post-assessment differences, including differences in functional status, the moderating variables that may affect outcome, discharge environment, and consumer satisfaction (including the SM/veteran, family, employer/Command, and referral source) (Helmick, 2010).

ACTION STATEMENT

Outcome measurement should be conducted to establish the effect of cognitive-communication interventions.

RECOMMENDATIONS

Outcome measurements should include standardized evaluation of discrete cognitive-communication skills, symptom status, and functional status.

1. Areas of objective testing and symptom reports that are measured post-rehabilitation should be consistent with those areas initially evaluated during the assessment phase.
2. Functional outcomes should be monitored on an ongoing basis. Functional areas that should be addressed in outcome assessment include:
   - Job performance (MOS, work, school);
   - Need for job re-designation and/or duty/work/school restrictions or limitations;

636

- Differential between pre-injury performance and current functional status;
- Performance on simulators (e.g., rifle, flight) and work trials;
- Quality of life;
- Community participation.

SLPs may benefit from collaboration with the IDT in the selection of outcome measurements that integrate cognitive-communication changes in the larger context of rehabilitation outcomes. In such cases, however, it may be difficult to establish a direct correlation between changes in specific cognitive-communication abilities and differences in global measures of function.

DISCUSSION

Analysis of the outcome measurements in cognitive-communication rehabilitation for mTBI is disadvantaged by the many unknown facts about the nature of blast-related mTBI and by the paucity of scientific evidence about the efficacy of cognitive-communication rehabilitation in both military and civilian mTBI. For these reasons, it is important to carefully describe the patients receiving cognitive rehabilitation, including identification of moderating variables, confounds, and co-morbidities of mTBI. Understanding which patients with mTBI respond to cognitive rehabilitation interventions and which do not is the key to advancing this field in medicine (Helmick, 2010).

Appendix: List of Acronyms

AD: Active Duty

ANCDS: Academy of Neurologic Communication Disorders and Sciences

ASHA: American Speech-Language-Hearing Association

CDC: Centers for Disease Control and Prevention

CONUS: continental United States

CPD: cognitive prosthetic device

CMG: Clinical Management Guidance

CSH: combat support hospital

CT: computed tomography

DAI: diffuse axonal injury

DCoE: Defense Centers of Excellence for Psychological Health and Traumatic Brain Injury

DoD: Department of Defense

DVBIC: Defense and Veterans Brain Injury Center

FST: forward surgical team

ICD-10: International Classification of Diseases, 10th edition

IDT: interdisciplinary team

IED: improvised explosive device

JC: The Joint Commission LRMC: Landstuhl Regional Medical Center, Germany

MACE: Military Acute Concussion Evaluation

MEB: Medical Evaluation Board

MOA: Memorandum of Agreement

MOS: military occupational specialty

MPT: Matching Person & Technology

MRI: magnetic resonance imaging

mTBI: mild traumatic brain injury

MTF: medical treatment facility

MVC: motor vehicle crash

NIH: National Institutes of Health

OEF: Operation Enduring Freedom

OIF: Operation Iraqi Freedom

OT: occupational therapist

OTSG: Office of The Surgeon General

PCS: post-concussion symptoms

PNS: VA Polytrauma Network Sites

POC: point of contact

PRC: Polytrauma Rehabilitation Centers

PSC: Polytrauma/TBI System of Care

PT: physical therapist

PTSD: post-traumatic stress disorder

SAC: Standardized Assessment of Concussion

SCI: spinal cord injury

SLP: speech-language pathology; speech-language pathologist

SM: service member

TBI: traumatic brain injury

VA: Department of Veterans Affairs

VAMC: VA Medical Center

VHA: Veterans Health Administration

VISN: Veterans Integrated Service Networks

WHO: World Health Organization

References

Adler, L., Leong, S., & Delgado, R. (1987). Drug-induced stuttering treated with propranolol. *Journal of Clinical Psychopharmacology, 7,* 115-116.

Alderfer, B. S., Arciniegas, D. B., & Silver, J. M. (2005). Treatment of depression following traumatic brain injury. *Journal of Head Trauma Rehabilitation, 20,* 544–562.

Ambrose, N. G., Cox, N. J., & Yairi, E. (1997). The genetic basis of persistence and recovery in stuttering. *Journal of Speech, Language, and Hearing Research 40,* 556-566.

American Congress of Rehabilitation Medicine. (1993). Definition of mild traumatic brain injury. *Journal of Head Trauma Rehabilitation, 8*(3), 86–87.

American Speech-Language-Hearing Association. (1987). The role of speech-language pathologists in the habilitation of cognitively impaired individuals: A report of the subcommittee on language and cognition. *American Speech-Language-Hearing Association, 29,* 53-55.

American Speech-Language-Hearing Association. (1991). *Guidelines for speech-language pathologists serving persons with language, socio-communication, and/or cognitive-communication impairments* [Guidelines]. Retrieved March 04, 2012 from www.asha.org/policy.

American Speech-Language-Hearing Association. (2003). *Rehabilitation of children and adults with cognitive-communication disorders after brain injury* [Technical Report]. Retrieved March 04, 2012 from www.asha.org/policy.

American Speech-Language-Hearing Association. (2004a). *Preferred Practice Patterns for the Profession of Speech-Language Pathology* [Preferred Practice Patterns]. Retrieved March 04, 2012 from www.asha.org/policy.

American Speech-Language-Hearing Association. (2004b). Admission/Discharge Criteria in Speech-Language Pathology [Guidelines]. Retrieved March 04, 2012 from www.asha.org/policy.

American Speech-Language-Hearing Association. (2005). *Knowledge and skills needed by speech-language pathologists providing services to individuals with cognitive-communication disorders* [Knowledge and Skills]. Retrieved March 04, 2012 from www.asha.org/policy.

American Speech-Language-Hearing Association (retrieved 14 Jun 2009). *Treatment efficacy summary: Cognitive-communication disorders resulting from traumatic brain injury.* Retrieved March 04, 2012 from http://www.asha.org/uploadedFiles/public/TESCognitiveCommunicationDisordersFromTBI.pdf.

ADA (Americans With Disabilities Act). ADA Amendments Act of 2008.

Aron, A., Melinat, E., Aron, E. N., Vallone, R. D., & Bator, R. J. (1997). The experimental generation of interpersonal closeness: A procedure and some preliminary findings. *Personality and Social Psychology Bulletin, 4,* 363-377.

Aronson, A. E., & Bless, D. M. (2009). *Clinical Voice Disorders* (4th ed.). New York: Thieme.

Bach-y-Rita, P. (2003). Late postacute neurologic rehabilitation: Neuroscience, engineering, and clinical programs. *Archives of Physical Medicine & Rehabilitation, 84,* 1100-1108.

Baddeley, A. (1992). Working memory. *Science, 255,* 556-559.

Baumgartner, J. (1999). Acquired psychogenic stuttering. In R. Curlee (Ed.), *Stuttering and Related Disorders of Fluency* (2nd ed., pp. 269-288). New York: Thieme.

Baumgartner, J., & Duffy, J. (1997). Psychogenic stuttering in adults with and without neurologic disease. *Journal of Medical Speech-Language Pathology, 5,* 75-95.

Belanger, H. G., Kretzmer, T., Yoash-Gantz, R., Pickett, T., & Tupler, L. A. (2009). Cognitive sequelae of blast-related versus other mechanisms of brain trauma. *Journal of the International Neuropsychological Society, 15(1),* 1–8.

Belanger, H. G., Uomoto, J. M., & Vanderploeg, R. D. (2009). The Veterans' health administration system of care for mild traumatic brain injury: Costs, benefits, and controversies. *Journal of Head Trauma Rehabilitation, 24(1),* 4-13.

Belanger, H. G., & Vanderploeg, R. D. (2005). The neuropsychological impact of sports-related concussion: A meta-analysis. *Journal of the International Neuropsychological Society, 11(4),* 345-357.

Bertoni, J. M., Schwartzman, R. J., Van Horn, G., & Partin, J. (1981). Asterixis and encephalopathy following metrizamide myelography: Investigations into possible mechanisms and review of the literature. *Annals of Neurology, 9,* 366-370.

Bigler, E. D. (2007). Anterior and middle cranial fossa in traumatic brain injury: Relevant neuroanatomy and neuropathology in the study of neuropsychological outcome. *Neuropsychology, 21,* 515-531.

Bond, W. S., Carvalho, M., & Foulkes, E. F. (1982). Persistent dysarthria with apraxia associated with a combination of lithium carbonate and haloperidol. *Journal of Clinical Psychiatry, 43,* 256-257.

Bordin, E. S. (1979). The generalizability of the psychoanalytic concept of the working alliance. *Psychotherapy: Theory, Research and Practice, 16(3),* 252-260.

Borg, J., Holm, L., Peloso, P. M., Cassidy, J. D., Carroll, L. J., von Holst, H.,...Yates, D. (2004). Non-surgical intervention and cost for mild traumatic brain injury: Results of the WHO collaborating centre task force on mild traumatic brain injury. *Journal of Rehabilitation Medicine, 19*, 805-816.

Brady, K. T., Killeen, T. K., Brewerton, T., & Lucerini, S. (2000). Comorbidity of psychiatric disorders and posttraumatic stress disorder. *Journal of Clinical Psychiatry, 61*(Suppl. 7), 22-32.

Brahm, K. D., Wilgenburg, H. M., Kirby, J., Ingalla, S., Chang, C. Y., & Goodrich, G. L. (2009). Visual impairment and dysfunction in combat-injured service members with traumatic brain injury. *Optometry and Vision Science, 86*(7), 817-825.

Brooks, N., McKinlay, W., Symington, C., Beattie, A., & Campsie, L. (1987). Return to work within the first seven years of severe head injury. *Brain Injury, 1*, 5-20.

Burgess, S., & Turkstra, L. S. (2006). Social skills intervention for adolescents with autism spectrum disorders: A review of the experimental evidence. *Evidence-Based Practice (EBP) Briefs, 1*, 1-20.

Burke, J. M., Danick, J. A., Bemis, B., & Durgin, C. J. (1994). A process approach to memory notebook training for neurologic patients. *Brain Injury, 8*(1), 71-81.

Canter G. (1971). Observations on neurogenic stuttering: A contribution to differential diagnosis. *British Journal of Disorders of Communication, 6*, 139-143.

Carroll, L. J., Cassidy, J. D., Holm, L., Kraus, J., & Coronado, V. G. (2004). Methodological issues and research recommendations for mild traumatic brain injury: The WHO collaborating centre task force on mild traumatic brain injury. *Journal of Rehabilitation Medicine, 36*(Suppl. 43), 113-125.

CDC (Centers for Disease Control and Prevention). (1999). National center for injury prevention and control. *Traumatic brain injury in the United States: A report to congress.* Atlanta, Georgia.

CDC (Centers for Disease Control and Prevention). (2003). National center for injury prevention and control. *Report to congress on mild traumatic brain injury in the United States: Steps to prevent a serious public health problem.* Atlanta, Georgia.

Chandler, D. (2006). Blast-related ear injury in current U.S. military operations. *The ASHA Leader, 11*, pp. 8, 9, 29.

Chiaravalloti, N. D., Christodoulou, C., Demaree, H. A., & DeLuca, J. (2003). Differentiating simple versus complex processing speed: Influence on new learning and memory performance. *Journal of Clinical and Experimental Neuropsychology, 25*(4), 489-501.

Cicerone, K. D. (1996). Attention deficits and dual task demands after mild traumatic brain injury. *Brain Injury, 10*(2), 79-90.

Cicerone, K. D. (2002). Remediation of 'working attention' in mild traumatic brain injury. *Brain Injury, 16*(3), 185-195.

Cicerone, K. D., & Azulay, J. (2007). Perceived self-efficacy and life satisfaction after traumatic brain injury. *Journal of Head Trauma Rehabilitation, 22*(5), 257-266.

Cicerone, K. D., Dahlberg, C., Kalmar, K., Lagenbahn, D. M., Malec, J. F., Bergquist, T. F.,...Morse, P. A. (2000). Evidence-based cognitive rehabilitation: Recommendations for clinical practice. *Archives of Physical Medicine and Rehabilitation, 81*(12), 1596-1615.

Cicerone, K. D., Dahlberg, C., Malec, J.F., Langenbahn, D. M., Felicetti, T., Kneipp, S.,...Cantanese, J. (2005). Evidence-based cognitive rehabilitation: Updated review of the literature from 1998 through 2002. *Archives of Physical Medicine and Rehabilitation, 86*, 1681-1692.

Cicerone, K. D., & Kalmar, K. (1995). Persistent concussion syndrome: The structure of subjective complaints after mild traumatic brain injury. *Journal of Head Trauma Rehabilitation, 10*(3), 1-17.

Cicerone, K. D., Langenbahn, D. M., Braden, C., Malec, J. F., Kalmar, K., Fraas, M.,...Ashman, T. (2011). Evidence-based cognitive rehabilitation: Updated review of the literature from 2003 through 2008. *Archives of Physical Medicine and Rehabilitation, 92*, 519-530.

Cicerone, K. D., Mott, T., Azulay, J., Sharlow-Galella, M. A., Ellmo, W. J., Paradise, S., & Friel, J. C. (2008). A randomized controlled trial of holistic neuropsychologic rehabilitation after traumatic brain injury. *Archives of Physical Medicine & Rehabilitation, 89*, 2239-2249.

Coelho, C., Ylvisaker, M., & Turkstra, L. (2005). Nonstandardized assessment approaches for individuals with traumatic brain injuries. *Seminars in Speech and Language, 26*(4), 223-241.

Comper, P., Bisschop, S. M., Carnide, N., & Tricco, A. (2005). A systematic review of treatments for mild traumatic brain injury. *Brain Injury, 19*(11), 863-880.

Cornis-Pop, M. (2008). The role of speech-language pathologists in the cognitive-communication rehabilitation of traumatic brain injury. *California Speech-Language Hearing Association Magazine, 38*(1), 14-18.

Cornis-Pop, M., Alligood, S., Beasley, P., Budd, L. V., Magee, J. T., Morris, P.,...Williams G. (1998). *A project-oriented approach to brain injury rehabilitation*. Presentation at Williamsburg, VA.

Corrigan, J. D., & Cole, T. B. (2008). Substance use disorders and clinical management of traumatic brain injury and posttraumatic stress disorder. *Journal of the American Medical Association, 300*(6), 720-721.

Cummings, L. (2007). Pragmatics and adult language disorders: Past achievements and future directions. *Seminars in Speech & Language, 28*, 96-110.

Dahlberg, C. A., Cusick, C. P., Hawley, L. A., Newman, J. K., Morey, C. E., Harrison-Felix, C. L., & Whiteneck, G. G. (2007). Treatment efficacy of social communication skills training after traumatic brain injury: A randomized treatment and deferred treatment controlled trial. *Archives of Physical Medicine and Rehabilitation, 88*, 1561-1573.

Darley, F. L., Aronson, A.E., & Brown, J.R. (1975). *Motor Speech Disorders*. Philadelphia: WB Saunders.

De Beaumont, L., Lassonde, M., Leclerc, S., & Théoret, H. (2007). Long-term and cumulative effects of sports concussion on motor cortex inhibition. *Neurosurgery, 61(2)*, 329-337.

DCoE(Defense Centers of Excellence)/DVBIC (Defense and Veterans Brain Injury Center) Consensus Conference on Cognitive Rehabilitation for Mild Traumatic Brain Injury (2009, June).

DePalma, R. G., Burris, D. G., Champion, H. R., & Hodgson, M. J. (2005) Blast Injuries. *New England Journal of Medicine, 352(13)*, 43-50.

Dikmen, S., Machamer, J., & Temkin, N. (2001). Mild head injury: Facts and artifacts. *Journal of Clinical and Experimental Neuropsychology, 23*, 729–738.

Draper, K., & Ponsford, J. (2008). Cognitive functioning ten years following traumatic brain injury and rehabilitation. *Neuropsychology, 22(5)*, 618-625.

Duffy, J. R. (2005). *Motor speech disorders: Substrates, differential diagnosis, and management* (2nd ed.). St. Louis, MO: Mosby.

Duffy, J. R. (2008). *Psychogenic speech disorders in people with suspected neurologic disease: Diagnosis & management.* Paper presented at the Annual Convention of the American Speech-Language-Hearing Association, Chicago.

Duffy, J. R. (2009). *Psychogenic speech disorders in people with possible neurologic disease: Substrates, diagnosis & management.* Grand Rounds on Traumatic Brain Injury. Brooke Army Medical Center, San Antonio.

Duffy, J. R., Manning, R. K., and Roth, C. R. (2011). *Acquired stuttering in post-deployed service members: Neurogenic or psychogenic.* Paper presented at the Annual Convention of the American Speech-Language-Hearing Association, San Diego.

Ehlhardt, L. A., Sohlberg, M. M., Kennedy, M., Coelho, C., Ylvisaker, M., Turkstra, L., & Yorkston, K. (2008). Evidence-based practice guidelines for instructing individuals with neurogenic memory impairments: What have we learned in the past 20 years? *Neuropsychological Rehabilitation, 18 (3)*, 300-342.

Etherton, J. L., Bianchini, K. J., Heinly, M. T., & Greve, K. W. (2006). Pain, malingering, and performance on the WAIS-III processing speed index. *Journal of Clinical and Experimental Neuropsychology, 28*, 1218-1237.

Fann, J. R., Katon, W. J., Uomoto, J. M., & Esselman, P. C. (1995). Psychiatric disorders and functional disability in outpatients with traumatic brain injuries. *The American Journal of Psychiatry,152*, 1493-1499.

Fann, J. R., Uomoto, J. M., & Katon, W. J. (2001). Cognitive improvement with treatment of depression following mild traumatic brain injury. *Psychosomatics, 42*, 48-54.

Fasotti, L., Kovacs, F., Eling, P. A. T. M., & Brouwer, W. H. (2000). Time pressure management as a compensatory strategy training after closed head injury. *Neuropsychological Rehabilitation, 10*, 47-65.

Fayen, M., Goldman, M. B., Moulthrop, M. A., & Luchins, D. J. (1988). Differential memory function with dopaminergic versus anticholinergic treatment of drug-induced extrapyramidal symptoms. *American Journal of Psychiatry, 145*, 483-486.

Felmingham, K. L., Baguley, I. J., & Green, A. S. (2004). Effects of diffuse axonal injury on speed of information processing following severe traumatic brain injury. *Neuropsychology, 18*, 564-571.

Frencham, K. A. R., Fox, A. M., & Mayberry, M. T. (2005). Neuropsychological studies of mild traumatic brain injury: A meta-analytic review of research since 1995. *Journal of Clinical and Experimental Neuropsychology, 27*, 334-351.

Galarneau, M. R., Woodruff, S. I., Dye, J. L., Mohrle, C. R., & Wade, A. L. (2008). Traumatic brain injury during Operation Iraqi Freedom: Findings from the United States Navy-Marine Corps Combat Trauma Registry. *Journal of Neurosurgery,108*(5), 950-957.

Gawande, A. (2004). Casualties of war—military care for the wounded from Iraq and Afghanistan. *New England Journal of Medicine, 351*, 2471-2475.

Gentilini, M., Nichell, P., & Schoenhube, R. (1989). Assessment of attention in mild head injury. In H.S. Levin, H.M. Eisenberg, A.L. Benton (Eds.), *Mild Head Injury (pp 162-175).* New York: Oxford.

Giovanello, K. S., & Verfaellie, M. (2001). Memory systems of the brain: A cognitive neuropsychological analysis. *Seminars in Speech and Language, 22*, 107-116.

Godfrey, H., & Shum, D. (2000). Executive functioning and the application of social skills following traumatic brain injury. *Aphasiology, 14*, 433-444.

Goodrich, G. L., Kirby, J., Cockerham, G., Ingalla, S. P., & Lew, H. L. (2007). Visual function in patients of a polytrauma rehabilitation center: A descriptive study. *Journal of Rehabilitation Research and Development, 44*(7), 929–936.

Guskiewicz, K. M., Marshall, S. W., Bailes, J., McCrea, M., Cantu, R. C., Randolph, C., & Jordan, B. D. (2005). Association between recurrent concussion and late-life cognitive impairment in retired professional football players. *Neurosurgery, 57*(4), 719-726.

Guthrie, S., & Grunhaus, L. (1990). Fluoxetine-induced stuttering. *Journal of Clinical Psychiatry 51*(2), 85.

Hambrick, J. P., Weeks, J. W., Harb, G. C., & Hemiberg, R. (2003) Cognitive-behavioral therapy for social anxiety disorder: Supporting evidence and future directions. *CNS Spectrums, 8*, 373-381.

Hartley, L. L. (1995). *Cognitive-communicative abilities following brain injury: A functional approach.* New York: Thomson Delmar Learning.

Helffenstein, D. A., & Wechsler, F. S. (1982). The use of interpersonal process recall (IPR) in the remediation of interpersonal and communication skill deficits in the newly brain-injured. *Clinical Neuropsychology, 4*, 139-143.

Helm-Estabrooks, N. (1999). Stuttering associated with acquired neurological disorders. In R. Curlee (Ed.), *Stuttering and related disorders of fluency* (2nd ed., pp. 255-268). New York: Thieme Medical Publishers.

Helmick, K. (2010). Cognitive rehabilitation for military personnel with mild traumatic brain injury and chronic post-concussional disorder: Results of April 2009 consensus conference. *NeuroRehabilitation, 26*, 239-255.

Hoffer, M. H. (2009). Meet Navy Captain Michael H. Hoffer Who is Someone You Should Know: Marine Corps Community for Marine Veterans. Retrieved March 04, 2012 from http://www.leatherneck.com/forums/showthread.php?t=76750.

Hoge, C. W., Goldberg, H. M., & Castro, C. A. (2009). Care of war Veterans with mild traumatic brain injury-flawed perspectives. *New England Journal of Medicine, 360*, 1588-1591.

Hoge, C. W., McGurk, D., Thomas, J. L., Cox, A. L., Engel, C. C., & Castro, C. A. (2008). Mild traumatic brain injury in U.S. soldiers returning from Iraq. *New England Journal of Medicine, 358*, 453-463.

IOM (Institute of Medicine). (2008). *Gulf War and Health: Vol. 7: Long-term consequences of traumatic brain injury.* Washington, DC: The National Academies Press.

IOM (Institute of Medicine). (2011). *Cognitive rehabilitation therapy for traumatic brain injury: Evaluating the evidence.* Washington, DC: The National Academies Press.

Iverson, G. L., Gaetz, M., Lovell, M. R., & Collins, M. W. (2004). Cumulative effects of concussion in amateur athletes. *Brain Injury. 18*(5), 433-443.

JCAHO (Joint Commission on Accreditation of Healthcare Organizations). (2004). *Disease-Specific Care Certification Manual.* Oakbrook Terrace, IL: Joint Commissions Resources.

Joint Committee on Interprofessional Relations Between the American Speech-Language-Hearing Association and Division 40 (Clinical Neuropsychology) of the American Psychological Association. (2007). *Structure and Function of an Interdisciplinary Team for Persons With Acquired Brain Injury.* Retrieved March 04, 2012 from www.asha.org/policy.

Kaschel, R., Della Sala, S., Cantagallo, A., Fahlbock, A., Laaksonen, R., & Kazen, M. (2002). Imagery mnemonics for the rehabilitation of memory: A randomised group controlled trial. *Neuropsychological Rehabilitation, 12*(2), 127-153.

Katz, D. I., Ashley, M. J., O'Shanick, G. J., & Connors, S. H. (2006). *Cognitive rehabilitation: The evidence, funding and case for advocacy in brain injury.* McLean, VA: Brain Injury Association of America.

Kennedy, M. R., & Coelho, C. (2005). Self-regulation after traumatic brain injury: A framework for intervention of memory and problem solving. *Seminars in Speech and Language, 26*(4), 242-255.

Kennedy, M. R., Coelho, C., Turkstra, L., Ylvisaker, M., Moore Sohlberg, M., Yorkston, K.,...Kan, P. F. (2008). Intervention for executive functions after traumatic brain injury: A systematic review, meta-analysis and clinical recommendations. *Neuropsychological Rehabilitation, 18*(3), 257-299.

King, K. A., Hough, M. S., Walker, M. M., Rastatter, M., & Holbert, D. (2006). Mild traumatic brain injury: Effects on naming in word retrieval and discourse. *Brain Injury, 20*(7), 725-732.

Kleim, J.A., & Jones, T.A. (2008. Principles of experience-dependent neural plasticity: Implications for rehabilitation after brain damage. *Journal of Speech Language and Hearing Research, 51*, S225-S239.

Knight J. (2008, June). *Considerations for treating PTSD within the context of cognitive impairments.* VA Polytrauma Conference, San Diego, CA.

Lange, R. T., Iverson, G. T., Franzen, M. D. (2009). Neuropsychological functioning following complicated vs. uncomplicated mild traumatic brain injury. *Brain Injury, 23*(2), 83-91.

Lannsjo, M., Geijjerstam, J. A., Johansson, U., Bring, J., & Borg, J. (2009). Prevalence and structure of symptoms at 3 months after mild traumatic brain injury in a national cohort. *Brain Injury, 23*, 213-219.

Lazare, A. (1981). Current concepts in psychiatry: Conversion symptoms. *New England Journal of Medicine, 305*(13), 745-748.

Lee, H. J., Lee, H. S., Kim, L., Lee, M. S., Suh, K. Y., & Kwak, D. I. (2001). A case of risperidone-induced stuttering. *Journal of Clinical Psychopharmacology, 21*(1), 115-116.

Lengenfelder, J., Schultheis, M. T., Al-Shihabi, T., Mourant, R., & DeLuca. J. (2002). Divided attention and driving: A pilot study using virtual reality technology. *Journal of Head Trauma Rehabilitation, 17*(1), 26-37.

Levin, H. S., Goldstein, F. C., & MacKenzie, E. J. (1997). Depression as a secondary condition following mild and moderate traumatic brain injury. *Seminars in Clinical Neuropsychology, 2*, 207-215.

Lew, H. L., Jerger, J. F., Guillory, S. B., & Henry, J. A. (2007). Auditory dysfunction in traumatic brain injury. *Journal of Rehabilitation Research and Development, 44*(7), 921-928.

Lew, H. L., Lin, P. H., Fu, J., Wang, S., Clark, D. J., & Walker, W. (2006). Characteristics and treatment of headache after traumatic brain injury. *American Journal of Physical Medicine and Rehabilitation, 85*(5), 619-627.

Lew, H. L., Poole, J. H., Vanderploeg, R. D., Goodrich, G. L., Dekelboum, S., Guillory, S. B.,....Cifu, D. X. (2007). Program development and defining characteristics of returning military in a VA polytrauma network site. *Journal of Rehabilitation Research and Development, 44*(7), 1027-1034.

Lezak, M. (2004). *Neuropsychological Assessment.* New York: Oxford.

Macciocchi, S. N., Barth, J. T., Littlefield, L., & Cantu, R. C. (2001). Multiple concussions and neuropsychological functioning in collegiate football players. *Journal of Athletic Training, 36*(3), 303-306.

MacLennan, D. L., & MacLennan, D. C. (2008). Assessing readiness for post-secondary education after traumatic brain injury using a simulated college experience. *NeuroRehabilitation, 23*, 521-528.

MacLennan, D. L., & Petska, K. (2008). Assessment and treatment of mild TBI. Presentation at the 3rd VA Polytrauma Conference, San Diego, California.

Mahr, G., & Leith,W. (1992). Stuttering after a dystonic reaction. *Psychosomatics, 31*, 465.

Malia, K., Law, P., Sidebottom, L., Bewick, K., Danziger, S., Schold-Davis, E., ...Vidaya, A. (2004). Recommendations for best practice in cognitive rehabilitation therapy: Acquired brain injury. The Society for Cognitive Rehabilitation, Inc.

Mateer, C. A. (1992). Systems of care for post-concussive syndrome. In L. J. Horn & N. Zasler (Eds.), *Rehabilitation of Post-Concussive Disorders*. Philadelphia: Henley & Belfus.

Mateer, C. A., & Sira, C. S. (2006). Cognitive and emotional consequences of TBI: Intervention strategies for vocational rehabilitation. *NeuroRehabilitation, 21*(4), 315-326.

McCrea, M. (2008). *Mild traumatic brain injury and postconcussion syndrome. The new evidence base for diagnosis and treatment*. New York: Oxford University Press.

McCrea, M., Guskiewicz, K. M., Marshall, S. W., Barr, W., Randolph, C., Cantu, R.,...Kelly, J. P. (2003). Acute effects and recovery time following concussion in collegiate football players. The NCAA Concussion Study. *Journal of the American Medical Association, 290*, 2556-2563.

McCrea, M., Kelly, J. P., & Randolph, C. (2000). *Standardized Assessment of Concussion (SAC): Manual for administration, scoring and interpretation* (3rd ed.). Waukesha, WI: Comprehensive Neuropsychological Services.

Medd, J., & Tate, R. L. (2000). Evaluation of an anger management therapy programme following acquired brain injury: A preliminary study. *Neuropsychological Rehabilitation, 10*, 185-201.

Meghji, C. (1994). Acquired stuttering. *Journal of Family Practice 39*, 325-326.

Melamed, S., Stern, M., Rahmani, L., Groswasser, Z., & Najenson, T. (1985). Attention capacity limitation, psychiatric parameters and their impact on work involvement following brain injury. *Scandinavian Journal of Rehabilitation Medicine, 12*, 21-26.

Meythaler, J. M., Peduzzi, J. D., Eleftheriou, E., & Novack, T. A. (2001). Current concepts: Diffuse axonal injury-associated traumatic brain injury. *Archives of Physical Medicine and Rehabilitation, 82*, 1461–1471.

Miller, P. S., Richardson, J. S., Jyu, C. A., Lemay, J. S., Hisock, M., & Keegan, D. L. (1988). Association of low serum anticholinergic levels and cognitive impairment in elderly presurgical patients. *American Journal of Psychiatry, 145*, 342-345.

Milton, S. (1988). Management of subtle cognitive-communication deficits. *Journal of Head Trauma Rehabilitation, 3*(2), 1-11.

Mittenberg, W., Canyock, E. M., Condit, D. Y., & Patton, C. (2001). Treatment of post-concussion syndrome following mild head injury. *Journal of Clinical & Experimental Neuropsychology, 23*, 829-836.

Mittenberg, W., DiGiulio, D. V., Perrin, S., & Bass, A. E. (1992). Symptoms following head injury: Expectations as etiology. *Journal of Neurology, Neurosurgery, & Psychiatry, 41*, 611-616.

Mittenberg, W., Tremont, G., Zielinski, R. E., Fichera, S., & Rayls, K. R. (1996). Cognitive-behavioral prevention of postconcussion syndrome. *Archives of Clinical Neuropsychology. 11(2)*, 139-145.

Montgomery, E. B., & Turkstra, L. S. (2003). Evidence-based practice: Let's be reasonable. *Journal of Medical Speech-Language Pathology, 11(2)*, ix-xii.

Moore, E. L., Terryberry-Spohr, L., & Hope, D. A. (2006). Mild traumatic brain injury and anxiety sequelae: A review of the literature. *Brain Injury, 20*, 117-132.

Moran, C., & Gillon, G. (2005). Inference comprehension of adolescents with traumatic brain injury: A working memory hypothesis. *Brain Injury, 19*, 743-751.

Munroe, J. (2005). Transitioning from the war zone: Information for veterans and those who care. Retreived March 04, 2012 from http://www.nami.org/Content/Microsites191/NAMI_Oklahoma/Home178/Veterans3/Veterans_Articles/15VetandFamilyInformationBooklet.pdf.

Murray, C. K., Reynolds, J. C., Schroeder, J. M., Harrison, M. B., Evans, O. M., & Hospenthal, D. R. (2005). Spectrum of care provided at an echelon II medical unit during Operation Iraqi Freedom. *Military Medicine, 170*, 516-530.

NIH (National Institutes of Health). (1999). NIH Consensus Development Panel on Rehabilitation of Persons with Traumatic Brain Injury. *Journal of the American Medical Association, 282(10)*, 974-983.

Nolin, P., Villemure, R., & Heroux, L. (2006). Determining long-term symptoms following mild traumatic brain injury: Method of interview affects self-report. *Brain Injury, 20(11)*, 1147-1154.

Norton, P. J., & Price, E. C. (2008). A meta-analytic review of adult cognitive-behavioral treatment outcome across the anxiety disorders. *Journal of Nervous and Mental Disease, 196*, 716-718.

Novack, T.A., Caldwell, S. G., Duke, L. W., Bergquist, T. F., & Gage, R. J. (1996). Focused versus unstructured intervention for attention deficits after traumatic brain injury. *Journal of Head Trauma Rehabilitation, 11*, 52-60.

Nurnberg, H. G., & Greenwald, B. (1981). Stuttering: An unusual side effect of phenothiazines. *American Journal of Psychiatry, 139*, 386-387.

Owens, B. D., Kragh, J. F., Wenke, J. C., Macaitis, J., Wade, C. E., & Holcomb, J. B. (2008). Combat wounds in Operation Iraqi Freedom and Operation Enduring Freedom. *Journal of Trauma, 64*, 295-299.

Pagulayan, K. F., Hoffman, J. M., Temkin, N. R., Machamer, J. E., & Dikmen, S. S. (2008). Functional limitations and depression after traumatic brain injury: Examination of the temporal relationship. *Archives of Physical Medicine and Rehabilitation, 89*, 1887–1892.

Parente, R., & Herrmann, D. (2002). *Retraining Cognition Techniques and Applications* (2ⁿᵈ ed.). Austin, Texas: Pro-ed.

Parente, R., & Stapleton, M. (1999). Development of a cognitive strategies group for vocational training after traumatic brain injury. *NeuroRehabilitation, 13,* 13-20.

Parry-Jones, B. L., Vaughan, F. L., & Cox, W. M. (2006). Traumatic brain injury and substance misuse: A systematic review of prevalence and outcomes research (1994-2004). *Neuropsychological Rehabilitation, 16(5),* 537-560.

Peppings, M. (1998). The value of group psychotherapy after brain injury: A clinical perspective. *Brain Injury Source, 2(1).*

Perkins, W.H. (1971). *Speech pathology: An applied behavioral science.* St. Louis: C.V. Mosby.

Ponsford, J., Whelan-Goodinson, R., & Bahar-Fuchs, A. (2007). Alcohol and drug use following traumatic brain injury: A prospective study. *Brain Injury, 21(13-14),* 1385-1392.

Ponsford,J., Willmott, C., Rothwell, A., Cameron, P., Kelly, A. M., Nelms, R., & Curran, C. (2002). Impact of early intervention on outcome following mild head injury in adults. *Journal of Neurology, Neurosurgery & Psychiatry, 73(3),* 330-2.

Ponsford, J., Willmott, C., Rothwell, A., Cameron, P., Kelly, A. M., Nelms, R.,…Kim, N. G. (2000). Factors influencing outcome following mild traumatic brain injury in adults. *Journal of the International Neuropsychological Society, 6(5),* 568-579.

Pontifex, M. B., O'Connor, P. M., Broglio, S. P., & Hilllman, C. H. (2009). The association between mild traumatic brain injury history and cognitive control. *Neuropsychologia, 47(14).*

Quemada, J.I., Cespedes, J. M., Exkerra. J., Ballesteros, J., Ibarra, N., & Urruticoechea, I. (2003). Outcome of memory rehabilitation in traumatic brain injury assessed by neuropsychological tests and questionnaires. *The Journal of Head Trauma Rehabilitation, 18,* 532-540.

Raskin, S. A., & Mateer, C. A. (2000). *Neuropsychological Management of Mild Traumatic Brain Injury.* New York: Oxford.

Rath, J. F., Simon, D., Langenbahn, D. M., Sherr, R. L., & Diller, L. (2003). Group treatment of problem-solving deficits in outpatients with traumatic brain injury: A randomised outcome study. *Neuropsychological Rehabilitation, 13(4),* 461-488.

Rebmann, M. J. & Hannon, R. (1995). Treatment of unawareness of memory deficits in adults with brain injury: Three case studies. *Rehabilitation Psychology, 40,* 279-287.

Resnik, L. J., & Allen, S. M. (2007). Using international classification of functioning, disability and health to understand challenges in community reintegration of injured veterans. *Journal of Rehabilitation Research and Development, 44*(7), 991-1006.

Rosenbek, J. C. (1984). Stuttering secondary to nervous system damage. In R.F. Curlee, and W.H. Perkins (Eds.), *Nature and treatment of stuttering: New directions* (pp. 31-48). San Diego: College Hill Press.

Roth, C., Aronson, A., & Davis, L. (1989). Clinical studies in psychogenic stuttering of adult onset. *Journal of Speech and Hearing Disorders, 54,* 634-646.

Roth, C., & Bibeau, R. (2011). *Post-deployment stuttering resulting from brain injury or stress?* Combat & Operational Stress Control Conference, San Diego.

Roth, C., & Manning, K. (2009). *Post-deployment stuttering resulting from brain injury or stress?* Paper presented at the Annual Convention of the American Speech-Language-Hearing Association, New Orleans.

Ruff, R. L., Ruff, S. S., & Wang, X. F. (2008). Headaches among Operation Iraqi Freedom/Operation Enduring Freedom veterans with mild traumatic brain injury associated with exposures to explosions. *Journal of Rehabilitation Research and Development, 45*(7), 941-952.

Ruff, R. M., & Jamora, C. W. (2009). Myths and mild traumatic brain injury. *Psychological Injury and Law, 2*: 34-42.

Ruh, D., Spicer, P., & Vaughan, K. (2009). Helping veterans with disabilities transition to employment. *Journal of Postsecondary Education & Disability 22*(1), 67-74.

Sarajuuri, J. M., Kaipio, M. L., Koskinen, S. K., Niemela, M. R., Servo, A. R., & Vilkki, J. S. (2005). Outcome of a comprehensive neurorehabilitation program for patients with traumatic brain injury. *Archives of Physical Medicine and Rehabilitation, 86*(12), 2296- 2302.

Sayer, N. A., Chiros, C. E., Sigford, B., Scott, S., Clothier, B., Pickett, T., & Lew, H. (2008). Characteristics and rehabilitation outcomes among patients with blast and other injuries sustained during the Global War on Terror. *Archives of Physical Medicine and Rehabilitation, 89,* 163-170.

Scherer, M. J., & Craddock, G. (2002). Matching Person and Technology (MPT) assessment process. *Technology and Disability, 14*(3), 125-131.

Schmitter-Edgecome, M., Fahy, J., Whelan, J., & Long, C. (1995). Memory remediation after severe closed head injury. Notebook training versus supportive therapy. *Journal of Consulting and Clinical Psychology, 63,* 484-489.

Scholten, J., & Walker, R. (2009, September). *Integrating pain management into TBI care across the spectrum of recovery.* 3rd Annual TBI Military Training Conference, Washington, D.C.

Schonberger, M., Humle, F., & Teasdale, T. W. (2006). Subjective outcome of brain injury rehabilitation in relation to the therapeutic working alliance, client compliance and awareness. *Brain Injury, 20*(12), 1271-1282.

Schonberger, M., Humle, F., & Teasdale, T. W. (2007). The relationship between clients' cognitive functioning and the therapeutic working alliance in post-acute brain injury rehabilitation. *Brain Injury, 21*(8), 825-836.

Sherer, M., Evans, C. C., Leverenz, J., Stouter, J., Irby, J. W., Lee, J. E., & Yablon, S. A. (2007). Therapeutic alliance in post-acute brain injury rehabilitation: Predictors of strength of alliance and impact of alliance on outcome. *Brain Injury, 21*(7), 663-672.

Silver, J. M., McAllister, T. W., Arciniegas, D. B. (2009). Depression and cognitive complaints following mild traumatic brain Injury. *American Journal of Psychiatry, 166*(6), 653-661.

Snell, D. L., Surgenor, L. J., Hay-Smith, E. J. C., & Siegert, R. J. (2009). A systematic review of psychological treatments for mild traumatic brain injury. *Journal of Clinical and Experimental Neuropsychology, 31*(1), 20-38.

Sohlberg, M.M. (2005). External aids for management of memory impairment. In W.M. High, A.M. Sander, M.A. Struchen, & K.A. Hart (Eds.), *Rehabilitation for traumatic brain injury.* New York: Oxford.

Sohlberg, M. M. (2009, January). Assistive technology for cognition: What every clinician needs to know. Paper presented at "Effective Practice of Audiology and Speech-Language Pathology for Operation Enduring Freedom (OEF) and Operation Iraqi Freedom (OIF) Veterans." Washington, D.C.

Sohlberg, M. M., Avery, J., Kennedy, M., Ylvisaker, M., Coelho, C., Turkstra, L., & Yorkston, K. (2003). Practice guidelines for direct attention training. *Journal of Medical Speech-Language Pathology, 11*(3), xix-xxxix.

Sohlberg, M. M., Ehlhardt, L., & Kennedy, M. (2005). Instructional techniques in cognitive rehabilitation: A preliminary report. *Seminars in Speech and Hearing, 26*(4), 268-279.

Sohlberg, M. M., Kennedy, M. R. T., Avery, J., Coelho, C., Turkstra, L., Ylvisaker, M., & Yorkston, K. (2007). Evidence-based practice for the use of external aids as a memory compensation technique. *Journal of Medical Speech-Language Pathology, 15*(1), xv-lii.

Sohlberg, M. M., & Mateer, C. (1989). The assessment of cognitive-communicative functions in head injury. *Topics in Language Disorders, 9*(2), 15-33.

Sohlberg, M. M., & Mateer, C.A. (2001). *Cognitive rehabilitation: An integrative neuropsychological approach.* New York: The Guilford Press.

Sohlberg, M. M., McLaughlin, K. A., Pavese, A., Heidrich, A., & Posner, M. I. (2001). Evaluation of Attention Process Training and brain injury education in persons with acquired brain injury. *Journal of Clinical and Experimental Neuropsychology, 22,* 656-676.

Sohlberg, M.M., & Turkstra, L.S. (2011). Optimizing cognitive rehabilitation: Effective instructional methods. New York: The Guilford Press.

Starkweather, C. W. (1987). *Fluency and Stuttering.* Englewood Cliffs, NJ: Prentice Hall.

Strasser, D. C., Falconer, J. A., Herrin, J. S., Bowen, S. E., Stevens, A., & Uomoto, J. (2005). Team functioning and patient outcomes in stroke rehabilitation. *Archives of Physical Medicine and Rehabilitation, 86,* 403-409.

Strasser, D. C., Uomoto, J. M., & Smits, J. (2008). The interdisciplinary team and polytrauma rehabilitation: Prescription for partnership. *Archives of Physical Medicine and Rehabilitation, 89,* 179-181.

Struchen, M, (2005). Social communication interventions. In W. M., High, A. M., Sander, M. A., Struchen, & K. A., Hart (Eds.), *Rehabilitation for traumatic brain injury.* New York: Oxford.

Stuss, D. T., Stethem, L. L., Hugenholtz, H., Picton, T., Pivik, J., & Richard, M. T. (1989). Reaction time after head injury: Fatigue, divided and focused attention, and consistency of performance. *Journal of Neurology, Neurosurgery and Psychiatry, 52,* 742-748.

Taber, K. H., Warden, D. L., & Hurley, R. A. (2006). Blast-related brain injury: What is known? *Journal of Neuropsychiatry and Clinical Neuroscience, 18,* 141-145.

Tanielian, T., & Jaycox, L. H. (2008). *Invisible wounds of war: Psychological and cognitive injuries, their consequences, and services to assist recovery.* Santa Monica, California: RAND Corporation.

Terrio, H., Brenner, L. A., Ivins, B. J. et al. (2009). Traumatic brain injury screening: Preliminary findings in a US Army Brigade Combat Team. *Journal of Head Trauma Rehabilitation, 24(1),* 14–23.

Thickpenny-Davis, K. L., & Barker-Collo, S. L. (2007). Evaluation of a structured group format memory rehabilitation program for adults following brain injury. *Journal of Head Trauma Rehabilitation, 22(5),* 303-313.

Thurman, D. J., Alverson, C., Dunn, K. A., Guerrero, J., & Sniezek, J. E. (1999). Traumatic brain injury in the United States: A public health perspective. *Journal of Head Trauma Rehabilitation, 14,* 602–615.

Togher, L., McDonald, S., Code, C., & Grant, S. (2004). Training communication partners of people with traumatic brain injury: A randomized controlled trial. *Aphasiology, 18,* 313-335.

Tombaugh, T. N., Rees, L., Stormer, P., Harrison, A. G., & Smith, A. (2007). The effects of mild and severe brain injury on speed of information processing as measured by the computerized tests of information processing (CTIP). *Archives of Clinical Neuropsychology, 22*, 25-36.

Tomblin, J. B., Morris, H. L., & Spriestersbach, D. C. (2000). *Diagnosis in Speech-Language Pathology* (2nd ed.). San Diego, CA: Singular Publishing Group.

Trudel, T. M., Nidiffer, F. D., & Barth, J. T. (2007). Community-integrated brain injury rehabilitation: Treatment models and challenges for civilian, military, and veteran populations. *Journal of Rehabilitation Research & Development, 44* (7), 1007-1016.

Tsaousides, T., & Gordon, W. A. (2009). Cognitive rehabilitation following traumatic brain injury: Assessment to treatment. *Mount Sinai Journal of Medicine, 76*, 173-181.

Turkstra, L. S. (2009, May). Pragmatic communication deficits in adolescents and adults. Presentation at the Twin Cities Speech-Language Pathologists Meeting. St. Louis Park, MN.

Turkstra, L., Coelho, C., & Ylvisaker, M., (2005). The use of standardized tests for individuals with cognitive-communication disorders. *Seminars in Speech and Language, 26*(4), 215-222.

Turkstra, L., & McCarty, J. (2006, November). Evidence based practice in traumatic brain injury: Assessment and intervention for cognitive communication disorders. Telephone Seminar sponsored by American Speech-Language Hearing Association.

Turkstra, L., Ylvisaker, M., Coelho, C., Kennedy, M., Sohlberg, M. M., Avery, J., et al. (2005). Practice guidelines for standardized assessment for persons with traumatic brain injury. *Journal of Medical Speech-Language Pathology, 13*(2), ix-xxxviii.

Uomoto, J. M., & Brockway, J. A. (1992). Anger management for brain injured patients and their family members. *Archives of Physical Medicine and Rehabilitation, 73*, 674-679.

Van Dam-Baggen, R., & Kraaimaat, F. (2000). Group social skills training or cognitive group therapy as the clinical treatment of choice for generalized social phobia? *Journal of Anxiety Disorders, 14*, 438-450.

Vanderploeg, R. D. (2000). The Interpretation Process. In R. D. Vanderploeg (Ed.), *Clinician's Guide to Neuropsychological Assessment (2nd ed.*, pp. 111-154). Hillsdale, NJ: Lawrence Erlbaum Assoc., Inc.

Vanderploeg, R. D., Belanger, H. G., & Curtiss, G. (2006). Mild traumatic brain injury: Medical and neurologic causality in modeling. In G. Young, A. Kane, & K. Nicholson (Eds.), *Psychological knowledge in court: PTSD, pain, & TBI* (pp. 297-307). New York: Springer-Verlag.

Vanderploeg, R. D., Belanger, H. G., & Curtiss, G. (2009). Mild traumatic brain injury and posttraumatic stress disorder and their association with health symptoms. *Archives of Physical Medicine and Rehabilitation, 90*(7), 1084-1093.

Vanderploeg, R. D., Curtiss, G., & Belanger, H. G. (2005). Long-term neuropsychological outcomes following mild traumatic brain injury. *Journal of the International Neuropsychological Society, 11*, 228-236.

Vanderploeg, R. D., Curtiss, G., Luis, C. A., & Salazar, A. M. (2007). Long-term morbidities following self-reported mild traumatic brain injury. *Journal of Clinical and Experimental Neuropsychology, 29*, 585–598.

Vasterling, J. J., Proctor, S. P., Amoroso, P., Kane, R., Heeren, T., & White, R. F. (2006). Neuropsychological outcomes of Army personnel following deployment to the Iraq war. Journal of the American Medical Association, 296(5), 519-529.

VA/DoD. (2009, April). *Clinical practice guideline for management of concussion/mild traumatic brain injury.*

Warden, D. (2006). Military TBI during the Iraq and Afghanistan wars. *Journal of Head Trauma Rehabilitation, 21*, 398–402.

Webster, S. & Scott, R. R. (1983). The effects of self-instructional training on attentional deficits following head injury. *Clinical Neuropsychology, 5*, 69-74.

Weiner, A. E. (1981). A case of adult onset of stuttering. *Journal of Fluency Disorders 6*, 181-186.

Wertz, R. T., Collins, M. J., Weiss, D., Kurtzke, J. F., Friden, T., Brookshire, R. H.,...Morley, G. (1981). Veterans Administration cooperative study on aphasia: A comparison of individual and group treatment. *Journal of Speech and Hearing Research, 24*, 580-594.

Whelan, B., Murdoch, B., & Bellamy, N. (2007). Delineating communication impairments associated with mild traumatic brain injury: A case report. *Journal of Head Trauma Rehabilitation, 22*(3), 192-197.

Wilson, B. A., Emslie, H. C., Quirk, K., & Evans. (2001). Reducing everyday memory and planning problems by means of a paging system: A randomized control crossover study. *Journal of Neurology, Neurosurgery, and Psychiatry, 70*, 477-482.

WHO (World Health Organization). (2008). *Primary Health Care Now More Than Ever.* Geneva, Switzerland.

Ylvisaker, M., & Feeney, T. J. (1996). Executive functions after traumatic brain injury: Supported cognition and self advocacy. *Seminars in Speech Language, 17*(3) 217-232.

Ylvisaker, M., Jacobs, H. E., & Feeney, T. (2003). Positive supports for people who experience behavioral and cognitive disability after brain injury: A review. *Journal of Head Trauma Rehabilitation, 18*, 7-32.

Ylvisaker, M., Turkstra, L.S., & Coelho, C. (2005). Behavioral and social interventions for individuals with traumatic brain injury: A summary of the research with clinical implications. *Seminars in Speech and Language, 26*(4), 256-257.

Zencius, A. H., Wesolowski, M. D., & Burke, W. H. (1990). A comparison of four memory strategies for brain-injured clients. *Brain Injury, 4,* 33–38.

ABBREVIATIONS AND ACRONYMS

A

A-DEM: Adult-Developmental Eye Movement
AAA: anticipation, action, analysis
ABC: Activities-Specific Balance Confidence (Scale)
ABI: acquired brain injury
ACeS: Activity Co-Engagement Self-Assessment
ACIS: Assessment of Communication and Interaction Skills
ADL: activity of daily living
ASHA NOMS: American Speech-Language-Hearing Association National Outcomes Measurement System
ASHA-FACS: American Speech Language and Hearing Association Functional Assessment of Communication Skills for Adults

B

BESS: Balance Error Scoring System
BESTest: Balance Evaluation Systems Test
biVABA: Brain Injury Visual Assessment Battery for Adults
BNT: Boston Naming Test
BPPV: benign paroxysmal positional vertigo
BRI: behavior rating index
BRIEF-A: Behavior Rating Inventory of Executive Function-Adult

C

c/mTBI: concussion/mild traumatic brain injury
CCT: Co-occurring Conditions Toolkit
CDP: computerized dynamic posturography
CLQT: Cognitive-Linguistic Quick Test
CMT: Contextual Memory Test
COPM: Canadian Occupational Performance Measure
COVD QOL: College of Optometrists in Vision Development Quality of Life Outcomes
CPAC: Chronister Pocket Acuity Chart
CRM: canalith repositioning maneuver

D

DA: Department of the Army
DAS: Dyadic Adjustment Scale
DCoE: Defense Centers of Excellence for Psychological Health and Traumatic Brain Injury
DCT: Discourse Comprehension Test
DEM: developmental eye movement
DGI: Dynamic Gait Index
DHI: Dizziness Handicap Inventory
DoD: Department of Defense
DVAT: Dynamic Visual Acuity Test

E

EET: Emotion Evaluation Test
ESS: Epworth Sleepiness Scale

F

FAVRES: Functional Assessment of Verbal Reasoning and Executive Strategies
FCM: functional communication measure
FGA: Functional Gait Assessment
FSS: Fatigue Severity Scale
FTSST: Five-Times-Sit-To-Stand Test

G

GAS: goal attainment scaling
GCS: Glasgow Coma Scale
GEC: Global Executive Composite
GRS: Guyatt's responsiveness statistic

H

HA: horizontal adjusted
HDI: Headache Disability Inventory
HiMAT: High-Level Mobility Assessment Tool
HRQOL: health-related quality of life
HSN: head-shaking nystagmus

I

IADL: instrumental activity of daily living
IAT: Illinois Agility Test
ICC: intraclass correlation coefficient
ICD-9-CM: *International Classification of Diseases, Ninth Revision, Clinical Modification*
ICF: International Classification of Functioning Disability and Health

J

JFLS: Jaw Functional Limitation Scale

L

LCQ: Latrobe Communication Questionnaire
LLATBI: Living Life After Brain Injury

M

M-CSM: Mortera-Cognitive Screening Measure
MAD: migraine-associated dizziness
MCT: Motor Control Test
mCTSIB: Modified Clinical Test of Sensory Interaction and Balance
MDC: minimal detectable change
MDIC: minimal clinically important differences
MI: metacognitive index
MPAI-4: The Mayo-Portland Adaptability Inventory–4
MSQ: Motion Sensitivity Quotient (Test)

N

NDI: Neck Disability Index
NPC: near point of convergence
NPRS: Numeric Pain Rating Scale
NSUCO: Northeastern State University College Of Optometry
NVR: Neurovision Rehabilitator
NVT: Neuro Vision Technology

O

OT: occupational therapist

P

PCS: post-concussion syndrome
PDA: personal digital assistant
PO: participation objective
PQRST: preview, question, read, summary, test
PS: participation subjective
PSFS: Patient-Specific Functional Scale
PTH: posttraumatic headache

R

RBANS: Repeatable Battery for the Assessment of Neuropsychological Status

RBMT: Rivermead Behavioral Memory Test
RBMT-E: Rivermead Behavioral Memory Test–Extended
RCI: reliable change index
RMDQ: Roland Morris Disability Questionnaire
RTW: return to work

S

SCATBI: Scales of Cognitive Ability for TBI
SCOLP: Speed and Capacity of Language Processing
SEM: standard error of measurement
SF-36: The Medical Outcomes Study 36-Item Short-Form Health Survey
SLP: speech-language pathologist
SLS: Single-Limb Stance (Test)
SM: service members
SMART: specific, measurable, achievable, realistic, and time-targeted
SO: significant other
SOT: Sensory Organization Test
SST: silly sentences test
STW: spot-the-word (test)

T

T2: National Center for Telehealth and Technology
TASIT: The Awareness of Social Inference Test
TBI: traumatic brain injury
TEA: Test of Everyday Attention
TMD: temporomandibular disorder
TMJ: temporomandibular joint
TUG: Timed Up and Go (test)

U

UVH: unilateral vestibular hypofunction
UVL: unilateral vestibular loss
UVL: unilateral vision loss

V

VADL: Vestibular Activities of Daily Living (scale)
VOR: vestibulo-ocular reflex

W

WART: Walking and Remembering Test
WHO: World Health Organization
WHOQOL-BREF: The World Health Organization Quality of Life–BREF
WJ III COG: Woodcock-Johnson III Tests of Cognitive Abilities

INDEX